STEROLS AND BILE ACIDS

New Comprehensive Biochemistry

Volume 12

General Editors

A. NEUBERGER
London

L.L.M. van DEENEN
Utrecht

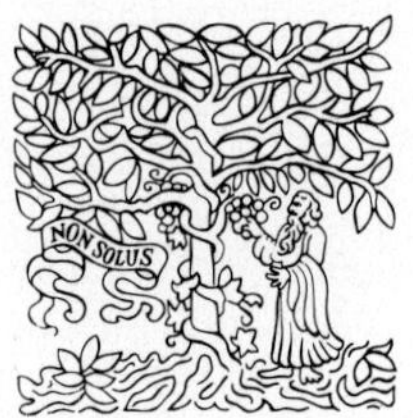

ELSEVIER
AMSTERDAM · NEW YORK · OXFORD

Sterols and Bile Acids

Editors

HENRY DANIELSSON [a] and JAN SJÖVALL [b]

[a] *Department of Pharmaceutical Biochemistry, University of Uppsala, Uppsala (Sweden) and* [b] *Department of Physiological Chemistry, Karolinska Institutet, Stockholm (Sweden)*

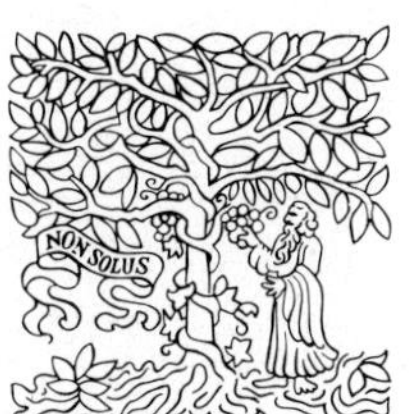

1985
ELSEVIER
Amsterdam · New York · Oxford

ISBN for the series: 0-444-80303-3
ISBN for the volume: 0-444-80670-9

Published by:

Elsevier Science Publishers B.V. (Biomedical Division)
P.O. Box 211
1000 AE Amsterdam
(The Netherlands)

Sole distributors for the U.S.A. and Canada:
Elsevier Science Publishing Company, Inc.
52 Vanderbilt Avenue
New York, NY 10017
(U.S.A.)

Library of Congress Cataloging-in-Publication Data
Main entry under title:

Sterols and bile acids.

(New comprehensive biochemistry; v. 12)
Includes bibliographies and index.
1. Sterols--Metabolism. 2. Bile acids--Metabolism.
I. Danielsson, Henry. II. Sjövall, Jan. III. Series.
[DNLM: 1. Bile Acids and Salts--metabolism. 2. Sterols
--metabolism. W1 NE372F v.12 / QU 95 S839]
QD415.N48 vol. 12 574.19′2 s [574.19′2431] 85-20620
[QB752.S75]
ISBN 0-444-80670-9 (U.S.)

Printed in The Netherlands

Preface

Sterols are essential components of all eukaryotic cells. Their function is structural, and by being precursors of hormones and bile acids they exert a regulatory function on metabolic processes. Cholesterol and its metabolism are of importance in human disease. Although the mechanisms are largely unknown, it can be surmised that abnormalities in the metabolism of sterols and bile acids are associated with cardiovascular disease and gallstone formation. Steroid hormones are vital for man, animals and plants. Disturbances in their production can have deleterious consequences.

This volume of New Comprehensive Biochemistry is entitled Sterols and Bile Acids. It includes fourteen chapters written by prominent scientists in the field. The large volume of material in the field of sterols and bile acids has necessitated a limitation of the areas covered. Chapters on steroid hormones have been excluded since this field requires a volume of its own. In spite of this it has not been possible to produce a book of some few hundred pages. Efforts have been made to condense the contributions of the individual authors, but the wealth of important information is such that a further reduction in size would seriously affect the value of the chapters to the reader.

It may be argued that there are important gaps in the contents of this volume. For instance, full discussions of the role of compartmentation of sterols and their metabolism, of the dynamics of cholesterol balance, etc. are lacking. We as editors take full responsibility for this. Our only excuse is that the material contained in the volume is already at the limit of what can be accommodated in a volume of New Comprehensive Biochemistry.

Although we have tried to make terminology, abbreviations, etc. reasonably uniform it will be apparent that there are differences between chapters, but hopefully not within a chapter. We have felt it more important to let the individualities of the authors be expressed.

It is our conviction that the eminent contributions in this volume, for which we are very grateful to our colleagues, will be of the value they deserve for all scientists in the field of sterol and bile acid research.

Uppsala and Stockholm
September 1985

Henry Danielsson
Jan Sjövall

H. Danielsson and J. Sjövall (Eds.), *Sterols and Bile Acids*

Contents

H. Danielsson and J. Sjövall (Eds.), *Sterols and Bile Acids*

CHAPTER 1

Biosynthesis of cholesterol

HANS C. RILLING [a] and LILIANA T. CHAYET [b]

[a] *Department of Biochemistry, University of Utah School of Medicine, Salt Lake City, UT 84108 (U.S.A.), and*
[b] *Departamento de Bioquimica, Facultad de Ciencias Basicas y Farmaceuticas, Universidad de Chile, Santiago (Chile)*

(I) Introduction

It is not possible to write a comprehensive review of cholesterol biosynthesis in the space allotted nor is it our desire to do so. Consequently, we have been selective as to what has been included and the list of references is far from exhaustive. We hope that no one will be offended by our choices. In addition, where appropriate, the stress has been on enzymes from liver. There are several recent and comprehensive reviews on cholesterol biosynthesis. Two books, one by Nes and McKean [1] and another by Gibbons, Mitropoulos and Myant [2] provide excellent and current reviews on the biosynthesis and function of cholesterol. In addition, about half of the chapters in a book edited by Porter and Spurgeon [3] deal with selected aspects of the biochemistry of sterologenesis and, taken as an aggregate, provide a comprehensive review of the subject. Also Schroepfer has published recently two reviews on cholesterol biosynthesis in *Annual Reviews of Biochemistry* [4,5].

Cholesterol is primarily restricted to eukaryotic cells where it plays a number of roles. Undoubtedly, the most primitive function is as a structural component of membranes. Its metabolism to bile acids and the steroid hormones is relatively recent in the evolutionary sense. In this chapter, the pathway of cholesterol biosynthesis will be divided into segments which correspond to the chemical and biochemical divisions of this biosynthetic route. The initial part of the pathway is the 3-step conversion of acetyl-CoA to 3-hydroxy-3-methylglutaryl-CoA (HMG-CoA). The next is the reduction of this molecule to mevalonate, considered to be the rate-controlling step in the biosynthesis of polyisoprenoids. From thence, a series of phosphorylation reactions both activate and decarboxylate mevalonate to isopentenyl pyrophosphate, the true isoprenoid precursor. After a rearrangement to the allylic pyrophosphate, dimethylallyl pyrophosphate, a sequence of 1′-4 condensations (head-to-tail) * between the allylic and homoallylic pyrophosphates leads to the synthesis of prenyl pyrophosphates which are requisite for the synthesis of the higher polyprenols such as cholesterol, dolichol, and coenzyme Q. For the synthesis of cholesterol, the polymerization is halted at the sesquiterpene level. Two molecules of the farnesyl pyrophosphate thus formed condense in a 1′-2-3 manner (head-to-head) producing presqualene pyrophosphate. After a reductive rearrangement of the carbon skeleton to squalene, an epoxidation leads to the formation of 2,3-oxidosqualene which then cyclizes to lanosterol. The final stages of sterologenesis involve the removal of 3 methyl groups from lanosterol and the migration and reduction of double bonds to give cholesterol. In higher organisms, this pathway is primarily restricted to the liver, small intestine, kidney, and endocrine organs. While other classes of cells do maintain the enzymes for this set of reactions, they depend upon the liver as a source of sterol.

Very early in the investigation of sterol biosynthesis it was established that acetate was the primary precursor. In 1942 Bloch and Rittenberg found that deutero-acetate could be converted to cholesterol in the intact animal in high yields [7]. This was in accord with the earlier observation of Sonderhoff and Thomas that the nonsaponifiable lipids from yeast (primarily sterol) were heavily labeled by the same substrate [8]. Degradation of the sterol molecule in the laboratories of both Bloch and Popjak showed that all of the carbon atoms of cholesterol were derived from acetate and that the labeling pattern of methyl and carboxyl carbons originating from acetate indicated that the molecule was isoprenoid in nature [9]. It was apparent then that sterols have as their fundamental building block, acetate, a molecule that resides at the center of intermediary metabolism.

(II) Source of acetyl-CoA

The synthesis of fatty acids and sterols in the liver cytosol depends upon a common pool of acetyl-CoA. This was demonstrated by Decker and Barth in a series of experiments utilizing perfused rat liver [10]. Lipid synthesis was measured by incorporation of tritium from $[^3H]H_2O$. They used (−)-hydroxycitrate to inhibit ATP-dependent citrate lyase and measured radioisotope incorporation into fatty acids and sterols as a function of the concentration of this inhibitor. A parallel decrease in incorporation into these two products was found as the concentration of (−)-hydroxycitrate in the perfusate was increased. Contrastingly, if radioisotopic acetate was used as the substrate in the perfusing medium, this inhibitor had relatively little effect on the rate of sterologenesis, a result that would be expected if the natural source of acetate was from the action of the cytoplasmic citrate lyase. Their experiments also demonstrated that the ratio of fatty acid synthesis to sterol synthesis in the liver of fed rats is about 10 : 1.

* The nomenclature used is described in ref. 6, p. 163.

The beginning stages of fatty acid as well as cholesterol biosynthesis are cytoplasmic processes. The initial substrate for both pathways is acetyl-CoA which is generated in the mitochondria primarily from glycolysis via pyruvate and pyruvate dehydrogenase or by the β-oxidation of fatty acids. Since mitochondrial membranes are impermeable to coenzyme A derivatives, other derivatives of acetate must be utilized to move the acetyl unit from the mitochondria to the cytoplasm. The major pathway involves citrate as the carrier. Citrate generated in the mitochondrion from acetyl-CoA and oxaloacetate moves to the cytosol, a process that is facilitated by the dicarboxylate transport system. In the cytosol, the citrate cleavage enzyme utilizes ATP and CoA to convert citrate to acetyl-CoA and oxaloacetate. The acetyl group is used for lipogenesis while the oxaloacetate is reduced to malate by NADH. Malate is then oxidized to pyruvate and CO_2 by NADP and the malic enzyme. This step affords NADPH-reducing equivalents for both lipogenesis and sterologenesis. Either malate or pyruvate can re-enter the mitochondrion.

Acetoacetate is another vehicle for transporting acetyl groups into the cytoplasm. This molecule, one of the end products of ketone body synthesis, is free to diffuse from the mitochondrion. When in the cytoplasm it can be activated to acetoacetyl-CoA by an ATP-dependent acetoacetyl-CoA synthetase. Edmonds' group has shown that the activity of this enzyme parallels the rate of cholesterologenesis in the livers of animals given a variety of dietary regimes [11]. Their data also indicate that this pathway furnishes as much as 10% of the carbon required for cholesterol biosynthesis.

Several other pathways have been postulated for the transport of acetyl units from the mitochondrion to the cytoplasm. One entails carnitine as a transporter, as it is for fatty acids, the other invoked free acetate. It is unlikely that either of these is significant [12].

(III) Acetyl-CoA acetyl transferase (EC 2.3.1.9)

The first enzyme in the pathway is acetoacetyl-CoA thiolase which catalyzes the condensation of two molecules of acetyl-CoA.

$$2\,CH_3{-}\overset{\overset{\displaystyle O}{\|}}{C}{-}S{-}CoA \rightleftharpoons CH_3{-}\overset{\overset{\displaystyle O}{\|}}{C}{-}CH_2{-}\overset{\overset{\displaystyle O}{\|}}{C}{-}S{-}CoA + CoASH$$

(1) Cellular location

There are two discrete locations of enzymes for the biosynthesis of acetoacetyl-CoA and HMG-CoA; one is mitochondrial and serves the purpose of generating ketone bodies (acetoacetate and 3-hydroxybutyrate). The other is cytoplasmic and provides precursors for isoprene units for the biosynthesis of cholesterol and other terpenoids.

Early in the study of the enzymology of the biosynthesis of HMG-CoA, there was some confusion as to whether these processes were physically separated within the cell. Studies by Lane and his collaborators [13] and by others [14] clearly indicated a duality of locus. The cytosolic enzyme, purified from avian liver [13], was found to have a molecular weight of 1.7×10^5 with 4 apparently identical subunits (41 000 by SDS gel electrophoresis). The cytosolic enzyme constituted 70% of total thiolase found in chicken liver.

(2) Enzymology

The equilibrium position of this reaction is 6×10^{-6} which is quite unfavorable for the synthesis of acetoacetyl-CoA. However, as will be pointed out below, when it functions in conjunction with the next enzyme in the sequence, synthesis is favored. The turnover number in the forward direction (as written) was found to be 1770 while that of the reverse was 54 000. The enzyme from mitochondria has two electrophoretically distinct forms, and the cytoplasmic enzyme could be clearly distinguished from the two mitochondrial proteins by the difference in their isoelectric points. Middleton surveyed many tissues from rat as well as selected tissues from ox and pigeon for both the cytoplasmic and the mitochondrial enzymes. The highest levels of the cytoplasmic enzyme were found in the liver, adrenal, brain of the neonate, and ileum [14,15]. There was an obvious positive correlation between sterol biosynthetic capacity and the distribution of this enzyme. The mitochondrial enzyme was found predominantly in heart, kidney, and liver. The cytosolic enzyme has also been highly purified from rat liver [16].

(3) Mechanism

Kinetic analysis indicated that the mechanism is ping-pong with an acyl enzyme intermediate [17]. Since Lynen had shown earlier that –SH-directed reagents inhibit the enzyme [18], it was assumed that an acyl-*S*-enzyme was an intermediate in the reaction. Suicide substrates for this enzyme have been prepared and tested against the protein isolated from heart mitochondria. The substrate analogs 4-bromocrotonyl-, 3-pentenoyl-, 3-butynoyl-, and 2-bromoacetyl-CoA all progressively and irreversibly inhibited the enzyme. Thus, 3-acetylenic CoA esters are effective site-specific inhibitors of this enzyme and a mechanism to account for this is shown in Fig. 1. This inactivation resulted in the formation of a stable thiol ether with the enzyme. Other enzymes with putative sulfhydryl groups in the catalytic site behave in a similar manner with acetylenic substrate analogs [19].

The enzyme could be inactivated by $NaBH_4$ in the presence of either acetoacetyl-CoA or acetyl-CoA. This observation strongly suggests that the reaction is through a Claisen condensation with an amine as the base and with an enzyme substrate ketimine as an intermediate [20]. A mechanism was postulated for the reaction as indicated in Fig. 2.

The stereochemistry of acetoacetyl-CoA thiolase was examined by utilizing

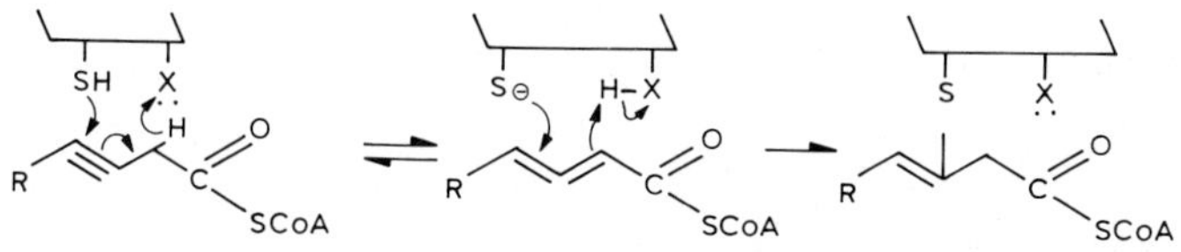

Fig. 1. The mechanism by which acetylenic analogs irreversibly inhibit acetyl-CoA acetyl transferase.

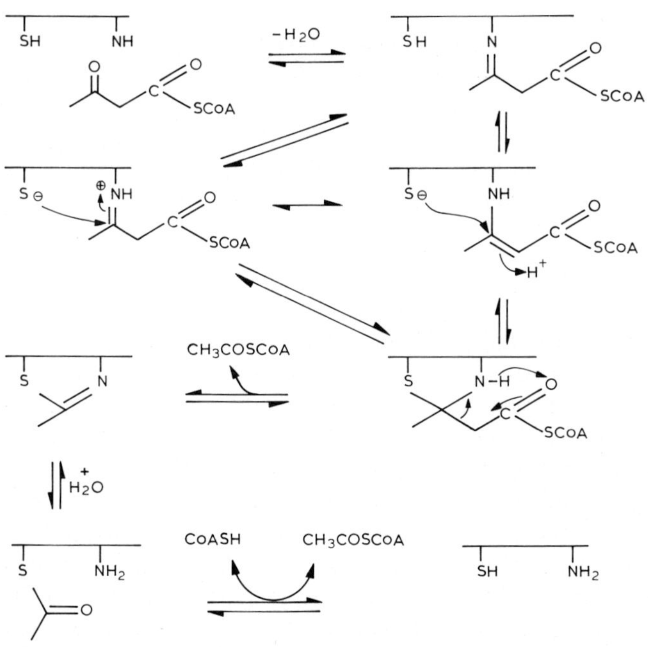

Fig. 2. A mechanism for the reaction catalyzed by acetyl-CoA acetyl transferase.

$(2S,3S)$-3-hydroxy[2-$^{2}H_1$,$^{3}H_1$]butyryl-CoA as substrate. It was cleaved by the enzyme and the resulting radioactive acetate examined for its chirality by standard procedures. The results demonstrated that the cleavage reaction (and presumably the condensation reaction) proceeds with inversion of the methylene group that becomes the methyl group on cleavage [21].

(IV) 3-Hydroxy-3-methylglutaryl-CoA synthetase (EC 4.1.3.5)

(1) Cellular location

3-Hydroxy-3-methylglutaryl-CoA synthetase, like the enzyme that precedes it, enjoys two subcellular locals.

$$CH_3-\overset{\overset{\displaystyle O}{\|}}{C}-S-CoA + CH_3-\overset{\overset{\displaystyle O}{\|}}{C}-CH_2-\overset{\overset{\displaystyle O}{\|}}{C}-S-CoA$$

$$\rightleftharpoons HO-\overset{\overset{\displaystyle O}{\|}}{C}-CH_2-\underset{\underset{\displaystyle CH_3}{|}}{\overset{\overset{\displaystyle OH}{|}}{C}}-CH_2-\overset{\overset{\displaystyle O}{\|}}{C}-S-CoA + CoASH$$

In the mitochondrion it participates in ketone body synthesis, while as a cytoplasmic enzyme it functions in cholesterol biogenesis [22].

(2) Enzymology

This enzyme has been extensively studied by Lane and his collaborators utilizing preparations from chicken liver as well as rat liver [22]. With chicken liver preparations, a number of forms of the enzyme were detected and purified. One was associated with the mitochondrial fraction and was presumably the enzyme of ketogenesis. Other, multiple forms were recovered from the cytosol. One of these was immunologically cross-reactive with the mitochondrial enzyme. Since this form of the cytosolic enzyme was also detected in tissues that do not have mitochondrial HMG-CoA synthetases, such as brain and heart, it seemed unlikely that they were dealing with a proteolytic artifact or a product precursor relationship between the different proteins. The other three cytosolic synthetases were immunologically related. The most abundant, synthetase II, constituted more than 60% of the cytosolic activity. This protein has a molecular weight of about 100 000 and is comprised of two subunits of identical molecular weight. Dissociation into monomers was easily accomplished by increasing the ionic strength. The other two cytoplasmic forms could be derived from the predominant form presumably by a minor modification such as a proteolytic cleavage or removal of a phosphate residue.

The level of the cytoplasmic proteins but not the mitochondrial form of the synthetase was governed by the dietary regime of the birds. Cholesterol feeding, which diminishes cholesterol synthesis, suppressed the activity level of the enzyme. Inclusion of cholestyramine in the diet, which elevates cholesterol synthesis, enhanced the activity of the enzyme. Unlike avian liver, rat liver cytosol contains a single HMG-CoA synthetase, suggesting that the multiple enzymes recovered from chicken liver are artifacts. The rat liver cytosolic enzyme is subject to repression by cholesterol feeding as well as by fasting; both procedures cause an 80% reduction in activity within 24 h. Also, since cholestyramine caused an enhanced level of the enzyme, the authors concluded that this enzyme might play a regulatory role in cholesterol biosynthesis [22].

Because of the poor equilibrium position of acetoacetyl-CoA synthetase, they tested the effect of the combined presence of acetoacetyl-CoA synthetase and HMG-CoA synthetase on the equilibrium between acetyl-CoA and HMG-CoA. At equilibrium slightly more than half of the acetyl-CoA had been converted to product. The position of the equilibrium is governed by the expression

$$K_{app} = \frac{[\text{HMG-CoA}][\text{CoA}]^2}{[\text{acetyl-CoA}]^3}$$

The K_{app} determined was 1.33. Thus, the overall equilibrium for the combined reactions favors cholesterol biosynthesis. An improved preparation of HMG-CoA synthetase from chicken liver mitochondria has been recently reported [23].

(3) Mechanism

The mechanism of this reaction was determined utilizing homogeneous protein isolated from mitochondria [24]. The enzyme catalyzes an exchange of acetyl groups between acetyl-CoA and several sulfhydryl-containing acceptors. The most effective acceptor was dephospho-CoA, with an exchange rate 50% of normal condensation. Cysteamine, the CoA analog used by Lynen to study fatty acid biosynthesis, also participated in the exchange reaction but at 25% of the normal reaction. The enzyme also catalyzes a slow hydrolysis of acetyl-CoA. These observations, plus the fact that the exchange reactions followed zero-order kinetics, led to the postulate that an enzyme-*S*-acetyl intermediate was involved in the reaction. Earlier, Stewart and Rudney had shown that the thiol ester carbonyl of acetyl-CoA gave rise to the free carboxyl of HMG-CoA [25], and it was postulated that the functionality on the enzyme responsible for hydrolysis was the group involved in acyl transfer.

Brief incubation of the enzyme at 0°C with radioactive acetyl-CoA led to the formation of acyl enzyme which could be isolated by chromatography on Sephadex [24]. The enzyme–substrate complex was then reacted with acetoacetyl-CoA with the concomitant formation of HMG-CoA. Further studies indicated that the functional group on the enzyme that accepted the acetyl residue was a cysteine sulfhydryl. 4′-Phosphopantetheine is known to accept acyl residues, but it was not found in this protein. The stoichiometry for acetylation was 0.7 acetyl groups per mole of enzyme; since it is a dimeric protein with apparently identical subunits, this observation is surprising. Thus, it is possible that the subunits perform different functions; for example, one could be regulatory. It is interesting to note that both the thiolase and HMG-CoA synthetase utilize acyl enzyme intermediates in their catalytic mechanisms.

In a later publication, another enzyme-bound intermediate involved in the reaction mechanism of HMG-CoA synthetase was reported [26]. On the assumption that acetylation of the enzyme by acetyl-CoA was the initial step in the reaction sequence, they felt that condensation with the second substrate, acetoacetyl-CoA,

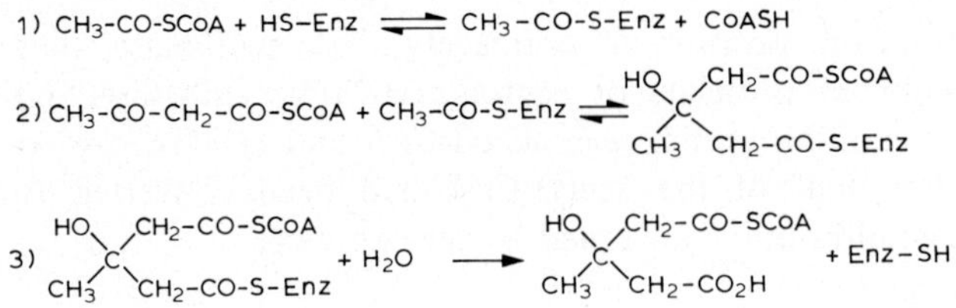

1) $CH_3\text{-}CO\text{-}SCoA + HS\text{-}Enz \rightleftharpoons CH_3\text{-}CO\text{-}S\text{-}Enz + CoASH$

2) $CH_3\text{-}CO\text{-}CH_2\text{-}CO\text{-}SCoA + CH_3\text{-}CO\text{-}S\text{-}Enz \rightleftharpoons (HO)(CH_3)C(CH_2\text{-}CO\text{-}SCoA)(CH_2\text{-}CO\text{-}S\text{-}Enz)$

3) $(HO)(CH_3)C(CH_2\text{-}CO\text{-}SCoA)(CH_2\text{-}CO\text{-}S\text{-}Enz) + H_2O \longrightarrow (HO)(CH_3)C(CH_2\text{-}CO\text{-}SCoA)(CH_2\text{-}CO_2H) + Enz\text{-}SH$

Fig. 3. A mechanism for the reaction catalyzed by 3-hydroxy-3-methylglutaryl-CoA synthetase.

would lead to the formation of HMG-CoA-*S*-enzyme as a second enzyme-bound intermediate. When acetylated enzyme was mixed with acetoacetyl-CoA at low temperatures in the presence of a mixture of ethanol and glycerol, this intermediate could be demonstrated. Perchloric acid was required to cleave the enzyme substrate adduct, indicating that the linkage was covalent. Pronase digestion of the intermediate gave *N*-HMG-cysteine. Since *S*-to-*N* migration occurs under these conditions, they concluded that the bonding to the enzyme was through the sulfur of cysteine. An isotope dilution method was used to evaluate the relative kinetic constants for the formation and utilization of the acetyl-*S*-enzyme moiety. With this technique the necessary requirements were met for the existence of covalent enzyme–substrate intermediate. The sequence of reactions leading to the formation of HMG-CoA are shown in Fig. 3.

The enzyme demonstrates partial selectivity for its acyl substrate since both acetyl-CoA and propionyl-CoA will react to give an acyl-*S*-enzyme species. However, only the acetyl-enzyme will react with acetoacetyl-CoA [23]. The enzyme will also bind other acyl groups such as a rather bulky spin-labeled CoA derivative, 3-carboxy-2,2,5,5-tetramethyl-1-pyrrolidinyloxyl-CoA, very tightly but not covalently in the acetyl-accepting site [27]. Interestingly, the enzyme will accept the thioether analog of acetoacetyl-CoA, 3-oxobutyl-CoA, to give as product a thioether analog of HMG-CoA. Because of the covalent linkage of one substrate and of product to the enzyme, a ping-pong mechanism would be anticipated and has been demonstrated for the mitochondrial enzyme [28].

(V) 3-Hydroxy-3-methylglutaryl-CoA reductase (EC 1.1.1.34)

The enzymes so far described are identical, with respect to the reactions catalyzed, to the enzymes that make ketone bodies. Since these pathways are physically separated within the cell, it would seem that regulation of sterol synthesis could reside in this region of the pathway. However, the key regulatory step in cholesterol biosynthesis is HMG-CoA reductase (Chapter 2). A book on this protein has been published recently [29], and among others Qureshi and Porter have also reviewed this enzyme [12]. Comments on this protein will be restricted to noting a few salient features that will enable the reader to progress without referring to other sources.

(1) Enzymology

There is a substantial variance in the literature concerning the molecular weight of HMG-CoA reductase. There was once a consensus that the enzyme had a molecular weight of approximately 52 000; however, when efforts are made to prevent proteolysis during isolation, the apparent molecular weight of the protomer was found to be 92 000. Indications are that the polymeric form of the enzyme has a molecular weight of 360 000 [30]. The observations that the reductase was a soluble protein probably resulted from proteolysis during extraction from the tissue. Evidence supporting this conclusion has come from immunotitration experiments which demonstrated that the microsomal enzyme and the "solubilized" species had the same antigen–antibody reactions [31]. In the absence of protease, the enzyme can only be solubilized with detergent. Thus, it is probably an integral membrane protein. It is possible that much of the protein is exposed to the cytosol while a noncatalytic portion is buried in the membrane. This situation is reminiscent of cytochrome P-450 reductase.

(2) Mechanism

HMG-CoA reductase catalyzes the reductive deacylation of its substrate to mevalonate and coenzyme A in a 2-step reaction with a stoichiometry of 2 moles of NADPH oxidized per mole of product formed.

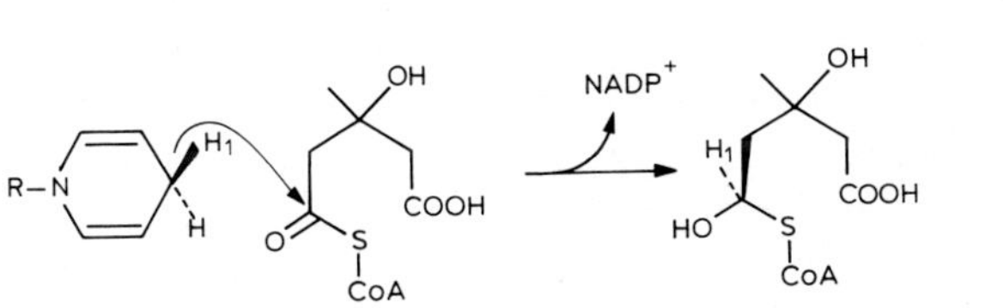

$$HO(CH_3)C(CH_2\text{-}COOH)(CH_2\text{-}CO\text{-}S\text{-}CoA) + 2\,NADPH + 2\,H^+ \rightleftharpoons HO(CH_3)C(CH_2\text{-}COOH)(CH_2\text{-}CH_2OH) + 2\,NADP^+$$

The optimum pH for the reaction is near 7. The enzyme is extremely sensitive to

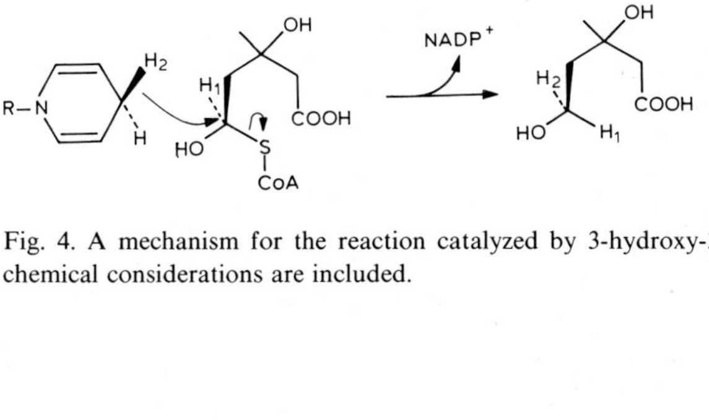

Fig. 4. A mechanism for the reaction catalyzed by 3-hydroxy-3-methylglutaryl-CoA reductase. Stereochemical considerations are included.

sulfhydryl-directed reagents, but the exact role of the free sulfhydryl remains unknown. Detailed kinetic mechanisms for the reaction have been determined for both the yeast and rat liver enzyme [12]. The overall reaction is essentially irreversible; however, the first portion has been studied in the reverse direction. The reaction takes place in 2 sequential reductive steps which have been studied by the standard techniques of product inhibition and dead-end inhibitors. The binding of substrates may be ordered with HMG-CoA adding first. A thiol hemiacetal complex between CoA and mevaldic acid is believed to be an intermediate in the reaction (Fig. 4). However, it has never been detected and must be tightly bound to the enzyme. It is also possible that mevaldic acid is the true substrate and that CoA acts as an allosteric activator.

The stereochemistry for all of the reductases that have been studied is the same. The 3-*S* enantiomer of HMG-CoA is the substrate utilized, and both of the hydrides originate as the pro-*R* hydrogen in the 4 position of the reduced pyridine nucleotide. The aldehydic intermediate is the (3*S*,5*R*)-thiohemi-acetal and is reduced by incorporation of a hydrogen into the 5-pro-*S* position of (3*R*)-mevalonate [30].

Relatively little information is available concerning the substrate specificity of vertebrate reductase. The requirement for NADPH is absolute, and little has been done to investigate the structural requirements of the substrate. The important features appear to be a terminal carboxyl group, a 3-hydroxyl, and a nonpolar substituent on the 3 position. Interestingly, the 3-ethyl analog is an effective substrate for the reductase from insects which synthesize juvenile hormone [30].

A number of substrate analogs have been synthesized and tested for inhibition of

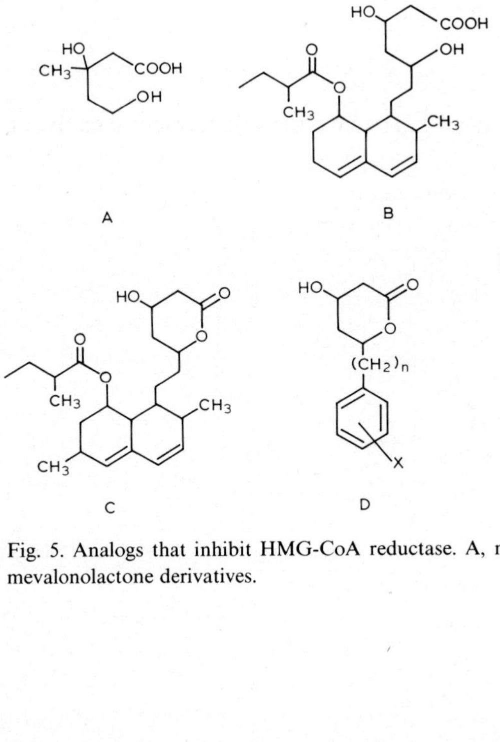

Fig. 5. Analogs that inhibit HMG-CoA reductase. A, mevalonic acid; B, compactin; C, mevinolin; D, mevalonolactone derivatives.

HMG-CoA reductase. Some are analogs of the isoprene precursor while others are NADP(H) analogs. Analogs such as mevinolin have been extremely useful in evaluating the role of the enzyme and in manipulating the concentration of the enzyme in vivo and finally in stabilizing HMG-CoA reductase during purification (for example, see ref. 32). Several effective competitive inhibitors and their structural similarities are shown in Fig. 5.

(3) Regulation

HMG-CoA reductase is a protein of the endoplasmic reticulum whose concentration is determined by rates of synthesis and degradation (Chapter 2). These, in turn, are governed by the amount of cholesterol in the cell. Cholesterol content is, in turn, influenced both by its rate of synthesis and a lipoprotein system that traffics in the intercellular movement of cholesterol. The liver is the principal organ of cholesterol biosynthesis. During growth, incorporation into membrane is an important fate for this molecule. However, in homeostasis the primary "fate" is conversion to bile acids or transport to other tissues via low-density lipoprotein. High-density lipoprotein also serves as a cholesterol carrier, and apparently serves to bring cholsterol from the peripheral tissues to the liver. The major route of loss is via bile acids and neutral sterols which are excreted from the liver via the bile. All eukaryotic cells have the capacity to synthesize cholesterol; however, most peripheral tissues depend upon the liver as a source and usually are shut down with respect to biosynthesis (cf. Chapter 5). It is not clear as to whether the affecting molecules are cholesterol or an oxidized derivative. Kandutsch and others [33] have shown that 25-hydroxycholesterol and many other oxidized sterols are extremely efficient in stopping the synthesis of the reductase as well as enhancing its degradation. In addition, phosphorylation of the protein, which inactivates it, may be important for short-term regulation of its activity [34].

Mevalonic acid was discovered by Folker's group at Merck, Sharpe, and Dohme. The initial isolation was based upon the fact that it acted as a growth factor, or vitamin, for a strain of bacteria [35]. Once the structure had been determined, it was apparent that the molecule might well be the isoprenoid precursor that had been sought for many years. Subsequent experiments demonstrated that the sole (or nearly so) fate of the molecule was polyisoprenoid synthesis. In examining the role of cofactors necessary for the synthesis of cholesterol from mevalonate, only ATP and NADPH were found to be required. Experiments with a solubilized preparation from yeast demonstrated that there were 3 phosphorylated intermediates that could be isolated. These were shown to be mevalonic-5-phosphate, mevalonic-5-pyrophosphate, and isopentenyl pyrophosphate [9]. These intermediates are derived from mevalonate in a sequence of phosphorylations, and the enzymes for all reactions have been obtained in homogeneous form. These enzymes, as well as the rest that lead to the synthesis of farnesyl pyrophosphate, are cytosolic proteins.

(VI) Mevalonate-5-phosphotransferase (EC 2.7.1.36)

The first enzyme of mevalonate metabolism, mevalonate kinase, has been partially purified from a variety of sources.

$$HO_2C{-}CH_2{-}\underset{\substack{|\\OH}}{\overset{\substack{CH_3\\|}}{C}}{-}CH_2{-}CH_2OH + ATP \overset{Mg^{2+}}{\rightleftharpoons} HO_2C{-}CH_2{-}\underset{\substack{|\\OH}}{\overset{\substack{CH_3\\|}}{C}}{-}CH_2{-}CH_2{-}OPO_3^{2-} + ADP$$

Pure protein has been isolated by Beytia and his collaborators with porcine liver as the source of the enzyme [36]. Recently, the preparation of this enzyme has been reviewed by Porter [37]. The molecular weight of the enzyme is 98 000 with an isoelectric point of 4.7. Subunit characterization of the protein has not been reported. By a combination of studies on the kinetics of the reaction which included product and dead-end inhibition measurements, they concluded that the reaction is sequential. Mevalonate is the first reactant and MgATP second. After phosphorylation of the isoprene precursor, mevalonate-5-phosphate is released followed by MgADP. There was a lack of exchange between MgATP and ADP or MVA and MVA-P which provided additional evidence for a sequential reaction [12]. Other studies had shown that both geranyl and farnesyl pyrophosphate were potent competitive inhibitors of the enzyme when MgATP was the variable substrate while these compounds were uncompetitive against mevalonate. These data suggest that the addition of substrates is ordered. In addition, evidence has been presented that a sulfhydryl group is important for the phosphorylation of mevalonate. A direct search for enzyme-bound intermediates was negative; i.e., preincubation of the protein with any of its substrates failed to reveal any linkage between enzyme and substrate. However, sulfhydryl-directed reagents were effective inhibitors, and their action could be prevented by the presence of either substrate [36]. It has been demonstrated that the enzyme catalyzes the phosphorylation of (3*R*)-mevalonate to (3*R*)-5-phosphomevalonate.

(VII) Phosphomevalonate kinase (EC 2.7.4.2)

The next reaction in the transformations of mevalonate is unusual in that the transfer of a phosphoryl entity from ATP to mevalonate-5-phosphate forms the

5′-pyrophosphoryl ester of mevalonate.

$$HO_2C-CH_2-\underset{\underset{OH}{|}}{\overset{\overset{CH_3}{|}}{C}}-CH_2-CH_2-OPO_3 + ATP$$

$$\xrightleftharpoons{Mg^{2+}} HO_2-C-CH_2-\underset{\underset{OH}{|}}{\overset{\overset{CH_3}{|}}{C}}-CH_2-CH_2-O-\underset{\underset{O^-}{|}}{\overset{\overset{O}{\|}}{P}}-O-\underset{\underset{O^-}{|}}{\overset{\overset{O}{\|}}{P}}-O^- + ADP$$

Usually, pyrophosphate esters are synthesized in one step by the direct transfer of pyrophosphate from a nucleotide triphosphate. The enzyme responsible for this reaction has been detected in a number of organisms and tissues. Purification to homogeneity has been achieved recently with pig liver as the source of the enzyme [38,39]. The protein is relatively small with a molecular weight of 22 000 and consists of a single polypeptide chain. A 1000-fold purification was required for purification to homogeneity, and the presence of sulfhydryl-containing compounds was essential during the purification procedure. ATP was found to be the only nucleotide that would serve as a phosphoryl donor. A number of divalent cations, Zn^{2+}, Mn^{2+}, and Co^{2+} as well as Mg^{2+}, which was about 2-fold better than any of the other ions, supported activity. A sulfhydryl group as well as a lysine are probably essential for catalytic activity, since the enzyme is inhibited by 5,5′-dithiobis(2-nitrobenzoate) as well as pyridoxal phosphate. The inhibition by pyridoxal phosphate was permanent if the mixture was reduced with $NaBH_4$ [40]. Kinetic analysis revealed that the mechanism is sequential with relatively high K_m values of 75 μM and 460 μM for phospho-mevalonate and ATP, respectively.

(VIII) Pyrophosphomevalonate decarboxylase (EC 4.1.1.33)

The enzyme catalyzes the simultaneous dehydration and decarboxylation of mevalonate-5-pyrophosphate to isopentenyl pyrophosphate.

$$HO_2C-CH_2-\underset{\underset{OH}{|}}{\overset{\overset{CH_3}{|}}{C}}-CH_2-CH_2-CH_2-O-\underset{\underset{O^-}{|}}{\overset{\overset{O}{\|}}{P}}-O-\underset{\underset{O^-}{|}}{\overset{\overset{O}{\|}}{P}}-O^- + ATP$$

$$\xrightarrow{Mg^{2+}} H_2C{=}\overset{\overset{CH_3}{|}}{C}-CH_2-CH_2-O-\underset{\underset{O^-}{|}}{\overset{\overset{O}{\|}}{P}}-O-\underset{\underset{O^-}{|}}{\overset{\overset{O}{\|}}{P}}-O^- + PO_4^{3-} + ADP + CO_2$$

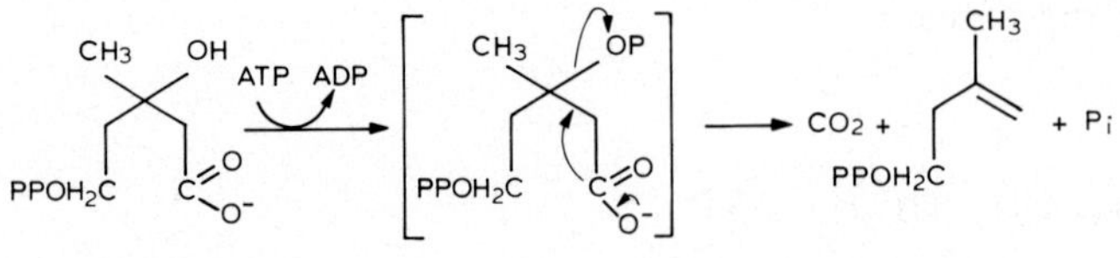

Fig. 6. The mechanism of pyrophosphomevalonate decarboxylase.

This enzyme has been isolated from a variety of tissues and purified to homogeneity from chicken liver [41,42]. The enzyme has a molecular weight of 85400 and is apparently composed of 2 identical subunits. It is absolutely specific for ATP and will accept either Mg^{2+} or Mn^{2+} as the divalent cation. Recently evidence has been presented that an arginyl residue is essential for catalytic activity [43]. Again, no evidence has been presented for any covalently linked enzyme–substrate intermediates.

Early studies were carried out with partially purified preparations from yeast and entailed the use of [3-^{18}O]mevalonate-5-pyrophosphate [44]. The labeled oxygen appeared in the orthophosphate that was cleaved from ATP indicating that this position in mevalonate had been phosphorylated during the course of the reaction. This observation suggested that 3-phospho-5-pyrophosphomevalonate might be a transient intermediate in the reaction. No such intermediate has been isolated and a concerted mechanism involving the transient formation of an ester linkage between phosphate and the 3-hydroxyl of 5-pyrophosphomevalonate has been proposed as is shown in Fig. 6. In this reaction the hydroxyl and carboxyl groups are eliminated in an anti-manner.

(IX) Isopentenyl pyrophosphate isomerase (EC 5.3.3.2)

(1) Enzymology

Isopentenyl pyrophosphate isomerase catalyzes the equilibrium between the Δ^2 and Δ^3 double bonds of a 3-methylbutenyl pyrophosphate (Fig. 7). This is the first enzyme in the biosynthesis of allylic pyrophosphates and is a cytoplasmic protein that has been detected in many tissues. Initial purification was reported from yeast [45] and a subsequent purification to homogeneity has been reported with pig liver as the source of protein [46]. There are some variances in the apparent molecular weight of this protein. One group [46] reported a molecular weight of 85000 while we found 22000 to be the value for the enzyme from the same source [47]. There is

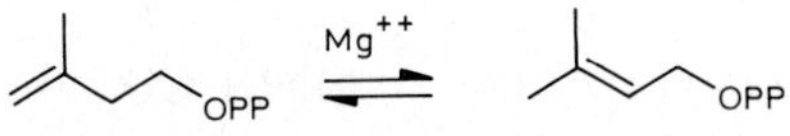

Fig. 7. The reaction catalyzed by isopentenyl pyrophosphate isomerase.

also a discrepancy in the number of different forms of the enzyme present in any tissue. The existence of several separable forms has been reported [48]; however, it has been the experience in one laboratory that the varying forms are the result of proteolysis during purification [47]. A homogeneous preparation of isomerase (M_r, 35 000) has also been obtained from the mold *Claviceps purpurea* [47]. Banthorp et al. [46] found the protein to be comprised of 2 similar subunits while the fungal enzyme is a single polypeptide [47].

The enzyme reversibly isomerizes the double bond of isopentenyl and dimethylallyl pyrophosphates with an equilibrium position of about 9 to 1 favoring the allylic compound. The apparent lability of this enzyme, which may be due to its sensitivity to proteases, has limited investigation of its catalytic properties. The stereospecificity was established in early investigations by the demonstration that the 2-pro-*R* hydrogen of the isopentenyl pyrophosphate was lost during isomerization while in the reverse direction the addition of a heavy isotope of hydrogen gave the 2-*R* enantiomer of isopentenyl pyrophosphate. The insertion of hydrogen for the conversion of isopentenyl pyrophosphate to dimethylallyl pyrophosphate is on the *re* face of the double bond, and the (*E*)-methyl of dimethylallyl pyrophosphate comes from C-2 of mevalonate which is C-4 in isopentenyl pyrophosphate [6,49,50]. This enzyme which has an absolute requirement for a divalent cation, either Mn^{2+} or Mg^{2+}, is inhibited by sulfhydryl-directed reagents and, in turn, is protected by free sulfhydryls [46]. However, definitive evidence for the role of an essential sulfhydryl is lacking. With the fungal enzyme, inhibition by iodoacetamide and 5,5′-dithiobis(2-nitrobenzoate) was also noted; however, the concentration of reagents, required to inhibit the enzyme, was greater than that necessary to titrate the sulfhydryl groups in the pure protein [51]. Thus, mechanisms for this reaction that postulate a role for a substrate–enzyme intermediate covalently bound through sulfur should be viewed with skepticism.

(2) Substrate specificity

Several studies with this enzyme have shown that many organic pyrophosphates inhibit this enzyme regardless of the source of protein. Of the most effective of these are geranyl and farnesyl pyrophosphate with K_i values of 10 μM for the avian enzyme. Inorganic pyrophosphate had a K_i of 2 μM [51]. Ogura probed the catalytic site of the enzyme from pumpkin fruit with substrate analogs, including inorganic pyrophosphate, allyl pyrophosphate, (*E*)-2-butenyl, neryl and geranyl pyrophosphates, all were about equally effective as inhibitors while the monophosphates were less effective [52]. These results indicate that the interaction of the pyrophosphate moiety with the enzyme is of major importance in substrate binding. It is somewhat surprising that the alkyl portion does not have a greater effect. Several analogs of isopentenyl pyrophosphate, 3-ethyl-3-butenyl and (*E*)-3-methyl-3-pentenyl pyrophosphate have been found to be substrates for the enzyme [53]. The second of these substrate analogs participates in a reversible isomerization with (*E*)-3-methyl-2-pentenyl pyrophosphate in a way expected for the 1,3 transposition of hydrogen

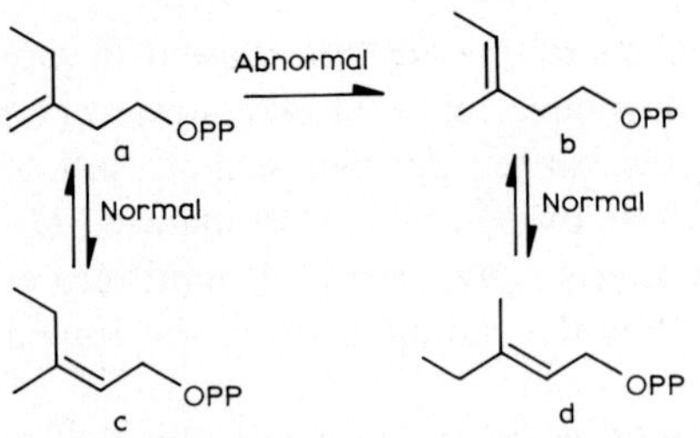

Fig. 8. The normal and abnormal isomerizations catalyzed by isomerase with substrate analogs.

based on the normal course of the reaction. The reactions of 3-ethyl-3-butenyl pyrophosphate were much more complex. One product was the isomer expected for the normal rearrangement, but the other, which was formed more rapidly, is homoallylic (Fig. 8). This aberrant isomerization must be due to distortion of the substrate in the catalytic site caused by the more bulky ethyl group. This distortion might bring the base required for removal of the allylic hydrogens in close contact with hydrogens on the ethyl group and cause their removal.

(3) Mechanism

Except for studies involved with characterization of the enzyme, there is little relevant material in the literature concerning the mechanism of the reaction. The incorporation of ^{3}H from water into isopentenyl pyrophosphate and dimethylallyl pyrophosphate has been determined. The exchange was substantially faster with isopentenyl pyrophosphate and the label was located primarily on C-4. The results were interpreted in terms of a mechanism in which a carbonium ion, formed by protonation, partitions between the two substrates and a covalent adduct with the enzyme (Fig. 9). A covalent substrate adduct was reported, but this undoubtedly resulted as an artifact of the experimental procedures used [6].

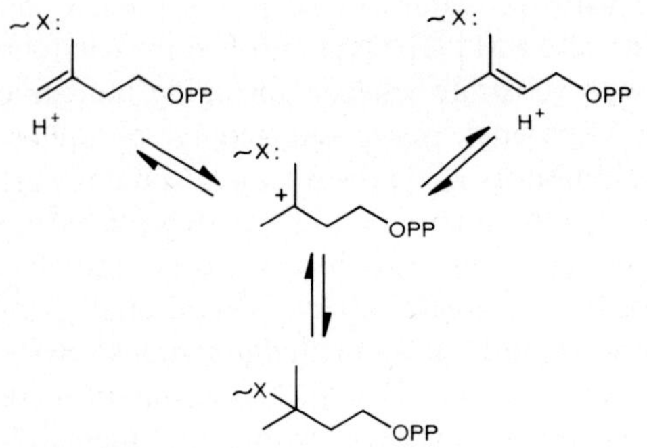

Fig. 9. Potential mechanisms for isomerase.

In more recent experiments, Satterwhite found that there was an isotope effect in $^{3}H^{+}$ uptake during conversion of isopentenyl pyrophosphate to dimethylallyl pyrophosphate [54]. The experiments utilized prenyltransferase to trap the allylic product as farnesyl pyrophosphate. With [4-^{14}C]isopentenyl pyrophosphate as an internal standard, a 4.6-fold discrimination against tritium was determined. The discrimination against deuterium was 2.8-fold in good agreement with the data obtained with tritium. This isotope effect was consistent with early data published on this reaction which had indicated a similar effect [55]. One interpretation is that the addition of a proton to C-4 is the rate-limiting step of this reaction and that a covalent H bond is broken during the transfer. An isotope effect was also found for removal of hydrogen from C-2 during the reaction [55]. It should be noted that isomerase does not transfer a hydrogen from C-2 to C-4 during the course of the reaction.

Satterwhite also investigated the effect of fluorine substitution for hydrogen in the substrate [54]. 2-Fluoro-isopentenyl pyrophosphate was converted to 2-fluoro-dimethylallyl pyrophosphate by isomerase at about 1% of the normal rate. Since only the *S* enantiomer of the racemic mixture is utilized by the enzyme, the remaining *R* enantiomer would be expected to be a competitive inhibitor. Consequently, the true velocity is not known. The tremendous resistance of 2- and 4-fluoro-hydroxy esters to elimination of substituents at C-3 practically eliminates the existence of a covalent enzyme–substrate intermediate. Also, since a much larger depression in rate would have been expected with the fluorine analog as substrate, a mechanism entailing the formation of a tertiary cationic intermediate, is also unlikely. A concerted hydrogenation dehydrogenation reaction has been suggested (Fig. 10).

(X) Prenyltransferase (EC 2.5.1.1)

(1) Enzymology

Prenyltransferase catalyzes the 1′-4 condensation between an allylic pyrophosphate and isopentenyl pyrophosphate in the presence of either Mg^{2+} or Mn^{2+}. The products are the next higher homolog of the allylic substrate, inorganic pyrophosphate and a proton (Fig. 11). Since the organic product is chemically identical to one of the substrates, it can be a polymerization reaction. In mammalian systems there are several end products for prenyltransferases; hence, there must be several enzyme systems. The enzymes for the biosynthesis of dolichols and/or the side chains of ubiquinone have not been isolated. The prenyltransferase for generating farnesyl

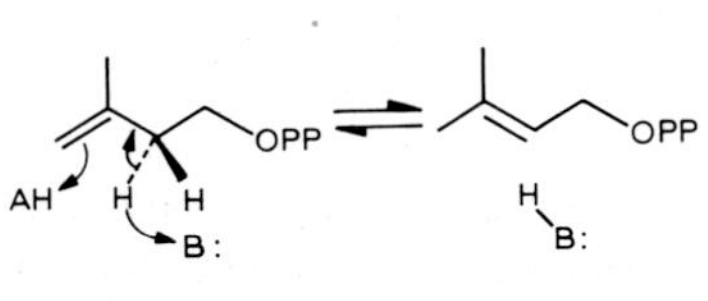

Fig. 10. A concerted hydrogenation–dehydrogenation reaction mechanism for isomerase.

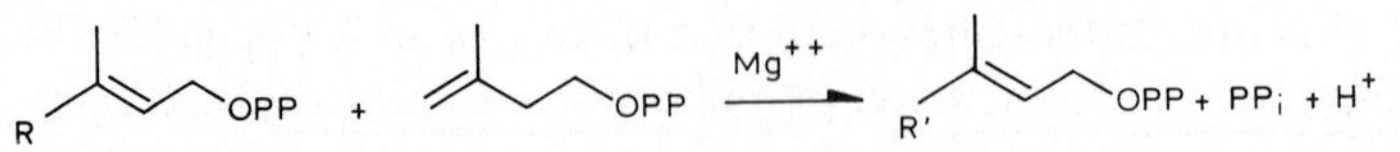

$$R\text{-}C(CH_3)\!=\!CH\text{-}CH_2\text{-}OPP + CH_2\!=\!C(CH_3)\text{-}CH_2\text{-}CH_2\text{-}OPP \xrightarrow{Mg^{++}} R'\text{-}C(CH_3)\!=\!CH\text{-}CH_2\text{-}OPP + PP_i + H^+$$

Fig. 11. The reaction catalyzed by prenyltransferase. $R = C_5H_9$; $R' = C_{10}H_{17}$.

pyrophosphate for squalene and sterol synthesis, and perhaps the side chain of cytochrome *a*, have been purified to homogeneity from a number of sources [6,56,57]. It is worth noting that *Z* as well as *E* prenols can be synthesized by the different prenyltransferases. The 2-pro-*S* hydrogen is removed by those that synthesize *Z* olefins while the 2-pro-*R* is removed by the enzymes that synthesize *E* olefins. This property has been used diagnostically for determining the stereochemistry of the product; however, one needs to retain reservations about its universality. The *si* face of the C-3–C-4 double bond of isopentenyl pyrophosphate is attacked, and the 1′-4 condensation reaction has been shown to occur with inversion of configuration of C-1 of the allylic substrate.

Farnesyl pyrophosphate synthetases have been isolated from yeast, *Phycomyces blakesleanus,* and livers of pig, chicken [6] and man [58]. All of the transferases have molecular weights of 75 000–85 000 and are comprised of two apparently identical subunits. These enzymes have relatively broad activity maxima at neutral pH, and the K_m values of substrates are around 0.5 μM. Evidence has been presented for the participation of an arginine and the presence of an essential sulfhydryl in the enzyme from human liver [57,58]. The chicken liver enzyme apparently lacks these features [6].

(2) Substrate binding

Since the enzyme from avian liver has been the most extensively studied, it will be considered in greater detail. It catalyzes 3 prenylation reactions, the condensation of both a C_5 and C_{10} allylic pyrophosphate with isopentenyl pyrophosphate to give farnesyl pyrophosphate. The third reaction between the C_{15} pyrophosphate and isopentenyl pyrophosphate proceeds at about 2% of the rate of others. Although the chemistry of these reactions is identical, the substrates utilized are not. Thus, it was possible that the subunits could be homogenous or heterogenous with respect to substrate specificity. Substrate-binding studies demonstrated that the subunits were identical. Each mole of enzyme bound 2 moles of either the C_5 or C_{10} allylic substrate in a competitive manner. The protein bound 4 moles of isopentenyl pyrophosphate, thus indicating that the allylic site would accommodate the homoallylic substrate while the converse was not true. The product, farnesyl pyrophosphate, competes for binding against the allylic substrates and, in the absence of a divalent cation to prevent catalysis, will compete against isopentenyl pyrophosphate for binding. Additional studies with 2-fluoro-farnesyl pyrophosphate, which is nonreactive, indicated that the presence of this farnesyl analog blocked the binding of both the allylic and homoallylic substrate. Apparently each subunit of the enzyme has an allylic and an isopentenyl pyrophosphate binding site [6].

The enzyme has an absolute requirement for a divalent cation, which could function in substrate binding, catalysis, or both. Radioactive Mn^{2+} did not bind appreciably in the absence of substrate. With substrate or product present, 2 moles of metal were bound per subunit. Metal ions (Mn^{2+} or Mg^{2+}) also enhanced the binding of substrates several-fold. Simultaneous binding of two unreactive fluorine analogs, one allylic the other homoallylic, did not enhance the binding of the metal ion. These experiments demonstrated that the metal ion is essential for catalysis and may not play an important role in substrate binding [6].

(3) Mechanism

The earliest studies relative to the mechanism was the stereochemical work of Conforth, Popjak, and their collaborators [49]. They concluded that there was an inversion of configuration at C-1 of the allylic substrate, consistent with a concerted process, the new carbon-to-carbon bond being formed as the carbon-to-oxygen bond is cleaved. They also felt that elimination of a proton from C-2 of the isopentenyl moiety would not be concerted with this, since suprafacial (same side) reactions are generally considered unfavorable. To circumvent this, a 2-stage mechanism involving an electron donor "X", with X being covalently linked to the initial condensation product, was proposed. The X residue is then lost simultaneously with elimination of the proton in an anti-mode (Fig. 12).

Reed found that crystalline prenyltransferase could solvolyze the allylic substrates. This reaction required inorganic pyrophosphate and had a velocity of about 2% of the normal reaction rate [6]. Examination of the allylic product, either dimethylallyl alcohol or geraniol, revealed that C-1 had inverted and the carbinol oxygen had come from water. Since the normal reaction involves inversion of C-1 and scission of C–O bond, the solvolysis seemed to be mimicking the normal reaction, with H_2O replacing the organic portion of isopentenyl pyrophosphate in the catalytic site. This indicates that ionization of the allylic pyrophosphate is the first event, followed by condensation to form a new bond, then a hydrogen elimination from C-2 of the former isopentenyl moiety. Thus, there is an ionization–condensation–elimination sequence of events.

Poulter and his group used another approach to demonstrate this mechanism [6].

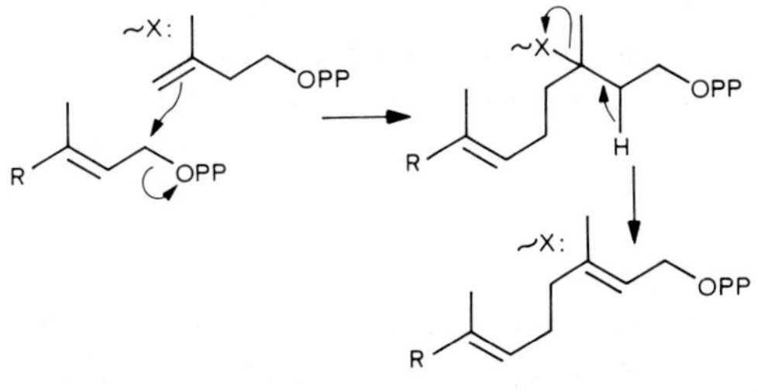

Fig. 12. The "X" mechanism for prenyltransferase.

TABLE 1
Relative reactivities of allylic systems in nucleophilic substitution reactions

Reactant	k
Dimethylallyl methanesulfonate	1.2
Geranyl methanesulfonate	1
(E)-3-Trifluoromethyl-2-buten-1-yl methanesulfonate	4×10^{-7}
(Z)-3-Trifluoromethyl-2-buten-1-yl methanesulfonate	4×10^{-7}
2-Fluorogeranyl methanesulfonate	4.4×10^{-3}

TABLE 2
Relative reactivities of allylic pyrophosphates in 1′-4 condensation reactions

Substrate	V_{max}
Dimethylallyl pyrophosphate	0.5
Geranyl pyrophosphate	1
(E)-3-Trifluoromethyl-2-buten-1-yl pyrophosphate	7×10^{-7}
(Z)-3-Trifluoromethyl-2-buten-1-yl pyrophosphate	1×10^{-6}
2-Fluorogeranyl pyrophosphate	8×10^{-4}

They replaced hydrogen atoms in the periphery of the C-2–C-3 double bond of the allylic pyrophosphate with fluorine. The electron-withdrawing effect of the fluorine should greatly retard the rate of the ionization step by depleting electron density in the allylic moiety. This effect would be much less on the rate of a nucleophilic displacement. If the rate-limiting step or partial rate-limiting step is the cleavage of the C–O bond of the allylic molecule, these fluorine-containing compounds would react more slowly during condensation. To determine the effects of fluorine substitution on the rates of ionization, model compounds were prepared and their rates of solvolysis determined. The results are shown in Tables 1 and 2.

Although these experiments made an S_N2 mechanism most unlikely, it was still possible that a developing positive charge at C-3 might be stabilized by an X group from the protein. Since the final step of this mechanism is the elimination of hydrogen from C-2 and X from C-3, the inclusion of fluorine at C-2 of isopentenyl pyrophosphate should trap any enzyme-bound intermediate. Two analogs, 2-fluoro- and 2,2′-difluoroisopentenyl pyrophosphate, effective competitive inhibitors of the enzyme, were tested but no enzyme-bound intermediate was detected [6].

(4) Kinetics

The kinetic analysis of this enzyme is difficult since isopentenyl pyrophosphate binds at both sides as does the product, inorganic pyrophosphate. In addition, farnesyl pyrophosphate interferes with binding of substrates at both sites. An early kinetic analysis by Holloway and Popjak [59] indicated an ordered bimolecular reaction, with geranyl pyrophosphate being the first substrate added and farnesyl pyrophosphate the first product to be released. More recently a detailed kinetic study by Laskovics et al. [60] showed inhibition by the homoallylic substrate. Also fluorogeranyl and fluoroisopentenyl pyrophosphates were used as dead-end inhibitors. However, differentiation between ordered and random sequential mechanisms was not possible because of the lack of specificity of both inhibitors and products.

To solve the problem of mechanism, trapping experiments were performed. In these experiments, the enzyme was preincubated with one substrate (radioactive), then the second added along with an excess of nonradioactive initial substrate [61]. Since any substrate trapped by the chase before dissociation from the enzyme would yield a product of high specific activity, it was possible to calculate the fraction of the first substrate that condenses before dissociation. With this technique, half of the allylic substrate and none of the homoallylic were trapped. Thus the mechanism is ordered with the allylic substrate binding first. At very short reaction times, a burst of synthesis of farnesyl pyrophosphate was observed followed by a steady-state rate that was 50 times slower. The burst was due to the formation of farnesyl pyrophosphate on the enzyme surface (catalytic site), while the slower steady state is the result of the product leaving the enzyme [61]. Recently, a free-energy study was reported which indicated that the cleavage of the pyrophosphate ester bond of geranyl pyrophosphate is a discrete step and yields a geranyl cation–pyrophosphate ion pair, which is the species that then reacts with the double bond of isopentenyl pyrophosphate [62]. This ion pair is sufficiently tight that there is no exchange between bridging oxygen and nonbridging oxygen in the

$$\begin{array}{c} \quad\quad O^- \\ \quad\quad | \\ -C-O-P- \\ \quad\quad | \\ \quad\quad O^- \end{array}$$

linkage of this pyrophosphate ester [63].

(5) Termination

Prenyltransferase is a polymerizing enzyme that stops after 2 condensation reactions (farnesyl pyrophosphate is an inefficient substrate). Some experiments gave an insight as to the mechanism of termination of the polymerization reaction [64]. As discussed above, inorganic pyrophosphate promotes the solvolysis of geranyl pyrophosphate to the parent alcohol. However, with farnesyl pyrophosphate as a substrate, the reaction was quite slow and a mixture of hydrocarbon and alcohols was recovered. This could be accounted for if, while binding in the allylic site, the tail of the hydrocarbon chain of farnesyl pyrophosphate was forced back over C-1 by the shape of the catalytic site, preventing isopentenyl pyrophosphate from binding in the catalytic site and excluding water for the solvolytic reaction as well. Also, the cation formed upon the ionization step would have time to rearrange before reacting with water and give it the opportunity to react intramolecularly with the C-10–C-11 double bond. Predicted cyclic sesquiterpenes were found, thus indicating that it is the size and shape of the allylic binding site that determines termination by the crowding out of an incoming isopentenyl pyrophosphate molecule [64].

(6) Analogs

The potential role of cholesterol in atherosclerosis has led to the synthesis of many substrate analogs for prenyltransferase that have been tested as inhibitors or substrates. Consequently, some topological aspects required for substrate binding are known. The pyrophosphate group is required for reaction. Dimethylallyl phosphate and geranyl phosphate inhibit the enzyme but do not participate in the condensation. The C-2–C-3 double bond is essential for reactivity and major changes in the vicinity of this bond destroy the analog's ability to interact with the protein. Fluorine is the only substitution permitted for hydrogen at C-2. C-3 must be disubstituted with alkyl groups. The methyl group at the *Z* configuration of C-3 can be substituted by short linear alkyl chains up to butyl. On the other hand, the enzyme will accept extensive modifications in the *E* position. More than 30 analogs have been reported [6]. For example, when the hydrocarbon chain in this position was extended up to 10 residues, the analogs were utilized by the enzyme. Two optima were found, one for dimethylallyl residue and one when the alkyl chain was 5 carbons longer; i.e., a geranyl analog [65].

Binding and reactivity at the isopentenyl pyrophosphate site are more stringent. For example, dimethylallyl pyrophosphate does not bind at this site. When the alkyl substituent at C-3 is varied from none to 3 carbons, only the methyl and the ethyl homologs participate. Functional substrates were obtained with an analog substituted with dimethyl at C-4 as well as one with an extra methyl at both C-4 and C-5. Two very unusual analogs, a cyclohexene and a cyclopentene derivative, also were reactive. If a single methylene is inserted between C-1 and C-3 of isopentenyl pyrophosphate, the product of the condensation of this analog with geranyl pyrophosphate had *Z* stereochemistry at the new C-3–C-4 double bond (Fig. 13).

Advantage was taken of this lack of specificity and several photoreactive substrate analogs were synthesized. One of these, *o*-azidophenethyl pyrophosphate, when photolyzed with avian prenyltransferase, gave extensive inactivation. Frag-

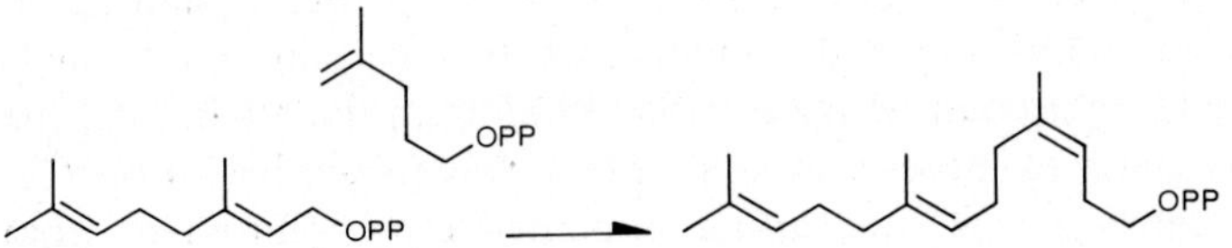

OPP
OPP
OPP

Fig. 13. The observed condensation between geranyl pyrophosphate and 4-methylpent-4-enyl pyrophosphate.

mentation of the derivatized protein with cyanogen bromide yielded 8 peptides, only one of which was labeled. Sequencing of this peptide revealed two rather broad regions associated with the photoaffinity label [66].

(XI) Squalene synthetase

(1) Enzymology

The conversion of farnesyl pyrophosphate to squalene is a 2-step process. First is the 1′-2-3 condensation of 2 farnesyl pyrophosphate molecules with the concomitant loss of a proton and inorganic pyrophosphate to form presqualene pyrophosphate [67,68].

$$\text{2 farnesyl pyrophosphate} \rightarrow \text{presqualene pyrophosphate} + PP_i + H^+$$

$$\text{Presqualene pyrophosphate} + NADPH + H^+ \rightarrow \text{squalene} + NADP + PP_i$$

The resulting cyclopropylcarbinyl pyrophosphate is reduced to squalene by NADPH. This is the "head-to-head" condensation of terpene biosynthesis. The absolute stereochemistry of presqualene pyrophosphate has been determined [69].

The enzymes necessary for the conversion of farnesyl pyrophosphate to squalene are called "squalene synthetase". The enzymes necessary for the two reactions have not been resolved nor has either been purified to a significant extent, and it is not yet certain if the two reactions are catalyzed by two discrete entities. Squalene synthetase has an absolute requirement for a divalent cation, Mg^{2+} and Mn^{2+} being the best. A reduced pyridine nucleotide (NADH or NADPH) is required for the reduction of presqualene pyrophosphate to squalene. Yeast microsomes with Mn^{2+} and no reduced pyridine nucleotide will form dehydrosqualene instead [70]. The conversion of farnesyl pyrophosphate to presqualene pyrophosphate is enhanced several-fold by the reduced pyridine nucleotide [71]. Also, some organic solvents as well as detergents increase this activity.

Apparently, squalene synthetase is a relatively small microsomal protein. The enzyme was solubilized from yeast microsomes by deoxycholate. If detergent was then removed, the microsomal proteins aggregated. If instead, the preparation was centrifuged in a sucrose gradient containing detergent, squalene synthetase sedimented with an $S_{20,w}$ of 3.3 in contrast to the 14.2 $S_{20,w}$ value reported earlier. Centrifugation failed to resolve the two catalytic activities of squalene synthetase [72].

The deoxycholate-solubilized squalene synthetase was also chromatographed on Sephadex G-200 and a Stokes radius of 40 Å was found for the enzyme. Again, the two catalytic activities were not resolved [72]. This value, along with the $S_{20,w}$, indicated a molecular weight of 55000 for the protein(s). This contrasts with much higher values reported earlier. Inclusion of certain phospholipids in the tubes used for collecting the chromatographic fractions greatly enhanced the recovery of activity.

(2) Kinetics

The kinetics of the overall reaction are controversial as might be expected since the substrate is water soluble while the intermediate and the product are not. What can be said is that under the right conditions there is stoichiometry between presqualene pyrophosphate, squalene and farnesyl pyrophosphate. In addition, since high concentrations of farnesyl pyrophosphate transitorily inhibit the second reaction, and NADPH stimulates the first, it can be concluded that the enzyme(s) has separate but closely related sites for the two reactions. These sites could be on one or two peptide chains [71].

(3) Analogs

A variety of substrate analogs have been tested with microsomal squalene synthetase, and these have served to determine some of the specificity parameters for binding and reacting in this system. The requirement for the pyrophosphate moiety is absolute since farnesyl monophosphate does not participate in the reaction. It is not known if the divalent cation requirement is for binding and/or catalysis [67].

Interaction with the hydrocarbon moiety is not as specific. The effect of the chain length has been studied by Ogura who demonstrated that replacement of either terminal methyl group of farnesyl pyrophosphate by ethyl yielded the corresponding bishomo squalene derivative [73]. More dramatically, geranylgeranyl pyrophosphate can serve as a substrate in a yeast system. The product lycopersene is a C_{40} homolog of squalene. However, shortening the chain length of the analog to C_{10} (geranyl) gives an inactive substrate [67]. This is interesting since geranyl pyrophosphate is an intermediate in farnesyl pyrophosphate synthesis while geranylgeranyl pyrophosphate only participates in a relatively minor pathway leading to the ubiquinone side chain.

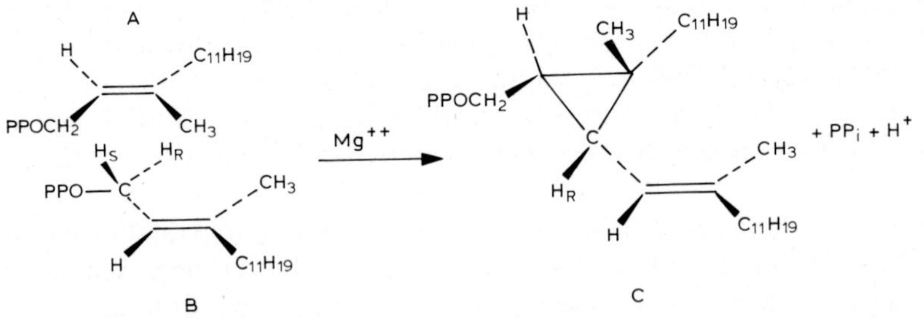

Fig. 14. The condensation between 2 molecules of farnesyl pyrophosphate (A, acceptor; B, donor). The product is presqualene pyrophosphate (C).

Ortiz de Montellano and collaborators tested a number of analogs of farnesyl pyrophosphate as substrates for squalene synthesis [74]. Three of these compounds served as substrates but only when farnesyl pyrophosphate was a co-reactant. The analogs were incorporated regiospecifically. Experiments with C-1 tritium-labeled analogs demonstrated that they occupied the acceptor site during the condensation reaction (see Fig. 14). A similar observation had been made with the analog 7-desmethylfarnesyl pyrophosphate. In these experiments it was estimated that the discrimination against the analog was 20-fold. Thus, the enzyme has been shown to be fairly selective, with the donor region being considerably more specific. Condensation was not seen with more extensive modifications in the vicinity of the C-2–C-3 and C-6–C-7 double bonds. It should be noted, because of the way these experiments were done, that they only rule out these analogs as donors and not as acceptors in the condensation reaction to form presqualene pyrophosphate [74]. The nonparticipating analogs were studied as inhibitors for this condensation reaction. The C-6–C-7 double bond is particularly important since compounds in which this is saturated are relatively ineffective inhibitors. Also, the 6,7-dihydro- and 6,7,10,11-tetrahydrofarnesyl pyrophosphates are unreactive in the condensation reaction as well as being relatively poor inhibitors [67].

A most interesting analog of presqualene containing a nitrogen adjacent to the cyclopropane ring has been prepared [75]. This compound failed to inhibit squalene synthesis in the absence of phosphate-containing buffer. However, in the presence of inorganic phosphate, moderate inhibition was found. If inorganic pyrophosphate was included, complete inhibition could be obtained. The authors suggested that the pyrophosphate salt of the amine duplicated the topological and electrostatic features of an ion pair involved in the rearrangement of presqualene pyrophosphate to squalene (Fig. 15).

(4) Mechanism

The 1′-2-3-condensation of two farnesyl pyrophosphate molecules results in the formation of a cyclopropane ring with 3 chiral centers. The C-2–C-3 double bond of one farnesyl unit which is attacked by the C-1 of another, retains the relative orientation of the substituents on the double bond. The alkyl group at C-3 of the cyclopropane ring is *trans* to the carbinyl carbon at C-1 of the ring. Popjak et al.

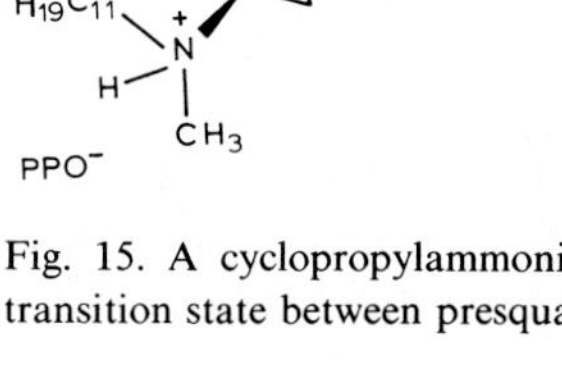

Fig. 15. A cyclopropylammonium analog of presqualene. As the pyrophosphate, it may resemble a transition state between presqualene pyrophosphate and squalene.

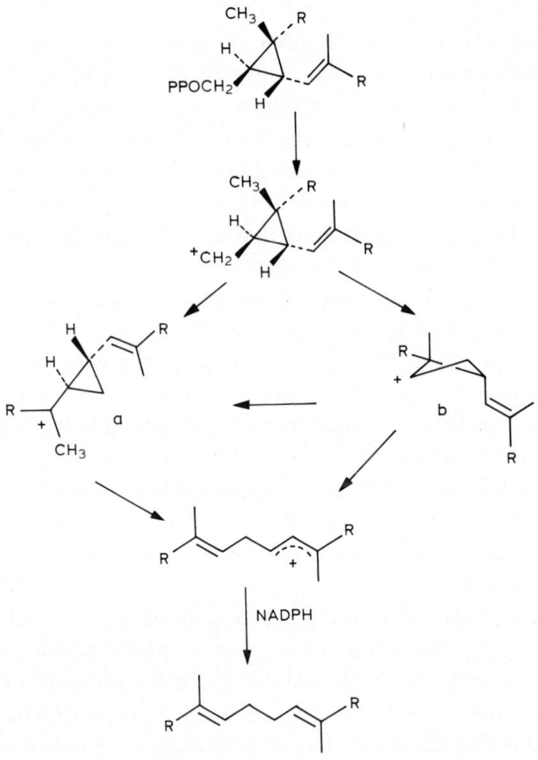

Fig. 16. Two possible pathways for rearrangements leading to the formation of squalene from presqualene pyrophosphate.

established the absolute configuration about the cyclopropane ring to be 1*R*, 2*R*, 3*R* by circular dichroism [69]. This is illustrated in Fig. 16.

During the condensation reaction, the donating farnesyl residue loses a proton (the pro-*S* hydrogen) at C-1 (cf. Fig. 14). This information, in conjunction with the known absolute configuration, indicates that the prenylation is at the 2-*si*, 3-*re* face of the acceptor. This indicated that C-1 of the donor farnesyl unit inverts [67].

The series of rearrangements leading from the cyclopropyl carbinyl system of presqualene pyrophosphate to squalene is complex; 5 bonds are made or broken during this rearrangement. As for presqualene pyrophosphate synthesis, no satisfactory enzymology for this transformation has been achieved. Therefore, conclusions about the sequence of rearrangements that lead from this cyclopropyl intermediate have come from model studies, principally in laboratories of Poulter and of Coates who have studied the solvolysis of C_{10} analogs of presqualene pyrophosphate [67]. Two pathways that progress from the presqualene analog to the 1′-1 product are shown in Fig. 16. Unfortunately, in the model studies the yield of the 1′-1 product was low, indicating that the enzyme plays an important role in directing the course of the reaction as might be antcipated. Poulter has suggested that the topology of the enzyme–substrate complex be maintained in the ion pair (carbonium ion–pyrophosphate) formed, since electrostatic attractions can govern the regiochemistry of the rearrangement [67]. Given the intermediate ions and $a + b$, the remaining process was regiospecific, giving good yields of the 1′-1 product. However, it is not possible to distinguish between the cyclopropyl or cyclobutyl cations as intermediates on the way to the final product. The stereochemistry of the conversion of the 1′-2-3 condensation has also been determined, and very interestingly, the net stereochemistry in the model system is the same as that for the biosynthesis of squalene [67].

(XII) Squalene epoxidase and cyclase

(1) Enzymology

The enzymic conversion of squalene to lanosterol proceeds through an oxygen-dependent epoxidation to form 2,3-oxidosqualene which then undergoes cyclization and rearrangement to lanosterol. The reaction requires microsomes, a supernatant fraction, NADPH, and O_2 and is not inhibited by CO, N_3, CN^-, NH_2OH, EDTA or *o*-phenanthroline [76]. The activity can be separated into microsomal and soluble fractions. The supernatant fraction could be replaced by FAD, a phospholipid and a soluble protein [77]. In turn, the phospholipid and the soluble protein can be replaced by Triton X-100 [78] which also solubilizes the epoxidase activity from the microsomes. The solubilized activity could be resolved by DEAE-cellulose chromatography into 2 components which, by recombination, gave epoxidase activity. These components were a NADPH-cytochrome *c* reductase and the epoxidase which is believed to be a flavoprotein with dissociable FAD. The reconstituted system is dependent on FAD, Triton X-100, O_2, and NADPH for activity. The involvement of a NADPH cytochrome *c* reductase was confirmed [79,80], but the exact nature of the epoxidase activity still remains uncertain. The participation of cytochrome P-450 can be discarded because its presence has not been demonstrated [78,81,82], and because of the lack of sensitivity of the reaction to inhibition by CO, CN, benzphetamine and aniline [80]. The participation of hemoprotein is improbable due to the fact that yeast mutants that do not have the respiratory cytochromes are able to synthesize lanosterol but not ergosterol [83,84]. The epoxidase has been purified (95%), has a molecular weight of around 51 000, and requires for activity NADPH-cytochrome *c* reductase, NADPH, and FAD.

The role of the cytoplasmic effectors is obscure since their effects disappear when the enzyme is solubilized by Triton X-100. The possible participation of the soluble protein factor (SPF) as a carrier for substrate inside the membrane has been explored (Chapter 3). The SPF has been shown not only to stimulate the conversion of externally added squalene and oxidosqualene but also to activate squalene epoxidase as well as 2,3-oxidosqualene cyclase when the substrate is membrane bound [85,86]. SPF has been purified and shown to promote the transfer of squalene from one population of microsomes to another [87,88]. Nevertheless, SPF has no

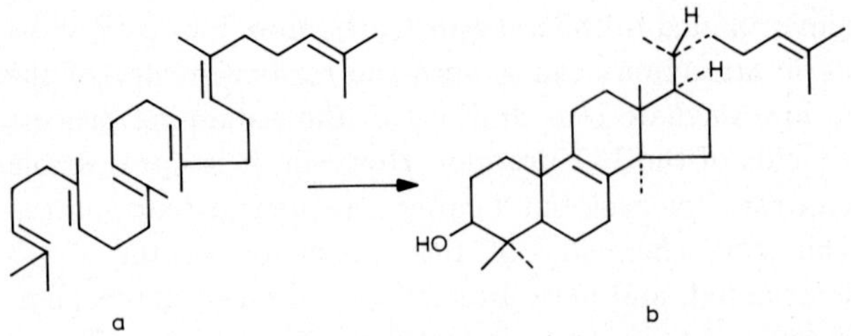

Fig. 17. The Woodward–Bloch scheme for the folding of squalene (a), for its conversion to lanosterol (b).

affinity for squalene or 2,3-oxidosqualene, nor for the microsomal membranes but only exhibits strong binding to anionic phospholipid vesicles [89].

(2) Mechanism

Squalene has been shown to assume the folding pattern of Woodward and Bloch in the cyclization process that forms sterols (Fig. 17). This was demonstrated by the labeling patterns of sterols derived from acetate and mevalonate [90,91]. There are several ways by which squalene can cyclize, consequently it is the precursor of several polycyclic terpenoids (Chapter 7). The product depends on the conformation squalene assumes in binding to the cyclase and the nature and position of the nucleophiles and bases on the enzyme. Mechanistically, squalene requires an electrophilic attack at C-3 for cyclization to occur. This can be accomplished by direct attack of a H^+ as in the cyclization that produces tetrahymanol and fernene or by

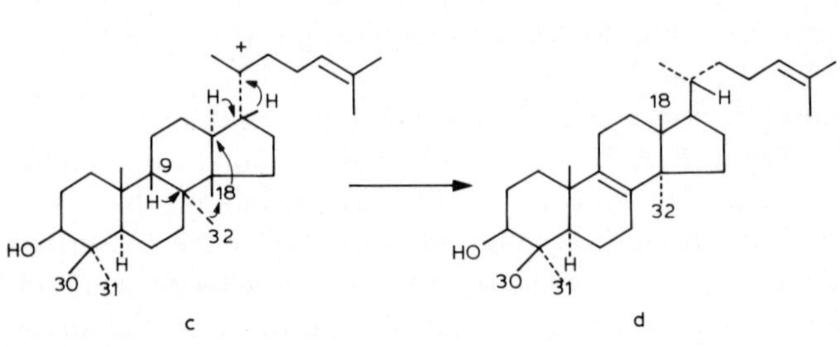

Fig. 18. The cyclization of 2,3-oxidosqualene (b) to the protosterol cation (c) and its subsequent rearrangement to lanosterol by a series of 1–2 shifts.

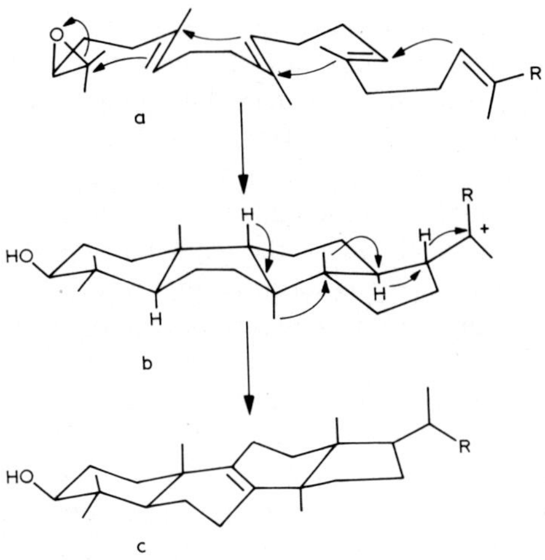

Fig. 19. The cyclization of 2,3-oxidosqualene (a), showing the folding in a *trans-syn-trans-anti-trans-anti* conformation that leads to the protosterol cation (b) and then to lanosterol (c).

electrophilic attack of a H^+ to a previously oxygenated species for the formation of the C-3 oxygenated steroids and triterpenes. After cyclization, a sequential neutralization of electrophilic centers by redistribution of electrons from neighboring double bonds occurs and finally the resulting cation is stabilized by a concerted 1,2 antiplanar migration of H and CH_3 with expulsion of H at C-9 to give lanosterol (see Fig. 18). For a detailed view on the chemistry and stereochemistry of the process, see ref. 1.

Initially, this process was thought to be concerted in nature, but it has been demonstrated that oxidation and cyclization are different steps by the synthesis and isolation of 2,3-oxidosqualene as an intermediate and the use of inhibitors of the cyclization reaction such as 2,3-iminosqualene [92]. The enzymes for the oxidation and cyclization differ in their susceptibility to solubilization by detergents. The partially purified cyclase (M_r 90 000) aggregates and is inactivated upon removal of the detergent. The oxidation is O_2 dependent while cyclization is anaerobic with no cofactors required.

It is accepted that triterpenoids in plants are formed through an all *trans-anti* conformation of squalene while lanosterol is formed through a *trans-syn-trans-anti-trans-anti* conformation to give the protosteroid cation (Fig. 19).

van Tamelen has shown that in the nonenzymic polycyclization of terminal epoxide derivatives, ring A is formed with anchimeric assistance of the neighboring double bond and that the complete annulation process is not fully concerted but would involve a series of conformationally rigid carbocyclic intermediates or ion pairs [93].

The driving force for the rearrangement comes in part from the relief of repulsive interactions in the protosteroid cation which are associated with ring B (twist-boat geometry) and its substituents especially the methyl group on C-8. Corey et al. [94] have shown that cyclization and rearrangements are distinct steps during lanosterol formation by using 2,3-oxido-10,15-bisnorsqualene which cyclizes to the corresponding protosteroid cation which is stabilized without rearrangement by deprotonation at C-20. This was confirmed by van Tamelen [95], who used 2,3-oxido-15-norsqualene to give the normal rearrangement product which lacked the methyl at C-13 of the steroid. The use of 20,21-dehydrooxidosqualene [96] as substrate that would lead to a very stable protosteroid cation gave, as product, a nonrearranged tetracyclic diol.

The process is known to be stereoselective; the *S* enantiomer of squalene epoxide is formed and only the C-20-*R* isomer of the steroids is formed. All steroids are formed through the protosteroid cation by elimination of protons at C-7, C-9, C-11, or C-19 to give lanostadienol, lanosterol, parkeol and cycloartenol, respectively. All have the same absolute configuration at C-5–C-10, the enzyme being responsible for enantiomeric selection.

Squalene epoxidase is not stringent in its substrate requirement but is sensitive to the overall structure of the substrate, showing little sensitivity to steric factors at the site of oxidation, and to the nucleophilic character of the double bond. However, it has impaired activity for analogs that are partially cyclized or are shortened by 2-isoprenoid units [97]. The products of the epoxidation reaction using 10,11-dihydrosqualene are the 2,3-oxide, 22,23-oxide, and 2,3,22,23-dioxide derivatives of the 10,11-dehydrosqualene [98], which again shows the lack of specificity of the epoxidase. The cyclase is also not specific since 2,3,22,23-dioxidosqualene can be converted to 24,25-oxidolanosterol in yeast and to 24,25-oxidocholesterol by liver [99,100]. The reaction catalyzed by the cyclase is initiated by an electrophilic attack of H^+ or a group in the enzyme to open the oxiran ring, giving rise to a carbocation. This has been recently shown with analogs like 2-aza-2,3-dihydrosqualene which proved to be a very strong inhibitor ($I_{50} = 1$ μM compared with $K_m = 250$ μM) of oxidosqualene α-amirin cyclase and oxidosqualene-cycloartenol cyclase [101] (see Fig. 20).

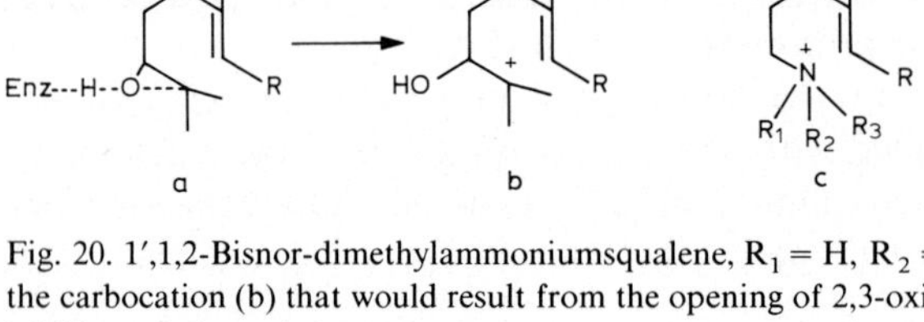

Enz---H--O--- R HO + R +N R R_1 R_2 R_3

a b c

Fig. 20. 1′,1,2-Bisnor-dimethylammoniumsqualene, $R_1 = H$, $R_2 = R_3 = CH_3$ (c), shown in comparison to the carbocation (b) that would result from the opening of 2,3-oxidosqualene (a) by a proton. C is a potent inhibitor of the cyclase.

(XIII) The conversion of lanosterol to cholesterol

(1) Sterol function

Sterols have several roles in eukaryotic cells, and probably the initial function was as a membrane component. In membranes, sterols serve to condense the phospholipids in the bilayer and at the same time they help to divide the membrane into two discrete phases, an outer more rigid zone and an inner fluid region (Chapter 6). The rigid portion of the sterol molecule serves to restrict the motion of the first 10–12 carbons of the fatty acyl chains of the phospholipids [102]. Bloch has examined the structure–function relationship of sterols by determining the microviscosity of phosphatidylcholine vesicles as a function of concentration as well as methyl substituents [103]. The findings indicated that the presence of a methyl group at C-14 has a marked effect on the microviscosity of sterols dissolved in a phospholipid bilayer, while the methyls at C-4 had a less profound effect on the bilayer. It is apparent that the first sterol to be synthesized, lanosterol, is not efficient in modifying the properties of membranes and that it is necessary to streamline the molecule by removing the methyl groups that protrude from the plane of the molecule. Again from an evolutionary standpoint it would seem that the modified sterols, the bile acids, the steroid hormones were derived from the basic membrane sterol, i.e. without the "extra" methyls at C-4 and C-14, rather than lanosterol. The double bond migration and saturation that occurs during the conversion of lanosterol to cholesterol must produce a much more subtle effect of the sterol on the properties of membranes.

(2) General aspects of enzymology

Nineteen discrete reactions are used to convert lanosterol to cholesterol. All of the enzymes necessary for these reactions are embedded in the microsomal membrane. Some of these proteins have been solubilized and purified. However, many questions of the mechanism and enzymology of these reactions remain to be answered.

Early in the study of cholesterol biosynthesis it was known that the methyl groups, upon removal appeared as CO_2 [104]. This conclusion has been revised since it is apparent that one of the three is removed as formate [105]. Reduced pyridine nucleotides and oxygen are required for the demethylation reactions; so it was concluded that monooxygenase(s) would be required for the initial hydroxylation. There are several possible mechanisms for the oxidation of the alcohol formed by oxygenation. The first mechanism considered was that the alcohol would be successively dehydrogenated, first by an alcohol dehydrogenase and then by an aldehyde dehydrogenase. This, however, is not the mechanism and further oxidations are catalyzed by monooxygenases [105]. There are two possible mechanisms for continued oxidation by monooxygenases. One would be that the carbinol carbon be hydroxylated again and the resulting hemiacetal decompose to the aldehyde. The second would be that the oxidant would directly abstract a hydrogen from the carbinol to give the aldehyde. It has not been possible to distinguish between these two mechanisms. In cholesterol biosynthesis, the carbon at C-14 (C-32) is not further oxidized and it leaves as formic acid. However, there is another oxidation of carbons C-30 and C-31 at C-4 to give the carboxylates. Again, the same two mechanisms are possible. The introduction of the double bond at C-5 also involves a monooxygenase and another one assists in the deformylation of C-32. In all, there are 10 oxidations by monooxygenases in the synthesis of cholesterol from lanosterol, some of which involve cytochrome P-450. For a general description of mechanisms of cytochrome P-450-catalyzed reactions the reader is referred to the review by White and Coon [106].

(3) The pathway

For the conversion of lanosterol to cholesterol, there are a number of excellent reviews that consider the sequence of events and the participants therein [1,2,5,105].

The enzymes responsible for the conversion of lanosterol to cholesterol, as were those for the conversion of farnesyl pyrophosphate to squalene and lanosterol, are all integral membrane-bound proteins of the endoplasmic reticulum. Many have resisted solubilization, some have been partially purified, and several have been obtained as pure proteins. As a consequence, much of the enzymological and mechanistic studies have been done on impure systems and one would anticipate a more detailed and improved understanding of these events as more highly purified enzymes become available. Many approaches have been taken to establish the biosynthetic route that sterols follow to cholesterol. Some examples are synthesis of potential intermediates, the use of inhibitors, both of sterol transformations and of the electron transfer systems, and by isotope dilution experiments. There is good evidence that the enzymes involved in these transformations do not have strict substrate specificity. As a result, many compounds that have been found to be converted to intermediates or to cholesterol may not be true intermediates. In addition, there is structural similarity between many of the intermediates so that alternate pathways and metabolites are possible. For example, it has been shown that side-chain saturation can be either the first or the last reaction in the sequence. Fig. 21 shows a most probable series of intermediates for this biosynthetic pathway.

(4) Decarbonylation at C-14

It is apparent that the first series of reactions involves the removal of the methyl on C-14 (C-32). This is initiated by hydroxylation of the methyl group by a cytochrome P-450. The involvement of cytochrome P-450 was demonstrated by the sensitivity of the reaction to CO. Squalene epoxidation and oxidation of the methyls at C-4 (C-30, C-31) are insensitive to this reagent. So when lanosterol and dihydrolanosterol accumulated in CO-poisoned liver preparations, the indications were clear that hydroxylation at C-32 was the first step in lanosterol metabolism [105]. In

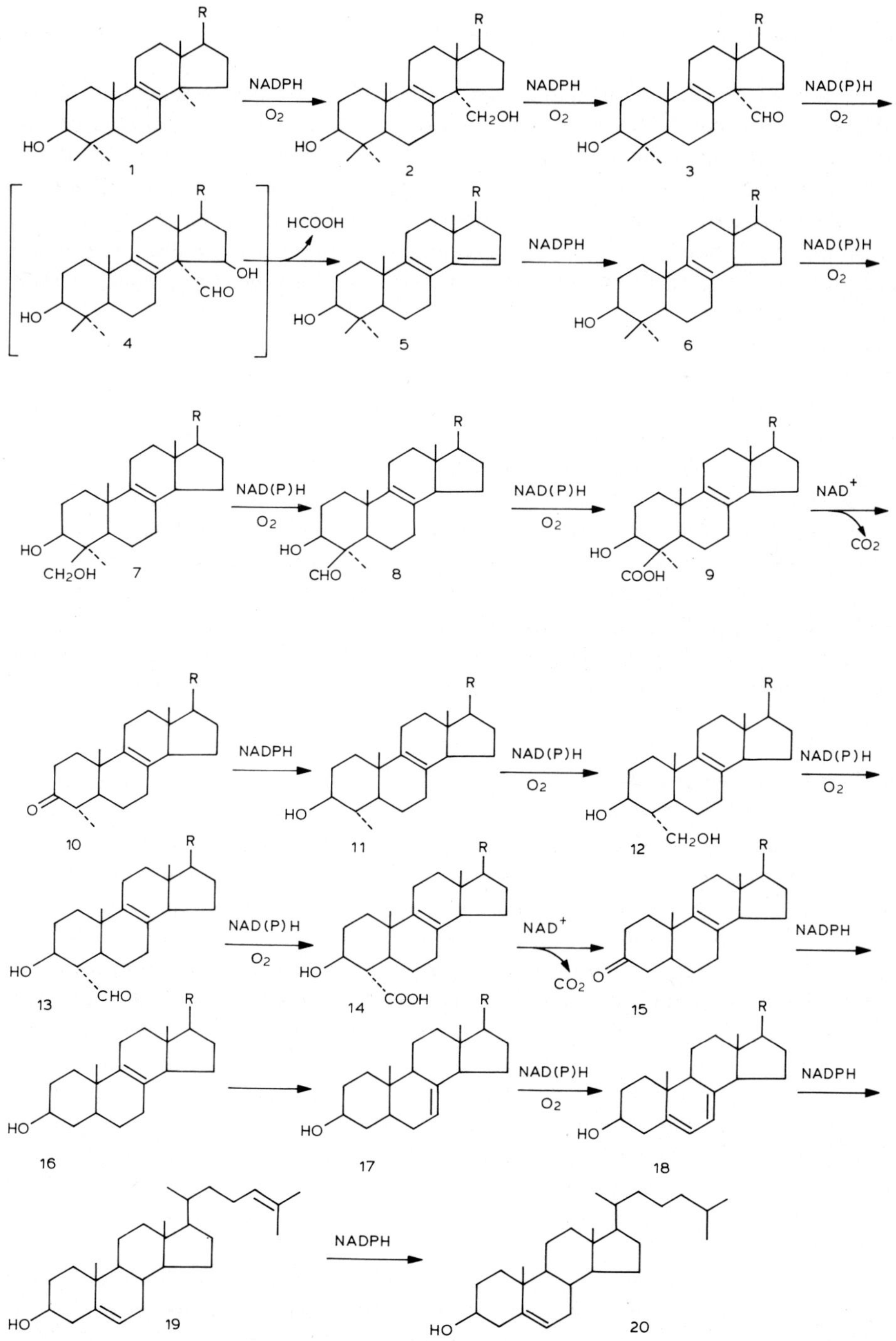

Fig. 21. The conversion of lanosterol to cholesterol.

addition, 32-hydroxylanosterol is efficiently converted to cholesterol as is the 14α-aldehyde.

Enzymes of lanosterol metabolism are enhanced in yeast grown semi-anaerobically. A cytochrome P-450 that bound lanosterol was isolated from this yeast and purified to near homogeneity. This purified (90%) cytochrome P-450 when incubated in the presence of dioxygen, NADPH, and pure NADPH-cytochrome P-450 reductase converted lanosterol to 4,4-dimethyl-cholesta-8,14,24-trien-3β-ol. This system was also inhibited by CO. The interesting point raised here is that, with nearly pure proteins, apparently one cytochrome P-450 is catalyzing three hydroxylation reactions [107].

As indicated, the oxidative demethylation of lanosterol in rat liver preparations is inhibited by CO. However, if 32-hydroxylanosterol is used as substrate, CO no longer inhibits. This indicates that in animals cytochrome P-450 catalyzes only the first oxidation and that other cytochromes are used in the subsequent steps. Apparently, the yeast and liver systems are different [5].

During the oxidative decarbonylation, the 15α-hydrogen is lost. Also, if squalene is converted to cholesterol in ^3H_2O, the 15 position of cholesterol is labeled. This led to the suggestion that C-15 was hydroxylated and that a 4,4-dimethyl-14α-formyl-cholest-7-ene-3β,15-diol was the substrate for the oxidative decarbonylation. Several 15α-hydroxy sterols have been tested as precursors. One did not work, the other was converted only poorly [105]. The double bond at C-14 is probably reduced as the next step since Δ^{14} sterols are rarely encountered. NADPH would be a probable reductant.

(5) Decarboxylation at C-4

It was originally postulated that the methyl groups at C-4 were removed as CO_2 – a suggestion that has proved to be correct. These groups are hydroxylated by a mixed-function oxidase which is NAD(P)H and O_2 dependent. First, the 4α-methyl is attacked, yielding the 4α-hydroxymethyl-4β-methyl sterol. This reaction is catalyzed by a methyl sterol oxidase which has been solubilized and partially purified in Gaylor's laboratory [108]. The same enzyme preparation will, with reduced pyridine nucleotide and dioxygen, oxidize the C-30 carbon to a carboxylic acid. The 4α-methyl-4β-hydroxymethyl-5α-cholestan-3β-ol is not a substrate for sterol biosynthesis while its epimer is [5]. The detailed mechanisms for the enzymatic removal of C-30 and C-31 are not fully understood. The initial reaction yields a 4α-hydroxymethyl sterol by inference; however, neither the isolation nor the enzymatic formation of a 4α-hydroxymethyl sterol has been demonstrated in animal tissues. This may well result from the fact that the hydroxylation reaction is the slow step in the demethylation process [5].

A somewhat contradictory report comes from Sprinson's group who solubilized a 4α-methyl oxidase from rat liver microsomes. Dioxygen was required as well as NAD(P)H and a cyanide-sensitive nonheme ion protein which they purified to homogeneity. A labile fraction which they could not purify was also required. Using

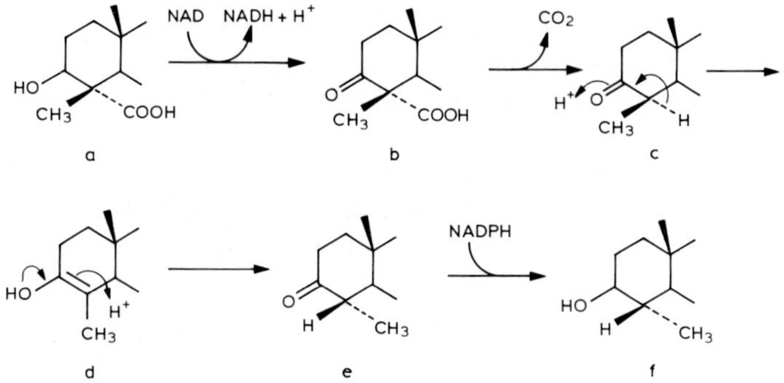

Fig. 22. A mechanism for demethylation at C-4.

monospecific antibodies against either cytochrome P-450 or cytochrome b_5, they could not obtain a significant inhibition of the oxygenation. The conclusion was that they had found a new redox protein involved in oxygenation of C-30 [109].

The alcohol once formed is oxidized by an NAD(P)H- and O_2-dependent oxygenase to the aldehyde and then to the carboxylic acid. The 4α-carboxylic acid is oxidized by an NAD^+-dependent enzyme to the 3-oxo-4α-carboxylic acid. This enzyme has been solubilized and purified from rat liver microsomes. The enzyme has a K_m of 7 μM for the sterol substrate and is maximally active at alkaline pH. The preparation was free of the hydroxylase activities and was uninfluenced by treatment with several phospholipases. It is not known whether the β-oxo acid formed decarboxylates spontaneously or enzymatically [105].

During decarboxylation, the 4β-methyl epimerizes to the more stable 4α position (see Fig. 22). This may simply be a part of the decarboxylation process where an intermediate proceeds to the most stable product or it may be guided by an enzyme. The driving force has been assumed to be relief of steric strain. The resulting monocarboxyketone is reduced to the corresponding alcohol by NADPH and 3-ketosteroid reductase. This enzyme is quite unstable, However, it has been purified from microsomes to some degree [110].

The product of the sequence of reactions outlined above is a 4α-methyl sterol which is then oxidized to the 4α-carboxysterol by a series of oxygenase reactions. It would be attractive if the same set of enzymes that oxidized the α-methyl of the dimethyl sterol did the same to the monomethyl sterol. Both activities travel together during the limited purification procedure, and both reactions appear to proceed at about the same rate [111]. Also, the partially purified ketoreductase used in the previous decarboxylation works well with the 4α-carboxysterol, and Gaylor has suggested that the α-face of the planar sterol is not involved in substrate binding in the catalytic process. The 4β-hydrogen epimerizes during this decarboxylation [105].

The saturation of the side-chain double bond and the migration of the nuclear double bond apparently occur during the later stages of cholesterol biosynthesis. The $\Delta^{8(9)}$ double bond migrates to the Δ^7 position with the assistance of a microsomal enzyme. This reaction requires no cofactors nor is oxygen involved. The specific activity is an order of magnitude greater than that of the 4-methyl sterol oxidase — an observation that accounts for the relative abundance of Δ^7-sterols in many tissues. Phospholipid was required for activity. The reaction is reversible, and during the conversion of the $\Delta^{8(9)}$- to Δ^7-sterol, a proton from solvent is incorporated at C-9 of the Δ^7-sterol and a hydrogen is lost from C-7 of the Δ^7-sterol in animals. With yeast microsomes, the 7α-hydrogen is lost during synthesis of the Δ^7-sterol. There is no hydride shift [105].

(6) Introduction of Δ^5

An oxidative *cis* elimination of the 5α- and 6α-hydrogens serves to insert the Δ^5 double bond into the sterol nucleus. The microsomal enzyme utilizes the Δ^7-sterol as a substrate. The enzyme is similar to 4-methyl sterol oxidase in that the proteins copurify through a limited purification. Both reactions require dioxygen and NAD(P)H, and the abstracted hydrogens appear as protons, indicating that there is not a direct transfer to pyridine nucleotide. Sensitivity of the dehydrogenation to cyanide and insensitivity towards CO indicates that a cytochrome other than cytochrome P-450 is involved. Early experiments had also indicated that compounds hydroxylated on C-5 or C-6 were not intermediates. Thus, hydroxylation–dehydration was not utilized as a mechanism for insertion of the double bond [105]. This is similar to the NADPH-, O_2-dependent desaturation of fatty acids. The enzyme has been solubilized from microsomal membranes and partially purified [111]. The purified oxidase fraction contained the oxidase, NADH-cytochrome b_5 reductase, and phospholipid but no cytochrome b_5 and was inactive by itself. Addition of pure cytochrome b_5 to the fraction containing the oxidase restored activity. This was in accord with earlier experiments which demonstrated that the Δ^7-sterol 5-desaturase could be inhibited by antibodies against cytochrome b_5. In this system, NADPH and cytochrome P-450 would also support the desaturation reaction, indicating that the desaturase may work either of two electron transfer systems and thus either NADH or NADPH would support dehydrogenation. The purification procedures used to separate Δ^7-sterol 5-desaturase from its electron carriers were the same as used with 4α-methyl sterol oxidase from its electron carriers. There is speculation, but no proof, that the enzymes may be the same [111].

The reduction of the Δ^7 bond NADPH is the next reaction in this pathway. The microsomal enzyme transfers a hydride ion from NADPH to the 7α position while the 8β-hydrogen comes from water [105]. The enzyme is readily detached from microsomes and has been purified to a significant extent [112]. It is inhibited by several drugs that block cholesterol synthesis such as AY-9944 and MER-29.

The final reaction in hepatic cholesterologenesis is the reduction of the Δ^{24} double bond, although under conditions when the oxidation of C-32 is blocked, it can be the first. It is obvious that the enzyme is not specific with respect to substrate. Yet, the stereochemistry of the reduction has received considerable attention and the stereospecific origin of each hydrogen atom has been determined. NADPH is the source of reductant [105].

Acknowledgement

Supported in part by a grant (AM13140) from the National Institutes of Health.

References

1 Nes, W.R. and McKean, M.L. (1977) Biochemistry of Steroids and Other Isoprenoids, University Park Press, Baltimore, MD.
2 Gibbons, G.F., Mitropoulos, K.A. and Myant, N.B. (1982) Biochemistry of Cholesterol, Elsevier Biomedical Press, Amsterdam.
3 Porter, J.W. and Spurgeon, S.L. (Eds.) (1981) Biosynthesis of Isoprenoid Compounds, Vol. 1, John Wiley, New York.
4 Schroepfer Jr., G.J. (1981) Annu. Rev. Biochem. 50, 585–621.
5 Schroepfer Jr., G.J. (1982) Annu. Rev. Biochem. 51, 555–585.
6 Poulter, C.D. and Rilling, H.C. (1981) in: Biosynthesis of Isoprenoid Compounds (Porter, J.W. and Spurgeon, S.L., Eds.) Vol. 1, pp. 161–224, John Wiley, New York.
7 Bloch, K. and Rittenberg, D. (1942) J. Biol. Chem. 145, 625–636.
8 Sonderhoff, R. and Thomas, H. (1937) Ann. Chem. 530.
9 Bloch, K. (1965) Science 150, 19–28.
10 Decker, K. and Barth, C. (1973) Mol. Cell. Biochem. 2, 179–188.
11 Bergstrom, J.D., Rohns, K.A. and Edmond, J. (1982) Biochem. Biophys. Res. Commun. 106, 856–862.
12 Qureshi, N. and Porter, J.W. (1981) in: Biosynthesis of Isoprenoid Compounds (Porter, J.W. and Spurgeon, S.L., Eds.) Vol. 1, pp. 47–94, John Wiley, New York.
13 Clinkenbeard, K.D., Sugiyama, T., Moss, J., Reed, W.D. and Lane, M.D. (1973) J. Biol. Chem. 248, 2275–2284.
14 Middleton, B. (1973) Biochem. J. 132, 731–737.
15 Middleton, B. (1973) Biochem. J. 132, 717–730.
16 Bergstrom, J.D. and Edmond, J. (1985) Methods Enzymol. 110, 3–9.
17 Middleton, B. (1974) Biochem. J. 139, 109–121.
18 Lynen, F. (1953) Fed. Proc. Am. Soc. Exp. Biol. 12, 683–691.
19 Ables, R.H. and Maycock, A.L. (1976) Acc. Chem. Res. 9, 313–319.
20 Holland, P.C., Clark, M.G. and Bloxham, D.P. (1973) Biochemistry 12, 3309–3315.
21 Willadsen, P. and Eggerer, H. (1975) Eur. J. Biochem. 54, 253–258.
22 Clinkenbeard, K.D., Sugiyama, T., Reed, D. and Lane, M.D. (1975) J. Biol. Chem. 250, 3124–3135.
23 Miziorko, H.M. (1985) Methods Enzymol. 110, 19–26.
24 Miziorko, H.M. (1975) J. Biol. Chem. 250, 5768–5773.
25 Steward, P.R. and Rudney, H. (1966) J. Biol. Chem. 241, 1222–1225.
26 Miziorko, H.M. and Lane, M.D. (1977) J. Biol. Chem. 252, 1414–1420.
27 Miziorko, H.M., Lane, M.D. and Weidman, S.W. (1979) Biochemistry 18, 399–403.
28 Page, M.A. and Tubbs, P.K. (1978) Biochem. J. 173, 925–928.
29 Sabine, J.R. (Ed.) (1983) 3-Hydroxy-3-Methylglutaryl Coenzyme A Reductase, CRC Press, Boca Raton, FL.
30 Rogers, D.H., Panini, S.R. and Rudney, H. (1983) in: 3-Hydroxy-3-Methylglutaryl Coenzyme A Reductase (Sabine, J.R., Ed.) pp. 57–75, CRC Press, Boca Raton, FL.
31 Edwards, P.A., Fogelman, A.M. and Tanaka, R.D. (1983) in: 3-Hydroxy-3-Methylglutaryl Coenzyme A Reductase (Sabine, J.R., Ed.) pp. 93–106, CRC Press, Boca Raton, FL.
32 Edwards, P.A., Lan, S.-F. and Fogelman, A.M. (1983) J. Biol. Chem. 258, 10219–10222.
33 Gibbons, G.F. (1983) in: 3-Hydroxy-3-Methylglutaryl Coenzyme A Reductase (Sabine, J.R., Ed.) pp. 153–168, CRC Press, Boca Raton, FL.

34 Beg, Z.H. and Brewer Jr., H.B. (1981) Curr. Topics Cell. Regul. 20, 139–184.
35 Folkers, K., Shunk, C.H., Linn, B.O., Robinson, F.M., Wittreich, P.E., Huff, J.W., Gilfillan, J.L. and Skeggs, H.R. (1959) in: Biosynthesis of Terpenes and Sterols (Wolstenholme, G.E.W. and O'Connor, M., Eds.) pp. 20–45, Little Brown and Co., Boston, MA.
36 Beytia, E., Dorsey, J.K., Marr, J., Cleland, W.W. and Porter, J.W. (1970) J. Biol. Chem. 245, 5450–5458.
37 Porter, J.W. (1985) Methods Enzymol. 110, 71–78.
38 Bazaes, S., Beytia, E., Jabalquinto, A.M., Solis de Ovando, F., Gomez, I. and Eyzaguirre, J. (1980) Biochemistry 19, 2300–2304.
39 Eyzaguirre, J. and Bazaes, S. (1985) Methods Enzymol. 110, 78–85.
40 Bazaes, S., Beytia, E., Jabalquinto, A.M., Solis de Ovando, R., Gomez, I. and Eyzaguirre, J. (1980) Biochemistry 19, 2305–2310.
41 Alvear, M., Jabalquinto, A.M., Eyzaguirre, J. and Cardemil, E. (1982) Biochemistry 21, 4645–4650.
42 Cardemil, E. and Jabalquinto, A.M. (1985) Methods Enzymol. 110, 86–92.
43 Jabalquinto, A.M., Solis de Ovando, F. and Cardemil, E. (1983) Unpublished observations cited in ref. 42.
44 Lindberg, M., Yuan, C., de Waard, H. and Bloch, K. (1962) Biochemistry 1, 182–188.
45 Agranof, B.W., Eggerer, H., Henning, U. and Lynen, F. (1960) J. Biol. Chem. 235, 326–332.
46 Banthorp, D.V., Doonan, S. and Gutowski, J.A. (1977) Arch. Biochem. Biophys. 184, 381–390.
47 Rilling, H.C. and Bruenger, E., Unpublished.
48 Sagami, H. and Ogura, K. (1983) J. Biochem. 94, 975–979.
49 Clifford, K., Cornforth, J.W., Mallaby, R. and Phillips, J. (1971) Chem. Commun. 1599–1600.
50 Popjak, G. and Cornforth, J.W. (1966) Biochem. J. 101, 553–568.
51 Chayet, L.T. and Rilling, H.C., Unpublished.
52 Ogura, K., Koyama, T., Shibuya, T., Nishino, T. and Seto, S. (1969) J. Biochem. 66, 117–118.
53 Koyama, T., Ogura, K. and Seto, S. (1973) J. Biol. Chem. 248, 8043–8051.
54 Satterwhite, D.M. (1979) Ph.D. Dissertation, University of Utah.
55 Shah, D.H., Cleland, W.W. and Porter, J.W. (1965) J. Biol. Chem. 240, 1946–1956.
56 Rilling, H.C. (1985) Methods Enzymol. 110, 145–152.
57 Barnard, G.F. and Popjak, G. (1981) Biochim. Biophys. Acta 661, 87–99.
58 Barnard, G.F. (1985) Methods Enzymol. 110, 155–167.
59 Holloway, P.W. and Popjak, G. (1967) Biochem. J. 104, 57–70.
60 Laskovics, F.M., Krafick, J.M. and Poulter, C.D. (1979) J. Biol. Chem. 254, 9458–9463.
61 Laskovics, F.M. and Poulter, C.D. (1981) Biochemistry 20, 1893–1901.
62 Poulter, C.D., Wiggins, P.L. and Le, A.T. (1981) J. Am. Chem. Soc. 103, 3926–3927.
63 Mash, E.A., Gurria, G.M. and Poulter, C.D. (1981) J. Am. Chem. Soc. 103, 3927–3929.
64 Saito, A. and Rilling, H.C. (1979) J. Biol. Chem. 254, 8511–8515.
65 Nishino, T., Ogura, K. and Seto, S. (1972) J. Am. Chem. Soc. 94, 6849–6853.
66 Brems, D.N. and Rilling, H.C. (1981) Biochemistry 20, 3711–3718.
67 Poulter, C.D. and Rilling, H.C. (1981) in: Biosynthesis of Isoprenoid Compounds (Porter, J.W. and Spurgeon, S.L., Eds.) Vol. 1, pp. 413–441, John Wiley, New York.
68 Altman, L.J., Kowerski, R.C. and Rilling, H.C. (1971) J. Am. Chem. Soc. 93, 1782–1783.
69 Popjak, G., Edmond, J. and Wong, S.-W. (1973) J. Am. Chem. Soc. 95, 2713–2714.
70 Nishino, T. and Katsuki, H. (1985) Methods Enzymol. 110, 373–375.
71 Agnew, W.S. and Popjak, G. (1978) J.Biol. Chem. 253, 4566–4573.
72 Agnew, W.S. and Popjak, G. (1978) J. Biol. Chem. 253, 4574–4583.
73 Ogura, K., Koyama, T. and Seto, S. (1972) J. Am. Chem. Soc. 94, 307–309.
74 Ortiz de Montellano, P.R., Wei, J.S., Vinson, W.A., Castillo, R. and Boparai, A.S. (1977) Biochemistry 16, 2680–2685.
75 Sandifer, R.M., Thompson, M.D., Gaughan, R.G. and Poulter, C.D. (1982) J. Am. Chem. Soc. 104, 7376–7378.
76 Yamamoto, S. and Bloch, K. (1970) J. Biol. Chem. 245, 1670–1674.
77 Tai, H.-H. and Bloch, K. (1972) J. Biol. Chem. 247, 3767–3773.

78 Ono, T. and Bloch, K. (1975) J. Biol. Chem. 250, 1571–1579.
79 Ono, T., Osaza, S., Hasegawa, F. and Bloch, K. (1977) Biochim. Biophys. Acta 486, 401–407.
80 Ono, T. and Imai, Y. (1965) Methods Enzymol. 110, 375–380.
81 Ono, T., Takahashi, K., Odani, S., Konno, H. and Imai, Y. (1980) Biochem. Biophys. Res. Commun. 96, 522–528.
82 Ono, T., Odani, S. and Nakazono, K. (1981) in: Oxygenases and Oxygen Metabolism (Nasaki, M. et al., Eds.) pp. 637–643, Academic Press, New York.
83 Band, M., Woods, R.A. and Haslam, J.M. (1974) Biochem. Biophys. Res. Commun. 56, 324–330.
84 Gollub, E.G., Trocha, P., Liu, P.K. and Sprinson, D.B. (1974) Biochem. Biophys. Res. Commun. 56, 471–477.
85 Saat, Y.A. and Bloch, K. (1976) J. Biol. Chem. 252, 5515–5560.
86 Gavey, K.J. and Scallen, T.J. (1978) J. Biol. Chem. 253, 5476–5483.
87 Friedlander, E.J., Caras, I.W., Liu, L.F.H. and Bloch, K. (1980) J. Biol. Chem. 255, 8042–8045.
88 Kojima, Y., Friedlander, E.J. and Bloch, K. (1981) J. Biol. Chem. 256, 7235–7239.
89 Caras, I.W., Friedlander, E.J. and Bloch, K. (1980) J. Biol. Chem. 3575–3580.
90 Cornforth, J.W., Gore, I.Y. and Popjak, G. (1957) Biochem. J. 65, 94–109.
91 Maudgal, R.K., Tchen, T.T. and Bloch, K. (1958) J. Am. Chem. Soc. 80, 2589–2590.
92 Corey, E.J., Ortiz de Montellano, P.R., Kin, K. and Dean, P.D.G. (1967) J. Am. Chem. Soc. 89, 2797–2799.
93 van Tamelen, E.E. and James, D.R. (1977) J. Am. Chem. Soc. 99, 950–952.
94 Corey, E.J., Ortiz de Montellano, P.R. and Yamamoto, K.B. (1968) J. Am. Chem. Soc. 90, 3284–3286.
95 van Tamelen, E.E., Hanzlik, R.P., Sharpless, K.B., Clayton, R.B., Richter, W.J. and Burlingame, A.L. (1968) J. Am. Chem. Soc. 90, 3284–3286.
96 Corey, E.J., Lin, K. and Yamamoto, H. (1969) J. Am. Chem. Soc. 91, 2132–2134.
97 van Tamelen, E.E. and Heys, J.R. (1975) J. Am. Chem. Soc. 97, 1252–1253.
98 Corey, E.J. and Russey, W.E. (1966) J. Am. Chem. Soc. 88, 4751–4752.
99 Field, R.B. and Holmlund, C.E. (1977) Arch. Biochem. Biophys., 180, 465–471.
100 Nelson, J.A., Steckbeck, S.R. and Spencer, T.A. (1981) J. Biol. Chem. 256, 1067–1068.
101 Rahier, A., Bouvier, P., Cattel, L., Narula, H. and Benveniste, P. (1983) Biochem. Soc. Trans. 11, 537–543.
102 Houslay, M.D. and Stanley, K.K. (1982) Dynamics of Biological Membranes, pp. 71–76, John Wiley, Chicester.
103 Bloch, K. (1981) in: Current Topics in Cellular Regulation (Estabrook, R.W. and Srere, P., Eds.) Vol. 18, pp. 289–299, Academic Press, New York.
104 Johnson, J.D. and Bloch, K. (1957) J. Am. Chem. Soc. 79, 1145–1149.
105 Gaylor, J.L. (1981) in: Biosynthesis of Isoprenoid Compounds (Porter, J.W. and Spurgeon, S.L., Eds.) Vol. 1, pp. 481–543, John Wiley, New York.
106 White, R.E. and Coon, M.J. (1980) Annu. Rev. Biochem. 49, 315–356.
107 Aoyama, Y. and Yoshida, Y. (1978) Biochem. Biophys. Res. Commun. 85, 28–34.
108 Fukishima, H., Grinstead, G.F. and Gaylor, J.L. (1981) J. Biol. Chem. 256, 4822–4826.
109 Maitra, U.S., Mohan, V.P., Kochi, H., Shankar, V., Adlersberg, M., Liu, K.-P., Ponticorvo, L. and Sprinson, D.B. (1982) Biochem. Biophys. Res. Commun. 108, 517–525.
110 Trzaskos, J.M., Bowen, W.D., Fisher, G.J., Billheimer, J.T. and Gaylor, J.L. (1982) Lipids 17, 250–256.
111 Grinstead, G.F. and Gaylor, J.L. (1982) J. Biol. Chem. 257, 13927–13944.
112 Dempsey, M.E. (1969) Methods Enzymol. 15, 501–514.

H. Danielsson and J. Sjövall (Eds.), *Sterols and Bile Acids*

CHAPTER 2

Control mechanisms in sterol uptake and biosynthesis

JOHN F. GILL Jr., PETER J. KENNELLY and VICTOR W. RODWELL

Department of Biochemistry, Purdue University, West Lafayette, IN 47907 (U.S.A.)

(I) Control of sterol uptake

(1) Plasma lipoproteins

Cholesterol, which is largely insoluble in aqueous media, travels through the blood circulation in the form of lipoprotein complexes. The plasma lipoproteins are a family of globular particles that share common structural features. A core of hydrophobic lipid, principally triacylglycerols (triglycerides) and cholesterol esters, is surrounded by a hydrophilic monolayer of phospholipid and protein (the apolipoproteins) [1–3]. Lipid–apolipoprotein interactions, facilitated by amphipathic protein helices that segregate polar from nonpolar surfaces [2,3], provide the mechanism by which cholesterol can circulate in a soluble form. In addition, the apolipoproteins modulate the activities of certain enzymes involved in lipoprotein metabolism and interact with specific cell surface receptors which take up lipoproteins by receptor-mediated endocytosis. Differences in the lipid and apolipoprotein compositions of plasma lipoproteins determine their target sites and classification based on buoyant density.

(a) Normal plasma lipoproteins

Four main classes of lipoproteins are present in normal human plasma (for reviews, see refs. 1–3). The largest of these, the chylomicrons (diameter 800–5000 Å, density < 0.95 g/ml; they remain at the origin during electrophoresis, Fig. 1), contain predominantly dietary triglycerides and a spectrum of apolipoproteins (Fig. 2). Chylomicrons are manufactured in the intestines from dietary lipids, secreted into the lymph, and subsequently enter the blood circulation. Since chylomicrons are too large to cross the vascular endothelium, they are degraded in plasma by the enzyme lipoprotein lipase which is present on the surface of endothelial cells that

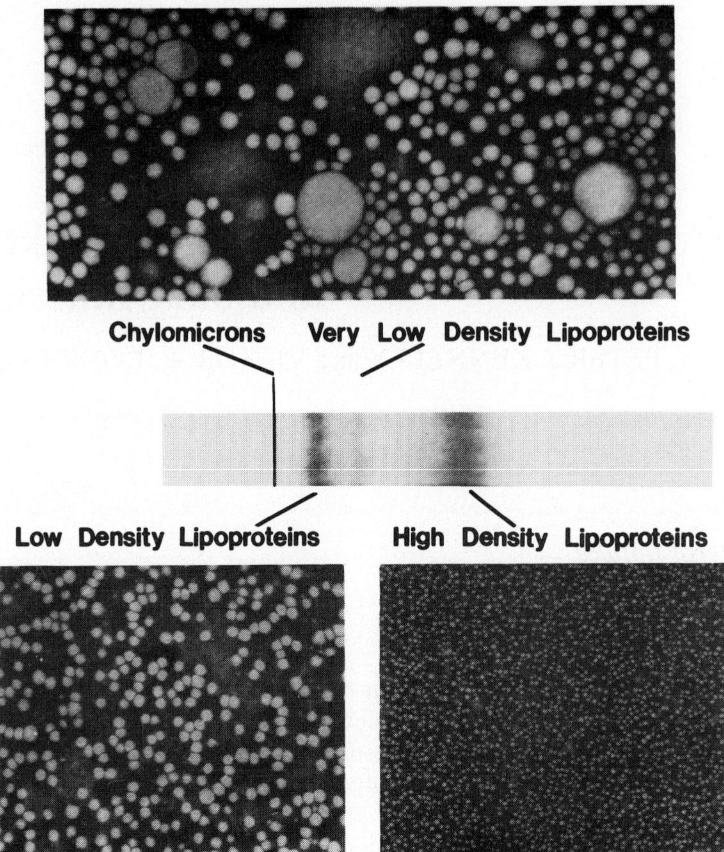

Fig. 1. Relative size and electrophoretic mobility of the major classes of human lipoproteins. Reproduced, with permission of the authors and publisher, from Mahley and Innerarity [12].

line the lumen of capillaries. Apolipoprotein CII (apo-CII) present on the chylomicrons activates the lipoprotein lipase, which liberates fatty acids and monoglycerides for adsorption by adjacent tissues [4]. A portion of the phospholipid and unesterified cholesterol is transferred to high-density lipoprotein (HDL) [5] and the depleted particle is released as a chylomicron remnant (diameter 300–800 Å). Chylomicron remnants, which retain two major apolipoproteins (apo-B and apo-E), are enriched in cholesterol esters and are rapidly cleared from plasma by the liver with a measured half-life of 4–5 min [2].

Very-low-density lipoproteins (VLDL) are large particles (diameter 300–900 Å, density range 0.95–1.006 g/ml, pre-β electrophoretic mobility, Fig. 1) in which triacylglycerols predominate. VLDL contain 8–10% protein (predominantly apo-B and apo-E, see Fig. 2) and 90–92% lipid (triacylglycerols 56%, phospholipids 19–21%, cholesterol and cholesterol esters 17% [6]). VLDL are synthesized in the

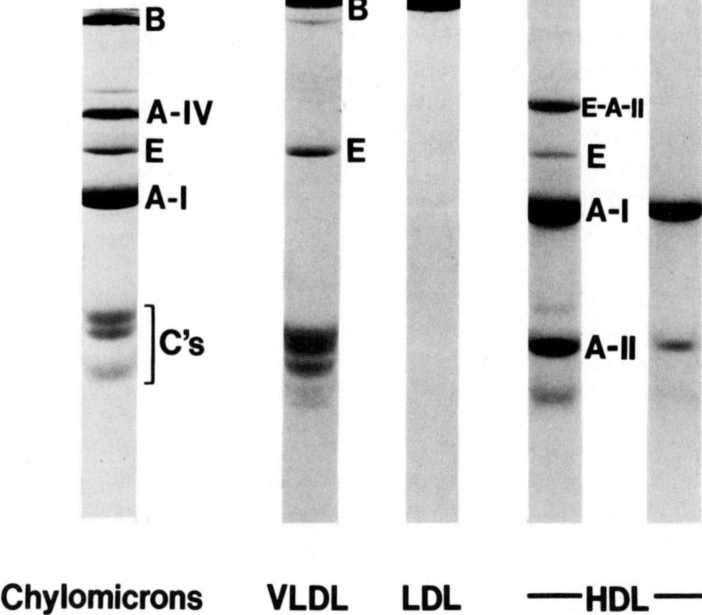

Fig. 2. The apoproteins of the major classes of lipoproteins separated on sodium dodecyl–polyacrylamide gels. Reproduced with permission of the authors and publisher, from Mahley and Innerarity [12].

liver and are believed to function in the distribution of triacylglycerols to peripheral tissues. VLDL are depleted of triacylglycerols by capillary lipoprotein lipase as described above for chylomicrons. A portion of the phospholipid and unesterified cholesterol of VLDL is transferred to HDL. Lipid depletion of VLDL involves a transition through lipoprotein particles of intermediate density (IDL) [7,8]. The cholesterol transferred to HDL is esterified by the interaction of HDL with the plasma enzyme lecithin-cholesterol acyltransferase (LCAT) [9]. Esterified cholesterol is then transferred back into IDL particles, which undergo further release of triglycerides and of all apolipoproteins except apo-B to form the smaller, spherical low-density lipoprotein (LDL) particles.

LDL (diameter 200–250 Å, density range 1.019–1.063 g/ml, β-electrophoretic mobility, Fig. 1) are often termed β-lipoproteins. LDL contain, by weight, 75% lipid (principally esterified cholesterol) and 25% protein which consists exclusively of apo-B (Fig. 2). LDL is the major vehicle for transport of cholesterol to peripheral tissues and normally accounts for about 70% of total plasma cholesterol [10]. LDL metabolism is of medical interest since there is a direct correlation between increased plasma LDL concentration and an increased incidence of atherosclerotic heart disease [11].

HDL, the smallest of the lipoprotein particles (diameter 80–120 Å, density range 1.063–1.210 g/ml, α-electrophoretic mobility, Fig. 1), constitute a heterogeneous class of lipoproteins that contain various subclasses of apolipoproteins (Fig. 2).

Apo-AI and apo-AII predominate, although under certain conditions HDL can acquire apo-E (Fig. 2). HDL contains, by weight, 50% protein and 50% lipid (phospholipid 47–51%, cholesterol 32%, triacylglycerols 10%). In addition to the previously mentioned lipid transfer functions, HDL appear to be involved in transport of cholesterol from peripheral tissues to the liver for excretion [12]. Recent interest in HDL metabolism has been stimulated by the observed correlation between increased plasma HDL levels and a lower incidence of atherosclerotic heart disease [11].

(b) Abnormal plasma lipoproteins

Abnormal lipoproteins are produced under various metabolic conditions. β-VLDL, a triglyceride-depleted, cholesterol-enriched form of VLDL, accumulates in the plasma of cholesterol-fed animals [13,14] or of humans with type III hyperlipoproteinemia [15]. In patients with this disease, the accumulation of β-VLDL is believed to be due to incomplete clearance of chylomicron remnants by the liver. Slow turnover of remnants allows them to accumulate cholesteryl esters and thus to evolve into β-VLDL particles [16,17]. β-VLDL (density < 1.006 g/ml, β-electrophoretic mobility) contain both apo-B and apo-E and may play a significant role in the formation of atherosclerotic foam cells [18].

Animals fed cholesterol-rich diets also accumulate HDL_c, a form of HDL that is believed to be produced when normal HDL acquire (1) abnormally high quantities of cholesterol (50% of their particle weight), and (2) apo-E from macrophages and smooth muscle cells [12]. The enriched cholesterol and apo-E content of HDL_c particles substantially increases their diameter (to 200 Å) and decreases their density such that HDL_c begins to physically resemble LDL. HDL_c are believed to function in transport of cholesterol from peripheral tissues to the liver for excretion [12].

(c) Chemically modified lipoproteins

Chemically modified lipoproteins, in particular modified LDL, have facilitated the identification of additional receptor-mediated systems for cholesterol uptake. Macrophages take up LDL modified by acetylation or related processes which increase negative charge [19–21] via a receptor system distinct from the LDL receptor (for reviews see refs. 12 and 22). Receptors which recognize LDL/dextran sulfate complexes [23] or which recognize cholesterol ester/protein complexes [24] are also present in macrophages. Although receptors for artificially modified lipoproteins have been identified in aortic foam cells and macrophages, it has not been possible to isolate a naturally occurring ligand for these receptors. This failure may reflect the rapid clearance of the physiological ligand since artificially modified lipoproteins are rapidly cleared in vivo [25].

(2) Cellular mechanisms of cholesterol uptake

The principal mechanism for cellular uptake of cholesterol involves receptor-mediated endocytosis of plasma lipoproteins. Brown and Goldstein elucidated the "LDL pathway" for LDL uptake and degradation using fibroblasts from normal human subjects and from patients with genetic defects in lipoprotein metabolism. Subsequently, receptor systems for the uptake of other plasma lipoproteins were identified. The generalized sequence of events involved in lipoprotein receptor-mediated endocytosis are:

(1) Lipoprotein binds to a specific receptor.

(2) The lipoprotein–receptor complex is internalized.

(3) Lipoprotein dissociates from the receptor and the receptor returns to the cell surface.

(4) Lipoprotein is degraded in lysosomes.

While these events were first described for LDL uptake, they may represent a general mechanism for receptor-mediated lipoprotein uptake by all lipoprotein receptors (for reviews, see refs. 10, 12, 22, 26 and 27).

(a) The LDL receptor and receptor-mediated endocytosis

Specific cell surface receptors which mediate LDL uptake have been identified in adipocytes, adrenal cortex, fibroblasts, leukocytes, liver, lymphocytes, macrophage-monocytes, ovaries, smooth muscle cells and testes. Table 1 summarizes certain properties of the LDL receptor. The LDL receptor appears to be a protein since (1) LDL-binding activity is destroyed by treatment with proteolytic enzymes [28,29], and (2) subsequent restoration of LDL-binding activity is blocked when protein synthesis is inhibited by cycloheximide [29]. Genetic evidence suggests that the LDL receptor is the product of a single gene locus. Fibroblasts from patients with receptor-negative homozygous familial hypercholesterolemia (FH) express no high-affinity LDL-binding activity. By contrast, fibroblasts from patients with heterozygous FH express about one-half of the receptor activity of normal fibroblasts [30,31].

LDL receptor purified from bovine adrenal cortex has an estimated molecular weight of 163 000 [32]. The receptor, which spans the plasma membrane and contains *N*- and *O*-linked carbohydrate chains [33], has an isoelectric point of 4.6, indicating that it has a net negative charge at physiological pH. Purified receptor has multiple binding affinity since 4 LDL particles can bind to 1 receptor molecule [34]. Binding appears to be functionally irreversible. The rate of spontaneous dissociation of LDL receptors at 4°C, a temperature that arrests internalization, is slow relative to the rate of internalization at 37°C [10].

Recognition of lipoproteins by the LDL receptor is believed to be due to the presence of apo-B and/or apo-E. The LDL receptor recognizes the apo-B-containing lipoproteins LDL and Lp(a), a modified form of LDL (Table 1). Modification of lysyl [35] or arginyl [36] residues of the apo-B portion of LDL blocks LDL binding. In addition, LDL is readily dissociated from the receptor by polyanions such as heparin and dextran sulfate [37]. Thus, LDL binding appears to involve strong ionic interactions between the negatively charged receptor and positively charged apolipoproteins. Binding of LDL to the LDL receptor also requires divalent cations [28,29] and appears to be temperature-dependent [37].

TABLE 1

Summary of lipoprotein receptors

Receptors	Cells or tissues	Lipoproteins bound	Ligands involved	Receptor regulation	Functional roles
LDL (apo-B, E)	Fibroblasts Smooth muscle cells Liver Adrenal cortex Ovaries Testes Adipocytes Lymphocytes Macrophage-monocytes	LDL HDL-with apo-E (HDL_c) VLDL Chylomicron remnants Lp(a) β-VLDL (cholesterol-induced)	Apo-B Apo-E	Regulated by delivery of lipoprotein cholesterol	Regulation of LDL levels Redistribution of cholesterol by apo-B and apo-E lipoproteins to various tissues Cholesterol utilized for membrane or hormone production
Apo-E (chylomicron remnant)	Liver	Chylomicron remnants HDL-with apo-E (HDL_c)	Apo-E	Not subject to marked down-regulation	Uptake of chylomicron remnants and cholesterol-loaded HDL-with-apo-E Delivery of cholesterol to the liver for excretion
β-VLDL	Macrophage	β-VLDL (from type III subjects and induced by cholesterol)	?	Poorly regulated	Potential role in foam cell production in atherogenesis Uptake of diet-induced lipoproteins (link between diet and atherosclerosis)
Chemically modified lipoprotein	Macrophage	Modified LDL	Charge-modified apo-B	Not regulated	Potential role in foam cell production in atherogenesis

Reproduced with permission of the authors and publishers, from Mahley and Innerarity [12].

The LDL receptor also recognizes apo-E-containing lipoproteins such as HDL_c, chylomicron remnants, β-VLDL, or VLDL from hypertriglyceridemic patients (Table 1). In fact, the LDL receptor has a 10–100-fold greater affinity for apo-E than for apo-B [38,39]. The presence of apo-E and/or apo-B does not always ensure recognition by the LDL receptor since chylomicrons and normal VLDL, which both contain apo-B and apo-E, are poorly recognized [40,41]. The lipid content of chylomicrons may impair receptor recognition by creating conformational changes which mask the apolipoprotein determinants. Alternatively, the presence of apo-C in these triglyceride-rich lipoproteins may oppose their recognition by hepatic LDL receptors [42].

LDL receptors are synthesized in the rough endoplasmic reticulum, travel to the Golgi apparatus and are then randomly inserted into the plasma membrane [26]. See Fig. 3 for the life cycle of receptors. At the cell surface, the receptors bind LDL and cluster into membranous invaginations which are coated on their internal surface with the protein clathrin. These "coated pit" regions have been visualized by electron microscopy using ferritin-coupled LDL [43]. Binding of ligand does not appear to induce the LDL receptor to enter coated pits since cells fixed with formaldehyde in the absence of ligand exhibit 70% of their LDL receptors in coated pits [43,44]. Rather, LDL receptors appear to cycle continuously to and from the cell

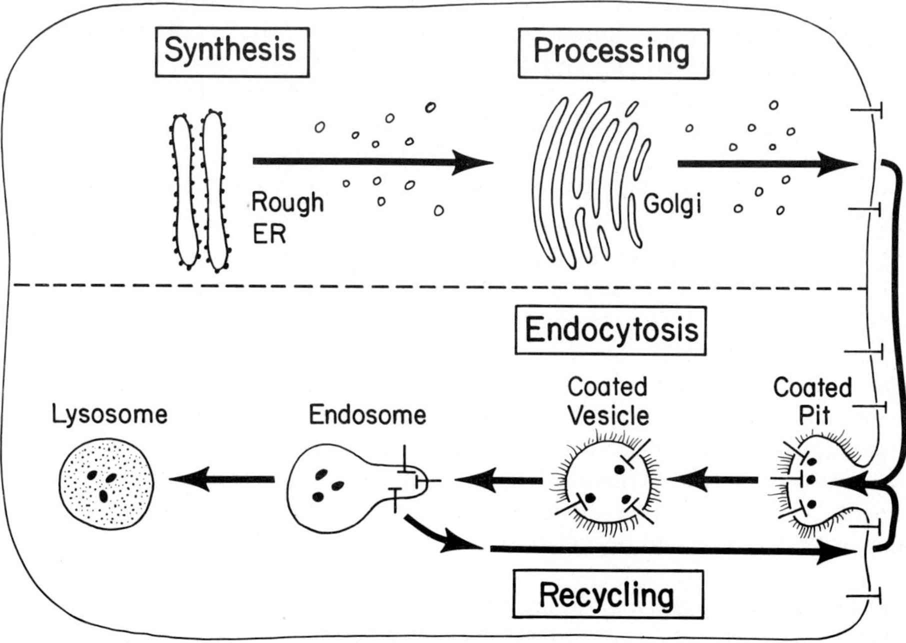

Fig. 3. The life cycle of cell surface receptors. Reproduced, with permission of the authors and publisher (copyright held by MIT), from Brown et al. [26].

surface. In the absence of LDL, receptors can be trapped internally when cells are treated with monensin, a carboxylic ionophore which disrupts the movement of intracellular vesicles [45]. It has been estimated that an LDL receptor can make an average of at least 150 round-trips to and from the cell surface without undergoing proteolytic degradation [46].

Receptor–LDL complexes are rapidly internalized (50% of bound LDL is internalized in 3 min at 37°C [37]) in clathrin-coated vesicles which rapidly shed their clathrin coats and fuse to form larger vesicles called endosomes. Endosomes are believed to be the sites for dissociation of LDL from its receptor since, following internalization, receptors return to the cell surface within 3 min, a time insufficient for the receptor–ligand complex to reach the lysosomes. A proposed mechanism for ligand dissociation involves endosome acidification, which is known to lower the pH of the endosome below 6 [47]. Many receptor–ligand complexes, including that of LDL, dissociate under these conditions. Once ligands have dissociated, the receptors may segregate into a small tubular out-pocketing of the endosome called CURL (compartment of uncoupling of receptor and ligand) as is the case for asialoglycoprotein receptors [48]. This model proposes that CURL buds off from the endosome and returns to the cell surface while the ligand-containing endosome migrates to the lysosome for subsequent fusion and ligand degradation.

Lysosomal degradation of LDL following endosome fusion [44] is suggested by the accumulation of undegraded LDL in cells exposed to chloroquine, a lysosomotrophic amine which blocks vesicular fusions [49,50]. In addition, the observed pH optimum (pH 4) for hydrolysis of [^{3}H]cholesterol linoleate in cell extracts [50] is consistent with hydrolysis of lipoprotein-derived cholesterol esters by lysosomal acid lipase. Lysosomal involvement in LDL degradation is underscored by the accumulation of cholesterol esters in lysosomes of cells from patients with Wolman syndrome or cholesterol ester storage disease, two conditions characterized by genetic defects in lysosomal acid lipase [50,51]. LDL that contain radioactively labeled lipid and protein have been used to show that LDL is delivered to lysosomes as an intact unit. [^{125}I]Monoiodotyrosine from labeled apo-B eventually appears in the culture medium while [^{3}H]cholesterol accumulates in cellular membranes [49]. Excess cholesterol is re-esterified by acyl-CoA : cholesterol acyltransferase (ACAT) and stored as cholesterol esters [49,50].

While the events in receptor-mediated lipoprotein uptake are best characterized for the LDL receptor, they probably are representative of common mechanisms for the receptor-mediated endocytosis of other lipoproteins as well as for many other nonlipoprotein ligands. Individual lipoprotein receptor systems appear to differ primarily with respect to the lipoproteins recognized and the regulatory events which follow internalization and degradation.

(b) Other receptor-mediated lipoprotein uptake mechanisms

Table 1 summarizes salient properties of other lipoprotein receptors.

(i) The Apo-E receptor. Apo-E receptors, present in the livers of dog, cat, rat, swine, and man [52,53], are responsible for the plasma clearance of chylomicron

remnants and HDL_c, but not for clearance of normal HDL or LDL [52,54,55]. Receptor–ligand recognition is thought to involve apo-E since chemical modification of lysyl or arginyl residues of apo-E significantly decreases the rate of HDL_c clearance by the liver [25]. A single high-affinity apo-E receptor is believed to take up both HDL_c and chylomicron remnants since in the perfused rat liver both lipoproteins mutually compete for the same binding sites and are endocytosed at the same rate [56,57]. Apo-E receptors are believed to function in the uptake by the liver of cholesterol-rich, apo-E-containing lipoproteins (e.g.: HDL_c) for the ultimate excretion of their cholesterol as bile acids.

(ii) The β-VLDL receptor. Despite their lack of LDL receptors, macrophages of patients with homozygous FH accumulate LDL-derived cholesterol esters as cytoplasmic droplets. The resulting cholesterol-bloated "foam cells" are notably present in atherosclerotic plaques and in xanthomas associated with the skin and tendons of body joints [1]. Systems for lipoprotein uptake distinct from the LDL receptor therefore must exist in macrophages.

The β-VLDL receptor has been identified on mouse peritoneal macrophages [13,14], foam cells associated with rabbit aortic atherosclerotic plaques [58], and human monocyte-derived macrophages [14]. Although β-VLDL can bind to LDL receptors, LDL do not compete with ^{125}I-labeled β-VLDL for uptake by mouse peritoneal macrophages [13,14]. In addition, monocytes from LDL receptor-negative FH patients or from normal subjects express equivalent numbers of β-VLDL receptors [14]. The β-VLDL receptors thus are distinct from LDL receptors. The β-VLDL receptor is also distinct from the receptors for chemically modified lipoproteins (see below).

β-VLDL is the only naturally occurring lipoprotein known to bind to macrophage lipoprotein receptors [22]. Receptor–ligand recognition is partially due to β-VLDL protein composition since chemical modification of β-VLDL apolipoproteins completely inhibits binding [59]. However, other apo-B- and apo-E-containing lipoproteins such as LDL and HDL_c are not taken up by macrophages [12]. β-VLDL from type III hyperlipoproteinemic patients or from dogs fed high cholesterol diets has been subdivided into fraction I (of intestinal origin; high cholesterol/protein ratio) and fraction II (hepatic in origin, lower cholesterol/protein ratio) [15]. Fraction I β-VLDL is preferentially taken up by macrophages as evidenced by its greater ability to stimulate cholesterol ester accumulation. The tissue of origin of apolipoproteins and the lipid/protein ratio of the lipoprotein thus appears to contribute to ligand recognition by the β-VLDL receptor.

Macrophage β-VLDL receptors may serve a "back-up" function in cholesterol clearance by facilitating removal of cholesterol-rich β-VLDL particles which accompany diet-induced hypercholesterolemia. When dog plasma cholesterol levels exceed 750 mg/dl, β-VLDL accumulate in plasma and macrophages accumulate cholesterol and cholesterol esters [60]. The association of these events suggests that β-VLDL may be taken up by macrophage β-VLDL receptors for the deposition of plasma cholesterol esters.

β-VLDL receptors are present on both human blood monocytes and on foam cells associated with rabbit aortic atherosclerotic plaques [14,58]. Because macrophages of the arterial wall are believed to originate from blood monocytes, the β-VLDL receptor may play a significant role in the cholesterol ester deposition associated with foam cell production in the genesis of atherosclerotic heart disease.

(iii) The acetyl-LDL receptor. The acetyl-LDL receptor was first detected using acetylated LDL, which is taken up by mouse peritoneal macrophages, resulting in a massive accumulation of cholesterol esters [19,61]. Other chemical modifications which increase the net negative charge on LDL (e.g.: acetoacetylation [20], maleylation [19], succinylation [19], or malondialdehyde treatment [21]) yield alternate ligands for the acetyl-LDL receptor. While acetyl-LDL receptors are present on macrophages from all sources so far tested, they are absent from most non-macrophage cells. One exception is freshly isolated human blood monocytes, which express both LDL and acetyl-LDL receptor acivities [19,21,62,63].

The acetyl-LDL receptor is distinct from the LDL receptor. Acetyl-LDL can be precipitated by antibody raised against LDL, yet is not taken up by the LDL receptor [64]. By contrast, LDL is taken up by macrophages only at a low rate without accumulation of cholesterol esters [19,61]. Unlike the LDL receptor, the acetyl-LDL receptor does not require divalent cations for uptake [19]. In addition, monocytes from normal subjects exhibit an acetyl-LDL receptor activity comparable to that of monocytes from patients with LDL receptor-negative homozygous FH.

Binding of modified LDLs to the acetyl-LDL receptor is due in part to their enhanced negative charge, and may involve both the number and spatial arrangement of these negative charges [62]. Consistent with this hypothesis is the observed inhibition of acetyl-LDL binding by high molecular weight polyanions such as polyinosinic acid or fucoidin, but not by low molecular weight polyanions such as GTP or ATP [19,62].

The acetyl-LDL receptor appears also to function in vivo. ^{125}I-Labeled acetyl-LDL administered intravenously is cleared within minutes by liver macrophages [19,25]. Simultaneous injection of fucoidin blocks hepatic uptake [19], consistent with the in vitro specificity. While the physiological ligand for the acetyl-LDL receptor is not known, cultured endothelial cells convert human LDL to a form with decreased electrophoretic ability (possibly due to increased negative charge) that is taken up by macrophage acetyl-LDL receptors [65].

(iv) The LDL–dextran sulfate complex receptor. Complexes of LDL with sulfated polysaccharides bind with high affinity to specific surface receptors on several types of macrophages [23,66–68], but not to cultured human fibroblasts [23]. These complexes enter macrophages as a single unit [23,69]. One important factor in uptake appears to be the size of the complex. High (MW 500 000), but not low molecular weight (MW 40 000) dextran sulfate effectively promotes LDL uptake [23]. Moreover, naturally occurring low molecular weight sulfated glycosaminoglycans such as heparin that form strong complexes with LDL [70] fail to stimulate LDL uptake [23].

LDL–dextran sulfate receptors appear to be distinct from both LDL and acetyl-LDL receptors. LDL–dextran complexes are taken up and degraded at the same rate in monocyte-derived macrophages from normal subjects or from patients with LDL receptor-negative homozygous FH [66]. In addition, uptake of LDL–dextran sulfate complexes is not inhibited by a concentration of polyinosinic acid that completely blocks acetyl-LDL uptake [23]. Since sulfated polysaccharides abound in the extracellular spaces of arterial walls [71], an attractive, but unproven, model for atherosclerotic foam cell production suggests that proteoglycan–LDL complexes form as LDL traverses the endothelium of arterial walls. These complexes may then be taken up by the LDL–dextran sulfate complex receptors of resident macrophages causing massive accumulation of cholesterol esters.

(v) The cholesteryl ester–protein complex receptor. Cholesteryl ester–protein (CEP) complexes appear to be large aggregates with a lipid and protein composition resembling that of LDL [24]. Mouse peritoneal macrophages, but not cultured human fibroblasts, possess receptors for internalization of CEP complexes isolated from atherosclerotic plaques of the human aorta [24]. However, CEP complexes isolated from liver or adrenal gland are not internalized [24]. Uptake of complexes by macrophages causes a marked increase in cholesterol esterification and in the accumulation of cholesteryl esters.

CEP receptors exhibit high ligand affinity and saturation kinetics for ligand binding. The protein portion of these complexes appears to participate in ligand–receptor interaction since protease treatment of aortic CEP complexes abolishes uptake [24]. Binding is competitively inhibited by polyanions in a pattern similar to the inhibition observed for the acetyl-LDL receptor [24]. However, the CEP receptor appears to be distinct from the acetyl-LDL receptor since their ligands do not mutually compete for uptake [24].

(c) Receptor-independent cholesterol uptake

In addition to high-affinity receptor-mediated uptake, cultured fibroblasts can take up LDL by receptor-independent bulk fluid pinocytosis (for a review of endocytosis, see ref. 72). LDL uptake by this process is non-saturable and is directly proportional to the concentration of LDL in the medium. Unlike receptor-dependent uptake, receptor-independent uptake of LDL is protease-insensitive and does not require divalent cations [28]. In addition, LDL entering cells through non-specific pinocytosis do not increase cellular cholesterol content or regulate cellular cholesterol synthesis or cholesterol esterification [28,73], possibly because the amount of LDL taken up may be insufficient to significantly expand cellular cholesterol pools.

When the rates of receptor-dependent and receptor-independent clearance of LDL were compared in hamster tissues, approximately 10% of total LDL clearance was found to be receptor-independent [74]. An average of over 90% of LDL uptake by liver, ovaries, adrenal glands, lung and kidney was receptor-dependent. However, receptor-independent clearance in spleen and intestine represented a large fraction (72% and 44%, respectively) of total clearance by these organs. This may reflect the presence of a larger number of phagocytic cells in the splenic pulp and the villous core of the intestine. Similarly, it has been calculated that in 1 day normal subjects can clear 45% of their plasma LDL [75–77] while patients with homozygous FH clear only 15% [75,76]. Because homozygous patients lack functional high-affinity LDL receptors, as much as one-third of the LDL clearance in man may be attributable to receptor-independent clearance.

The precise contribution of bulk fluid endocytosis to plasma LDL clearance is complicated by recent observations concerning low-affinity LDL receptors. These have been identified in fibroblasts from patients with homozygous FH previously thought to be receptor-negative [78] and possibly in macrophages derived from human monocytes [79]. LDL uptake by FH fibroblasts exhibits saturation kinetics. However, K_m for LDL is 4–7 times greater than that for the LDL receptor. The mechanism of LDL internalization and degradation by the low-affinity receptor appears to be identical to that of the high-affinity LDL receptor. Low-affinity LDL receptor-mediated endocytosis also appears to mediate the regulatory events typical of high-affinity LDL uptake. While characterization is still preliminary, the implication is that low-affinity receptor-mediated endocytosis of LDL may become important in delivery of cholesterol to cells when elevated plasma LDL concentrations saturate high-affinity uptake.

(3) Regulation of receptor-mediated sterol uptake

The regulatory events which result from the receptor-mediated uptake and degradation of LDL in cultured human fibroblasts are shown in Fig. 4. These events can be described in the context of cyclic changes that occur in cultured human fibroblasts in response to the absence or presence of LDL (see Fig. 5). When LDL is

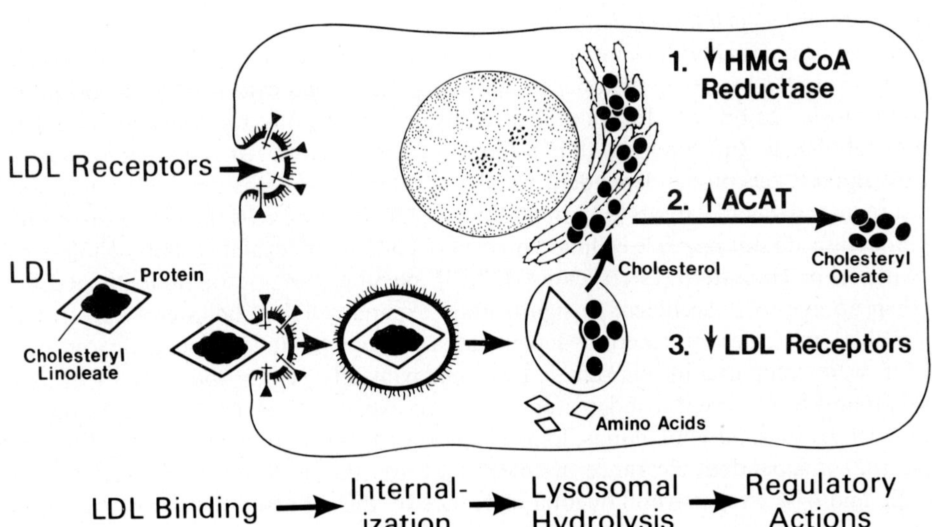

Fig. 4. Sequential steps in the LDL pathway in cultured human fibroblasts. Reproduced, with permission of the authors and publisher, from Brown and Goldstein [80].

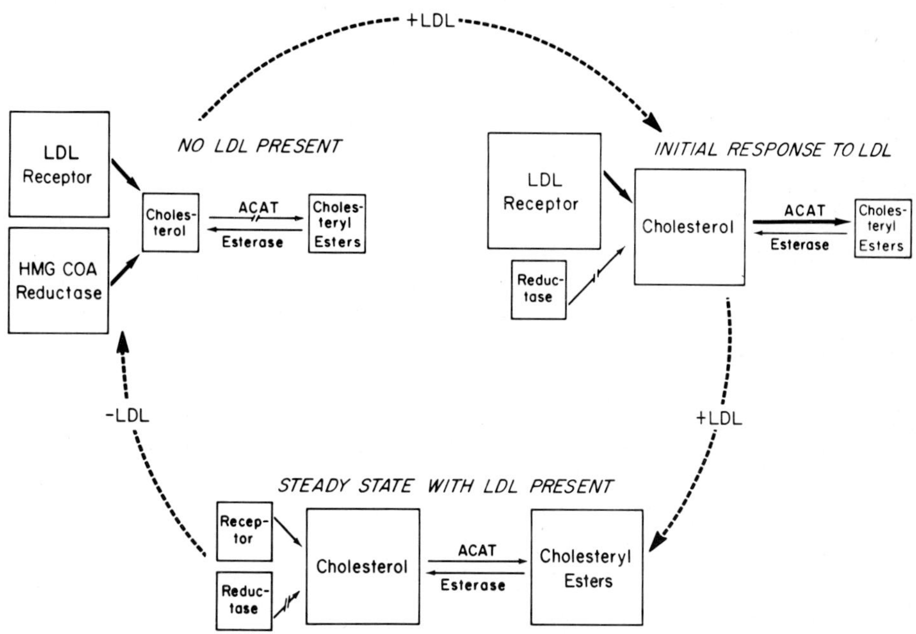

Fig. 5. Cyclic changes in cholesterol metabolism that occur in cultured human fibroblasts when LDL is removed from the culture medium (−LDL) and is subsequently returned to the medium (+LDL). The relative level of each constituent is indicated by the size of the square. Reproduced, with permission of the authors and publishers, from Goldstein and Brown [10].

absent both 3-hydroxy-3-methylglutaryl-coenzyme A (HMG-CoA) reductase, the rate-limiting enzyme for cholesterol synthesis [81–83], and the number of LDL receptors attain maximal levels while acyl-CoA : cholesterol acyltransferase (ACAT), which esterifies free cholesterol with oleate or palmitoleate, declines to basal levels. Under these conditions, de novo synthesis of cholesterol and hydrolysis of pre-existing cholesteryl esters supply sufficient cholesterol for survival.

Exposure of cholesterol-starved cells to LDL is followed by massive buildup of intracellular free cholesterol pools. HMG-CoA reductase is suppressed, shutting down cellular cholesterol synthesis [84,85]. ACAT is stimulated as much as 500-fold by a process that apparently is independent of protein synthesis [86]. Subsequently, the number of LDL receptors declines dramatically with a calculated half-life of 15–20 h [29,31]. Since the rate of decline under conditions which block protein synthesis is comparable to the LDL-mediated rate of decline [29,87], down-regulation may be due to suppression of receptor synthesis. Excess cholesterol is esterified and stored in the cytoplasm as cholesteryl esters. A steady-state characterized by large cholesteryl ester and free cholesterol pools and by basal levels of both HMG-CoA reductase and LDL receptors is ultimately attained. This regulatory mechanism allows cells to control their rate of cholesterol uptake, synthesis, and storage in response to the available supply of lipoprotein cholesterol.

HMG-CoA reductase activity and LDL receptor levels always appear to change in the same direction in cells exposed to different levels of LDL. Similarly, a mutant line of Chinese hamster ovary (CHO) cells exposed to delipidated serum expresses low levels of both HMG-CoA reductase and LDL receptor activities compared to normal cells [88]. Taken together, this evidence suggests coordinate expression of these two activities.

While the LDL pathway for control of cholesterol uptake was elucidated using cultured cells, it also appears to be functional in vivo. The pattern of regulation depicted in Fig. 5 has been confirmed in freshly isolated blood leukocytes and lymphocytes [89–92]. In addition, administration of 4-aminopyrazolepyrimidine, a drug which suppresses lipoprotein release from animal liver [93], elevates HMG-CoA reductase levels and cholesterol synthesis in non-hepatic tissues [94,95]. These observations are consistent with the hypothesis that non-hepatic cells exhibit a low rate of cholesterol synthesis because they utilize cholesterol synthesized by the liver and present in the plasma lipoproteins [96].

Regulation associated with the receptor-mediated uptake of lipoproteins by the apo-E receptor of liver is somewhat limited. While there is a marked suppression of HMG-CoA reductase activity and cholesterol synthesis [97], liver apo-E receptors are not drastically down-regulated [12] as are LDL receptors in non-hepatic tissues.

The only receptor-mediated uptake process regulated in macrophages involves suppression of β-VLDL receptors. This suppression only occurs after extensive cholesterol ester accumulation and can be induced by either β-VLDL or chemically modified LDL [13]. Lipoprotein uptake by all known receptor systems in macrophages causes a marked stimulation of ACAT activity which results in the massive accumulation of cholesteryl ester droplets in the cytoplasm [13]. Free cholesterol can be excreted from the macrophage if cholesterol-accepting lipoproteins such as HDL are present. The uncontrolled uptake and deposition of cholesteryl esters in macrophages is believed to be the key to formation of the foam cells which are associated with atherosclerosis.

(4) Diseases related to receptor-mediated cholesterol uptake

Elucidation of the LDL pathway benefited from analysis of fibroblasts from patients with genetic mutations affecting different portions of the pathway. Many significant insights into the pathway resulted from the study of fibroblasts from patients with familial hypercholesterolemia (FH). Two other diseases were important in identifying the lysosomes as the site of LDL degradation. The effects of each mutation on the LDL pathway appear in Table 2.

(a) Homozygous FH, receptor-negative and receptor-defective

The clinical pathology associated with both receptor-negative and receptor-defective forms of homozygous FH include (1) plasma LDL levels elevated from 6- to 10-fold above normal, (2) xanthomas resulting from the accumulation of free and esterified cholesterol in the interstitial spaces and within skin and tendon macro-

TABLE 2

Expression in growing fibroblasts of naturally occurring mutations affecting steps in the LDL pathway [a]

Mutation	Typical plasma LDL-cholesterol concentration (mg/dl)	Amount of [^{125}I]LDL bound to cell surface receptor	Events in the LDL pathway in fibroblasts measured at saturating levels of LDL (% normal)					
			Rate of internalization of receptor-bound [^{125}I]LDL	Rate of lysosomal hydrolysis		Regulatory events		
				[^{125}I]LDL	[^{3}H]Cholesteryl linoleate-labeled LDL	Suppression of HMG-CoA reductase in 6 h	Activation of cholesteryl ester formation in 6 h	Suppression of LDL receptor activity in 48 h
Normal	125	100 (150 ng/mg)	100 (600 ng/h/mg)	100 (600 ng/h/mg)	100 (300) pmoles/h/mg)	100 (98)	100 (500-fold increase)	100 (90)
Homozygous familial hypercholesterolemia	625							
Receptor-negative		< 2	< 2	< 2	< 2	< 2	< 1	–
Receptor-defective		10	10	10	10	50	10	–
Internalization defect		100	< 2	< 2	< 2	< 2	< 1	< 2
Heterozygous familial hypercholesterolemia	300							
Receptor-negative		50	50	50	50	50	50	50
Wolman syndrome	Normal	100	100	100	< 2	10	1	5
Cholesteryl ester storage disease	Moderately elevated	100	100	100	5	30	10	10

[a] Reproduced with permission of the authors and publisher, from Goldstein and Brown [10].

phages, and (3) severe atherosclerosis resulting in myocardial infarction as early as 18 months of age. The autosomal mutations associated with FH appear to result in disruption of post-translational processing events associated with LDL maturation (for a review see refs. 26 and 98). Receptor-negative fibroblasts express LDL receptors at a level less than 2% that of normal cells [28,37,43,99], while fibroblasts from receptor-defective patients express 5–20% of normal receptor levels [100–102]. Because homozygous FH cells are unable to take up LDL with high affinity, cholesterol needs must be satisfied by increasing de novo cholesterol synthesis [103,104].

(b) Heterozygous FH

Fibroblasts from patients with the heterozygous form of both receptor-negative and receptor-defective FH express one-half the number of normal LDL receptors [30,31] and these patients clear LDL at one-half the normal rate. Thus, plasma LDL concentrations are only 2–4-fold above normal. This moderate increase in plasma LDL results in a progressive development of atherosclerosis, which may result in myocardial infarction between ages 30 and 60 [16].

(c) Homozygous FH, internalization-defective

Fibroblasts from these patients express the normal number of surface LDL receptors which exhibit normal binding capacity. Moreover, immunodetection of LDL receptors analyzed by two-dimensional isoelectric focusing and sodium dodecyl sulfate polyacrylamide gel electrophoresis revealed that internalization-defective receptors are indistinguishable from those of normal cells [105]. Despite the presence of the normal number of intact receptors, fibroblasts from these patients are unable to take up LDL by receptor-mediated endocytosis. The mutation thus appears to be in some aspect of the receptor internalization mechanism [87]. Clinical symptoms resemble those of receptor-negative or receptor-defective FH.

(d) Wolman syndrome

Patients with this autosomal recessive mutation are deficient in the lysosomal acid lipase that hydrolyzes cholesteryl esters and triglycerides derived from plasma lipoproteins [106]. This deficiency results in the accumulation of cholesteryl esters in the lysosomes of all body tissues [16,107]. Wolman syndrome patients usually do not survive the first year of life.

(e) Cholesteryl ester storage disease

Cholesteryl ester storage disease is a less severe form of Wolman syndrome in which a residual amount (1–5%) of lysosomal acid lipase activity is expressed [108,109]. Patients with this disease may survive until young adulthood.

(II) *Control of sterol biosynthesis*

The biosynthesis of sterols takes place via the protracted sterol/isoprenoid biosynthetic pathway (Chapter 1). Although the major portion of the carbon flux through this pathway is normally directed into sterols, several branches exist leading to the production of other isoprenoid compounds needed by the cell, such as ubiquinone, dolichol and isopentenyl adenine. Total carbon flux is regulated through the enzymes of the early, or common, portion of the pathway of which the most important is HMG-CoA reductase. Distribution of carbon between the various end products is regulated at later stages of the pathway.

Because of its predominant role in the regulation of sterol biosynthesis, the first portion of this section will be devoted to the regulation of HMG-CoA reductase. The second portion will review current knowledge of other control points whose importance and roles have been less extensively studied and are less well understood.

(1) *Mammalian HMG-CoA reductase*

(a) *Rate-limiting step in sterol biosynthesis*

The enzyme HMG-CoA reductase catalyzes the reductive deacylation of HMG-CoA to mevalonate by two molecules of NADPH (Chapter 1). In most tissues this can be considered the first committed step in sterol/isoprenoid biosynthesis. Under most of the physiological conditions studied, this reaction is the rate-limiting step for sterol biosynthesis [81–83]. Evidence for this includes:

(1) Mevalonate, the product of the HMG-CoA reductase reaction, is incorporated into sterols at a rate far faster than is acetate, which forms acetyl-CoA and hence proceeds through HMG-CoA reductase to sterols [110].

(2) Carbon flux through HMG-CoA reductase into mevalonate and the rate of sterol biosynthesis correlate closely under various lighting and feeding conditions which cause these rates to vary over 100-fold [81].

(3) Sterol biosynthesis and HMG-CoA reductase activity, but not conversion of mevalonate to sterols, exhibit diurnal rhythms [111].

(4) Numerous effectors (sterols, sterol derivatives, hormones, hormonal second messengers, lipoproteins, dietary components, drugs, lighting, conditioning and stress) produce quantitatively and temporally equivalent changes in HMG-CoA reductase activity and sterol biosynthesis in animals, tissue slices and primary and continuously cultured cells.

(b) *Distribution*

HMG-CoA reductase activity has been detected in mammals, birds, insects, reptiles, fish, higher plants, moulds, yeast and bacteria [112]. HMG-CoA reductase probably is present in any life form capable of synthesizing isoprenoids. In mammals, HMG-CoA reductase activity has been detected in many tissues (Table 3). The highest quantities are present in liver and intestine, which together provide 2/3–3/4

TABLE 3

Mammalian tissues in which HMG-CoA reductase activity has been detected

Adrenal gland	Intestine	Mammary gland
Aortic smooth muscle	Kidney	Ovary
Brain	Leukocytes	Skin
Brown fat	Liver	Spermatocytes
Glial cells	Lung	Spleen
Hair root	Lymphocytes	Testis
Hepatomas	Lymphoid tissue	Vascular endothelium
	Macrophages	

of the whole body's cholesterol biosynthetic capacity [113]. HMG-CoA reductase is also present in several lines of cultured mammalian cells.

Within mammalian cells, HMG-CoA reductase activity is associated almost exclusively with the microsomal membrane fraction [114]. Cell fractionation studies [114,115] and the pronounced proliferation of the smooth endoplasmic reticulum in a cell line which overproduces HMG-CoA reductase 500-fold [116] indicate that the majority of the enzyme resides in the smooth endoplasmic reticulum. An exception is the adrenal gland, in which a major fraction is associated with mitochondria [117,118].

(c) Diurnal rhythm and developmental pattern

Rat liver HMG-CoA reductase activity exhibits a complex series of changes in the fetal and newborn rat before reaching a stable basal level in the adult [119]. Cholesterol synthesis undergoes a similar pattern of fluctuations [120,121], indicating that during development the rate of sterol biosynthesis is controlled at the level of HMG-CoA reductase [82]. The final mean level of HMG-CoA reductase activity achieved in adult rats is influenced by both neonatal sex imprinting under the influence of gonadal hormones [122] and the diet of the nursing mother [123].

In both rats [82] and chicks [124] a diurnal rhythm of HMG-CoA reductase activity and sterol biosynthesis develops in liver and intestine after the first week of life (Fig. 6). The amplitude of the rhythm is greatest in liver, where the ratio of peak to nadir activity can reach 10 to 1. In the intestines, a ratio of 2 or 3 to 1 is observed. With the exception of mammary gland [126] and possibly adrenal gland [127] and other secretory tissues, most extrahepatic tissues exhibit no diurnal rhythm in HMG-CoA reductase. During suckling, the livers of newborn rats exhibit an inverted rhythm. Peak activity occurs in the middle of the light period rather than the middle of the dark period, as is typical for the adult [119]. Following weaning, a normal phasing of the rhythm becomes established [119]. Since newborn rats suckle during daylight while adult rats feed during darkness, such an inversion is consistent with the concept that feeding and activity patterns play important roles in the development and maintenance of the rhythm. Feeding itself, however, is not the trigger for the diurnal increase. In livers of meal-fed rats, the rise in HMG-CoA reductase activity precedes the time when feeding begins [128]. The rhythm also

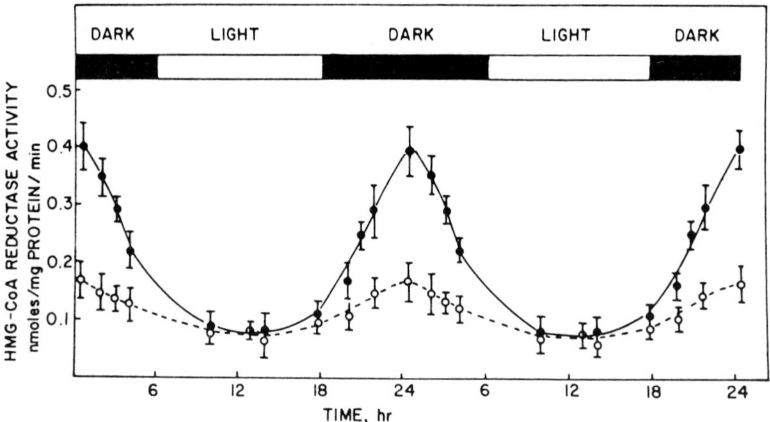

Fig. 6. Diurnal rhythm of HMG-CoA reductase activity of liver (●) and of ileal crypt cells (○). Data are mean values ±S.D. for 4–9 determinations at each time. Reproduced, with permission of the authors and publisher, from Shefer et al. [125].

persists during continual light or darkness, indicating that neither light nor darkness itself serves as trigger [129]. In addition, liver HMG-CoA reductase activity of lactating rats exhibits a normally phased diurnal rhythm while that of the mammary gland simultaneously exhibits an inverted rhythm [126]. In rats, hypophysectomy abolishes the diurnal rhythm [130], as does streptozotocin-induced diabetes [131]. In both cases, administration of the appropriate hormone restores the diurnal rhythm in HMG-CoA reductase activity [131,132]. Our present understanding is that the diurnal rhythm of HMG-CoA reductase is under hormonal control and results from the complex interplay of hormones that include insulin, glucagon, glucocorticoids, prolactin (for the mammary gland [133]) and triiodothyronine whose levels vary in response to long-term feeding and activity patterns [131,132].

(d) Regulation of HMG-CoA reductase protein levels

In general, most changes in HMG-CoA reductase activity arise, at least in part, from alterations in the quantity of HMG-CoA reductase protein. Investigations using antibodies, protein synthesis inhibitors, and activity assays measuring total, phosphatase-activated HMG-CoA reductase activity [134,135], have revealed that many effectors of HMG-CoA reductase activity do so, at least in part, by altering HMG-CoA reductase protein levels (see Table 4). The diversity of effectors which trigger these alterations is matched by the apparent complexity of the mechanisms by which they act. Effectors have been observed to alter the levels of HMG-CoA reductase protein by changing the rate of its synthesis, its degradation, or both.

Certain effectors alter the level of HMG-CoA reductase mRNA [137,138]. Others appear to alter as yet unidentified post-transcriptional events [146,155,163–166] such as mRNA translation [166], mRNA degradation, or the glycosylation of nascent HMG-CoA reductase polypeptides [167,168]. Some compounds may affect both

TABLE 4

Effectors known to alter HMG-CoA reductase protein levels

Effector	Animal, tissue or cell type examined	Direction of alteration	Refs.
Diurnal light cycling			
Dark period	Rat and chicken	+	82
Light period	liver/intestine	−	82
Feeding regimens			
Cholesterol	Rat	−	127, 136
Cholestyramine	Rat	+	127, 136
Cholestyramine + mevinolin [a]	Rat	+	137, 138
High carbohydrate + low fat	Rat	−	139
Fasting	Rat	−	83
Stress	Rat	+	83
Cyclic monoterpene injection	Rat	−	140
Mevalonolactone [b]	Fibroblasts	−	141
Cholesterol	Hepatoma tissue culture cells	−	142
Oxygenated sterols	CHO [c] cells	−	143, 144
Bile acids	Cultured intestinal mucosa	−	145
Whole serum	Hepatoma tissue culture cells	−	142
Lipid-depleted serum	Hepatoma tissue culture cells	+	146
Lipoproteins			
HDL	Vascular endothelial cells	+	147
HDL_2	Fibroblasts	−	148
HDL_3	Fibroblasts	+	148
LDL	Rat/CHO [c] cells	−	127, 143
Streptozoticin diabetes	Rat intestine and liver	+	149
Hormones			
Insulin	Rats/hepatocytes	+	150, 151
Glucagon	Rats/hepatocytes	−	150, 152
Glucocorticoids	Adrenalectomized rats	+	153
Prolactin	Mammary gland explants	+	133
Epinephrine	Hepatocytes	+	154
Norepinephrine	Hepatocytes	+	151
Triiodothyronine	Hypophysectomized rats	+	130
Lecithin infusion	Rat	+	155
Triton WR-1339 injection	Rat	+	156
Compactin [a]	Fibroblasts	+	157
Dexamethasone	Rats/cultured cells	+	158
Clofibrate	L cells	−	159
Dichloroacetate	Rat	−	160

[a] Mevinolin [161] and compactin [162] (structures given in Chapter 1) are two inhibitors of HMG-CoA reductase activity with similar properties. Both are fungal metabolites which are competitive inhibitors of HMG-CoA reductase with low K_is of about 1 nM.

[b] Mevalonolactone was used instead of the anion, mevalonate, because only the former is permeable to mammalian cells.

[c] CHO, Chinese hamster ovary.

TABLE 5

Mechanisms implicated in the control of HMG-CoA reductase protein levels

Mechanism	Effector(s)	Cell type	Refs.
Increased levels of HMG-CoA reductase mRNA	Cholestyramine ± mevinolin in diet	Rat liver	137, 138
Decreased levels of HMG-CoA reductase mRNA	Cholesterol in diet	Rat liver	138
	LDL	UT-1 CHO cells	170
Increased efficiency of a post-transcriptional event	Lecithin mesophase injections	Rat liver	155
	Compactin	HTC cells	146
	Compactin	Hepatocytes	163
	Lipoprotein-poor serum	Lymphocytes	164, 165
Decreased efficiency of a post-translational event	25-Hydroxycholesterol	Myeloblasts	166
Amplification of the HMG-CoA reductase gene	Compactin [a]	UT-1 CHO cells	169
Increased degradation rate of HMG-CoA reductase protein	25-Hydroxycholesterol	CHO cells	171
	Mevalonolactone	CHO cells	171
	Mevalonolactone	Rat hepatocytes	172
Decreased degradation rate of HMG-CoA reductase protein	Mevinolin	CHO cells	173

[a] This required severe selection pressure involving selective killing of cells by stepwise increases in the level of compactin in the growth media.

transcriptional and post-transcriptional events. In a cell line selected for its resistance to compactin, a potent inhibitor of HMG-CoA reductase, a several hundred-fold overproduction of the enzyme occurs with an accompanying 15-fold gene amplification [169]. A normal physiological role for this gene amplification is doubtful, however, since it resulted from several steps of selective killing with compactin and therefore represents a response to selective pressure of extreme severity.

Table 5 summarizes the mechanisms implicated thus far in the control of HMG-CoA reductase protein levels and the effector responsible for the alteration. The accelerated degradation of HMG-CoA reductase induced in CHO cells by incubation with 25-hydroxycholesterol was abolished by prior treatment of cells with cycloheximide or puromycin, suggesting that the mechanism for accelerating degradation requires the synthesis of one or more other proteins possessing short half-lives [171].

Regulation of HMG-CoA reductase protein levels is mechanistically complex and subject to "multivalent feedback control" [141]. The following lines of evidence indicate that HMG-CoA reductase responds to multiple regulatory signals which exert independent, cumulative effects:

(1) Sterols only partially suppress HMG-CoA reductase in cultured fibroblasts. Complete suppression requires both lipoprotein-supplied sterols and mevalonolactone [157].

(2) HDL plus compactin added to cultured vascular epithelial cells induces higher levels of HMG-CoA reductase than either present alone [174].

(3) Induction of HMG-CoA reductase produced by exposure of cultured vascular epithelial cells to HDL is reversed by addition of LDL, but LDL does not reverse the induction by compactin [174].

The identity of the multiple signals which regulate HMG-CoA reductase levels has yet to be established. One of these appears to be a sterol or sterol derivative. The second appears to be mevalonate or one of its metabolites [141]. Leading candidates for the sterol signal(s) are oxygenated derivatives of cholesterol. These are present in the circulation and many are potent suppressors of HMG-CoA reductase levels [175–177]. A candidate for the regulatory metabolite of mevalonate is isopentenyl adenine. Compactin added to baby hamster kidney-21 cells completely inhibits both DNA synthesis and cell proliferation [178]. Added mevalonolactone relieved this inhibition, but added sterols did not. Isopentenyl adenine also relieved compactin inhibition, and did so 100–200 times more effectively than did mevalonolactone [178].

To summarize, many effectors which regulate sterol biosynthesis through control of HMG-CoA reductase do so by mechanisms that involve changes in the level of HMG-CoA reductase protein. These mechanisms involve alteration of the rate of HMG-CoA reductase synthesis, HMG-CoA reductase degradation, or both. Control of the rate of HMG-CoA reductase synthesis is complex, since changes in both the levels of its mRNA and the efficiency of post-transcriptional processes have been observed. Full induction or suppression of HMG-CoA reductase occurs only in response to changes both in the level of a sterol or sterol derivative and of mevalonate or one of its metabolites. Changes in the level of either alone result in changes in HMG-CoA reductase protein levels of a smaller magnitude. This phenomenon has been termed multivalent feedback regulation.

(e) Modulation of HMG-CoA reductase activity

The catalytic activity of existing HMG-CoA reductase molecules may be regulated, or modulated, in vitro by several mechanisms. However the physiological significance of these mechanisms has, in most instances, yet to be established. One exception is the reversible inactivation–reactivation of HMG-CoA reductase that accompanies its covalent phosphorylation–dephosphorylation [179].

(i) Phosphorylation–dephosphorylation. HMG-CoA reductase is inactivated by covalent phosphorylation by the γ-phosphate of ATP, a reaction catalyzed by HMG-CoA reductase kinase [180,181]. Phosphorylated HMG-CoA reductase is reactivated by dephosphorylation, a reaction catalyzed by HMG-CoA reductase phosphatase [182,183]. Multiple HMG-CoA reductase kinases and phosphatases are present in rat liver tissue. Analysis of phosphorylated HMG-CoA reductase by tryptic digestion indicates that it contains multiple, structurally distinct phosphoryl-

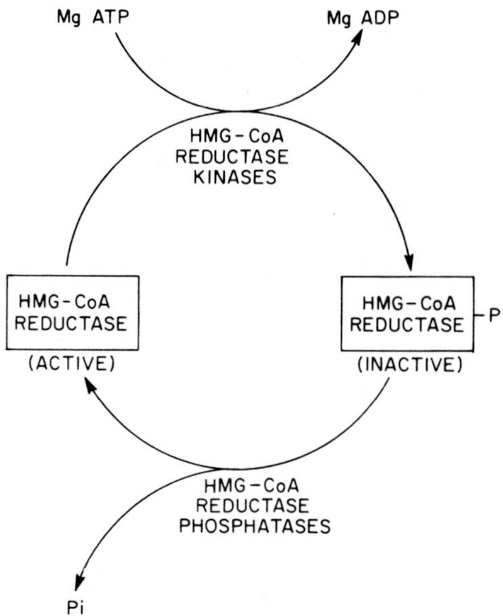

Fig. 7. Binary circuit mechanism for the modulation of HMG-CoA reductase activity by phosphorylation–dephosphorylation. Redrawn from Gibson and Ingebritsen [187].

ation sites [184,185]. These structurally distinct phosphorylation sites may also be functionally distinct, since it has been observed that full reactivation of HMG-CoA reductase by HMG-CoA reductase phosphatases can be achieved with only partial (approximately 50%) release of its protein-bound phosphate [182].

The discovery that HMG-CoA reductase activity can be controlled or modulated in vitro by phosphorylation–dephosphorylation led to the proposal that HMG-CoA reductase activity is regulated in vivo by a binary circuit [186] or cascade [187] mechanism which controls the proportion of the enzyme present in an active, dephosphorylated form in response to physiological stimuli (Fig. 7). The following evidence demonstrates the operation of this cascade mechanism in vivo:

(1) The proportion of HMG-CoA reductase in the active form in rat liver tumors (53–73%) is much higher than in normal rat liver (10–20%) [188].

(2) When rat hepatocytes are treated with insulin, glucagon or cAMP, the proportion of HMG-CoA reductase in the active, dephosphorylated form, but not HMG-CoA reductase protein levels, rapidly shifts. Insulin increases, and cAMP or glucagon decreases, the fraction of HMG-CoA reductase in an active, dephosphorylated form. These shifts are paralleled by changes in the rate of cholesterol synthesis [152].

(3) Bicarbonate ion added to rat ileal epithelial cells induces a rapid decrease in the proportion of HMG-CoA reductase in the active, dephosphorylated form which is reflected in a corresponding decrease in the rate of cholesterol biosynthesis [189].

(4) In rats fed cholesterol or mevalonolactone the proportion of hepatic HMG-

CoA reductase in the active, dephosphorylated form decreases within only 20 min, whereas HMG-CoA reductase protein levels begin to decline 60 min after feeding [190–192].

(5) The drug dichloroacetate, which lowers serum cholesterol levels in rats, decreases the proportion of hepatic HMG-CoA reductase in the active, dephosphorylated form within an hour after administration [160].

(6) Administration of glucagon, which lowers HMG-CoA reductase activity, to rats fed ^{32}P-phosphate increases the amount of radioactive phosphate bound to HMG-CoA reductase compared to controls [193].

(7) The activities of HMG-CoA reductase kinase [152] and HMG-CoA reductase phosphatase [194] rapidly respond to hormones and hormonal second messengers in a manner consistent with the observed changes in HMG-CoA reductase activity.

Regulation of HMG-CoA reductase activity by reversible phosphorylation–dephosphorylation thus allows cells to almost instantaneously alter the rate of sterol biosynthesis in response to physiological stimuli. Long-term adjustments (hours or days) are regulated by the quantity of HMG-CoA reductase protein.

(ii) Other potential mechanisms. A second potential mechanism for modulation of HMG-CoA reductase activity involves alterations in the lipid composition of microsomal membranes. According to this model, changes in the cholesterol content of microsomal membranes alter the catalytic efficiency of HMG-CoA reductase by changing membrane fluidity [195]. Evidence favoring such a mechanism includes:

(1) Chicks fed cholesterol exhibit increased hepatic microsomal cholesterol levels and decreased HMG-CoA reductase activity [196]. In addition, incubation of rat liver microsomes with serum increases their cholesterol content and decreases their HMG-CoA reductase activity in a concentration-dependent manner [197].

(2) Feeding rats cholesterol or cholestyramine alters both the K_m and the Arrhenius activation energies for microsomally bound, but not for solubilized, HMG-CoA reductase [198].

The changes in activity and/or properties of HMG-CoA reductase reported above are, however, accompanied by large changes in enzyme quantity typical of such feeding regimens. These would appear to overshadow any effects due to membrane compositional changes. However, the hypothesis that cholesterol directly feedback-inhibits its own synthesis by altering the catalytic activity of HMG-CoA reductase remains attractive since newly synthesized cholesterol appears preferentially in the smooth endoplasmic reticulum that harbors HMG-CoA reductase [115].

It has also been proposed that lipids, lipid metabolites and cytosolic lipid-binding proteins interact to regulate sterol biosynthesis [199] (see also Chapter 3). Under this model, the accumulation in cells of certain lipids or free lipid intermediates inhibits sterol biosynthetic enzymes. The level of the binding protein for a particular lipid would determine the threshold concentration of lipid needed to produce inhibition [199]. Such a mechanism would allow coordination between the biosynthesis of sterols and other lipids. Fatty acyl-CoAs and Z-protein, the fatty acyl-CoA-binding protein, may modulate HMG-CoA reductase activity [199–201] since physiological concentrations of fatty acyl-CoAs inhibit the activity of both microsomally bound [201,202] and solubilized [201] HMG-CoA reductase. This inhibition is prevented by addition of cytosol [201] or of purified Z-protein [200]. Thus, variations in the levels of Z-protein and fatty acyl-CoAs could potentially modulate HMG-CoA reductase activity. Many treatments known to affect sterol metabolism and HMG-CoA reductase activity (e.g. fasting, clofibrate feeding, or alloxan-induced diabetes) alter the level of Z-protein [200,203,204]. In addition, Z-protein is present in only very low levels in differentiated tumors, a cell type characterized by defective regulation of sterol biosynthesis [205]. Further investigation is needed, however, to determine whether the observed changes in Z-protein levels under these conditions represent the functioning of a regulatory mechanism.

Other naturally occurring substances that inhibit HMG-CoA reductase activity in vitro include rat milk [119], rat bile [119], oxidized glutathione [206,207] and iron plus a cytosolic iron-binding protein [208,209]. Although such observations suggest potential regulatory roles for these substances, physiological evidence supporting this is lacking.

(2) Other sites of control

HMG-CoA reductase functions as the major control point for sterol biosynthesis under most physiological conditions. However, regulation is not achieved solely through changes in the quantity and activity of HMG-CoA reductase. Several other enzymes are also subject to and function in regulatory control.

(a) Early sites of control

Alterations in the levels of each of the enzymes of the early, or common portion of the sterol/isoprenoid biosynthetic pathway (acetyl-CoA → isopentenyl pyrophosphate) have been observed in response to certain physiological stimuli. These alterations usually parallel those in HMG-CoA reductase. For example:

(1) HMG-CoA reductase and HMG-CoA synthase activities decrease in parallel in hypocholesterolemic rats infused with LDL [127].

(2) HMG-CoA reductase, HMG-CoA synthase, acetoacetyl-CoA thiolase and mevalonate kinase activities all increase when CHO cells are incubated in delipidated serum [210]. However, the rise in HMG-CoA reductase activity precedes that of these other enzymes [210].

(3) Mevalonate kinase and mevalonate pyrophosphate decarboxylase activities of skin fibroblasts respond in parallel to altered serum lipoprotein levels [211].

(4) Mevalonate kinase and mevalonate phosphate kinase activities both decrease in rats fed cholesterol [211].

(5) Mevalonate kinase activity increases in fibroblasts incubated with insulin or with democolcine, an inhibitor of LDL binding [211].

In at least one circumstance, however, sterol/isoprenoid biosynthesis is regulated by mechanisms independent of HMG-CoA reductase. When HeLa cells are exposed to dexamethasone, sterol biosynthesis and HMG-CoA synthase activity decrease, but HMG-CoA reductase activity increases [212,213]. This suggests that under these conditions sterol biosynthesis is controlled by regulation of HMG-CoA synthase.

To summarize, it appears that some regulatory control is exerted over several enzymes of the early portion of the sterol/isoprenoid biosynthetic pathway. The changes in these early enzymes usually parallel those in HMG-CoA reductase and probably represent a cellular conservation process rather than a mechanism for biosynthetic control [82]. The temporal relationship between the change in HMG-CoA reductase activity and that of other early enzymes when CHO cells are incubated in delipidated medium supports this hypothesis [210]. However, it also appears that, under certain circumstances, regulation of these enzymes can serve as a mechanism for control of sterol biosynthesis.

(b) Later sites of control

Reactions in the sterol/isoprenoid biosynthetic pathway located after the branch point intermediate farnesyl pyrophosphate regulate the distribution of common precursor molecules. Examples include:

(1) Biosynthesis of sterols and of dolichol are independently controlled in developing rat brain [214], in maturing mouse spermatocytes [215] and in mouse spleen cells during phenylhydrazine-induced erythropoiesis [216].

(2) Sterol and dolichol biosynthesis of cultured L cells exhibit differing sensitivities to 25-hydroxycholesterol [217].

(3) Compactin, a potent inhibitor of HMG-CoA reductase activity, inhibits biosynthesis of sterols, but not of ubiquinone, in heterozygous FH patients [218].

(4) Sterol and ubiquinone biosynthesis in fibroblasts exhibit differing sensitivities to LDL [219].

The identity of the sites responsible for regulating the distribution of intermediates between branches is presently unknown. Interpretation of available evidence is complicated by our incomplete understanding of the late steps of sterol biosynthesis (see Chapter 1). Experiments using various inhibitors of sterol biosynthesis have implicated the following as potential regulatory sites:

(1) NADPH-dependent 3-ketosterol reductase [200].
(2) Conversion of 4,4-dimethyl-Δ^8-cholestanol to C_{27} sterols [220].
(3) Conversion of 7-dehydrocholesterol to cholesterol [220].
(4) Sterol demethylation [126,221].
(5) Conversion of lanosterol to 24,25-dihydrolanosterol [222].

The emerging picture is that when sterol biosynthesis is suppressed, gross changes in the carbon flux through the sterol/isoprenoid biosynthetic pathway are mediated by HMG-CoA reductase. This decreases the supply of biosynthetic intermediates available for non-sterol products, which normally are synthesized in far smaller quantity than are sterols. To assure a sufficient supply of these intermediates for needed non-sterols such as dolichol and ubiquinone, later steps in the sterol/isoprenoid biosynthetic pathway are also down-regulated [141].

Acknowledgements

We wish to thank Libby Eberly for the preparation of this manuscript and our colleagues Michael Beach and Tuajuanda Jordan for their many helpful suggestions.

References

1 Havel, R.J., Goldstein, J.L. and Brown, M.S. (1980) in: Metabolic Control and Disease (Bondy, P.K. and Rosenberg, L.E., Eds.) pp. 393–494, Saunders, Philadelphia, PA.
2 Scanu, A.M. and Landsberger, F.R. (Eds.) (1980) Ann. N.Y. Acad. Sci. 348, 1–434.
3 Jackson, R.L., Morrisette, J.D. and Gotto Jr., A.M. (1976) Physiol. Rev. 56, 259–316.
4 Brown, M.S., Kovanen, P.T. and Goldstein, J.L. (1981) Science 212, 628–635.
5 Havel, R.J. (1957) J. Clin. Invest. 36, 848–854.
6 Skopski, V.W. (1972) in: Blood Lipids and Lipoproteins; Quantitation, Composition and Metabolism (Nelson, G.J., Ed.) pp. 471–583, Wiley, New York.
7 Bilheimer, D.W., Eisenberg, S. and Levy, R.I. (1972) Biochim. Biophys. Acta 260, 212–221.
8 Levy, R.I., Bilheimer, D.W. and Eisenberg, S. (1971) in: Plasma Lipoproteins (Smellie, R.M.S., Ed.) pp. 3–17, Academic Press, New York.
9 Grundy, S.M. and Mok, H.Y.I. (1976) Metabolism 25, 1225–1239.
10 Goldstein, J.L. and Brown, M.S. (1977) Annu. Rev. Biochem. 46, 897–930.
11 Heiss, G., Johnson, N.J., Reiland, S., Davis, D.E. and Tyroler, H.A. (1980) Circulation 62, 116–136.
12 Mahley, R.W. and Innerarity, T.L. (1983) Biochim. Biophys. Acta 737, 197–222.
13 Goldstein, J.L., Ho, Y.K., Brown, M.S., Innerarity, T.L. and Mahley, R.W. (1980) J. Biol. Chem. 255, 1839–1848.
14 Mahley, R.W., Innerarity, T.L., Brown, M.S., Ho, Y.K. and Goldstein, J.L. (1980) J. Lipid Res. 21, 970–980.
15 Fainaru, M., Mahley, R.W., Hamilton, R.L. and Innerarity, T.L. (1982) J. Lipid Res. 23, 702–714.
16 Brown, M.S., Goldstein, J.L. and Fredrickson, D.S. (1983) in: Metabolic Basis of Inherited Disease (Stanbury, J.B., Wyngaarden, J.B., Fredrickson, D.S., Goldstein, J.L. and Brown, M.S., Eds.) pp. 655–671, McGraw-Hill, New York.
17 Mahley, R.W. (1982) Med. Clin. N. Am. 66, 375–402.
18 Pitas, R.E., Innerarity, T.L. and Mahley, R.W. (1983) Arteriosclerosis 3, 2–12.
19 Goldstein, J.L., Ho, Y.K., Basu, S.K. and Brown, M.S. (1979) Proc. Natl. Acad. Sci. (U.S.A.) 76, 333–337.
20 Mahley, R.W., Innerarity, T.L., Weisgraber, K.H. and Oh, S.Y. (1979) J. Clin. Invest. 64, 743–750.
21 Fogelman, A.M., Shechter, I., Seager, J., Hokom, M., Child, J.S. and Edwards, P.A. (1980) Proc. Natl. Acad. Sci. (U.S.A.) 77, 2214–2218.
22 Brown, M.S. and Goldstein, J.L. (1983) Annu. Rev. Biochem. 52, 223–261.
23 Basu, S.K., Brown, M.S., Ho, Y.K. and Goldstein, J.L. (1979) J. Biol. Chem. 254, 7141–7146.
24 Goldstein, J.L., Hoff, H.F., Ho, Y.K., Basu, S.K. and Brown, M.S. (1981) Arteriosclerosis 1, 210–226.
25 Mahley, R.W., Weisgraber, K.H., Innerarity, T.L. and Windmueller, H.G. (1979) Proc. Natl. Acad. Sci. (U.S.A.) 76, 1746–1750.
26 Brown, M.S., Anderson, R.G.W. and Goldstein, J.L. (1983) Cell 32, 663–667.
27 Goldstein, J.L., Anderson, R.G.W. and Brown, M.S. (1979) Nature (London) 279, 679–685.
28 Goldstein, J.L. and Brown, M.S. (1974) J. Biol. Chem. 249, 5153–5162.
29 Brown, M.S. and Goldstein, J.L. (1975) Cell 6, 307–316.
30 Brown, M.S. and Goldstein, J.L. (1974) Science 185, 61–63.
31 Goldstein, J.L., Sobhani, M.K., Faust, J.R. and Brown, M.S. (1976) Cell 9, 195–203.
32 Schneider, W.J., Goldstein, J.R. and Brown, M.S. (1980) J. Biol. Chem. 255, 11442–11447.

33 Cummings, R.D., Kornfeld, S., Schneider, W.J., Hobgood, K.K., Tolleshaug, H., Brown, M.S. and Goldstein, J.L. (1983) J. Biol. Chem. 258, 15261–15273.
34 Innerarity, T.L., Kempner, E.S., Hui, D.Y. and Mahley, R.W. (1981) Proc. Natl. Acad. Sci. (U.S.A.) 78, 4378–4382.
35 Weisgraber, K.H., Innerarity, T.L. and Mahley, R.W. (1978) J. Biol. Chem. 253, 9053–9062.
36 Mahley, R.W., Innerarity, T.L., Pitas, R.E., Weisgraber, K.H., Brown, J.H. and Gross, E. (1977) J. Biol. Chem. 252, 7279–7287.
37 Goldstein, J.L., Basu, S.K., Brunschede, G.Y. and Brown, M.S. (1976) Cell 7, 85–95.
38 Mahley, R.W. and Innerarity, T.L. (1977) J. Biol. Chem. 252, 3980–3986.
39 Innerarity, T.L. and Mahley, R.W. (1978) Biochemistry 17, 1440–1447.
40 Florén, C.H., Albers, J.J., Kudchodkar, B.J. and Bierman, E.L. (1981) J. Biol. Chem. 256, 425–433.
41 Redgrave, T.G. (1970) J. Clin. Invest. 49, 465–471.
42 Windler, E., Chao, Y.S. and Havel, R.J. (1980) J. Biol. Chem. 255, 5475–5480.
43 Anderson, R.G.W., Goldstein, J.L. and Brown, M.S. (1976) Proc. Natl. Acad. Sci. (U.S.A.) 73, 2434–2438.
44 Anderson, R.G.W., Brown, M.S. and Goldstein, J.L. (1977) Cell 10, 351–364.
45 Basu, S.K., Goldstein, J.L., Anderson, R.G.W. and Brown, M.S. (1981) Cell 24, 493–502.
46 Brown, M.S., Anderson, R.G.W., Basu, S.K. and Goldstein, J.L. (1981) Cold Spring Harbor Symp. Quant. Biol. 46, 713–721.
47 Tycko, B. and Maxfield, F.R. (1982) Cell 28, 643–651.
48 Geuze, H.J., Slot, J.W., Strous, G.J.A.M., Lodish, H.F. and Schwartz, A.L. (1983) Cell 32, 277–287.
49 Brown, M.S., Dana, S.E. and Goldstein, J.L. (1975) Proc. Natl. Acad. Sci. (U.S.A.) 72, 2925–2929.
50 Goldstein, J.L., Dana, S.E., Faust, J.R., Beaudet, A.L. and Brown, M.S. (1975) J. Biol. Chem. 250, 8487–8495.
51 Brown, M.S., Sobhani, M.K., Brunschede, G.Y. and Goldstein, J.L. (1976) J. Biol. Chem. 251, 3277–3286.
52 Mahley, R.W., Hui, D.Y., Innerarity, T.L. and Weisgraber, K.H. (1981) J. Clin. Invest. 68, 1197–1206.
53 Carrella, M. and Cooper, A.D. (1979) Proc. Natl. Acad. Sci. (U.S.A.) 76, 338–342.
54 Sherrill, B.C. and Dietschy, J.M. (1978) J. Biol. Chem. 253, 1859–1867.
55 Hui, D.Y., Innerarity, T.L. and Mahley, R.W. (1981) J. Biol. Chem. 256, 5646–5655.
56 Sherrill, B.C., Innerarity, T.L. and Mahley, R.W. (1980) J. Biol. Chem. 255, 1804–1807.
57 Shelburne, F., Hanks, J., Meyers, W. and Quarfordt, S. (1980) J. Clin. Invest. 65, 652–658.
58 Pitas, R.E., Innerarity, T.L. and Mahley, R.W. (1983) Arteriosclerosis 3, 2–12.
59 Innerarity, T.L. and Mahley, R.W. (1980) in: Drugs Affecting Lipid Metabolism (Fumagalli, R., Kritchevsky, D. and Paoletti, R., Eds.) pp. 53–60, Elsevier/North-Holland Biomedical, Amsterdam.
60 Mahley, R.W. (1979) Atheroscler. Rev. 5, 1–34.
61 Brown, M.S., Goldstein, J.L., Krieger, M., Ho, Y.K. and Anderson, R.G.W. (1979) J. Cell Biol. 82, 597–613.
62 Brown, M.S., Basu, S.K., Falck, J.R., Ho, Y.K. and Goldstein, J.L. (1980) J. Supramol. Struct. 13, 67–81.
63 Traber, M.G. and Kayden, H.J. (1980) Proc. Natl. Acad. Sci. (U.S.A.) 77, 5466–5470.
64 Basu, S.K., Goldstein, J.L., Anderson, R.G.W. and Brown, M.S. (1976) Proc. Natl. Acad. Sci. (U.S.A.) 73, 3178–3182.
65 Henriksen, T., Mahoney, E.M. and Steinberg, D. (1981) Proc. Natl. Acad. Sci. (U.S.A.) 78, 6499–6503.
66 Knight, B.L. and Soutar, A.K. (1982) Eur. J. Biochem. 125, 407–413.
67 Traber, M.G., Defendi, V. and Kayden, H.J. (1981) J. Exp. Med. 154, 1852–1867.
68 Fogelman, A.M., Seager, J., Haberland, M.E., Hokom, M., Tanaka, R. and Edwards, P.A. (1982) Proc. Natl. Acad. Sci. (U.S.A.) 79, 922–926.
69 Kielian, M.C. and Cohn, Z.A. (1982) J. Cell Biol. 93, 875–882.
70 Iverius, P.-H. (1972) J. Biol. Chem. 247, 2607–2613.

71 Srinivasan, S.R., Dolan, P., Radhakishnamurthy, B., Pargaonkar, P.S. and Berenson, G.S. (1975) Biochim. Biophys. Acta 388, 58–70.
72 Silverstein, S.C., Steinman, R.M. and Cohn, Z.A. (1977) Annu. Rev. Biochem. 46, 669–722.
73 Brown, M.S., Faust, J.R. and Goldstein, J.L. (1975) J. Clin. Invest. 55, 783–793.
74 Spady, D.K., Bilheimer, D.W. and Dietschy, J.M. (1983) Proc. Natl. Acad. Sci. (U.S.A.) 80, 3499–3503.
75 Bilheimer, D.W., Goldstein, J.L., Grundy, S.M. and Brown, M.S. (1975) J. Clin. Invest. 56, 1420–1430.
76 Simons, L.A., Reichl, D., Myant, N.B. and Mancini, M. (1975) Arteriosclerosis 21, 283–298.
77 Packard, C.J., Third, J.L.H.C., Shepherd, J., Lorimer, A.R., Morgan, H.G. and Lawrie, T.D.V. (1976) Metabolism 25, 995–1006.
78 Semenkovich, C.F., Otlund Jr., R.E., Levy, R.A. and Osa, S.R. (1982) J. Biol. Chem. 257, 12857–12865.
79 Fogelman, A.M., Hokom, M.M., Haberland, M.E., Tanaka, R.D. and Edwards, P.A. (1982) J. Biol. Chem. 257, 14081–14086.
80 Brown, M.S. and Goldstein, J.L. (1979) Proc. Natl. Acad. Sci. (U.S.A.) 76, 3330–3337.
81 Dietschy, J.M. and Brown, M.S. (1974) J. Lipid Res. 15, 508–516.
82 Rodwell, V.W., Nordstrom, J.L. and Mitschelen, J.J. (1976) Adv. Lipid Res. 14, 1–74.
83 Brown, M.S., Goldstein, J.L. and Dietschy, J.M. (1979) J. Biol. Chem. 254, 5144–5149.
84 Brown, M.S., Dana, S.E. and Goldstein, J.L. (1973) Proc. Natl. Acad. Sci. (U.S.A.) 70, 2162–2166.
85 Brown, M.S., Dana, S.E. and Goldstein, J.L. (1974) J. Biol. Chem. 249, 789–796.
86 Goldstein, J.L., Dana, S.E. and Brown, M.S. (1974) Proc. Natl. Acad. Sci. (U.S.A.) 71, 4288–4292.
87 Brown, M.S. and Goldstein, J.L. (1976) Cell 9, 663–674.
88 Chin, J. and Chang, T.Y. (1981) J. Biol. Chem. 256, 6304–6310.
89 Fogelman, A.M., Edmond, J., Polito, A. and Popják, G. (1973) J. Biol. Chem. 248, 6928–6929.
90 Fogelman, A.M., Edmond, J., Seager, J. and Popják, G. (1975) J. Biol. Chem. 250, 2045–2055.
91 Williams, C.D. and Avigan, J. (1972) Biochim. Biophys. Acta 260, 413–423.
92 Ho, Y.K., Brown, M.S., Bilheimer, D.W. and Goldstein, J.L. (1976) J. Clin. Invest. 58, 1465–1474.
93 Henderson, J.F. (1963) J. Lipid Res. 4, 68–74.
94 Balasubramanian, S., Goldstein, J.L., Faust, J.R. and Brown, M.S. (1976) Proc. Natl. Acad. Sci. (U.S.A.) 73, 2564–2568.
95 Anderson, J.M. and Dietschy, J.M. (1976) Science 193, 903–905.
96 Brown, M.S. and Goldstein, J.L. (1976) Science 191, 150–154.
97 Lakshmanan, M.R., Muesing, R.A. and LaRosa, J.C. (1981) J. Biol. Chem. 256, 3037–3048.
98 Tolleshaug, H., Goldstein, J.L., Schneider, W.J. and Brown, M.S. (1982) Cell 30, 715–724.
99 Brown, M.S. and Goldstein, J.L. (1974) Proc. Natl. Acad. Sci. (U.S.A.) 71, 788–792.
100 Breslow, J.L., Spaulding, D.R., Lux, S.E., Levy, R.I. and Lees, R.S. (1975) New Engl. J. Med. 293, 900–903.
101 Brown, M.S. and Goldstein, J.L. (1976) New Engl. J. Med. 294, 1386–1390.
102 Goldstein, J.L., Dana, S.E., Brunschede, G.Y. and Brown, M.S. (1975) Proc. Natl. Acad. Sci. (U.S.A.) 72, 1092–1096.
103 Goldstein, J.L. and Brown, M.S. (1976) Curr. Top. Cell Regul. 11, 147–181.
104 Goldstein, J.L. and Brown, M.S. (1973) Proc. Natl. Acad. Sci. (U.S.A.) 70, 2804–2808.
105 Beisiegel, U., Schneider, W.J., Brown, M.S. and Goldstein, J.L. (1982) J. Biol. Chem. 257, 13150–13156.
106 Patrick, A.D. and Lake, B.D. (1969) Nature (London) 222, 1067–1068.
107 Patrick, A.D. and Lake, B.D. (1973) in: Lysosomes and Storage Diseases (Hers, H.G. and VanHoof, F., Eds.) pp. 453–473, Academic Press, New York.
108 Burke, J.A. and Schubert, W.K. (1972) Science 176, 309–310.
109 Sloan, H.R. and Fredrickson, D.S. (1972) J. Clin. Invest. 51, 1923–1926.
110 Shapiro, D.J. and Rodwell, V.W. (1971) J. Biol. Chem. 246, 3210–3216.
111 Back, P., Hamprecht, B. and Lynen, F. (1969) Arch. Biochem. Biophys. 133, 11–21.
112 Brown, W.B. and Rodwell, V.W. (1980) in: Dehydrogenases Requiring Nicotinamide Coenzymes (Jeffrey, J., Ed.) pp. 232–272, Birkhäuser Verlag, Basel.

113 Turley, S.D., Andersen, J.M. and Dietschy, J.M. (1981) J. Lipid Res. 22, 551–559.
114 Goldfarb, S. (1972) FEBS Lett. 24, 153–155.
115 Mitropoulos, K.A., Venkatesan, S., Balasubramaniam, S. and Peters, T.J. (1978) Eur. J. Biochem. 82, 419–429.
116 Chin, D.J., Luskey, K.L., Anderson, R.G.W., Faust, J.R., Goldstein, J.L. and Brown, M.S. (1982) Proc. Natl. Acad. Sci. (U.S.A.) 79, 1185–1189.
117 Lehoux, J.-G., Tan, L. and Preiss, B. (1977) Gen. Comp. Endocrinol. 33, 133–138.
118 Preiss, B. and Lehoux, J.-G. (1979) Biochem. Biophys. Res. Commun. 88, 1140–1146.
119 McNamara, D.J., Quackenbush, F.W. and Rodwell, V.W. (1972) J. Biol. Chem. 247, 5805–5810.
120 Ballard, F.J. and Hanson, R.W. (1967) Biochem. J. 102, 952–958.
121 Wróbel, J., Boguslawski, W., Michalska, L. and Niemiro, R. (1973) Int. J. Biochem. 4, 565–568.
122 Carlson, S.E., Mitchell, A.D., Carter, M.L. and Goldfarb, S. (1980) Biochim. Biophys. Acta 633, 154–161.
123 Reiser, R., Henderson, G.R. and O'Brien, B.C. (1977) J. Nutr. 107, 1131–1138.
124 Ramirez, H., Alejandre, M.J. and Garcia-Peregrin, E. (1982) Lipids 17, 434–436.
125 Shefer, S., Hauser, S., Lapar, V. and Mosbach, E.H. (1972) J. Lipid Res. 13, 571–573.
126 Gibbons, G.F., Pullinger, C.R., Munday, M.R. and Williamson, D.H. (1983) Biochem. J. 212, 843–848.
127 Balasubramaniam, S., Goldstein, J.L. and Brown, M.S. (1977) Proc. Natl. Acad. Sci. (U.S.A.) 74, 1421–1425.
128 Dugan, R.E., Slakey, L.L., Briedis, A.V. and Porter, J.W. (1972) Arch. Biochem. Biophys. 152, 21–27.
129 Huber, J., Latzin, S., Langguth, O., Brauser, B., Gabel, V.P. and Hamprecht, B. (1973) FEBS Lett. 31, 261–265.
130 Ness, G.C., Dugan, R.E., Lakshmanan, M.R., Nepokroeff, C.M. and Porter, J.W. (1973) Proc. Natl. Acad. Sci. (U.S.A.) 70, 3839–3842.
131 Nepokroeff, C.M., Lakshmanan, M.R., Ness, G.C., Dugan, R.E. and Porter, J.W. (1974) Arch. Biochem. Biophys. 160, 387–393.
132 Dugan, R.E., Ness, G.C., Lakshmanan, M.R., Nepokroeff, C.M. and Porter, J.W. (1974) Arch. Biochem. Biophys. 161, 499–504.
133 Middleton, B., Hatton, J. and White, D.A. (1982) J. Biol. Chem. 256, 4827–4834.
134 Huber, J., Guber, W., Müller, O.A., Latzin, S., Ganser, H. and Hamprecht, B. (1974) Hoppe-Seyler's Z. Physiol. Chem. 355, 669–674.
135 Philipp, B.W. and Shapiro, D.J. (1979) J. Lipid Res. 20, 588–593.
136 Kleinsek, D.A., Jabalquinto, A.M. and Porter, J.W. (1980) J. Biol. Chem. 255, 3918–3923.
137 Clarke, C.F., Edwards, P.F., Lan, S.-F., Tanaka, R.D. and Fogelman, A.M. (1983) Proc. Natl. Acad. Sci. (U.S.A.) 80, 3305–3308.
138 Liscum, L., Luskey, K.L., Chin, D.J., Ho, V.K., Goldstein, J.L. and Brown, M.S. (1983) J. Biol. Chem. 258, 8450–8455.
139 Stacpoole, P.W., Harwood Jr., H.J. and Varnado, C.E. (1983) Biochem. Biophys. Res. Commun. 113, 888–894.
140 Clegg, R.J., Middleton, B., Bell, G.D. and White, D.A. (1982) J. Biol. Chem. 257, 2294–2299.
141 Brown, M.S. and Goldstein, J.L. (1980) J. Lipid Res. 21, 505–517.
142 Bell, J.J., Sargeant, T.E. and Watson, J.A. (1976) J. Biol. Chem. 251, 1745–1758.
143 Chang, T.-Y., Limanek, J.S. and Chang, C.C.Y. (1981) J. Biol. Chem. 256, 6174–6180.
144 Sinensky, M., Torget, R. and Edwards, P.A. (1981) J. Biol. Chem. 256, 11774–11779.
145 Gebhard, R.L. and Cooper, A.D. (1978) J. Biol. Chem. 253, 2790–2796.
146 Kirsten, E.S. and Watson, J.A. (1974) J. Biol. Chem. 249, 6104–6109.
147 Cohen, D.C., Massoglia, S.L. and Gospadarowicz, D. (1982) J. Biol. Chem. 257, 9429–9437.
148 Daerr, W.H., Gianturco, S.H., Patsch, J.R., Smith, L.C. and Gotto Jr., A.M. (1980) Biochim. Biophys. Acta 619, 287–301.
149 Young, N.L., Saudek, C.D., Walters, L., Lapeyrolerie, J. and Cheng, V. (1982) J. Lipid Res. 23, 831–838.
150 Dugan, R.E., Baker, T.A. and Porter, J.W. (1982) Eur. J. Biochem. 125, 497–503.

151 Edwards, P.A., Lemongello, D. and Fogelman, A.M. (1979) J. Lipid Res. 20, 2–7.
152 Ingebritsen, T.S., Geelen, M.J.H., Parker, R.A., Evenson, K.J. and Gibson, D.M. (1979) J. Biol. Chem. 254, 9986–9989.
153 Mitropoulos, K.A. and Balasubramaniam, S. (1976) Biochem. J. 160, 49–55.
154 Edwards, P.A. and Gould, R.G. (1974) J. Biol. Chem. 249, 2891–2896.
155 Jakoi, L. and Quarfordt, S.H. (1974) J. Biol. Chem. 249, 5840–5844.
156 Kuroda, M., Tanzawa, K., Tsujita, Y. and Endo, A. (1977) Biochim. Biophys. Acta 489, 119–125.
157 Brown, M.S., Faust, J.R. and Goldstein, J.L. (1978) J. Biol. Chem. 253, 1121–1128.
158 Lin, R.C. and Snodgrass, P.J. (1982) Biochim. Biophys. Acta 713, 240–250.
159 Kaneko, I., Hazama-Shimada, Y., Kuroda, M. and Endo, A. (1977) Biochem. Biophys. Res. Commun. 76, 1207–1213.
160 Stacpoole, P.W., Harwood Jr., H.J., Varnado, C.E. and Schneider, M. (1983) J. Clin. Invest. 72, 1575–1585.
161 Alberts, A.W., Chen, J., Kuron, G., Hunt, V., Huff, J., Hoffman, C., Rothrock, J., Lopez, M., Joshua, H., Harris, E., Patchett, A., Monaghan, R., Currie, S., Stapley, E., Albers-Schonberg, G., Hirshfield, J., Hoogsteen, K., Liesch, J. and Springer, J. (1980) Proc. Natl. Acad. Sci. (U.S.A.) 77, 3957–3961.
162 Endo, A., Kuroda, M. and Tanzawa, K. (1976) FEBS Lett. 72, 323–326.
163 Koizumi, J., Mabuchi, H. and Takeda, R. (1982) Biochem. Biophys. Res. Commun. 108, 240–246.
164 Krone, W., Betteridge, D.J. and Galton, D.J. (1979) Biochim. Biophys. Acta 574, 361–365.
165 Krone, W. and Schettler, G. (1980) Atherosclerosis 36, 423–426.
166 Tanaka, R.D., Edwards, P.A., Lan, S.-F. and Fogelman, A.M. (1983) J. Biol. Chem. 258, 13331–13339.
167 Brown, D.A. and Simoni, R.D. (1983) J. Lipid Res. 24, 1405.
168 Volpe, J.J. and Goldberg, R.I. (1983) J. Biol. Chem. 258, 9220–9226.
169 Luskey, K.L., Faust, J.R., Chin, D.J., Brown, M.S. and Goldstein, J.L. (1983) J. Biol. Chem. 258, 8462–8469.
170 Chin, D.J., Luskey, K.L., Faust, J.R., MacDonald, R.J., Brown, M.S. and Goldstein, J.R. (1982) Proc. Natl. Acad. Sci. (U.S.A.) 79, 7704–7708.
171 Chen, H.W., Richards, B.A. and Kandutsch, A.A. (1982) Biochim. Biophys. Acta 712, 484–489.
172 Edwards, P.A., Lan, S.-F., Tanaka, R.D. and Fogelman, A.M. (1983) J. Biol. Chem. 258, 7272–7275.
173 Sinensky, M. and Vogel, J. (1983) J. Biol. Chem. 258, 8547–8549.
174 Cohen, D.C., Massoglia, S.L. and Gospodarowicz, D. (1982) J. Biol. Chem. 257, 11106–11112.
175 Estermann, A.L., Baum, H., Javitt, N.B. and Darlington, G.J. (1983) J. Lipid Res. 24, 1304–1309.
176 Kandutsch, A.A., Chen, H.W. and Heiniger, H.-J. (1978) Science 201, 498–501.
177 Schroepfer Jr., G.J. (1981) Annu. Rev. Biochem. 50, 585–621.
178 Quesney-Huneeus, V., Galick, H.A., Siperstein, M.D., Erickson, S.K., Spencer, T.A. and Nelson, J.A. (1983) J. Biol. Chem. 258, 378–385.
179 Ingebritsen, T.S. and Gibson, D.M. (1980) in: Recently Discovered Systems of Enzyme Regulation by Reversible Phosphorylation (Cohen, P., Ed.) Mol. Aspects Cell. Regul., Vol. 1, pp. 63–93, Elsevier, Amsterdam.
180 Beg, Z.H., Stonik, J.A. and Brewer Jr., H.B. (1979) Proc. Natl. Acad. Sci. (U.S.A.) 76, 4375–4379.
181 Harwood Jr., H.J., Brandt, K.G. and Rodwell, V.W., J. Biol. Chem., 259, 2810–2815.
182 Brown, W.E. and Rodwell, V.W. (1983) Biochim. Biophys. Acta 751, 218–229.
183 Gil, G., Sitges, M. and Hegardt, F.G. (1981) Biochim. Biophys. Acta 663, 211–221.
184 Font, E., Sitges, M. and Hegardt, F.G. (1982) Biochem. Biophys. Res. Commun. 105, 705–710.
185 Keith, M.L., Kennelly, P.J. and Rodwell, V.W. (1983) J. Protein Chem. 2, 209–220.
186 Nordstrom, J.L., Rodwell, V.W. and Mitschelen, J.J. (1977) J. Biol. Chem. 252, 8924–8934.
187 Gibson, D.M. and Ingebritsen, T.S. (1978) Life Sci. 23, 2649–2664.
188 Feingold, K.R., Wiley, M.H., Moser, A.H. and Siperstein, M.D. (1983) Arch. Biochem. Biophys. 226, 231–241.
189 Panini, S.R. and Rudney, H. (1980) J. Biol. Chem. 255, 11633–11636.
190 Arebalo, R.E., Hardgrave, J.E., Noland, B.J. and Scallen, T.J. (1980) Proc. Natl. Acad. Sci. (U.S.A.) 77, 6429–6433.
191 Arebalo, R.E., Hardgrave, J.E. and Scallen, T.J. (1981) J. Biol. Chem. 256, 571–574.

192 Arebalo, R.E., Tormanen, C.D., Hardgrave, J.E., Noland, B.J. and Scallen, T.J. (1982) Proc. Natl. Acad. Sci. (U.S.A.) 79, 51–55.
193 Beg, Z.H., Stonik, J.A. and Brewer Jr., H.B. (1980) J. Biol. Chem. 255, 8541–8545.
194 Gibson, D.M., Parker, R.A., Stewart, C.E. and Evenson, K.J. (1982) Adv. Enzyme Regul. 20, 263–283.
195 Sabine, J.R. and James, M.J. (1976) Life Sci. 18, 1185–1192.
196 Ramirez, H., Alejandre, M.J., Segovia, J.L. and Garcia-Peregrin, E. (1981) Lipids 16, 552–554.
197 Mitropoulos, K.A., Venkatesan, S., Reeves, B.E.A. and Balasubramaniam, S. (1981) Biochem. J. 194, 265–271.
198 Mitropoulos, K.A. and Venkatesan, S. (1977) Biochim. Biophys. Acta 489, 126–142.
199 Trzaszkos, J.M. and Gaylor, J.L. (1983) Biochim. Biophys. Acta 751, 52–65.
200 Grinstead, G.F., Trzaszkos, J.M., Billheimer, J.T. and Gaylor, J.L. (1983) Biochim. Biophys. Acta 751, 41–51.
201 Lehrer, G., Panini, S.R., Rogers, D.H. and Rudney, H. (1981) J. Biol. Chem. 256, 5612–5619.
202 Faas, F.H., Carter, W.J. and Wynn, J.O. (1978) Biochim. Biophys. Acta 531, 158–166.
203 Fleischner, G., Meijer, D.K.F., Levine, W.G., Gatmaitan, Z., Gluck, R. and Arias, I.M. (1975) Biochem. Biophys. Res. Commun. 67, 1401–1407.
204 Renaud, G., Foliot, A. and Infante, R. (1978) Biochem. Biophys. Res. Commun. 80, 327–334.
205 Mishkin, S., Morris, H.P., Murthy, P.V.N. and Halperin, M.L. (1977) J. Biol. Chem. 252, 3626–3628.
206 Dotan, I. and Schechter, I. (1982) Biochim. Biophys. Acta 713, 427–434.
207 Dotan, I. and Schechter, I. (1983) Arch. Biochem. Biophys. 226, 401–410.
208 Menon, A.S., Devi, S.V. and Ramasarma, T. (1982) Biochem. Biophys. Res. Commun. 109, 619–625.
209 Ramasarma, T., Paton, B. and Goldfarb, S. (1981) Biochem. Biophys. Res. Commun. 100, 170–176.
210 Chang, T.-Y. and Limanek, J.S. (1980) J. Biol. Chem. 255, 7787–7795.
211 Mitchell, E.D. and Avigan, J. (1981) J. Biol. Chem. 256, 6170–6173.
212 Johnson, D., Cavenee, W.K., Ramachandran, C.K. and Melnykovych, G. (1979) Biochim. Biophys. Acta 572, 188–192.
213 Ramachandran, C.K., Gray, S.L. and Melnykovych (1978) Arch. Biochem. Biophys. 199, 205–211.
214 James, M.J. and Kandutsch, A.A. (1980) Biochim. Biophys. Acta 619, 432–435.
215 Potter, J.E.R., Millette, C.F., James, M.J. and Kandutsch, A.A. (1981) J. Biol. Chem. 256, 7150–7154.
216 Potter, J.E.R., James, M.J. and Kandutsch, A.A. (1981) J. Biol. Chem. 256, 2371–2376.
217 James, M.J. and Kandutsch, A.A. (1979) J. Biol. Chem. 254, 8442–8446.
218 Mabuchi, H., Haba, T., Tatami, R., Miyamoto, S., Sakai, Y., Wakasugi, T., Watanabe, A., Koizumi, J. and Takeda, R. (1981) New Engl. J. Med. 305, 478–482.
219 Faust, J.R., Goldstein, J.L. and Brown, M.S. (1979) Arch. Biochem. Biophys. 192, 86–99.
220 Noland, B.J., Arebalo, R.E., Hansbury, E. and Scallen, T.J. (1980) J. Biol. Chem. 255, 4282–4289.
221 Havel, C., Hansbury, E., Scallen, T.J. and Watson, J.A. (1979) J. Biol. Chem. 254, 9573–9582.
222 Pinkerton, F.D., Izumi, A., Anderson, C.M., Miller, L.R., Kisic, A. and Schroepfer Jr., G.J. (1982) J. Biol. Chem. 257, 1929–1936.

H. Danielsson and J. Sjövall (Eds.), *Sterols and Bile Acids*

CHAPTER 3

Participation of sterol carrier proteins in cholesterol biosynthesis, utilization and intracellular transfer

TERENCE J. SCALLEN and GEORGE V. VAHOUNY

Department of Biochemistry and Department of Medicine, School of Medicine, University of New Mexico, Albuquerque, NM 87131, and Department of Biochemistry, George Washington University School of Medicine and Health Sciences, Washington, DC 20037 (U.S.A.)

(I) Introduction

Cholesterol and many of its biosynthetic precursors are highly insoluble in aqueous media. Yet, cholesterol biosynthesis, utilization and intracellular transfers occur in environments which involve both aqueous and nonaqueous components. For example, the enzymes involved in the conversion of squalene to cholesterol, the conversion of cholesterol to cholesterol esters, and the conversion of cholesterol to 7α-hydroxycholesterol are associated with the endoplasmic reticulum (microsomes). The conversion of cholesterol to pregnenolone, an essential first step in steroid hormone biosynthesis, occurs in mitochondria. In addition, transfers of cholesterol from cytoplasmic lipid inclusion droplets through the cytosol to the mitochondria are essential for steroid hormone production.

As will be described in this chapter, a highly specific system is present within the cell, i.e., sterol carrier proteins, which is capable of binding sterols (or squalene) and transporting them to specific enzyme sites involved in cholesterol biosynthesis and utilization.

Previous investigations from several laboratories have demonstrated that both microsomal membranes and the cytosolic fraction from rat liver are required for the biological synthesis of cholesterol [1–4]. Specifically, the following conversions have been reported to require both microsomes and cytosol: acetate to cholesterol [4]; squalene to cholesterol [1]; squalene-2,3-oxide to lanosterol [3]; lanosterol to cholesterol [1,5]; Δ^7-cholestenol to cholesterol [6]; lanosterol to dihydrolanosterol [7]; various 4,4-dimethyl sterols to cholesterol [8]; and 7-dehydrocholesterol to cholesterol [9,10].

Investigations conducted in our laboratory [3] and by Ritter and Dempsey [11] resulted in the proposal that a sterol carrier protein, present in rat liver cytosol, was required for the conversion of squalene to cholesterol by liver microsomal enzymes. Later, it was shown that rat liver cytosol contains two proteins which are required for the microsomal conversion of squalene to cholesterol [5,12]. Sterol carrier $protein_1$ (SCP_1) participates in the microsomal conversion of squalene to lanosterol, while sterol carrier $protein_2$ (SCP_2) participates in the microsomal conversion of lanosterol to cholesterol. In addition, SCP_2 also participates in key steps in the utilization of cholesterol as well as in the intracellular transfer of cholesterol between cellular organelles.

(II) Sterol carrier protein$_1$ (SCP$_1$)

(1) Purification and characterization of SCP$_1$

SCP_1 participates in the enzymatic conversion of squalene to lanosterol by rat liver microsomes (cf. Chapter 1). It has been purified both in our laboratory [13] and by Ferguson and Bloch [14]. In Dr. Bloch's laboratory, the protein has been called "supernatant protein factor" or SPF [14–20]. It is a single polypeptide chain with a molecular weight of approximately 47000 dalton [14] (Table 1). The protein has an acidic p*I*. Recent evidence suggests that SCP_1 and SPF are one and the same protein [21].

(2) Substrate specificity

By means of high resolution chromatographic techniques and mass spectrometry, it was shown that the major product (90%) formed when squalene was incubated with purified SCP_1, microsomes and cofactors (NADPH and FAD) was lanosterol [13]. While SCP_1 specifically activated the enzymatic conversion of squalene to lanosterol by liver microsomal membranes, it was not capable of activating reactions subsequent to the formation of lanosterol. Thus, the microsomal conversion of

TABLE 1

Characteristics of sterol carrier $protein_1$ (SCP_1) and sterol carrier $protein_2$ (SCP_2)

Protein	M_r	p*I*	Substrate specificity
SCP_1	47000 [a]	6.74 [a]	Squalene → lanosterol [13]
SCP_2	13500 [b]	~ 8.6 [b]	1. Lanosterol → cholesterol [21] 2. Reactions utilizing cholesterol as substrate [22,30,33] 3. Intracellular cholesterol transport [30,33]

[a] See ref. 14; called supernatant protein factor.
[b] See ref. 21.

4,4-dimethyl-Δ^8-cholestenol to C_{27} sterols or of 7-dehydrocholesterol to cholesterol were not activated [13] nor the conversion of cholesterol to cholesterol ester [22].

For SCP_1 to activate enzymatic reactions involving squalene and squalene-2,3-oxide, it was essential that microsomal membrane-bound enzymes be present. SCP_1 was catalytically inactive when it was incubated with squalene and cofactors in the absence of microsomes [13].

The conversion of farnesyl pyrophosphate to squalene marks the transition from water-soluble to water-insoluble intermediates in the biosynthesis of cholesterol. When the effect of liver cytosol or SCP_1 on the conversion of farnesyl pyrophosphate to squalene was investigated, neither rat liver cytosol nor partially purified SCP_1 had any significant effect on this conversion [23]. Therefore, microsomal squalene synthetase performs its catalytic function without responding to the mediating effect of any specific soluble protein.

(3) Participation of SCP_1 in the conversion of enzymatically generated, microsome-bound squalene to sterol

Although it had been demonstrated that SCP_1 was required for the conversion of squalene to lanosterol by rat liver microsomal membranes [13], these studies had the disadvantage that squalene was added exogenously to the incubations in an organic solvent mixture (dioxane : propylene glycol, 2 : 1). We therefore devised a method to study sterol synthesis from squalene without addition of organic solvents or detergents. Radioactive farnesyl pyrophosphate was used to enzymatically generate squalene, in situ, by the microsomal membranes [24]. This was done by anaerobic incubation conditions which prevent utilization of the squalene. The generated squalene was found to be firmly bound to the microsomes. The microsome-bound [^{3}H]squalene was then incubated in the presence or absence of rat liver cytosol or partially purified SCP_1. The results showed a marked enhancement of sterol synthesis when either cytosol or SCP_1 was added [24]. Fig. 1 shows that with increasing amounts of SCP_1 added, increasing amounts of squalene are converted to lanosterol.

These results demonstrate that SCP_1 is required for the conversion of squalene to lanosterol, even when squalene is enzymatically generated in situ bound to the microsomal membranes [24]. Furthermore, the results show excellent correspondence between experiments in which small quantities (less than 2 vol%) of organic solvent are used to add squalene to enzyme incubations [2,3,12,13] and experiments in which no organic solvent is employed.

Morin and Srikantaiah [25] have also demonstrated that squalene can be added to enzyme incubations in the form of a squalene–phospholipid liposome. Conversion of squalene, presented in this manner, to lanosterol also requires SCP_1.

(4) Properties of SCP_1

SCP_1 activity is enhanced by anionic phospholipid [15]. SPF has an absolute requirement for anionic phospholipid [14], e.g., phosphatidylserine. This is explained

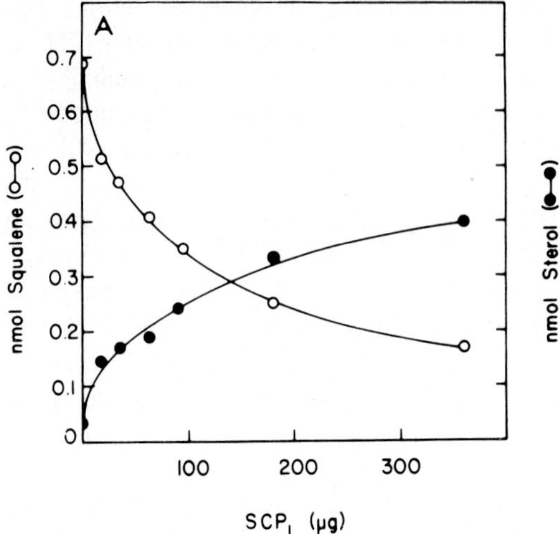

Fig. 1. Conversion of microsome-bound [^{14}C]squalene to sterol as a function of partially purified SCP_1 concentration. Microsome-bound [^{14}C]squalene was enzymatically generated from [1,5,9-^{14}C]farnesyl pyrophosphate [23]. Additional experimental details are described in ref. 24.

by the acetone : water fractionation procedure used in the purification of SPF. SCP_1 purification does not utilize solvent fractionation. Therefore, endogenous phospholipid which may be important in squalene binding would be retained. This preparative difference may be important in explaining the fact that SCP_1 binds squalene [12,13] while SPF does not [19], although binding of squalene by purified SPF in the presence of anionic phospholipid has not been evaluated. It has, however, been demonstrated that SPF does bind anionic phospholipids [19].

Substantial evidence supports a carrier role for SCP_1: (a) SCP_1 can bind squalene, and the complex is active [12,13]; (b) lanosterol formation is a hyperbolic function of SCP_1 protein concentration [13]; also, the velocity of lanosterol formation is a linear function of the velocity of lanosterol formed per mg of SCP_1 (Kim, I. and Scallen, T.J., unpublished data); (c) SCP_1, by itself, is catalytically inactive [13]; (d) the requirement for a specific soluble protein is seen only after the appearance of the first water-insoluble intermediate in cholesterol biosynthesis, i.e., squalene [23,24]; (e) no substantial effect of purified SCP_1 is observed on the energy of activation associated with the microsomal enzyme-catalyzed conversion of squalene to lanosterol (Gavey, K.L. and Scallen, T.J., unpublished data); (f) SCP_1 is required for squalene epoxidation only as long as the epoxidase is bound to the microsomal membrane; when the epoxidase is solubilized by detergent (Triton X-100), the detergent is capable of replacing SCP_1 [13,16]; (g) SCP_1 (SPF) promotes the transfer of squalene from one microsome population to another [20].

This last-mentioned finding is similar to the stoichiometric transfer of cholesterol between organelles by SCP_2, described later in this chapter. The experimental design of Friedlander et al. [20] should allow an examination of the stoichiometry of squalene binding and net mass transfer between populations of microsomal membranes in the presence of SCP_1. These studies should further define the quantitative aspects of squalene transfer by SCP_1.

(III) Sterol carrier protein$_2$ (SCP_2)

(1) Participation of SCP_2 in cholesterol biosynthesis

(a) General remarks

Sterol carrier protein$_2$ (SCP_2) participates in the enzymatic conversion of lanosterol to cholesterol by rat liver microsomal enzymes.

This is a complex enzymatic process which may involve as many as 20 steps [26] (Chapter 1). Available evidence, some of which is detailed below, is consistent with the conclusion that SCP_2 acts as a carrier for all of the intermediates involved in this pathway between lanosterol and cholesterol.

(b) Purification and characterization of SCP_2

SCP_2 was first separated from SCP_1 when rat liver cytosol was subjected to gel filtration [12]. A 4-step procedure for the purification of SCP_2 from rat liver cytosol was then developed by Noland et al. [21]. After the first step (55°C for 1 min), a blue dextran/Sepharose 4B affinity column was utilized, followed by a third step employing Sephadex G-75 (superfine) gel filtration. The final step was an ion exchange column (CM-cellulose), eluting purified SCP_2 at 30 mM potassium phosphate, pH 6.8. The resulting SCP_2 was approximately 1300-fold purified, when compared to the original rat liver cytosol.

Basic, acidic and SDS–polyacrylamide gel systems all revealed a single migrating band for purified SCP_2, as did analytical isoelectric focusing which showed a single band with pI of about 8.6. In addition, it was possible to recover SCP_2 activity from gels following polyacrylamide gel electrophoresis [21]. A precise correspondence was observed between the absorbance of the single protein band and SCP_2 activity, as measured by activation of the microsomal conversion of 7-dehydrocholesterol to cholesterol.

As determined by SDS–polyacrylamide gel electrophoresis, purified SCP_2 has a molecular weight of 13 500 (Table 1).

SCP_2 has also been purified by Trzaskos and Gaylor [27] as well as by Wirtz and coworkers [28]. The purification factor obtained by Wirtz and coworkers was also about 1300-fold. This factor has been confirmed by means of an enzyme-linked immunosorbent assay [29]. The apparently higher purification factor obtained on high-performance liquid chromatography (HPLC) by Trzaskos and Gaylor [27] is probably caused by oxidation of the protein to a disulfide dimer due to the absence of a sulfhydryl reagent during HPLC [29].

(c) Substrate specificity

Purified SCP_2 is capable of activating the microsomal conversion of 4,4-dimethyl-Δ^8-cholestenol to C_{27} sterols and of activating the microsomal conversion of 7-dehydrocholesterol to cholesterol [21]. Also, activity has been shown for other substrates such as lanosterol and desmosterol (Hansbury, E. and Scallen, T.J., unpublished data) and for Δ^7-cholestenol [27]. However, purified SCP_2 is not capable of significantly activating the microsomal conversion of squalene to lanosterol. Thus, there is no overlap in substrate specificity between SCP_2 and SCP_1.

(d) Kinetic studies

Fig. 2 shows the results of an experiment in which the activity of purified SCP_2 was measured using the conversion of 7-dehydrocholesterol to cholesterol by rat liver microsomes as the assay procedure. The assay was similar to that previously described [21] except the concentrations of microsomes and SCP_2 were increased 5-fold by reducing the incubation volume. Fig. 2A shows that the velocity of cholesterol formation is a hyperbolic function of the amount of SCP_2 protein present. In Fig. 2B, the velocity of cholesterol formation is plotted as a function of the velocity of cholesterol formed per mg of purified SCP_2. The X intercept of this plot yields the theoretical specific activity for purified SCP_2 at infinite dilution. The Y intercept is the maximum rate for the reaction in the presence of SCP_2 under the particular experimental conditions employed. The slope of the line is negative, and therefore, the absolute value of the slope is equal to the amount of SCP_2 giving half-maximal velocity. It is significant that a straight line is obtained when cholesterol formation is plotted as a function of cholesterol formed per mg SCP_2. The specific activity obtained for SCP_2 is 70 000 nmoles cholesterol formed/2 h/mg purified SCP_2. This value, obtained with the microassay, is 5-fold higher than that obtained previously [21] with the standard assay and is due to the 5-fold higher concentration of microsomes in the incubation mixture.

A similar kinetic approach has been used to measure the specific activity of rat liver cytosol or of protein fractions obtained during the purification of SCP_2 [21]. As with purified SCP_2, the velocity of cholesterol formed is a hyperbolic function of the amount of cytosol protein present. As before, a straight line is obtained when the velocity of cholesterol formation is plotted as a function of cholesterol formed per mg of rat liver cytosol [21]. The purification factor for SCP_2 can be calculated from: X intercept for rat liver cytosol/X intercept for purified SCP_2. Using this approach [21], a purification factor of 1300–1400-fold was obtained.

This mathematical approach was also used to examine the effect of cytosol and purified SCP_2 on the conversion of 4,4-dimethyl-Δ^8-cholestenol to C_{27} sterol by rat liver microsomes. As above, a straight line was obtained for both cytosol and SCP_2 when the velocity of C_{27} sterol formation was plotted as a function of C_{27} sterol formed per mg of SCP_2 (or cytosol). Again, the ratio of X intercepts gave the purification factor for purified SCP_2 compared to cytosol. The purification factor for 4,4-dimethyl-Δ^8-cholestenol was similar to that obtained for 7-dehydrocholesterol [21].

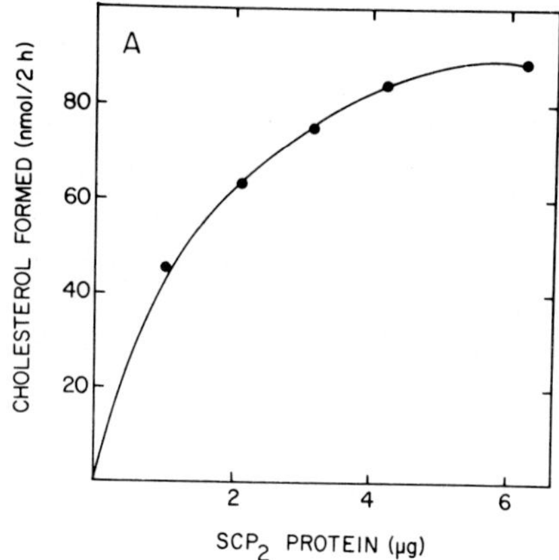

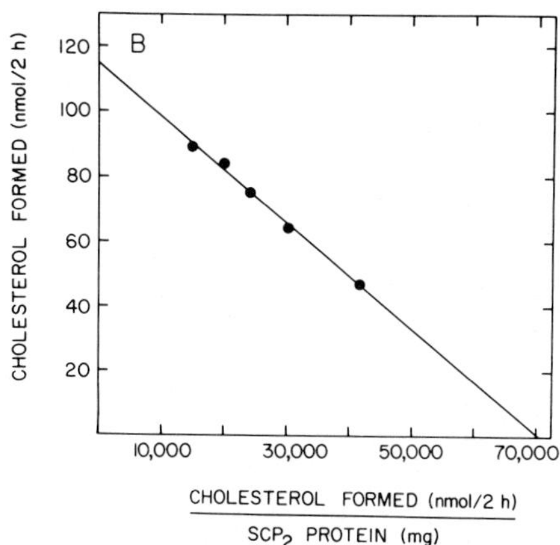

Fig. 2. Activity of homogeneous SCP_2 as measured in the activation of the conversion of 7-dehydrocholesterol to cholesterol by rat liver microsomes. Incubations were conducted as described [21] except that the incubation volume was 0.6 ml. (A) Cholesterol formed is plotted as a function of SCP_2 protein. (B) Cholesterol formed is plotted as a function of cholesterol formed per mg of SCP_2.

This mathematical procedure is, to the best of our knowledge, the first procedure to be described for the quantitative kinetic analysis of a carrier protein in an enzyme reaction [21].

(e) Anti-SCP_2 IgG

An antibody against rat liver SCP_2 has recently been prepared in rabbits [30]. Immunoelectrophoresis of this anti-SCP_2 IgG and homogeneous SCP_2 gave single immunoprecipitation arcs with anti-SCP_2 IgG, while no reaction occurred with control IgG. Rat liver cytosol gave a single immunoprecipitation arc with anti-SCP_2

IgG which was in the same position (basic p*I*) as that obtained with homogeneous SCP_2. No reaction occurred with control IgG.

The ability of anti-SCP_2 IgG to neutralize SCP_2 activity was assessed by assaying activation of the liver microsomal conversion of 7-dehydrocholesterol to cholesterol [30]. Treatment of rat liver cytosol with anti-SCP_2 IgG resulted in complete loss of the activating activity present in the cytosol for this enzyme reaction (SCP_2 activity). By contrast, similar treatment of the cytosol with control rabbit IgG had no significant effect on the microsomal conversion of 7-dehydrocholesterol to cholesterol.

(2) Participation of SCP_2 in cholesterol utilization

(a) Cholesterol esterification

Gavey et al. [22] studied the participation of SCP_2 in the conversion of cholesterol to cholesterol ester (acyl-CoA cholesterol acyl transferase, ACAT) by rat liver microsomes. The effect of rat liver cytosol on the conversion of [4-^{14}C]cholesterol to cholesterol ester was examined as a function of cytosol protein added. In the absence of cytosol, microsomes formed 1.0 nmole of labeled cholesterol ester/mg microsomal protein/2 h. The addition of rat liver cytosol to the microsomes produced a marked, concentration-dependent, increase in the amount of exogenously added [4-^{14}C]cholesterol that was converted to cholesterol ester. Specifically, with the addition of 37.6 mg of cytosol to the microsomes, 12.9 nmoles of labeled cholesterol ester/mg microsomal protein/2 h were formed. When cytosol was incubated with [4-^{14}C]cholesterol in the absence of microsomes, no cholesterol esters were formed.

To determine whether SCP_2 was actually the protein in liver cytosol which is involved in activating the microsomal conversion of cholesterol to cholesterol ester, purified SCP_2, in varying amounts, was added to the incubations in lieu of cytosol (Fig. 3). The amount of cholesterol ester formed by the microsomes was a hyperbolic function of the amount of SCP_2 added. In the incubations containing the greatest amount of SCP_2 (35 μg), 28.5 nmoles of cholesterol ester/mg microsomal protein/2 h were formed, while microsomes without added SCP_2 produced only 0.2 nmole. This experiment demonstrates a striking enhancement of cholesterol ester formation in the presence of pure SCP_2. Neither fatty-acid-free albumin nor partially purified SCP_1 was capable of activating the microsomal conversion of cholesterol to cholesterol ester.

Although the effect of SCP_2 was most clearly seen with exogenously added cholesterol, it was also demonstrated when [1-^{14}C]oleoyl-CoA was the labeled substrate and the incorporation of labeled oleate, using endogenous microsomal cholesterol as substrate, into cholesterol ester was determined. Furthermore, although it was determined that microsomes could bind large amounts of cholesterol in the absence of SCP_2, the bound cholesterol was ineffective as a substrate for microsomal ACAT. However, the microsomally bound cholesterol became an effective substrate for the enzyme upon the addition of SCP_2 [22]. This was true whether the cholesterol was bound to the microsomes via small quantities of organic solvent

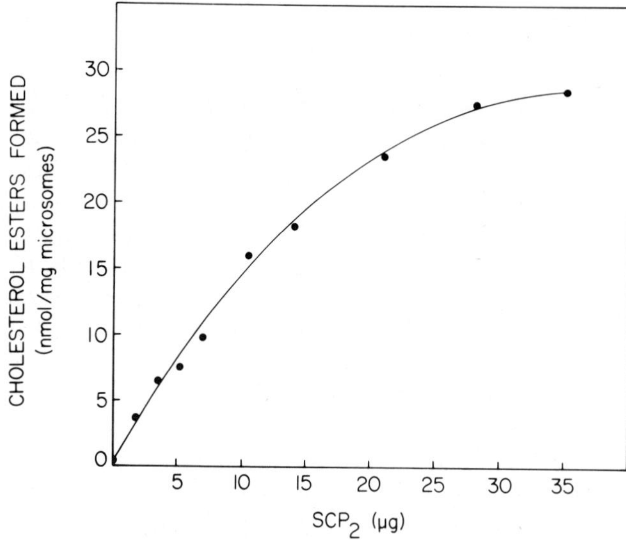

Fig. 3. The effect of purified SCP_2 on rat liver microsomal cholesterol ester biosynthesis, using [4-^{14}C]cholesterol as substrate. The microsomal conversion of cholesterol to cholesterol esters was conducted as described [22].

(dioxane : propylene glycol, 2 : 1) or via cholesterol : lecithin liposomes (Gavey, K.L. and Scallen, T.J., unpublished data).

These results demonstrate that SCP_2 participates in the microsomal conversion of cholesterol to cholesterol ester. It is quite possible that SCP_2 participates in the delivery of either exogenous (dietary) or endogenous (microsomally bound) cholesterol to ACAT which is bound to the endoplasmic reticulum.

(b) Cholesterol 7α-hydroxylase

The conversion of cholesterol to 7α-hydroxycholesterol is the first step and the major regulatory step in bile acid formation (Chapter 9).

SCP_2 significantly enhances 7α-hydroxycholesterol formation by rat liver microsomes, utilizing either endogenous microsomal membrane cholesterol as substrate, or exogenously supplied cholesterol (lipoprotein or cholesterol : phospholipid liposomes) [31, and Sanghvi, Scallen and Vahouny, unpublished data]. Also, preliminary experiments conducted in collaboration with the laboratory of Dr. G.S. Boyd, showed a concentration-dependent increase in the microsomal conversion of [4-^{14}C]cholesterol to 7α-hydroxycholesterol by SCP_2. This observation is consistent with the earlier findings of a protein fraction obtained from rat liver cytosol, which stimulated microsomal 7α-hydroxylation of [4-^{14}C]cholesterol [32] (see also Chapter 9).

These results are consistent with the conclusion that SCP_2 provides a physiological means for providing cholesterol to cholesterol 7α-hydroxylase and thus modulating its activity by regulating the availability of substrate.

(3) Participation of SCP_2 in intracellular cholesterol transfer

(a) SCP_2 is required for cholesterol transport from adrenal lipid droplets to mitochondria

The major substrate reservoir for adrenal steroid biosynthesis is from cholesterol residing as cholesterol esters in cytoplasmic lipid inclusion droplets. These lipid droplets are a storage depot for cholesterol in the cell and provide a ready source of substrate following hydrolysis of the esters by a hormone-sensitive enzyme. Initial studies demonstrated that incubations of lipid droplets, prelabeled with [4-^{14}C]cholesterol, and adrenal mitochondria did not result in significant transfer of cholesterol to mitochondria or conversion of the cholesterol to pregnenolone. The addition of rat adrenal cytosol to incubations containing the lipid droplets and adrenal mitochondria significantly improved the conversion of [4-^{14}C]cholesterol to labeled pregnenolone.

We investigated the effect of homogeneous rat liver SCP_2 on this process [33]. As shown in Fig. 4, the utilization of lipid droplet cholesterol for pregnenolone formation by adrenal mitochondria was dramatically increased by the addition of homogeneous SCP_2. This effect was concentration dependent, and it was not mimicked by the addition of albumin.

In order to determine the mechanism of this enhanced utilization of droplet cholesterol, the effect of SCP_2 on individual steps of the sterol transfer process and of mitochondrial utilization was tested. The ability of pure SCP_2 to bind unesterified cholesterol from lipid droplets was determined by incubation of lipid droplets with SCP_2 for 20 min at 37°C, followed by subsequent analysis of the levels of isotopic cholesterol remaining with the reisolated lipid droplets and that bound to SCP_2 in the droplet-free subnatant fraction. There was a linear increase in the amount of subnatant radioactivity with increasing amounts of SCP_2 added to the lipid droplets

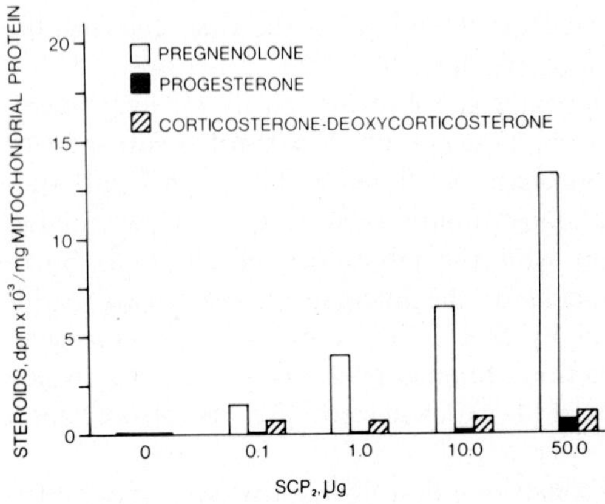

Fig. 4. Effect of SCP_2 on mitochondrial production of steroids from [4-^{14}C]cholesterol presented in adrenal lipid droplets. Experimental details are described in ref. 33.

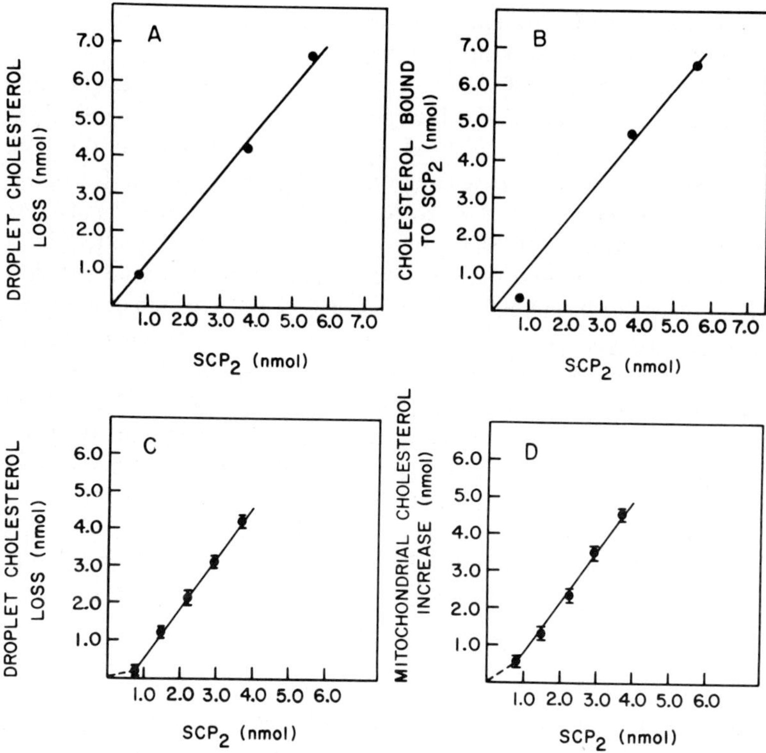

Fig. 5. Stoichiometric relationship between cholesterol mass transfer and SCP_2. In A and B, the effect of SCP_2 on net cholesterol mass released from adrenal lipid droplets and binding of cholesterol to SCP_2 in the droplet-free subnatant is shown. The small amount of cholesterol transfer which occurred in the absence of SCP_2 has been subtracted. In C and D, the effect of SCP_2 on the depletion of cholesterol from the lipid droplets and the accumulation of cholesterol mass in aminoglutethimide-treated mitochondria is shown. Experimental details are described in ref. 33.

with a linear correlation coefficient of 0.997 [33]. With 50 μg of SCP_2, 27% of the labeled cholesterol present in the lipid droplet became bound to SCP_2 in the subnatant, while with bovine serum albumin only 3% of the cholesterol was solubilized. It is important to note that the pure SCP_2 used in these studies did not contain any endogenous lipid [33].

In order to establish that the binding and solubilization of lipid droplet cholesterol by SCP_2 actually represented a net transfer, the changes in unesterified cholesterol mass for the lipid droplet and subnatant SCP_2 fractions were assessed following incubations at various levels of SCP_2. These data (Fig. 5A and B)were comparable to those obtained using isotopic cholesterol [33] and allowed calculation of the stoichiometry of binding between cholesterol and SCP_2. As shown in these studies, there is a clear stoichiometric relationship between the molar ratio of cholesterol depletion from the lipid droplets (Fig. 5A) or subnatant cholesterol accumulation

(Fig. 5B) to the quantity of SCP_2 present. This molar ratio was 1.02 ± 0.14. Thus, the stoichiometry of binding between cholesterol and SCP_2 is 1/1.

SCP_2-mediated mass transfer of cholesterol to, and accumulation in, mitochondria was assessed by utilizing mitochondria which were unable to produce pregnenolone [33]. This was achieved by incubating lipid droplets and mitochondria with aminoglutethimide (AG), and adding increasing increments of SCP_2. Lipid droplets and mitochondria were reisolated and assessed for changes in cholesterol mass. As shown in these studies, addition of SCP_2 in increasing amounts resulted in a progressive linear depletion of unesterified cholesterol mass from the lipid droplets (Fig. 5C) and a parallel linear increase in cholesterol mass associated with the mitochondria (Fig. 5D). By contrast, addition of albumin did not result in significant changes in either lipid droplet or mitochondrial cholesterol mass.

From the data shown (Fig. 5C and D), the molar ratio of cholesterol depletion from the lipid droplets or cholesterol accumulating in mitochondria to the quantity of SCP_2 added was 1.01 ± 0.05. Thus, the stoichiometry of transport of cholesterol from lipid droplets to AG-blocked mitochondria, conducted by SCP_2, is 1/1.

These studies demonstrate the carrier role of SCP_2 in the stoichiometric mass transfer of cholesterol from preformed physiological stores (cytoplasmic lipid inclusion droplets) to and into mitochondria for the initiation of steroid hormone synthesis.

(b) Identification of adrenal SCP_2

Since adrenal mitochondria contain endogenous cholesterol, we tested the effect of SCP_2 on the production of pregnenolone in the absence of cytoplasmic lipid droplets. The addition of increasing increments of hepatic SCP_2 to adrenal mitochondria resulted in a linear increase in pregnenolone production by adrenal mitochondria [30]. At 50 μg of SCP_2 added, pregnenolone formation was increased by 9-fold. At levels of SCP_2 beyond 50 μg, there was little further effect. A similar response was obtained by the addition of adrenal cytosol at levels of up to 10 mg of protein/ml.

We next examined the question of whether adrenal cytosol contained a protein similar to hepatic SCP_2 which was responsible for the marked stimulation of mitochondrial pregnenolone production [30]. Aliquots of authentic SCP_2 and adrenal cytosol were treated with either control rabbit IgG (IgG_c) or with anti-SCP_2 IgG (IgG_i). The data (Table 2) show that the IgG preparations alone had little effect on mitochondrial pregnenolone production. The presence of 20 μg of SCP_2 resulted in a 3.7-fold increase in pregnenolone production, while addition of adrenal cytosol (1.5 mg of protein) caused an almost 3-fold increase in hormone production. Treatment of SCP_2 with the preimmune IgG preparation caused a slight but significant decrease in the ability of SCP_2 to stimulate pregnenolone production. However, treatment of SCP_2 with anti-SCP_2 IgG (IgG_i) resulted in an immunoprecipitate and completely abolished the stimulatory effect of SCP_2 on mitochondrial pregnenolone production. When adrenal cytosol was treated with preimmune control IgG (IgG_c), no precipitate occurred and the resulting preparation still retained the ability to enhance

TABLE 2

Pregnenolone production by adrenal mitochondria

Additions to mitochondria	Pregnenolone production (% control)
None	100
Control IgG_c	110 ± 12
Anti-SCP_2 IgG_i	88 ± 5
SCP_2 (20 μg)	385 ± 22
SCP_2 treated with IgG_c	298 ± 9
SCP_2 treated with IgG_i	98 ± 6
Adrenal cytosol (1.47 mg)	280 ± 6
Cytosol treated with IgG_c	257 ± 10
Cytosol treated with IgG_i	94 ± 2

IgG_c, preimmune rabbit serum IgG; IgG_i, anti-SCP_2 rabbit serum IgG. The IgG fractions contained 160 μg protein. Immunotitrations and mitochondrial incubations were conducted as described [30]. Results are expressed as percentage of control $\pm$S.E.

mitochondrial pregnenolone production. This capacity, however, was completely lost following treatment of the cytosol with immune IgG (anti-SCP_2 IgG) raised against authentic rat or pig liver SCP_2.

The stimulation of mitochondrial pregnenolone production by adrenal cytosolic fractions has been observed repeatedly [34–38], but has not been adequately characterized. A heat-stable protein preparation has been obtained from adrenal cytoplasm [39] and has been reported to stimulate cholesterol side-chain cleavage by acetone powders of adrenal mitochondria [40]. Cholesterol-binding properties of cytosolic fractions from the adrenal and testis [41] and from ovary [41,42] have also been reported.

The results presented above (Table 2) clearly demonstrate that the enhancement of mitochondrial pregnenolone production by adrenal cytosol is completely abolished following treatment of the cytosol with a rabbit IgG preparation raised against homogeneous rat liver SCP_2. These data are entirely consistent with the earlier reports [33,34,43,44] and demonstrate the presence of a protein in adrenal cytosol which is either identical to, or which has antigenic determinants compatible with, hepatic SCP_2. Wayne et al. [37] have recently reported on a purified preparation of bovine adrenal cytosol which stimulates cholesterol side-chain cleavage by a reconstituted system and which has a molecular weight slightly less than 15 000 dalton. The electrophoretic pattern of this preparation closely approximates that of homogeneous rat liver SCP_2.

(c) SCP_2 facilitates the translocation of cholesterol from the outer to the inner mitochondrial membrane

Aminoglutethimide (AG) blocks cholesterol access to cytochrome P-450 (scc = side-chain cleavage system) by binding to the active site of the enzyme [46,47], but

TABLE 3

Effects of aminoglutethimide (AG) and SCP_2 on mitochondrial pregnenolone production and mitoplast cholesterol

Additions to mitochondria	Pregnenolone (% control)	Mitoplast cholesterol (% control)
None	100	100
AG (0.75 mM)	19 ± 2	77 ± 7
AG + SCP_2 (20 μg)	19 ± 2	132 ± 19

Following 30-min incubations of adrenal mitochondrial suspensions with the indicated additions, aliquots were taken for pregnenolone radioimmunoassay, and the remainder was subjected to preparation of the mitoplast fraction of mitochondria. For additional experimental details see ref. 30.

does not appear to affect translocation of cholesterol to the inner mitochondrial membrane where the hemoprotein is located [46]. To assess the effect of SCP_2 on the redistribution of mitochondrial cholesterol and on pregnenolone production, mitochondria were isolated from the adrenals of unstimulated rats and were incubated in the presence of AG (0.75 mM) and SCP_2 [30]. Aliquots were removed for pregnenolone assay, and the reisolated mitochondria were subjected to digitonin treatment, preparation of mitoplasts, and analysis of unesterified cholesterol and protein content.

As shown in Table 3, the direct incubation of isolated mitochondria with AG resulted in an 81% inhibition of pregnenolone production and a small but significant decrease in cholesterol associated with the mitoplast fraction. Addition of SCP_2 to this preparation did not improve pregnenolone production; however, the cholesterol content of the mitoplast fraction of these mitochondria was significantly greater than that associated with mitoplasts from AG-treated mitochondria in the absence of SCP_2. These data show that SCP_2 can affect redistribution of mitochondrial cholesterol from the outer mitochondrial membrane to the inner mitochondrial membrane (step 1 in Fig. 6), but does not directly improve the AG-blocked interaction of the cholesterol with cytochrome P-450_{scc} (step 2, Fig. 6). Previously, we showed that SCP_2 does not affect the release of pregnenolone (step 3, Fig. 6) from adrenal mitochondria [33].

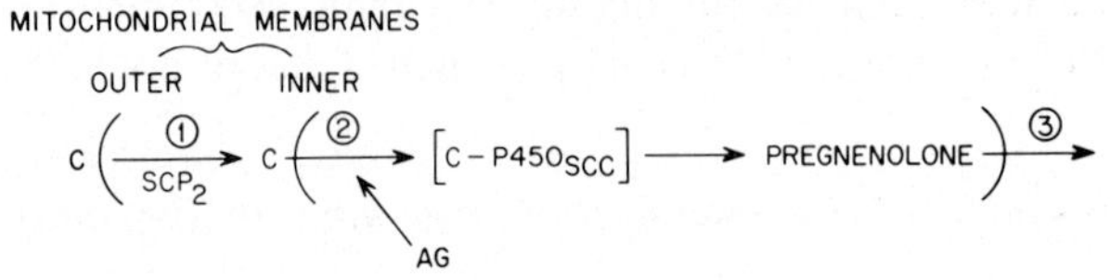

Fig. 6. SCP_2 translocates cholesterol from the outer to the inner membrane in adrenal mitochondria. Reaction 1, transmembrane translocation of cholesterol; reaction 2, interaction of cholesterol with cytochrome P-450_{scc}; reaction 3, removal of pregnenolone. C, cholesterol; AG, aminoglutethimide.

(4) Comparison of SCP_2 with other low molecular weight proteins

(a) Fatty-acid-binding protein (FABP)

Table 4 examines the amino acid composition of purified SCP_2 [21] and compares it with the amino acid compositions of 3 other preparations of interest [47–49]. The most abundant amino acid in purified SCP_2 is lysine, which accounts for 14 mole%. Since the isoelectric point for SCP_2 is approximately 8.6, it follows that a substantial portion of the glutamic and aspartic acid residues are amidated. Also of interest is the finding that SCP_2 contains no arginine or tyrosine, and only small amounts (perhaps 1 residue each) of histidine and tryptophan.

SCP_2 amino acid composition is compared in Table 4 with the protein preparation of Dempsey [47]. As can be seen, marked differences exist in the amino acid compositions of these two proteins, particularly in the quantities of threonine, alanine, valine and leucine. Also, the leucine/isoleucine ratio for SCP_2 was 2.04, while for the protein preparation of Dempsey it was 0.76. In addition, while arginine and tyrosine were present in the Dempsey protein preparation, none of these amino acids was found in SCP_2. The correlation coefficient between SCP_2 and the Dempsey protein preparation is 0.736. Clearly, SCP_2 and the protein isolated by Dempsey and coworkers are separate and distinct proteins.

TABLE 4

Amino acid compositions of SCP_2 and other low molecular weight proteins of interest

	SCP_2 [a]	Dempsey protein [b]	FABP [c]	CM_2 [d]
Asp(n)	10.8	8.9	8.7	10.4
Thr	3.6	9.4	9.4	3.7
Ser	6.0	3.6	4.8	6.2
Glu(n)	11.1	13.6	13.1	11.1
Pro	3.4	1.6	1.6	3.6
Gly	11.5	10.2	9.6	11.8
Ala	9.1	1.6	1.7	9.1
1/2 Cys	1.1	1.0	1.7	1.7
Val	4.8	9.5	9.1	4.6
Met	3.2	5.4	5.3	3.8
Ileu	4.9	6.7	6.6	4.4
Leu	10.0	5.1	4.8	8.8
Tyr	0.0	2.3	2.5	0.0
Phe	5.6	4.7	4.7	5.1
Lys	14.0	13.4	13.0	15.7
His	0.4	1.6	1.5	0.0
Arg	0.0	1.7	1.8	0.0
Try	0.6	0.0	0.0	0.0

[a] See ref. 21.
[b] See ref. 47.
[c] See ref. 48.
[d] See ref. 49.

The amino acid composition of purified SCP_2 is also compared in Table 4 with the amino acid composition of FABP [48]. Marked differences exist in the abundance of threonine, alanine, valine and leucine. The correlation coefficient between SCP_2 and FABP is 0.732. Clearly, SCP_2 and FABP are separate and distinct proteins. Furthermore, there is no immunological cross-reactivity between SCP_2 and FABP, in an extremely sensitive enzyme-linked immunosorbent assay procedure.

As seen in Table 4 the amino acid compositions of the Dempsey protein preparation [47] and FABP [48] are virtually identical. The correlation coefficient is 0.997. It is clear that the Dempsey protein preparation is identical to FABP [21,27,47,48].

When the release of cholesterol from adrenal cytoplasmic lipid inclusion droplets was measured as a function of either SCP_2 or FABP concentration, there was a concentration-dependent release of cholesterol from the lipid inclusion droplets with SCP_2, but not with FABP [50]. When pregnenolone production was measured there was a concentration-dependent formation of pregnenolone from endogenous mitochondrial cholesterol with SCP_2, but not with FABP. In contrast, FABP, but not SCP_2, induced a substantial increase in the release of labeled arachidonate from adrenal cytoplasmic lipid inclusion droplets, prelabeled with [1-^{14}C]arachidonate [50].

The question remained as to why SCP activity has been attributed to the Dempsey protein preparation [47] which has been demonstrated to be identical to FABP. The answer to this question is given by the conditions employed in the in vitro assay [47] which utilizes 15 vol% of propylene glycol [51]. Fig. 7A and B shows the results of an experiment in which the microsomal conversion of 7-dehydrocholesterol to cholesterol was measured with varying amounts of either SCP_2 or FABP. In Fig. 7A the standard assay procedure [21,30], which uses 1.6 vol% of organic solvent, shows marked activity for purified SCP_2 in activating the conversion of 7-dehydrocholesterol to cholesterol by rat liver microsomes. When the assay procedure of [47] is employed (preincubation for 15 min at 37°C and with approximately 15 vol% of propylene glycol present), the activity of purified SCP_2 is markedly inhibited. When a similar comparison was conducted with FABP (Fig. 7B), no SCP activity was observed as long as only small amounts of organic solvents (1.6 vol%) were used as in the standard SCP_2 microassay [51]. However, when 15 vol% propylene glycol was used as in [47], small amounts of SCP activity were detected with FABP, but only at levels of protein far greater than for SCP_2. A similar phenomenon was observed for bovine serum albumin, i.e., no SCP activity was observed with the standard SCP_2 assay; however, small amounts of SCP-like activity were observed when BSA was preincubated with 15 vol% propylene glycol prior to the addition of microsomes.

Since FABP is not capable of releasing cholesterol from adrenal lipid droplets or stimulating the utilization of endogenous mitochondrial cholesterol for pregnenolone production (see above), it is clear that FABP is not involved as a sterol carrier protein in a physiological sense [50]. Consistent with this finding is the observation of Mishkin et al. [52] that FABP does not bind sterol. It is also clear that the

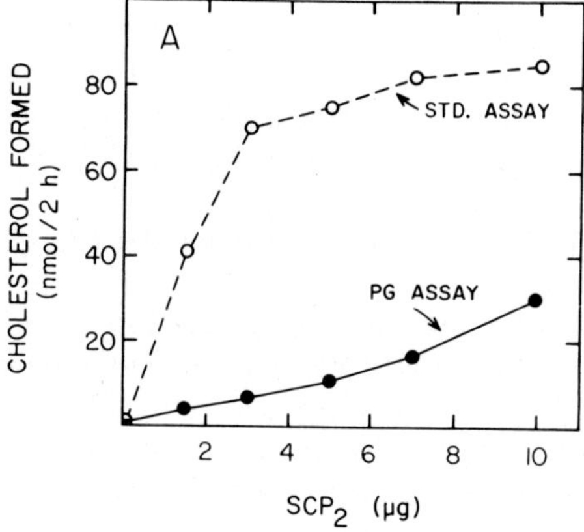

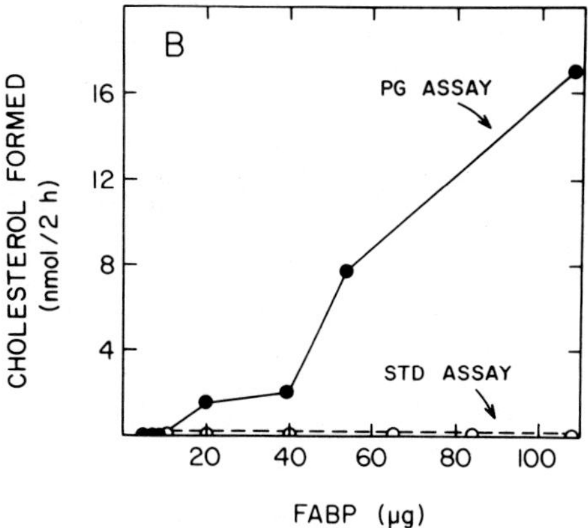

Fig. 7. Comparison of the capacity of SCP_2 and FABP to activate the microsomal conversion of 7-dehydrocholesterol to cholesterol. The standard (std.) assay procedure uses 1.6 vol% of dioxane/propylene glycol, 2:1, for substrate introduction [21]. The other assay, which contains propylene glycol (PG) (15 vol%), was conducted as described [47]. (A) The standard assay is compared with the assay containing 15 vol% propylene glycol (PG) for SCP_2. (B) The standard assay is compared with the assay containing 15 vol% propylene glycol (PG) for FABP.

physiologically relevant asays employed in the reconstituted adrenal systems correlate well with the rat liver microsomal assay in which small quantities of organic solvent are used for substrate addition. However, significant difficulties occur when propylene glycol in high concentration is used in the assay procedure [47]. Similar problems are observed when Tween 80 (0.05%) is present during assay (unpublished data). Therefore, it is not desirable to use detergent as a substrate vehicle as described [53].

(b) Nonspecific phospholipid exchange protein

In Table 4 the amino acid composition of purified SCP_2 is also compared with the amino acid composition of a protein described as a nonspecific phospholipid exchange protein (CM_2) [49]. The amino acid compositions of SCP_2 and CM_2 are nearly identical. The correlation coefficient is 0.992 [21].

We have confirmed the finding [54] that SCP_2 has in vitro phospholipid exchange activity assayed using a microsomal–liposome exchange system. But since a liposome is an artificial acceptor/donor, does this finding have physiological meaning? We examined this question by using a physiological donor, i.e., adrenal cytoplasmic lipid inclusion droplets. The lipid inclusion droplets were incubated with SCP_2 and the mass of lipids released from the lipid droplets was measured. The results (unpublished data) show that cholesterol was the only lipid released from the lipid droplet in the presence of SCP_2. Phospholipid, cholesterol ester, triglyceride, and free fatty acid were not released from the cytoplasmic lipid droplets by SCP_2.

These findings strongly support the conclusion that SCP_2 does not play a role in the physiological transfer of lipids other than sterols. The recent findings of Nichols

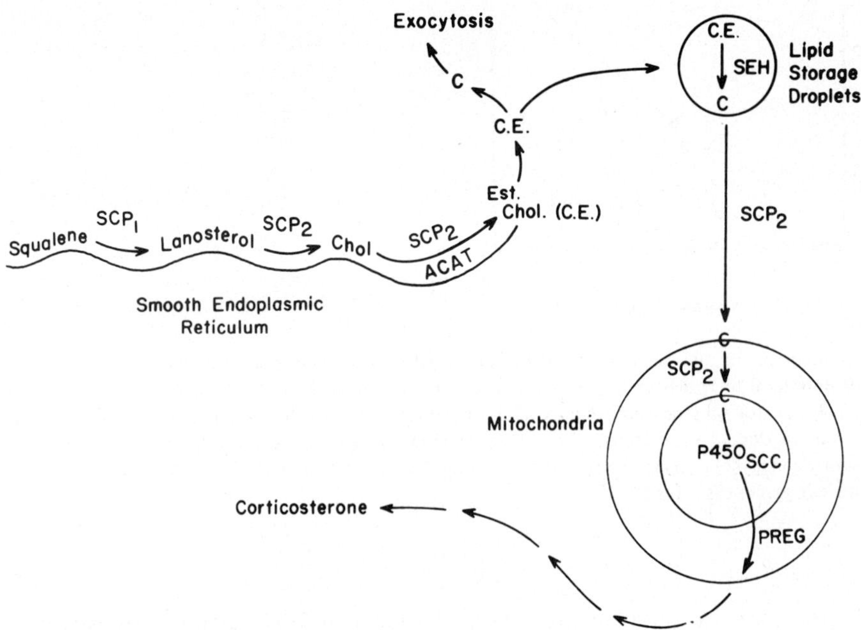

Fig. 8. A schematic diagram showing cellular processes known to require SCP_2. The reactions in cholesterol biosynthesis and esterification have been shown for liver. The reactions involving cholesterol transport from cytoplasmic lipid inclusion droplets to mitochondria have been demonstrated in endocrine tissues. Chol and C, cholesterol; ACAT, acyl-CoA:cholesterol acyl transferase; C.E., cholesterol ester; SEH, sterol ester hydrolase (hormone-dependent); P-450_{scc}, cytochrome P-450 cholesterol side-chain cleavage enzyme; PREG, pregnenolone.

and Pagano [55] demonstrate that, even in the in vitro liposomal assay, phospholipid is not bound by the protein but, instead, the protein facilitates dissociation of phospholipid at the liposomal surface. Also, the finding that the protein is relatively nonspecific as to the nature of the phospholipid exchanged in the liposomal assay [54] suggests strongly that this in vitro procedure does not reflect in vivo events. If SCP_2 facilitated the nonspecific exchange of a variety of phospholipids in vivo, this would be inconsistent with the known asymmetry of phospholipid distribution within the cell [56].

(IV) The participation of sterol carrier proteins in intracellular cholesterol metabolism

Fig. 8 is a schematic diagram of a cell which shows the known sites in which sterol carrier proteins are involved in cholesterol biosynthesis, utilization and intracellular transfer. SCP_1 participates in the conversion of squalene to lanosterol and SCP_2 participates in the conversion of lanosterol to cholesterol, the conversion of cholesterol to cholesterol ester by ACAT, and probably also in the conversion of cholesterol to 7α-hydroxycholesterol. SCP_2 transfers cholesterol from cytoplasmic lipid inclusion droplets to mitochondria in the adrenal and SCP_2 also translocates cholesterol from the outer to the inner mitochondrial membrane.

Significant progress has been made concerning the participation of sterol carrier proteins in cholesterol biosynthesis, utilization and intracellular transfer. It is anticipated that in the coming years research will focus not only on additional aspects of intracellular sterol transfer, but also on the molecular mechanisms involved in the binding of sterols to SCP_2.

Acknowledgements

It is a pleasure to acknowledge the important contributions of several scientists who made key contributions to this endeavor; Mrs. Billie Noland, the purification of SCP_2 as well as many other phases of this work; Dr. Kathleen Gavey, the effect of SCP_2 on ACAT and many of the studies on SCP_1; Dr. M.V. Srikantaish, purification of SCP_1; and Dr. Ron Chanderbhan, the effect of SCP_2 on adrenal cholesterol transport. We also thank Dr. Robert Ockner and Dr. Nathan Bass, University of California San Francisco, for samples of purified FABP.

References

1 Tchen, T.T. and Bloch, K. (1957) J. Biol. Chem. 226, 921–930.
2 Scallen, T.J., Dean, W.J. and Schuster, M.W. (1968) J. Biol. Chem. 243, 5202–5206.
3 Scallen, T.J., Schuster, M.W. and Dhar, A.K. (1971) J. Biol. Chem. 246, 224–230.
4 Bucher, N.L.R. and McGarrahan, K. (1956) J. Biol. Chem. 222, 1–15.

5 Johnson, R.C. and Shah, S.N. (1974) Arch. Biochem. Biophys. 164, 502–510.
6 Frantz Jr., I.D., Davidson, A.G., Dulitt, E. and Mobberley, M.L. (1959) J. Biol. Chem. 234, 2290–2294.
7 Avigan, J., Goodman, D.S. and Steinberg, D. (1963) J. Biol. Chem. 238, 1283–1286.
8 Gibbons, G.F. (1974) Biochem. J. 144, 59–68.
9 Kandutsch, A.A. (1962) J. Biol. Chem. 237, 358–362.
10 Dempsey, M.E. (1968) Ann. N.Y. Acad. Sci. 148, 631–646.
11 Ritter, M.C. and Dempsey, M.E. (1971) J. Biol. Chem. 246, 1536–1539.
12 Scallen, T.J., Srikantaiah, M.V., Seetharam, B., Hansbury, E. and Gavey, K.L. (1974) Fed. Proc. 33, 1733–1746.
13 Srikantaiah, M.V., Hansbury, E., Loughran, E.D. and Scallen, T.J. (1976) J. Biol. Chem. 251, 5496–5504.
14 Ferguson, J.B. and Bloch, K. (1977) J. Biol. Chem. 252, 5381–5385.
15 Tai, H.-H. and Bloch, K. (1972) J. Biol. Chem. 247, 3767–3773.
16 Ono, T. and Bloch, K. (1975) J. Biol. Chem. 250, 1571–1579.
17 Saat, Y.A. and Bloch, K. (1976) J. Biol. Chem. 251, 5155–5160.
18 Caras, I.W. and Bloch, K. (1979) J. Biol. Chem. 254, 11816–11821.
19 Caras, I.W., Friedlander, E.J. and Bloch, K. (1980) J. Biol. Chem. 255, 3575–3580.
20 Friedlander, E.J., Caras, I.W., Houlin, L.F. and Bloch, K. (1980) J. Biol. Chem. 255, 8042–8045.
21 Noland, B.J., Arebalo, R.E., Hansbury, E. and Scallen, T.J. (1980) J. Biol. Chem. 255, 4282–4289.
22 Gavey, K.L., Noland, B.J. and Scallen, T.J. (1981) J. Biol. Chem. 256, 2993–2999.
23 Gavey, K.L. and Scallen, T.J. (1978) J. Biol. Chem. 253, 5470–5475.
24 Gavey, K.L. and Scallen, T.J. (1978) J. Biol. Chem. 253, 5476–5483.
25 Morin, R.J. and Srikantaiah, M.V. (1980) J. Lipid Res. 21, 1143–1147.
26 Frantz Jr., I.D. and Schroepfer Jr., G.J. (1967) Annu. Rev. Biochem. 36, 691–726.
27 Trzaskos, J.M. and Gaylor, J.L. (1983) Biochim. Biophys. Acta 751, 52–65.
28 Poorthius, B.J.H.M., Glazta, J.F.C., Akeroyd, R. and Wirtz, K.W.A. (1981) Biochim. Biophys. Acta 665, 256–261.
29 Teerlink, T. (1983) Ph.D. Thesis, University of Utrecht.
30 Vahouny, G.V., Chanderbhan, Noland, B.J., Irwin, D., Dennis, P., Lambeth, J.D. and Scallen, T.J. (1983) J. Biol. Chem. 258, 11731–11737.
31 Sanghvi, A., Grassi, E., Bartman, C., Lester, R., Galli Kienle, M. and Galli, G. (1981) J. Lipid Res. 22, 720–724.
32 Craig, I.F., Boyd, G.S., McLeod, R.J. and Suckling, K.E. (1979) Biochem. Soc. Trans. 7, 967–969.
33 Chanderbhan, R., Noland, B.J., Scallen, T.J. and Vahouny, G.V. (1982) J. Biol. Chem. 257, 8928–8934.
34 Mahaffee, D., Reitz, R.C. and Ney, R.L. (1974) J. Biol. Chem. 249, 227–233.
35 Farese, R.V. (1967) Biochemistry 6, 2052–2065.
36 Ray, P. and Strott, C.A. (1981) Life Sci. 28, 1529–1534.
37 Wayne, P.A., Greenfield, N.J. and Lieberman, S. (1983) Proc. Natl. Acad. Sci. (U.S.A.) 80, 1877–1881.
38 Pedersen, R.C. and Brownie, A.C. (1983) Proc. Natl. Acad. Sci. (U.S.A.) 80, 1882–1886.
39 Kan, K.W. and Ungar, F. (1973) J. Biol. Chem. 248, 2868–2875.
40 Kan, K.W., Ritter, M.C., Ungar, F. and Dempsey, M.E. (1972) Biochem. Biophys. Res. Commun. 48, 423–429.
41 Lefevre, A., Morera, A.M. and Saea, J.M. (1978) FEBS Lett. 89, 287–292.
42 Chanderbhan, R., Tanaka, T., Strauss, J.F., Irwin, D., Noland, B.J., Scallen, T.J. and Vahouny, G.V. (1983) Biochem. Biophys. Res. Commun. 117, 702–709.
43 Simpson, E.R. (1979) Mol. Cell. Endocrinol. 13, 213–228.
44 Crivello, J.F. and Jefcoate, C.R. (1980) J. Biol. Chem. 255, 8144–8151.
45 Hall, P.F., Charpponnier, C., Nakamura, M. and Gabbiani, G. (1979) J. Biol. Chem. 254, 9080–9084.
46 O'Hare, M.J. and Neville, A.M. (1973) J. Endocrinol. 56, 537–549.
47 Dempsey, M.E., McCoy, K.E., Baker, H.N., Vafiadou, A.D., Lorsbach, T. and Howard, J.B. (1981) J. Biol. Chem. 256, 1867–1873.
48 Ockner, R.K., Manning, J.A. and Kane, J.P. (1982) J. Biol. Chem. 257, 7872–7878.

49 Bloj, B., Hughes, M.E., Wilson, D.B. and Zilversmit, D.B. (1978) FEBS Lett. 96, 87–89.
50 Vahouny, G.V., Chanderbahn, R., Noland, B.J., Bass, N.M., Ockner, R.K. and Scallen, T.J. (1984) Fed. Proc., 43, 2824.
51 Scallen, T.J., Noland, B.J., Gavey, K.L., Bass, N.M., Ockner, R.K. and Vahouny, G.V. (1984) Fed. Proc., 43, 2825.
52 Mishkin, S., Stein, L., Gatmaitan, Z. and Arias, I.M. (1972) Biochem. Biophys. Res. Commun. 47, 997–1003.
53 Ishibashi, T. and Bloch, K. (1981) J. Biol. Chem. 256, 12962–12967.
54 Bloj, B. and Zilversmit, D.B. (1977) J. Biol. Chem. 252, 1613–1619.
55 Nichols, J.W. and Pagano, R.E. (1983) J. Biol. Chem. 258, 5368–5371.
56 Rothman, J.E. and Lenard, J. (1977) Science 195, 743–753.

H. Danielsson and J. Sjövall (Eds.), *Sterols and Bile Acids*

CHAPTER 4

Biosynthesis, function and metabolism of sterol esters

ALAN JONES and JOHN GLOMSET

Departments of Medicine and Biochemistry, and Regional Primate Research Center, University of Washington, Seattle, WA 98195 (U.S.A.)

(I) Introduction

The blood and tissues of animals typically contain not only unesterified cholesterol (UC), but also cholesterol esters (CE). Most of the CE are formed from long-chain fatty acids such as palmitic acid, oleic acid, linoleic acid, or arachidonic acid, but small amounts of cholesterol sulfate (CS) and cholesterol glucuronide also are present. The aim of this chapter is to provide a brief overview of the biochemistry, physiology, and pathology of these esters as an introduction to the field of CE research. The primary focus will be on long-chain fatty acid esters because much more is known about them than about other CE. However, current knowledge of the biochemistry of CS will be reviewed as well.

(II) Distribution and physical properties of cholesterol esters

The distribution of UC and CE in 22 rat tissues is shown in Table 1. It will be seen that CE comprise only about one-eighth of the total body cholesterol, and that long-chain fatty acid esters of cholesterol predominate over CS. It is clear also that long-chain fatty acid esters of cholesterol are distributed very unevenly among different tissues. They are essentially absent from erythrocytes and are present in only extremely low amounts in tissues of the nervous system. On the other hand, they are present in relatively high amounts in the adrenal, ovaries and blood plasma, and the liver, too, can be relatively rich in CE.

Table 2 shows that UC and long-chain fatty acid esters of cholesterol are also distributed unevenly among the membranes and organelles of individual cells. (No information is available about the intracellular distribution of CS or cholesterol

TABLE 1

Tissue distribution of UC, CE, and CS in the rat [a]

Shown are the concentrations of UC and CE in 22 tissues as mg of sterol/g wet weight of tissue (columns 1 and 3). Also shown are the amounts of UC and CE found in each of the tissues of the rat relative to the total UC and CE of the whole animal (columns 2 and 4). Thus, although the concentration of UC in muscle is quite low (0.62 mg/g tissue wt.), the total mass of muscle harbors the largest single reservoir of UC (16.90% of the animal's total UC). Similarly, although the skin has a low concentration of CE (0.26 mg/g tissue), it contains the most CE of any tissue (25.47% of total animal CE). Column 5 identifies those tissues that contain particularly high proportions of UC (nerve tissue and erythrocytes) or CE (adrenal, ovary and plasma), suggesting specific roles in the cholesterol cycle for these tissues. Column 6 illustrates the markedly different tissue distribution of CS, an amphipathic molecule. The kidney and liver contain the largest portion of CS, organs that do not contain particularly large proportions of either UC or CE. That portion of CS in spermatozoa, although small, may be critically important in the normal functioning of spermatozoa. In many tissues, CS has been detected but is present in such small amounts that quantitation has not been attempted

Tissue	UC (mg/g tissue) (1)	Tissue UC as a percentage of total animal UC (2)	CE [b] (mg/g tissue) (3)	Tissue CE [b] as a percentage of total animal CE [b] (4)	CE [b]/UC (w/w) (5)	CS (mg/100 g tissue) (6)
Plasma	0.19	0.38	0.59	8.72	3.14	< 0.5
Bile	–	–	–	–	–	< 0.5
Red cell	1.45	2.30	0	0	0	~ 1.0
Stomach	2.29/2.4	0.73	0.05/0.1	0.12	0.02	[c]
Intestine	1.84	3.96	0.09	1.40	0.05	[c]
Colon	1.80	0.83	0.02	0.07	0.01	–
Liver	1.55	6.15	0.85	24.67	0.55	< 6.0
Spleen	3.72	0.52	0.05	0.05	0.01	–
Kidney	3.31/5.5	2.39	0.03/0.5	0.15	0.01	< 20.0
Lung	3.84/4.4	1.28	0.20/0.2	0.48	0.05	–
Skin	0.88/1.3	12.07	0.26/0.6	25.47	0.29	[c]
Hair	3.29	7.49	1.35	22.50	0.41	–
Adipose	0.54	3.42	0.05	2.23	0.09	–
Heart	1.12	0.31	0.02	0.03	0.01	–
Muscle	0.62	16.90	0.01	2.50	0.02	–
Testes	1.53/2.3	1.01	0.07/0.1	0.32	0.04	~ 1.0
Spermatozoa	–	–	–	–	–	1.0
Seminal plasma	–	–	–	–	–	0.5
Adrenal	4.5	–	38.8	–	8.62	[c]
Ovary	3.6	–	7.3	–	2.03	–
Bone	0.27	2.45	0.05	3.42	0.19	–
Bone marrow	2.58	4.87	0.09	1.25	0.03	–
Brain	16.39	6.83	0.02	0.06	0.001	[c]
Spinal cord	40.30	6.06	0.01	0.02	0.0003	[c]
Sciatic nerve	36.40	8.29	0.08	0.13	0.002	[c]
Sum	–	88.24	–	93.59	–	
Total rat (mg)		439.0/341 g rat		60.0/341 g rat	0.14	

[a] From refs. 1 and 2.

[b] Cholesterol esterified to fatty acid.

[c] Detected qualitatively but not quantitated.

TABLE 2
Intracellular distribution of UC and CE

Illustrated are the concentration of UC and CE within each organelle and the percentage of UC and CE within each organelle relative to the total amount of UC and CE within the cell. Column 2 values should be viewed cautiously, as there is some question of the amount of contamination of cellular fractions by plasma membrane [3], an organelle containing the largest amount of UC within the cell. Thus, plasma membrane UC may be much closer to 80% and other organelle UC much lower than indicated here. Column 4 reflects the virtual insolubility of CE within phospholipid membranes [4,5], and that most cellular CE appears to be contained within lipid droplets. Column 5 shows an apparent selective accumulation of UC within plasma membrane and mitochondria, and of CE within lipid droplets

Organelle	UC (mg/g protein) (1)	Organelle UC as a percentage of total cellular UC (2)	CE (mg/g protein) (3)	Organelle CE as a percentage of total cellular CE (4)	CE/UC (w/w) (5)
Golgi complex [a]	45.4	–	25.6	–	0.56
Golgi complex [b]	44.7	–	26.3	–	0.59
Mitochondria [b]	7.8	22.2	0.2	–	0.03
Plasma membrane [a]	117.8	43.5/80.0	10.2	–	0.09
Endoplasmic reticulum [b]	47.7	34.4	5.3	–	0.11
Lipid droplets [c]	–	13.1	–	64.1	4.89
Lipid droplets [d]	–	< 38.4	–	> 61.7	> 5.67
Nuclei [d]	–	7.0	–	–	–

[a] Rat liver.
[b] Rat kidney.
[c] Human aorta.
[d] Rat adrenal.
From refs. 3, 4, 6–10.

glucuronide.) UC is found mainly in membranes, and is concentrated particularly in the plasma membrane [3]. In contrast, long-chain fatty acid esters of cholesterol are found mainly in fat droplets in the cytoplasm. Similarly, in blood plasma lipoprotein UC appears to be associated primarily with the phospholipids of the lipoprotein particle surface, whereas the bulk of the CE is found in the particle core [10].

Studies of the physical properties of UC, reviewed in Chapter 6 of this volume, have contributed much to our understanding of the role of this lipid in membranes and lipoprotein surfaces. The shape and polarity of UC promote its association with the phospholipids of membranes and lipoproteins, and this association has important effects on membrane fluidity and permeability. The physical properties of long-chain fatty acid esters of cholesterol, on the other hand, differ strikingly from those of UC, and cause these esters to be largely excluded from phospholipid bilayers and monolayers and to aggregate instead in oil droplets.

Long-chain fatty acid esters of cholesterol are much bulkier than is UC, and lack a polar hydroxyl group. They do not become hydrated in the presence of water, and are essentially water insoluble. When mixed with water they form a floating oil phase, unlike UC, which forms a film [11]. They mix with phospholipids only in very low proportions (= 2 mole%) [5,12]. Film balance studies have suggested that higher proportions of CE lead to the formation of a second oil phase whose character depends somewhat on the fatty acid composition of the CE. At physiologic temperatures it tends to be liquid crystalline exhibiting both liquid and solid crystal properties. Liquid crystalline CE in an oil phase can equilibrate with CE that is present in a surrounding film of phospholipid. This makes it accessible to enzymes and transfer proteins at the lipid–water interface [6].

CE oil phases in cells or in lipoproteins almost always contain some triacylglycerol (TG). Physical studies of artificially prepared mixtures of CE and TG have indicated that the presence of more than 5% TG is sufficient to abolish the liquid crystalline character of CE. A two-phase system is thus created that is comprised on the one hand of solid CE and on the other of liquid CE and TG. CE oil phases in cells or lipoproteins also typically contain some UC. Most of the UC in oil droplets or lipoproteins is, however, present with phospholipid in a thin film that also contains a small amount of CE and TG [13,14].

(III) Enzymes and proteins that mediate the formation, transport, and hydrolysis of cholesterol esters

Enzymes and proteins that synthesize, transport, and hydrolyze CE are found both inside and outside of cells. In most cases, the intracellular and extracellular enzymes use entirely different cofactors, and have different pH optima. The enzymes found within cells typically include both a CE-synthesizing enzyme, acyl-CoA : cholesterol acyltransferase (ACAT), and 2 or 3 CE-degrading enzymes: acid CE hydrolase (CEH), neutral CEH, and possibly a mitochondrial CEH. Blood plasma and the extracellular fluid, on the other hand, contain only a CE-synthesizing enzyme, lecithin : cholesterol acyltransferase (LCAT), and a CE transfer protein (CETP). Finally, pancreatic juice contains a CE-degrading enzyme, pancreatic CEH. Each of these very different proteins is discussed below, with the exception of pancreatic CEH, which is discussed in Chapter 5.

(1) Acyl-CoA : cholesterol acyltransferase (EC 2.3.1.26)

Nearly all animal cells contain an enzyme that can catalyze the formation of long-chain fatty acid esters of cholesterol. This enzyme, ACAT, is associated with the endoplasmic reticulum [15,18] and appears to be an integral membrane protein [16,19]. It catalyzes the following reaction:

$$\text{fatty acyl-CoA} + \text{UC} \xrightarrow{\text{ACAT}} \text{CE} + \text{CoA}$$

The reaction requires no known cofactors, and appears to be essentially irreversible. It seems to occur on the surface of the endoplasmic reticulum membrane (Fig. 1).

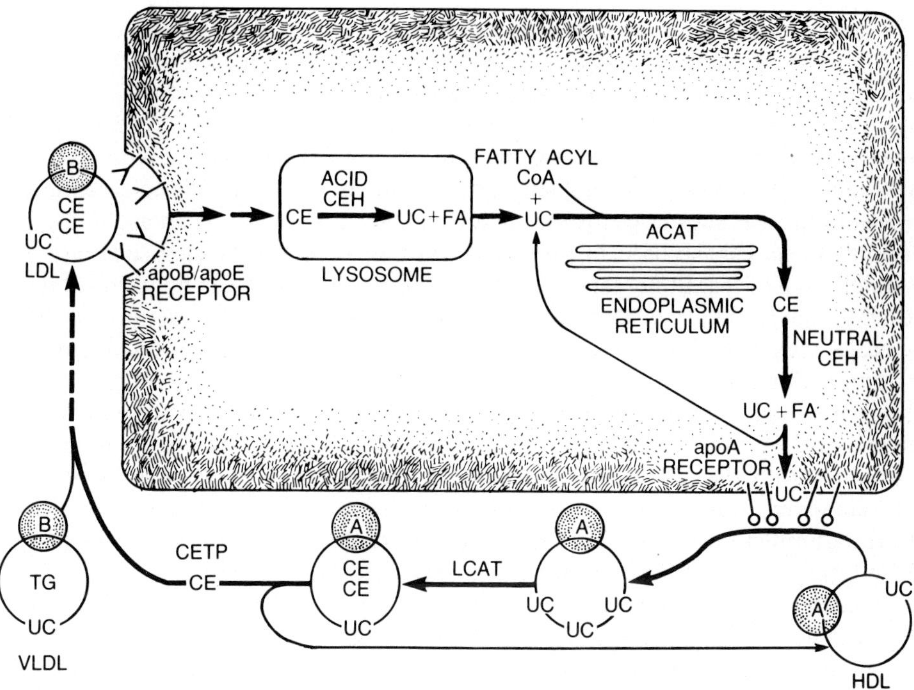

Fig. 1. The cycle of CE from plasma through a fibroblast-like cell. LDL containing CE bind to apo B/E receptors on the cell surface, whereupon the lipoprotein–receptor complexes are internalized by endocytosis. The lipoprotein CE is then hydrolyzed within lysosomes by an acid CEH. The UC and fatty acids (FA) released diffuse through the lysosomal membrane to the cytoplasm, where they may be re-esterified by the ACAT reaction on the endoplasmic reticulum. The CE accumulates in fat droplets by an unknown mechanism or it can be hydrolyzed to UC and FA by neutral CEH in a futile cycle involving successive re-esterification (ACAT) and hydrolysis (neutral CEH) reactions. Ultimately, UC may be utilized for membrane formation and/or excreted from the cell. To be excreted, an appropriate extracellular acceptor – here shown as HDL – may bind to receptors on the cell surface, which specifically recognize apo A, and thereafter adsorb UC from the cell surface. HDL UC may then be esterified by LCAT to form CE which may be transferred by CETP to VLDL as the HDL returns to the circulation. VLDL thus acquire CE and eventually become converted to LDL, completing the cycle.

This membrane contains both the enzyme and its fatty acyl-CoA and UC substrates, which are in equilibrium with fatty acyl-CoA and UC found elsewhere in the cell. Most of the CE formed from these membrane-associated substrates separates from the membrane in an unknown manner to form lipid droplets within the cytoplasm [20].

ACAT activity can be assayed in vitro by incubating microsomes (fragments of endoplasmic reticulum formed during tissue homogenization) with radioactive substrates and then isolating and counting the radioactive CE that are generated by the reaction. Most investigators add radioactive fatty acyl-CoA in the presence of an equimolar concentration of fatty-acid-poor albumin to the incubation mixtures and rely on the microsomal membranes themselves as a source of unlabeled, endogenous UC [16–18]. Albumin is used as a carrier because each molecule of the protein contains 2 high-affinity fatty-acyl-binding sites that can bind fatty acyl-CoA reversibly. In the presence of albumin, amounts of fatty acyl-CoA that would ordinarily have a disruptive, detergent-like action on the microsomal membrane bind reversibly instead to the fatty-acyl-binding sites of albumin and are gradually released in low concentrations as substrates for the ACAT reaction. Alternatively, an acyl-CoA-generating system can be used to provide a constant source of labeled substrate. For example, 1-oleoylcarnitine, carnitine acyltransferase, and CoA can be included in the reaction mixture [21]. Values obtained upon assaying ACAT activity in vitro typically vary from 60 to 200 pmoles of CE formed per milligram of microsomal protein per minute.

In vitro assay systems can also be used to show that ACAT uses oleoyl-CoA and palmitoyl-CoA preferentially as substrates [15,16,22]. This specificity is in good agreement with the fatty acid composition typically found upon analysis of tissue CE. However, some tissues, such as the rat adrenal, ovary, and testis, are rich in polyunsaturated fatty acids, raising the possibility that these tissues may contain an ACAT enzyme with a different fatty acid specificity [23].

Relatively little is known about the physical properties of ACAT. Enzyme activity has been solubilized from different tissues and reconstituted into lipid vesicles, but has been purified only partially [24,25]. Even the kinetics and mechanism of the ACAT reaction are poorly understood. As in the case of most enzymes involved in lipid metabolism, kinetic constants are difficult to determine because the substrates are water insoluble and membrane associated [26]. Moreover, systematic efforts to identify the active site of the enzyme through the use of active site-directed reagents have yet to be made. Such efforts might be worthwhile even at this stage of investigation of the enzyme because the use of radioactive, site-directed reagents might allow identification of the enzyme protein.

Because so little is known about the enzyme protein, information about the regulation of ACAT activity in cells is incomplete. Studies of the molecular biology of the enzyme must await enzyme purification. Nevertheless, several potential aspects of enzyme regulation have been explored. One of these is related to the phospholipid composition of microsomal membranes. Reconstitution experiments using solubilized ACAT preparations and different phospholipids have suggested that ACAT activity may be inhibited by acidic phospholipids such as phosphatidylserine [24]. Furthermore, experiments using modified microsomes have suggested that the fatty acid composition of membrane phospholipids may be important. For example, when dioleoylphosphatidylcholine (dioleoyl PC) or 1-palmitoyl-2-linoleoyl PC was substituted for native microsomal phospholipids by incubation with synthetic phospholipid vesicles and phospholipid exchange protein, ACAT activity increased [27]. In contrast, substitution of dilineoyl PC for native microsomal phospholipids inhibited ACAT activity [27].

Evidence has also been obtained that ACAT activity may be regulated by the content of UC in microsomal membranes. Thus, feeding cholesterol to monkeys and rats leads within 12–18 hours to both a 50% increase in the UC content of liver microsomes and a 2–3-fold increase in ACAT activity. Similar results were obtained in experiments in which hyperlipidemic very-low-density lipoproteins (VLDL) or acetyl low-density lipoproteins (LDL) were used to increase the content of cholesterol in hepatoma cells and human skin fibroblasts. In other experiments [16,20,28,29], incubation of microsome preparations with lipoproteins, UC-rich liposomes, or UC added in acetone or in detergent led to a 50–300% increase in ACAT activity. Finally, experiments with ACAT that was first solubilized, then partially purified and reconstituted into UC : PC liposomes showed that the enzyme activity increased with increasing content of UC up to a molar ratio of 0.4 : 1 [25,30], though a ratio of 0.8 : 1 led to enzyme inhibition [31].

ACAT may also be activated by covalent phosphorylation. Studies with microsomal ACAT that was incubated with Mg^{2+} and ATP showed an increase in activity, and a further increment in activity upon addition of a supernatant fraction from liver cells [32]. This type of activation seems similar to that observed with HMG-CoA reductase [33].

(2) Cholesterol ester hydrolase (EC 3.1.1.13)

Within the body there are 3 and possibly 4 separate enzymes that can hydrolyze long-chain fatty acid esters of cholesterol. These CEH catalyze the reversible reaction shown below:

$$\mathrm{CE} + \mathrm{H_2O} \rightleftharpoons \mathrm{UC} + \text{fatty acid}$$

Two intracellular enzymes, acid and neutral CEH, will be discussed in this section. Less is known about a third enzyme, which is apparently located in mitochondria [34].

(a) Acid CEH

Acid CEH has an optimum pH of 4.5 and is located within lysosomes (Fig. 1). Like many lipolytic enzymes, it is water soluble whereas its substrate is not. For this reason, devising a reliable assay method is difficult, and results should be viewed with caution [26,35]. Recently developed conditions found to yield satisfactory linearity with both time of incubation and enzyme concentration are: 12.7 μM cholesteryl oleate, dispersed in 1.27 mM egg PC; 50 mM acetate buffer; 2.0 mM sodium taurocholate; 0.005% digitonin; pH 3.9 [36]. In aortic cells these conditions gave an apparent K_m of 1.5 μM for cholesteryl oleate. It should be noted, however, that the nature, physical form, and molecular organization of the CE and associated molecules can have a critical effect on the activity of any preparation of CEH [37]. Rat liver acid CEH, for example, shows K_ms of 15.3, 14.3, and 7.3 μM for cholesteryl oleate when the latter is present in vesicles, micelles, and emulsions, respectively [35].

The same enzyme has been purified 120-fold with a 5% recovery of activity; the preparation was estimated to be about 90% pure. The molecular weight was estimated by sodium dodecyl sulfate (SDS)–polyacrylamide gel electrophoresis and gel filtration to be 60 000 [38].

The hydrolytic activity of acid CEH toward CE appears to have no specificity as to the nature of the fatty acyl ester [39]. Furthermore, the enzyme appears to hydrolyze emulsions of TG, and the ratio of the enzyme's activity toward cholesteryl oleate and TG remains the same during enzyme purification [38], suggesting that acid CEH may be a single polypeptide with a fairly broad spectrum of activity. Consistent with this possibility, the activities toward CE and TG show identical inhibition patterns, fractionation and anion-exchange behavior, and thermal inactivation patterns [38]. It should be noted that a separate, highly specific TG hydrolase (EC 3.1.1.3) is known to be present in rat liver [38].

The acid CEH reaction requires no known cofactors, and no physiological inhibitors have been described. However, regulation of acid CEH activity can be achieved in vitro by varying assay concentrations of UC and oleic acid, both of which inhibit enzyme activity [35]. In addition, there is evidence for enzyme regulation in vivo in concert with the regulation of other lysosomal hydrolases [40]. One factor known to affect acid CE activity in certain tissues is thyroid hormone [40,41]. Experimentally induced hypothyroidism in rats causes both hypercholesterolemia and reduced acid CEH activity in liver, muscle, skin, and fat pads. Subsequent treatment with L-triiodothyronine restores the acid CEH activity of these tissues to normal. Finally, a correlation between acid CEH activity and cyclic adenosine monophosphate (cAMP) has been reported recently. Hajjar and coworkers [42] found that PGI_2 (prostacyclin), 8-keto-$PGF_{1\alpha}$, and 6-keto-PGE_1 all enhanced smooth muscle cell acid CEH activity 4-fold, though PGE_1 and PGE_2 had no effect. Furthermore, the increased acid CEH activity was correlated with increased concentrations of cAMP. This interesting observation clearly deserves further study.

(b) Neutral CEH

Neutral CEH activity (optimum pH 7.5) is found in the cytoplasm of most cells (Fig. 1). It has been assayed in vitro at 37°C, pH 6.6, using mixed micelles containing radioactive cholesteryl oleate, PC, and sodium taurocholate [43]. Other research has demonstrated that cholesteryl oleate, presented in an acetone dispersion, yields submaximum rates of hydrolysis [44,45].

Neutral CEH has been purified 2000-fold from bovine adrenal cortex [46], and is very similar to the hormone-sensitive lipase of rat adipose tissue [44,47,48]. Both activities increase in response to ACTH via a cAMP-dependent protein kinase [42,44,47,49]. Both have an apparent molecular weight of 84 000 as determined by SDS–polyacrylamide gel electrophoresis and show identical activities toward different substrates including CE and TG. Finally, both are inhibited by NaF, Hg^{2+}, and diisopropylfluorophosphate, and show identical peptide proteolytic degradation patterns [44,47].

It appears, however, that regulation of neutral CEH activity may occur by different mechanisms in different cells. Some macrophages, for example, show cAMP-dependent activation of neutral CEH, just as the adrenal does [46,47,50,51]. But rabbit alveolar macrophages and thioglycollate-elicited mouse peritoneal macrophages show no evidence of this activity [49]. Mobilization of cholesterol from intracellular CE stores in these rabbit and mouse cells may depend on decreased cholesterol esterification due to loss of UC to extracellular acceptors.

Because none of these hydrolases has been purified to homogeneity, virtually nothing is known of their regulation at the transcriptional or translational level.

(3) Lecithin : cholesterol acyltransferase (EC 2.3.1.43)

LCAT is a plasma enzyme, of hepatic origin, that can catalyze the formation of plasma lipoprotein CE (for an excellent recent review, see Marcel [52]):

$$\mathrm{PC + UC} \xrightarrow{\mathrm{LCAT}} \mathrm{lysoPC + CE}$$

The cholesterol esterification reaction is thought to occur primarily on the surface of high-density lipoproteins (HDL) where both of the lipid substrates and one or more apolipoprotein activators are located (Fig. 2A). The enzyme presumably binds transiently to the same surface, and catalyzes the transfer of a fatty acyl group mainly from the C-2 position of PC to the 3β-hydroxyl group of UC. Because linoleic acid, arachidonic acid, and oleic acid usually predominate in the C-2 position, the CE formed are rich in these fatty acids. Once formed, the CE for the most part leave the lipoprotein surface. They partition into the core of the HDL or are transferred to other lipoproteins by the plasma CETP (see later). Meanwhile, the lysoPC formed by the LCAT reaction equilibrates with other lipoproteins and particularly with albumin. These changes in distribution of CE and lysoPC presumably account for the fact that the reaction is essentially irreversible.

LCAT activity can be demonstrated in plasma by incubating freshly obtained blood plasma for 30–45 min at 37°C and measuring changes in the concentrations of the reaction substrates or products. Alternatively, radioactive UC, PC, or UC–PC vesicles can be incubated with plasma, and the formation of radioactive CE can be measured. Because LCAT has been purified essentially to homogeneity [53–55] and antibodies to it have been developed [56], it is now possible to measure the concentration of the enzyme protein in plasma by immunoassay [56].

Studies of highly purified preparations of LCAT have provided important information about its properties and the factors that influence its activity. An acidic glycoprotein of 60–65 kDa, it contains a variable number of sialic acid residues [57]. Sulfhydryl reagents such as *N*-ethylmaleimide inhibit the enzyme, suggesting that one or more free sulfhydryl groups are required for its activity.

Purified preparations of LCAT show phospholipase A_2 activity, cholesterol-esterifying activity, or PC : lysoPC acyltransferase activity, depending on the reaction conditions. The first two activities are seen only in the presence of apolipoprotein AI (apo AI), apolipoprotein CI (apo CI), or apolipoprotein AIV (apo AIV) [58],

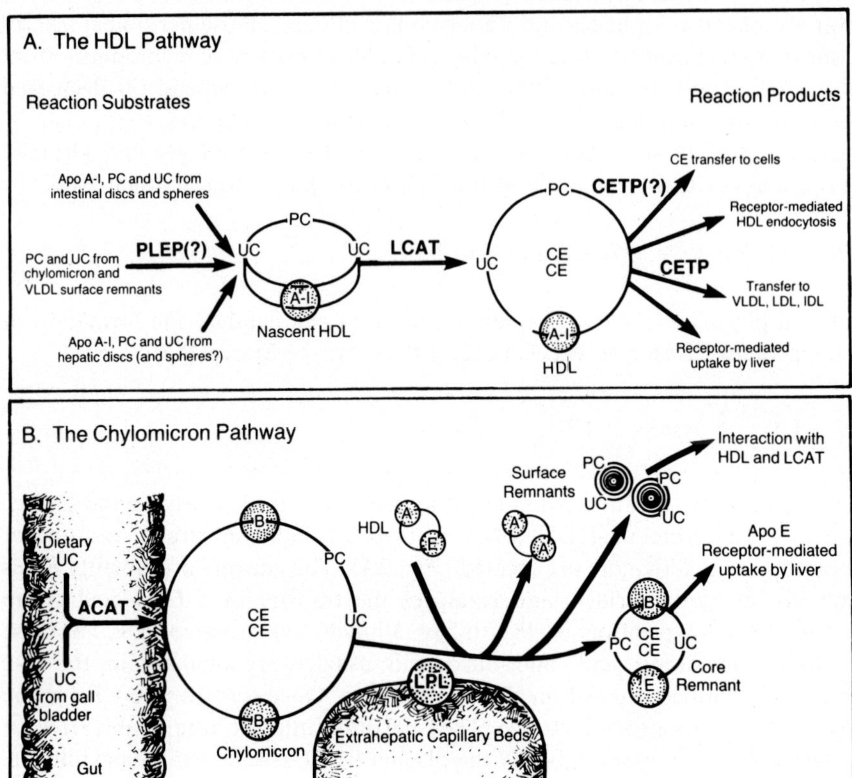

Fig. 2. Two principal pathways for CE transport exist in plasma and are distinguished by the lipoprotein species that carry CE. (A) Pathway involving nascent HDL discs and spheres containing UC, PC, and apo AI (A-1). The intestine can synthesize all 3 components and secrete them as nascent HDL, as can the liver. Nascent HDL can also form from the excess surface components of large chylomicrons and VLDL whose core lipids have been removed by lipolysis. PC may be added to HDL by the action of phospholipid exchange protein (PLEP) while UC is added via diffusion from the surfaces of plasma lipoproteins and plasma membranes. The HDL discs and spheres serve as substrates for the LCAT reaction, and change shape as the newly formed CE move to the lipoprotein particle core. CE formed by the LCAT reaction seem to have 4 potential fates: they may transfer directly to cells without lipoprotein internalization and degradation, a mechanism only poorly understood; CETP may transfer CE to other lipoproteins; the entire HDL particle may bind to an apo AI receptor and be internalized and degraded within lysosomes; or HDL that contain apo E may bind to an apo E receptor and be internalized and degraded. (B) Pathway involving formation of chylomicron CE by ACAT in the gut. Chylomicrons contain apo B, apo A, PC and UC in addition to core CE and a large amount of TG (not shown). In the plasma chylomicron, apo A is exchanged for HDL apo E, and TG, which forms the bulk of the chylomicron core, is hydrolyzed by lipoprotein lipase. This leads to a diminution in core volume, whereupon the chylomicron surface wrinkles, and surface remnants of UC and PC bud off to interact with HDL and LCAT as shown in A. The core remnant of chylomicron lipolysis, consisting of apo B, apo E, PC, UC and core CE, is then rapidly cleared from the plasma by hepatic receptors for apo E. The CE thus taken up by the liver is hydrolyzed by lysosomal acid CEH.

whereas PC : lysoPC acyltransferase activity has been demonstrated so far only in the presence of LDL.

LCAT shows phospholipase A_2 activity when incubated with apo AI and PC in the absence of UC, but even small amounts of UC effectively block this activity and promote cholesterol esterification. When apo AI, PC, and UC are present together in vesicles, optimal rates of cholesterol esterification occur at a molar ratio of PC : UC of about 4 : 1 [59]. On the other hand, recent work with artificially prepared, discoidal particles containing the same components [60] has shown that similar rates of cholesterol esterification occur across a wide range of relative UC contents.

Normally, LCAT acts primarily if not solely on plasma lipoproteins, and cholesterol esterification is clearly the principal reaction catalyzed. Furthermore, it has been recognized for many years that HDL play a special role in the esterification process. Nevertheless, questions still exist about the identity of the specific lipoprotein substrates of the reaction and about the factors that regulate the flow of the enzyme's lipid substrates and products in the plasma.

The HDL found in normal plasma include a large number of lipid–protein complexes. Some of these are presumably nascent lipoproteins that have appeared only recently in plasma, but most probably have circulated in plasma for varying periods of time under the influence of LCAT and other plasma lipoproteins (Fig. 2A). When freshly obtained plasma is incubated with LCAT, only a few of the HDL appear to react directly with the enzyme. The results of early HDL subfractionation experiments that employed gel filtration [61] suggested that the reactive HDL are very small. Subsequent studies with ultracentrifugation [62] showed that LCAT acts on HDL of *d* 1.125–1.21 g/ml (HDL_3), but not on HDL of *d* 1.063–1.125 g/ml (HDL_2), whereas more recent experiments with affinity chromatography have led to the proposal [63] that LCAT acts only on a very small lipoprotein complex comprised of apolipoprotein D (apo D), apo AI, UC, and PC. Meanwhile, other experiments with presumptive nascent HDL [64,65] have indicated that both large, disc-shaped HDL and small, spherical HDL can act effectively as substrates of the enzyme. It can be concluded, therefore, that LCAT acts only on certain species of HDL even though the number and precise composition of these species remain to be established.

Another conclusion supported by experiments in several laboratories is that the action of LCAT on HDL has several indirect effects on other plasma lipoproteins and also, potentially, on cell membranes. First, as the enzyme converts HDL UC directly to CE, UC from other sources such as VLDL, LDL or erythrocyte membranes transfers to the HDL. This transfer of UC to HDL appears not to be mediated directly by LCAT or any other plasma protein. Second, a CETP that can mediate either CE exchange or net transfer can transport the CE formed by the LCAT reaction from HDL to other plasma lipoproteins. Third, the lysoPC formed by the LCAT reaction transfers to other lipoproteins and especially to albumin, as mentioned previously. Finally, it is conceivable that the LCAT reaction may indirectly promote net transfer reactions involving PC, since CETP and other proteins present in plasma can transfer this lipid among lipoproteins [66].

Though LCAT has been purified to apparent homogeneity, and genetic linkage studies have suggested that its gene is located on chromosome 16 [67], studies of the molecular biology of the enzyme have yet to be done. Moreover, most investigators who have studied the regulation of the enzyme have sought to measure the effects of dietary perturbations on its overall activity in plasma, or have attempted to identify changes in this activity in different pathological conditions. No attempts have been made so far to correlate such perturbations or pathological conditions with changes in the concentration of enzyme protein as measured by immunoassay.

(4) Plasma cholesterol ester transfer protein

CETP is a plasma protein of unknown origin that transfers CE from one lipoprotein or artificially prepared bilayer to another (Fig. 2A). In addition to CE, the protein may also transfer other lipids such as TG or PC. It has been referred to as lipid transfer complex (LTC) [68,69], esterified cholesterol transfer/exchange protein (ECTEP) [70], CE transfer protein (CETP) [71], and lipid transfer fraction (LTP-1) [72]. The original observations regarding plasma CE transfer activity were made nearly 20 years ago [73], but even today the literature is confusing and incomplete and no generally accepted recent review is available.

CETP activity can be measured in vitro by a variety of methods, conditions, and substrates, but a common method is to monitor the transfer of [^{14}C]CE between HDL and LDL. The donor and receptor lipoproteins are separated by heparin–$MnCl_2$ precipitation and aliquots are counted [66,72]. CETP activity is determined by the difference between CE transfer with and without CETP. Fielding and coworkers [74] have devised an equally useful method, measuring CE transfer from cholesterol–lecithin liposomes to sphingomyelin–cholesterol liposomes.

CETP has been purified to apparent homogeneity from the $1.21 < d < 1.25$ g/ml fraction or the $d > 1.21$ g/ml fraction of plasma; its molecular weight has been estimated by SDS–polyacrylamide gel electrophoresis and gel filtration to be about 64000 [66,69]. It is an acidic protein (p*I* 5.0) that shows CE, TG, and PC transfer activities [60,63,68]. Because all three activities distribute similarly when the transfer protein fraction is exposed to a variety of ultracentrifugation and chromatographic separation procedures, they seem to depend on a single protein. However, several investigators have successfully dissociated CE and TG transfer activities in the same protein fraction using thiol-group inhibitors such as ethylmercurithiosalicylate [72] or parachloromercuriphenyl sulfonate [68,75]. Thus, the transfer protein may contain functionally different activities.

Several investigators have studied the physiological relation between these activities under a variety of in vitro conditions. Zilversmit and colleagues [68] demonstrated that transfer of CE from reconstituted lipoproteins to small, unilamellar vesicles proceeded on an equimolar, reciprocal basis with TG transfer. However, Fielding and coworkers [74] clearly showed that CETP can mediate the net transfer of CE in the complete absence of TG. Generating CE by co-incubating LCAT, A-1 and UC–PC liposomes, they found that CE accumulated up to a finite limit that was

[95,96]. Alternatively, CETP can be used to label lipoprotein CE by exchange [89]. Once the lipoproteins are labeled, they can be infused into whole animals, incorporated into organ perfusion media, or added to cells in culture; then uptake of CE into cells can be studied. In another approach, receptor-negative or receptor-deficient cells can be used to study the role of specific receptors in mediating the uptake of lipoprotein CE [97], patient lipoproteins containing abnormal apolipoproteins can be studied [98], or the apolipoprotein moieties of lipoproteins can be modified selectively to either increase [98] or decrease [99] lipoprotein uptake by adsorptive endocytosis. The role of lysosomal acid CEH in hydrolyzing the CE of internalized lipoproteins can be studied by using cells from patients afflicted with inborn deficiencies that affect this enzyme [100], or by using drugs such as chloroquine to raise the intralysosomal pH and thereby block the activity of the acid CEH [101]. The roles of ACAT and neutral CEH in metabolizing cytoplasmic CE can be studied by artificially loading the cells with cholesterol [98], by depleting the cells of cholesterol through incubation of the cells with phospholipid liposomes or a mixture of HDL and LCAT [76], or by adding hormones to steroidogenic cells to induce CE hydrolysis and steroid hormone synthesis [102].

(a) Fibroblasts

Studies of this type have provided evidence for several different cellular pathways of CE metabolism (see also Chapter 2). A major pathway, typical of cells such as fibroblasts [97], is shown schematically in Fig. 1. Plasma lipoproteins that contain CE and apolipoproteins B and/or E adsorb to specific apolipoprotein receptors on the cell surface, and are subsequently internalized by receptor-mediated endocytosis. Endocytotic vesicles containing the lipoproteins then fuse with lysosomes, whose enzymes catalyze lipoprotein hydrolysis. Lysosomal acid CEH catalyzes the hydrolysis of lipoprotein CE. The UC released then transfers across the lysosomal membrane and becomes available for synthetic processes within the cell. Excess UC entering the cytoplasm is converted into CE by the ACAT reaction, but can be released upon demand through the action of neutral CEH.

Studies of cells in culture have provided considerable information about the control of this pathway [97]. In early studies, cultured skin fibroblasts were maintained for 24 h in a medium containing lipoprotein-deficient serum. These cells showed increased binding of LDL to cell surface receptors and increased HMG-CoA reductase activity. When LDL were added to the medium, binding, uptake, and degradation of the LDL followed. LDL CE were hydrolyzed, and decreased levels of both HMG-CoA reductase and the apo B/E receptor were seen. Furthermore, increased formation of cholesteryl oleate could be demonstrated. In subsequent studies, modified LDL with a net positive charge were used. These "cationized" LDL were internalized by a mechanism that did not depend on the apo B/E receptor, and that led to a substantial increase in cell cholesterol [103]. Under these conditions there was again increased synthesis of cholesteryl oleate. These findings support two principal conclusions: (1) plasma lipoprotein CE is an important source of cholesterol for fibroblasts and similar cells; and (2) the formation of intracellular

CE by the ACAT reaction contributes to cellular mechanisms that buffer the content of UC in intracellular membranes.

(b) Cells that form steroid hormones

Cells that respond to pituitary hormones and other hormones by forming and secreting steroid hormones show several modifications of the basic pathway of CE metabolism seen in fibroblasts. First, some steroidogenic cells can use HDL CE in addition to or in preference to LDL CE as a source of exogenous cholesterol. These cells include rat adrenal, testis, and granulosa cells [104–107] as well as cells of the human corpus luteum [108]. They appear to have high-affinity receptors for HDL that differ from the apo B/E receptor. The HDL receptors presumably mediate the uptake of HDL CE, though the precise mechanism of this uptake remains to be clarified. Adsorptive endocytosis and degradation of the entire HDL particle may not be involved because Gwynne and Hess [88] have reported that the amount of HDL CE taken up by rat adrenal cells exceeds the amount of HDL apolipoprotein degraded. A second difference between steroidogenic cells and fibroblasts relates to the control of lipoprotein receptor levels. Both the apo B/E receptor and the HDL receptor can apparently be regulated by pituitary hormones [109–112]. A third difference relates to the control of the steady-state levels of intracellular CE. Steroidogenic cells clearly store greater amounts of CE than non-steroidogenic cells do (Table 1), which raises an important question about the mechanisms that control the content of CE in cells. These mechanisms are still largely obscure. A fourth difference between steroidogenic cells and fibroblasts is related to the mobilization of intracellular CE for use in steroid hormone production. The CE of some steroidogenic cells is hydrolyzed in response to external hormone stimulation [88,113]. As mentioned earlier, hormones such as ACTH seem to promote activation of neutral CEH by a cAMP-dependent phosphorylation mechanism. The UC released is then transferred to mitochondria which initiate steroid hormone biosynthesis [114] (see also Chapter 3).

(c) Macrophages

Another cell that shows a modified pathway of CE metabolism is the macrophage [115]. Macrophages have specialized receptors that bind abnormal, CE-rich lipoproteins such as "B VLDL"; lipoproteins that have been chemically modified; or lipoproteins that are complexed with other molecules. Via these receptors they can take up large amounts of lipoprotein-bound UC and CE. In addition, macrophages can take up dead or damaged cells by phagocytosis. Neither process seems to be regulated by the intracellular content of cholesterol or cholesterol-related compounds. For this reason, large amounts of intracellular cholesterol can accumulate. CE that is taken up is hydrolyzed within lysosomes by acid CEH. The UC that is released accumulates in the lysosome [116] or enters the cytoplasm, where it is re-esterified by ACAT. When massive amounts of CE are formed by the ACAT reaction and accumulate in lipid droplets, "foam cells" result, i.e. the cells appear to be filled with foam when fixed, extracted with organic solvents, stained, and examined under a microscope. Such cells can be seen in the skin and arteries of patients who have some forms of hyperlipidemia [117]. They are not seen normally, however, because the content of cholesterol in macrophages is usually balanced by HDL-dependent mechanisms that promote removal of UC from the cells. CE formed by the ACAT reaction is hydrolyzed by neutral CEH, whereupon the released UC is removed through interaction with extracellular HDL as shown in Fig. 1. In addition, overloading of macrophages with cholesterol apparently stimulates the synthesis and secretion of apo E-containing nascent HDL by a separate pathway [115]. These HDL contain both phospholipid and UC, and can be seen in peripheral lymph [118]. Once they enter plasma, they presumably participate in reactions involving LCAT and CETP, as described earlier.

(d) Hepatocytes

Hepatocytes show even more complicated pathways of CE metabolism than macrophages do. As discussed elsewhere (see Chapter 2), they play a key role in sterol metabolism because they possess receptors that can bind and mediate the internalization of chylomicron remnants [99], VLDL remnants [99], LDL [99], and HDL [99,119]. In addition, they secrete HDL and VLDL into the plasma, and in some species the VLDL can contain appreciable amounts of CE [120]. Hepatocytes also secrete LCAT into the plasma and thus control the formation of CE by this enzyme [121]. Finally, they convert UC into bile acids and secrete both UC and bile acids into the bile.

Control of these mechanisms occurs at several levels. The uptake of VLDL remnants and LDL by the apo B/E receptor has been shown to be linked to the excretion of biliary UC and bile acids [122], whereas the formation of intracellular CE by the ACAT reaction seems to be inversely proportionate to the excretion of the same bile components [123]. The uptake of chylomicron remnants does not seem to be related to bile formation and excretion. Instead, when large amounts of remnant CE enter hepatocytes, as is seen in some species in diet-induced hypercholesterolemia, the CE is hydrolyzed within lysosomes, then reformed by the ACAT reaction and recirculated in the plasma as VLDL CE. Less is known about the control of LCAT secretion by the liver. In rats and in humans the activity of LCAT in the plasma seems to be linked not only to the transport of cholesterol, but also to the transport of essential fatty acids [124].

(V) Cholesterol sulfate

CS is an amphipathic molecule that partitions easily into biological membranes. Because the sulfate moiety has a pK_a of 3.3, CS is ionized under physiological conditions [125]. It is found in small amounts in blood plasma and in seminal plasma, in bile and urine, and in tissues such as the liver, kidney, and skin (Table 1) [126]. It is found in larger amounts in feces [126].

Cholesterol sulfurylation is catalyzed by steroid sulfotransferase(s) according to the following reaction [127]:

$$3'\text{-phosphoadenosine } 5'\text{-phosphosulfate (PAPS)} + \text{cholesterol} \rightarrow \text{CS} + \text{PAP}$$

Enzyme activity is present in liver, and exhibits some steroid specificity [128]. The measured K_m for cholesterol is 0.02 mM [128]. Appreciable amounts of steroid sulfotransferase activity have also been found in adult mammalian adrenals, testes, and ovaries [129].

Hydrolysis of CS is catalyzed by steroid sulfatase, which is found in several tissues including the skin and is a component of microsomal membrane preparations [129]. For a review of the metabolism of CS, see Roberts and Lieberman [128].

Several physiologic roles for CS have been postulated. First, it has been suggested that the presence of CS in erythrocytes (about 700 μg of CS are present in 100 ml erythrocytes [125]) stabilizes the erythrocyte membrane [130]. Thus, CS was found to reduce hemolysis up to 56% in hypotonic solutions, whereas several other steroid sulfates and cholesterol conjugates were devoid of antihemolytic activity [125]. Furthermore, the presence of CS had a critical influence on the disc shape of erythrocytes in hypotonic solution; without CS, erythrocytes tended to become spherical and extend spicules [131]. A second postulated role of CS relates to spermatozoa. It has been suggested that CS stabilizes the membranes of these cells and that it may provide a structural trigger for capacitation [132,133]. Thus, CS is present in spermatozoa (15 $\mu g/10^9$ cells) as well as in seminal plasma, and appears to be concentrated in the acrosomal region [132]. On the other hand, sterol sulfatase activity is present in the human female reproductive tract [133]. There is no direct evidence, however, that CS contributes to the sperm membrane modification reactions that occur in association with fertilization.

A third physiological role postulated for CS involves the stratum corneum of the skin. CS is present in this layer, and apparently contributes to the intercellular lipid [134]. It may promote cellular adhesion in the stratum corneum because a 5-fold increase in CS content has been found in a form of X-linked ichthyosis characterized by steroid sulfatase deficiency [135,136].

Finally, CS may serve as a precursor of pregnenolone sulfate in human fetal adrenal mitochondria. It is converted to pregnenolone sulfate at a rate of 1.7 nmoles/min/mg protein [137].

In view of the special physical properties of CS and its ability to interact with membranes, it would seem to deserve more attention than it has received to date.

(VI) Cholesterol esters and disease

A complete description of all diseases that affect the metabolism of CE would be well beyond the scope of this chapter. However, several inborn errors involving CE have already been mentioned because of the information they have provided concerning the roles of specific enzymes, apolipoproteins, and receptors in CE metabolism. Several other disorders also deserve special attention. For example, a number of different diseases are known to lead to the demyelination of nerves [138,139]. These diseases affect the local metabolism of cholesterol in the nervous system because UC accounts for about 40% of the lipid of the myelin sheath. This UC is released by the demyelination process and is then converted to CE, which accumulates intracellularly in lipid droplets. Though the CE appears to be formed by the action of ACAT, the precise mechanisms involved remain to be clarified. Further studies would be of interest because the formation of CE that accompanies demyelination seems to provide yet another example of the role of CE in buffering the content of UC in cell membranes.

The accumulation of large amounts of intracellular CE is not always solely the result of UC overloading. In adrenoleukodystrophy, an inborn error that affects cells in the central nervous system and the adrenal gland [140], large amounts of intracellular CE accumulate, apparently the result of overloading by very-long-chain, saturated fatty acids. The fatty acids, predominantly 25 and 26 carbon atoms in length, seem to be incorporated slowly into CE by the ACAT reaction, but are released even more slowly by neutral CEH [141]. The difference between the rates of formation and hydrolysis of the very-long-chain fatty esters of cholesterol apparently accounts for the trapping of these esters within cells.

A disease that clearly merits special attention is atherosclerosis. It is characterized by focal accumulations of smooth muscle cells, macrophages, extracellular matrix, and extra- and intracellular lipid in the intima of arteries [142]. The principal lipid that accumulates is CE, and foam cells rich in this lipid are typically seen. Furthermore, atherosclerosis commonly occurs in individuals who show increased concentrations of lipoprotein CE in the plasma, and is particularly common in individuals who lack apo B/E receptors or show apo E abnormalities that cause pronounced hypercholesterolemia [143,117]. For all of these reasons, and because lesions similar to those seen in humans can be produced by feeding cholesterol-rich diets to experimental animals [144], it is worth considering the possibility that high concentrations of CE may in some way induce the disease. For example, an increased content of CE in arterial endothelial cells, arterial smooth muscle cells, or in macrophages might compromise important cell functions. The formation of intracellular, CE-rich fat droplets would necessarily be accompanied by the formation of a new intracellular lipid surface. Intracellular enzymes and proteins might bind to this surface, and this might alter the metabolism and function of cell organelles. Alternatively, the cholesterol overload reflected by the increased intracellular content of CE might be more critical. Such an overload would presumably be accompanied by down-regulation of receptors such as the apo B/E receptor, and this might limit the cellular uptake of important lipoprotein components such as antioxidants, fat-soluble vitamins, and essential fatty acids. Possibilities such as these would seem to deserve critical examination.

(VII) Conclusion

The information regarding CE that has been reviewed in this chapter can be summarized as follows:

First, the physical properties of CE differ greatly from those of UC, and clearly account for differences between the distribution of CE and UC within cells and in plasma lipoproteins.

Second, different pathways of CE metabolism involving different enzymes and substrates, exist in the blood plasma and in tissues.

Third, a major pathway in the plasma, involving plasma lipoproteins, LCAT, and CETP, appears to serve at least 3 major functions: (1) it provides a mechanism for buffering the content of UC in plasma membranes; (2) it contributes to receptor-dependent mechanisms that provide cholesterol and probably also essential fatty acids to peripheral cells; and (3) it is part of a mechanism for transporting excess cholesterol from peripheral cells to the liver.

Fourth, various modifications of a cellular pathway of CE metabolism involving plasma lipoprotein CE, apolipoprotein receptors associated with the cell surface, a lysosomal CEH, an intracellular ACAT, and a cytoplasmic, neutral CEH, can contribute to several cell functions. These functions include the synthesis of cell membranes, steroid hormones, or bile acids as well as the specialized scavenger functions of macrophages.

Finally, many fundamental questions related to the metabolism and function of CE remain to be answered. Virtually nothing is known regarding the molecular biology of any of the enzymes or transfer proteins involved in the metabolism of CE. Indeed, many of these enzymes have not even been purified to homogeneity. Furthermore, the close association between disordered CE metabolism and atherosclerosis suggests that the accumulation of CE may affect cellular function in ways that have yet to be explored.

References

1 Andersen, J.M. and Dietschy, J.M. (1978) J. Biol. Chem. 253, 9024–9032.
2 D'Hollander, F. and Chevallier, F. (1969) Biochim. Biophys. Acta 176, 146–162.
3 Lange, Y. and Ramos, B.V. (1983) J. Biol. Chem. 258, 15130–15134.
4 Small, D.M. (1977) J. Colloid Interface Sci., 58, 581–602.
5 Hamilton, J.A. and Small, D.M. (1982) J. Biol. Chem. 257, 7318–7321.
6 Smaby, J.M., Baumann, W.J. and Brockman, H.L. (1979) J. Lipid Res. 20, 789–795.
7 Wattenberg, B.W. and Silbert, D.F. (1983) J. Biol. Chem. 258, 2284–2289.
8 Smith, E.B., Evans, P.H. and Downham, M.D. (1967) J. Atheroscler. Res. 7, 171–186.
9 Moses, H.L., Davis, W.W., Rosenthal, A.S. and Garren, L.D. (1969) Science 163, 1203–1205.
10 Goodman, D.S. (1965) Physiol. Rev. 45, 747–839.
11 Small, D.M. (1968) J. Amer. Oil Chemists' Soc. 45, 108–119.
12 Gorrison, H., Mackay, A.L., Wassall, S.R., Valic, M.I., Tulloch, A.P. and Cushley, R.J. (1981) Biochim. Biophys. Acta 644, 266–272.
13 Kroon, P.A. (1981) J. Biol. Chem. 256, 5332–5339.

14 Sklar, L.A., Craig, I.F. and Pownall, H.J. (1981) J. Biol. Chem. 256, 4286–4292.
15 Spector, A.A., Mathur, S.N. and Kaduce, T.L. (1979) Prog. Lipid Res. 18, 31–53.
16 Lichtenstein, A.H. and Brecher, P. (1980) J. Biol. Chem. 255, 9098–9104.
17 Erickson, S.K., Shrewsbury, M.A., Brooks, C. and Meyer, D.J. (1980) J. Lipid Res. 21, 930–941.
18 Mitropoulos, K.A., Balasubramaniam, S., Venkatesan, S. and Reeves, B.E.A. (1978) Biochim. Biophys. Acta 530, 99–111.
19 Kaduce, T.L., Schmidt, R.W. and Spector, A.A. (1978) Biochem. Biophys. Res. Commun. 81, 462–468.
20 Rothblat, G.H., Naftulin, M. and Arbogast, L.Y. (1977) Proc. Soc. Exp. Biol. Med. 155, 501–506.
21 Haugen, R. and Norum, K.R. (1976) Scand. J. Gastroent. 11, 615–621.
22 Helgerud, P., Petersen, L.B. and Norum, K.R. (1982) J. Lipid Res. 23, 609–618.
23 Longcope, C. and Williams, R.H. (1963) Endocrinology 72, 735–741.
24 Mathur, S.N. and Spector, A.A. (1982) J. Lipid. Res. 23, 692–701.
25 Doolittle, G.M. and Chang, T.-Y. (1982) Biochemistry 21, 674–679.
26 Brockerhoff, H,. and Jensen, R.G. (1974) Lupolytic Enzymes, pp. 10–24, Academic Press, San Francisco, CA.
27 Mathur, S.N., Simon, I., Lokesh, B.R. and Spector, A.A. (1983) Biochim. Biophys. Acta 751, 401–411.
28 Hashimoto, S. and Dayton, S. (1979) Biochim. Biophys. Acta 573, 354–360.
29 Billheimer, J.T., Tavani, D. and Nes, W.E. (1981) Anal. Biochem. 111, 331–335.
30 Doolittle, G.M. and Chang, T.-Y. (1982) Biochim. Biophys. Acta 713, 529–537.
31 Suckling, K.E., Boyd, G.S. and Smellie, C.G. (1982) Biochim. Biophys. Acta 710, 154–163.
32 Suckling, K.E., Stange, E.F. and Dietschy, J.M. (1983) FEBS Lett. 151, 111–116.
33 Gavey, K.L., Trujillo, D.L. and Scallen, T.J. (1983) Proc. Natl. Acad. Sci. (U.S.A.) 80, 2171–2174.
34 Tuckey, R.C. and Stevenson, P.M. (1980) Biochim. Biophys. Acta 618, 501–509.
35 Lundberg, B., Klemets, R. and Lovgren, T. (1979) Biochim. Biophys. Acta 572, 492–501.
36 Haley, N.J., Fowler, S. and deDuve, C. (1980) J. Lipid Res. 21, 961–969.
37 Bhat, S.G. and Brockman, H.L. (1981) J. Biol. Chem. 256, 3017–3023.
38 Brown, W.J. and Sgoutas, D.S. (1980) Biochim. Biophys. Acta 617, 305–317.
39 Brecher, P., Pyun, H.Y. and Chobanian, A.V. (1978) Biochim. Biophys. Acta 530, 112–123.
40 DeMartino, G.N. and Goldberg, A.L. (1978) Proc. Natl. Acad. Sci. (U.S.A.) 75, 1369–1373.
41 Severson, D.L. and Fletcher, T. (1981) Biochim. Biophys. Acta 675, 256–264.
42 Hajjar, D.P., Minick, C.R. and Fowler, S. (1983) J. Biol. Chem. 258, 192–198.
43 Kothari, H.V. (1975) Lipids 10, 322–330.
44 Fredrikson, G., Strålfors, P., Nilsson, N.O. and Belfrage, P. (1981) J. Biol. Chem. 256, 6311–6320.
45 Severson, D.L. and Fletcher, T. (1982) Atherosclerosis 41, 1–14.
46 Cook, K.G., Lee, F.-T. and Yeaman, S.J. (1981) FEBS Lett. 132, 10–14.
47 Cook, K.,G. and Yeaman, S.J. (1982) Eur. J. Biochem. 125, 245–249.
48 Lee, F.-T. and Yeaman, S.J. (1980) Biochem. Soc. Trans. 8, 728–729.
49 Khoo, J.C., Mahoney, M. and Steinberg, D. (1981) J. Biol. Chem. 256, 12659–12661.
50 Brown, M.S., Ho, Y.K. and Goldstein, J.L. (1980) J. Biol. Chem. 255, 9344–9352.
51 Ho, Y.K., Brown, M.S. and Goldstein, J.L. (1980) J. Lipid Res. 21, 391–398.
52 Marcel, Y.L. (1982) Adv. Lipid Res. 19, 85–136.
53 Doi, Y. and Nishida, T. (1981) Methods Enzymol. 71, 753–767.
54 Chung, J., Abano, D.A., Fless, G.M. and Scanu, A.M. (1979) J. Biol. Chem. 254, 7456–7464.
55 Albers, J.J., Cabana, V.G. and Stahl, Y.D.B. (1976) Biochemistry 15, 1084–1087.
56 Albers, J.J., Adolphson, J.L. and Chen, C.-H. (1981) J. Clin. Invest. 67, 141–148.
57 Doi, Y. and Nishida, T. (1983) J. Biol. Chem. 258, 5840–5846.
58 Steinmetz, A. and Utermann, G. (1983) Arteriosclerosis 3, 495a.
59 Fielding, C.J., Shore, V.G. and Fielding, P.E. (1972) Biochim. Biophys. Acta 270, 513–518.
60 Jonas, A. and McHugh, H.T. (1983) J. Biol. Chem. 258, 10335–10340.
61 Glomset, J.A., Janssen, E.T., Kennedy, R. and Dobbins, J. (1966) J. Lipid Res. 7, 639.
62 Fielding, C.J. and Fielding, P.E. (1971) FEBS Lett. 15, 355–358.

63 Fielding, P.E. and Fielding, C.J. (1980) Proc. Natl. Acad. Sci. (U.S.A.) 77, 3327–3330.
64 Glomset, J.A., Mitchell, C.D., King, W.C., Applegate, K.R., Forte, T., Norum, K.R. and Gjone, E. (1980) Ann. N.Y. Acad. Sci. 348, 224–243.
65 Chen, C., Applegate, K., King, W.C., Glomset, J.A., Norum, K.R. and Gjone, E. (1984) J. Lipid Res. 25, 269–282.
66 Tall, A.R., Abreu, E. and Shuman, J. (1983) J. Biol. Chem. 258, 2174–2180.
67 Glomset, J.A., Norum, K.R. and Gjone, E. (1983) in: The Metabolic Basis of Inherited Disease (Stanbury, J.G., Wyngaarden, J.B., Fredrickson, D.S., Goldstein, J.L. and Brown, M.S., Eds.) 5th Edn., pp. 643–654, McGraw-Hill, New York.
68 Morton, R.E. and Zilversmit, D.B. (1983) J. Biol. Chem. 258, 11751–11757.
69 Ihm, J., Quinn, D.M., Busch, S.J., Chataing, B. and Harmony, J.A.K. (1982) J. Lipid Res. 23, 1328–1341.
70 Barter, P.J., Hopkins, G.J. and Calvert, G.D. (1982) Biochem. J. 208, 1–7.
71 Morton, R.E. and Zilversmit, D.B. (1981) Biochim. Biophys. Acta 663, 350–355.
72 Albers, J.J., Tollefson, J.H., Chen, C.-H. and Steinmetz, A. (1984) Arteriosclerosis 4, 49–59.
73 Nichols, A.V. and Smith, L. (1965) J. Lipid Res. 6, 206–210.
74 Chajek, T., Aron, L. and Fielding, C.J. (1980) Biochemistry 19, 3673–3677.
75 Hopkins, G.J. and Barter, P.J. (1982) Metabolism 31, 78–81.
76 Fielding, C.J. and Fielding, P.E. (1982) Med. Clin. N. Am. 66, 363–373.
77 Young, P.M. and Brecher, P. (1981) J. Lipid Res. 22, 944–954.
78 Albers, J.J., Cheung, M.C., Ewens, S.L. and Tollefson, J.H. (1981) Atherosclerosis 39, 395–409.
79 Morton, R.E. and Zilversmit, D.B. (1981) J. Biol. Chem. 256, 11992–11995.
80 Bisgaier, C.L. and Glickman, R.M. (1983) Annu. Rev. Physiol. 45, 625–636.
81 Drevon, C.A., Lilljeqvist, A.C., Schreiner, B. and Norum, K.R. (1979) Atherosclerosis 34, 207.
82 Forester, G.P., Tall, A.R., Bisgaier, C.L. and Glickman, R.M. (1983) J. Biol. Chem. 258, 5938–5943.
83 Kane, J.P. (1983) Annu. Rev. Physiol. 45, 637–650.
84 Minari, O. and Zilversmit, D.B. (1963) J. Lipid Res. 4, 424–436.
85 Schumaker, V. and Adams, G. (1970) J. Theoret. Biol. 26, 89–91.
86 Patsch, J.R., Botto, A.M., Olivecrona, T. and Eisenberg, S. (1978) Proc. Natl. Acad. Sci. (U.S.A.) 75, 4519–4523.
87 Oram, J.F., Brinton, E.A. and Bierman, E.L. (1983) J. Clin. Invest. 72, 1611–1621.
88 Gwynne, J.T. and Hess, B. (1980) J. Biol. Chem. 255, 10875–10883.
89 Fleisher, L.N., Tall, A.R., Witte, L.D. and Cannon, P.J. (1983) Adv. Prostagland. Thromb. Leuko. Res. 11, 475–480.
90 Glomset, J. and Norum, K. (1973) Adv. Lipid Res. 11, 1–65.
91 Herbert, P.N., Assman, G., Gotto Jr., A.M. and Fredrickson, D.S. (1983) in: The Metabolic Basis of Inherited Disease (Stanbury, J.B., Wyngaarden, J.B., Fredrickson, D.S., Goldstein, J.L. and Brown, M.S., Eds.) 5th Edn., pp. 589–621, McGraw-Hill, New York.
92 Vassilis, I.Z., Lees, A.M., Lees, R.S. and Breslow, J.L. (1982) J. Biol. Chem. 257, 4978–4986.
93 Gordon, J.I., Sims, H.G., Lentz, S.R., Edelstein, C., Scanu, A.M. and Strauss, A.W. (1983) J. Biol. Chem. 258, 4037–4044.
94 Schaefer, E.J., Kay, L.L., Zech, L.A. and Brewer Jr., H.B. (1982) J. Clin. Invest. 70, 934–945.
95 Krieger, M., Brown, M.S., Faust, J.R. and Goldstein, J.L. (1978) J. Biol. Chem. 253, 4093–4101.
96 Stein, O., Halperin, G. and Stein, Y. (1980) Biochim. Biophys. Acta 620, 247–260.
97 Goldstein, J.L. and Brown, M.S. (1977) Annu. Rev. Biochem. 46, 897–930.
98 Goldstein, J.L., Ho, Y.K., Basu, S.K. and Brown, M.S. (1979) Proc. Natl. Acad. Sci. (U.S.A.) 76, 333–337.
99 Mahley, R.W. and Innerarity, T.L. (1983) Biochim. Biophys. Acta 737, 197–222.
100 Brown, M., and Goldstein, J. (1976) Science 191, 150–154.
101 Goldstein, J.L., Brunscheide, G.Y. and Brown, M.S. (1975) J. Biol. Chem. 250, 7854–7862.
102 Anderson, J.M. and Dietschy, J.M. (1978) J. Biol. Chem. 253, 9024–9032.
103 Brown, M.S., Deuel, T.F., Basu, S.K. and Goldstein, J.L. (1978) J. Supramol. Struc. 8, 223–234.
104 Chen, Y.-D.I., Kraemer, F.B. and Reaven, G.M. (1980) J. Biol. Chem. 255, 9162–9167.

105 Schreiber, J.R., Nakamura, K. and Weinstein, D.B. (1982) Endocrinology 110, 55–63.
106 Gwynne, J.T., Mahaffee, D., Brewer Jr., H.B. and Ney, R.L. (1976) Proc. Natl. Acad. Sci. (U.S.A.) 73, 4329–4333.
107 Carr, B.R., Porter, J.C., MacDonald, P.C. and Simpson, E.R. (1980) Endocrinology 107, 1034–1040.
108 Ohashi, M., Carr, B.R. and Simpson, E.R. (1982) Endocrinology 110, 1477–1482.
109 Gwynne, J.T. and Hess, B. (1978) Metab. Clin. Exp. 27, 1593–1600.
110 Kovanen, P.T., Schneider, W.J., Hillman, G.M., Goldstein, J.L. and Brown, M.S. (1979) J. Biol. Chem. 254, 5498–5505.
111 Faust, J.R., Goldstein, J.L. and Brown, M.S. (1977) J. Biol. Chem. 252, 4861–4871.
112 Bruot, B.C., Weist, W.G. and Collins, D.C. (1982) Endocrinology 110, 1572–1578.
113 Freeman, D.A. and Ascoli, M. (1982) J. Biol. Chem. 25, 14231–14238.
114 Boyd, G.S. (1980) in: Hormones and Cell Regulation (Dumont, J. and Nunez, J., Eds.) Vol. 4, pp. 197–222, Elsevier, Amsterdam.
115 Brown, M.S. and Goldstein, J.L. (1983) Annu. Rev. Biochem. 52, 223–261.
116 Tall, A.R. and Small, D.M. (1980) Adv. Lipid Res. 17, 1–51.
117 Bierman, E.L. and Glomset, J.A. (1985) in: Williams Textbook of Endocrinology (Foster, D. and Wilson, J., Eds.) 7th Edn., pp. 1108–1136. Saunders, Philadelphia, PA.
118 Dory, L., Sloop, C.H., Boquet, L.M., Hamilton, R.L. and Roheim, P.S. (1983) Proc. Natl. Acad. Sci. (U.S.A.) 80, 3489–3493.
119 Bachorik, P.S., Franklin, F.A., Virgil, D.G. and Kwiterovich Jr., P.O. (1982) Biochemistry 21, 5675–5684.
120 Drevon, C.A., Engelhorn, S.C. and Steinberg, D. (1980) J. Lipid Res. 21, 1065–1071.
121 Simon, J.B. and Boyer, J.L. (1970) Biochim. Biophys. Acta 218, 549–551.
122 Brown, M.S. and Goldstein, J.L. (1983) J. Clin. Invest. 72, 743–747.
123 Del Pozo, R., Nervi, F., Covarrubias, C. and Ronco, B. (1983) Biochim. Biophys. Acta 753, 164–172.
124 Glomset, J.A. (1979) in: Prog. Biochem. Pharmacol. (Paoletti, R., Ed.) Vol. 15, pp. 41–66, Karger, Basel.
125 Bleau, G., Bodley, F.H., Longpre, J., Chapdelaine, A. and Roberts, K.D. (1974) Biochim. Biophys. Acta 352, 1–9.
126 Moser, H.W., Moser, A.B. and Orr, J.C. (1966) Biochim. Biophys. Acta 116, 146–155.
127 Banerjee, R.K. and Roy, A.B. (1966) Mol. Pharmacol. 2, 56–66.
128 Roberts, K.D. and Lieberman, S. (1970) in: Chemical and Biological Aspects of Steroid Conjugation (Bernstein, S. and Solomon, S., Eds.) pp. 219–290, Springer, New York.
129 Farooqui, A.A. (1981) Adv. Lipid Res. 18, 159–202.
130 Lalumiere, G., Longre, J., Trudel, J., Chapdelaine, A. and Roberts, K.D. (1975) Biochim. Biophys. Acta 394, 120–128.
131 Bleau, G., Lalumiere, G., Chapdelaine, A. and Roberts, K.D. (1975) Biochim. Biophys. Acta 375, 220–223.
132 Langlais, J., Zollinger, M., Plante, L., Chapdelaine, A., Bleau, G. and Roberts, K.D. (1981) Proc. Natl. Acad. Sci. (U.S.A.) 78, 7266–7270.
133 Lalumiere, G., Bleau, G., Chapdelaine, A. and Roberts, K.D. (1976) Steroids 27, 247–260.
134 Grayson, S. and Elias, P.M. (1982) J. Invest. Dermatol. 78, 128–135.
135 Shapiro, L.J., Weiss, R., Webster, D. and France, J.T. (1978) Lancet 1, 70–72.
136 Williams, M.L. and Elias, P.M. (1981) J. Clin. Invest. 68, 1404–1410.
137 Mason, J.I. and Hemsell, P.G. (1982) Endocrinology 111, 208–213.
138 Ludwin, S.K. (1981) in: Demyelinating Disease: Basic and Clinical Electrophysiology (Waxman, S.G. and Ritchie, J.M., Eds.) pp. 123–168, Raven, New York.
139 Lampert, P.W. (1978) Am. J. Pathol. 91, 176–197.
140 Molzer, B., Bernheimer, H., Budka, H., Pilz, P. and Toifl, K. (1981) J. Neurol. Sci. 51, 301–310.
141 Ogino, T. and Suzuki, K. (1981) J. Neurochem. 36, 776–779.
142 Ross, R. and Glomset, J.A. (1976) New Engl. J. Med. 295, 369–375, 420–425.
143 Goldstein, J.L. and Brown, M.S. (1977) Metabolism 26, 1257–1275.
144 Faggiotto, A., Ross, R. and Harker, L. (1984) Arteriosclerosis 4, 323–341.

H. Danielsson and J. Sjövall (Eds.), *Sterols and Bile Acids*

CHAPTER 5

Cholesterol absorption and metabolism by the intestinal epithelium

EDUARD F. STANGE * and JOHN M. DIETSCHY **

Department of Internal Medicine, University of Texas Health Science Center at Dallas, Southwestern Medical School, Dallas, TX 75235 (U.S.A.)

(I) Introduction

Cholesterol is essential for most mammalian cells where it is utilized either as a major structural component of membranes or as a substrate for the synthesis of more specialized sterols. Because of this critical role, mechanisms exist for maintaining cholesterol balance across the body so that the rate of sterol acquisition essentially equals the rate of sterol degradation and excretion, even under circumstances where there may be marked daily variation in the content of cholesterol in the diet. The intestinal mucosa plays a critical role in maintaining this balance since it is (1) the only site for absorption of dietary cholesterol, (2) one of the major organs involved in the de novo synthesis of cholesterol, and (3) essentially the only organ involved in the excretion of cholesterol and its metabolites [1,2]. The central role of the intestinal epithelial cell in cholesterol metabolism is summarized in Fig. 1. Dietary lipids, including cholesterol, triglycerides and fat-soluble vitamins, are partially digested in the intestinal lumen by various pancreatic enzymes and combine with bile acids to form mixed micelles (MM) [3]. After passive uptake into the epithelial cell, the free fatty acids and partial glycerides are synthesized back to triglycerides while the sterol enters one or more pools of cholesterol within the cell. Most of the triglyceride, along with a variable portion of the cholesterol, is then incorporated into the chylomicron (CM) and ultimately delivered to the vascular

* Current address: Eduard F. Stange, M.D., Department Innere Medizin, Steinhoevelstr. 9, 79 Ulm, F.R.G.

** Send correspondence to: John M. Dietschy, M.D., Department of Internal Medicine, University of Texas Health Science Center at Dallas, 5323 Harry Hines Boulevard, Dallas, TX 75235, U.S.A. Telephone: (214) 688-2150.

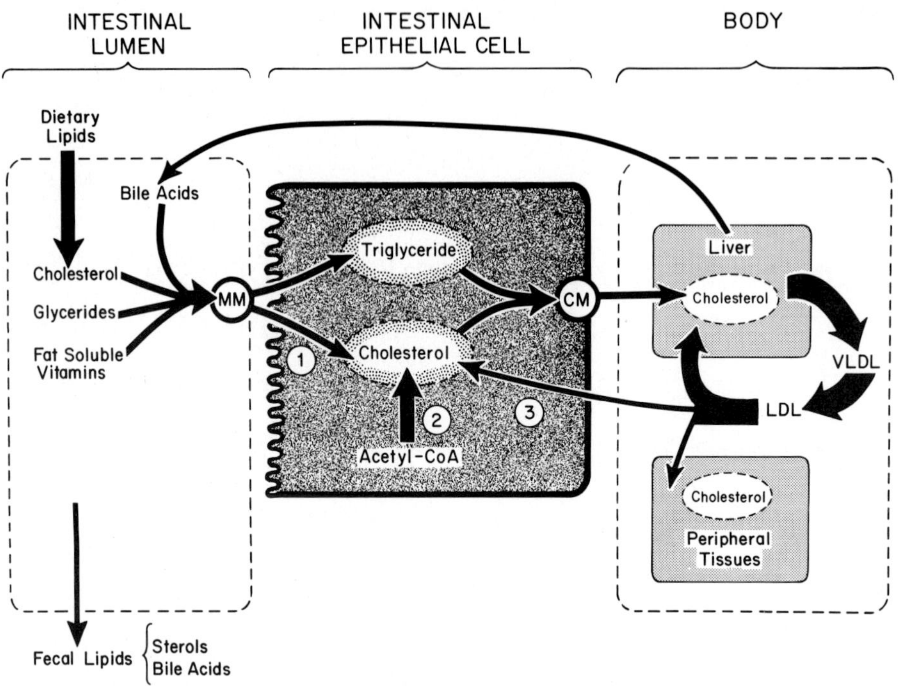

Fig. 1. Overall scheme for cholesterol balance across the intestinal epithelial cell. After digestion, lipids in the intestinal lumen combine with bile acids to form mixed micelles (MM) that promote uptake into the intestinal epithelial cell. Within the intestinal cell, triglyceride and cholesterol, along with specific apoproteins, are synthesized into the chylomicron (CM) which, ultimately, delivers much of the triglyceride to peripheral organs and most of the cholesterol to the liver. Also shown in this diagram are the 3 major sources for epithelial cell cholesterol including (1) uptake from the lumen, (2) synthesis from acetyl-CoA and (3) uptake of low-density lipoproteins (LDL) by both receptor-dependent and receptor-independent mechanisms.

space. Much of triglyceride carried in this lipoprotein particle is removed in peripheral tissues under the influence of the enzyme lipoprotein lipase [4] while most of the cholesterol is delivered to the liver in the chylomicron remnant which is bound to specific receptors on this organ and taken up intact [5–7]. This cholesterol, along with sterol synthesized locally in the hepatocyte, is then incorporated into very-low-density lipoproteins (VLDL) which are metabolized, in turn, to low-density lipoproteins (LDL) [8]. The LDL is then taken up and degraded by a variety of tissues by both receptor-dependent and receptor-independent processes [2], and of these tissues, the liver and intestine appear to be quantitatively most important [9,10].

From these brief considerations, it is apparent that the pool(s) of cholesterol in the intestinal epithelial cell subserve(s) at least two very different functions. On the one hand, the epithelium must have a constant supply of cholesterol for membrane synthesis and differentiation since the mucosal surface is constantly renewing itself. On the other hand, cholesterol also must be available for incorporation into the surface coat of chylomicrons during active triglyceride absorption. As also apparent in Fig. 1, this (these) intracellular pool(s) of sterol is (are) derived from at least 3 sources: (1) the uptake of molecular cholesterol from the diet; (2) the synthesis of cholesterol from acetyl-CoA; and (3) the receptor-dependent and receptor-independent uptake of LDL–cholesterol. This chapter will review how each of these pathways is regulated under a variety of circumstances so as to maintain cholesterol homeostasis across the intestinal epithelium.

(II) Absorption of cholesterol

Luminal cholesterol, derived from either the diet or from bile, represents one of the most important sources of sterol reaching the mucosal cell pool of cholesterol. The general features of how lipids, including cholesterol, are absorbed from the gastrointestinal tract have been reviewed in detail elsewhere [3,11,12, Chapter 14]. Generally, such molecules are taken up by passive mechanisms so that the rate of absorption is equal to the product of the chemical activity of a given lipid in the bulk luminal fluid adjacent to the intestinal microvilli and the passive permeability coefficient of that same lipid [13]. Since both the solubility and the passive permeability coefficient vary markedly among the different types of lipids, there are significant differences in the rates at which substances like fatty acids and sterols are taken up into the intestinal epithelium. Thus, as illustrated in Fig. 2, the logarithm of the passive permeability coefficient increases linearly with the hydrophobicity of the fatty acids and sterols in a given series (solid line, panel A). In contrast, the logarithm of the maximum solubility of these same molecules decreases with increasing hydrophobicity (dashed line, panel A). Since increasing hydrophobicity has a much greater effect in reducing maximum solubility than in increasing the passive permeability coefficient, the maximum rate of absorption (calculated as the product of these two values) decreases with increasing hydrophobicity (solid line, panel B) [11,14,15]. Under in vivo conditions, there is an even greater discrepancy between the maximum rates of absorption of the more hydrophilic medium and short-chain-length fatty acids and cholesterol than indicated by these quantitative considerations. This is due to the fact that the bulk solution of the intestinal contents, where digestion takes place, is separated from the microvillus border by layers of unstirred water and mucus (Fig. 3). Since these layers are not subject to gross mixing, molecules must move from the bulk solution to the limiting membrane of the intestine by diffusion. For molecules that are very hydrophobic and that have very high passive permeability coefficients, such as cholesterol, the rate of movement into the cytosolic compartment is much faster than the rate of diffusion from the bulk solution up to the microvillus interface. The rate of absorption of such molecules, therefore, is said to be diffusion, and not membrane, limited. Since the effect of such diffusion barriers increases with the hydrophobicity of the lipid molecule (and, hence, its passive permeability coefficient) the presence of these unstirred layers further reduces the rate of intestinal uptake of hydrophobic lipids

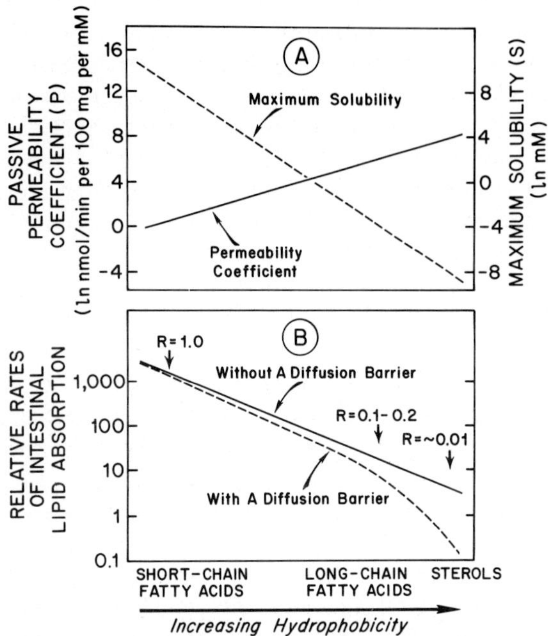

Fig. 2. The relationship of the hydrophobicity of different lipid molecules to their rates of absorption. Panel A shows the logarithm of the maximum solubility and passive permeability coefficient for a series of fatty acids and sterols of increasing hydrophobicity. The product of these two values for any given lipid yields the maximum rate of absorption of that lipid in the intestine both in the absence and presence of a diffusion barrier, as shown in panel B. The values of R show the ratios of the maximum rates of absorption of different lipids in the presence and absence of the diffusion barrier [15].

such as the longer-chain-length fatty acids and cholesterol (dashed line, panel B, Fig. 2) [13].

As also illustrated in Fig. 3, however, the presence of bile acid micelles overcomes this diffusion barrier resistance by delivering large amounts of the lipids directly to the aqueous–microvillus interface. Hence, the presence of bile acid micelles enhances the rate of lipid absorption, and the magnitude of this effect is directly related to the hydrophobicity of the lipid under study. This is best seen in Fig. 2 where the presence of a micellar phase in the intestinal contents can be viewed as overcoming unstirred layer resistance so that the dashed line in panel B is moved upward to merge with the solid line. It should be noted that in so doing, the rate of cholesterol absorption may be increased 100-fold and long-chain-length fatty acid absorption may be increased by 5–10-fold while there may be essentially no effect of the bile acids on the absorption of the more hydrophilic, shorter-chain-length fatty acids.

Thus, in the normal intestine with an intact enterohepatic circulation of bile acids, it is the product of the maximum solubility of the various lipids and their respective passive permeability coefficients that primarily dictates the rates of uptake into the intestinal mucosa. Hence, over 100 g of medium- and long-chain-length fatty acids

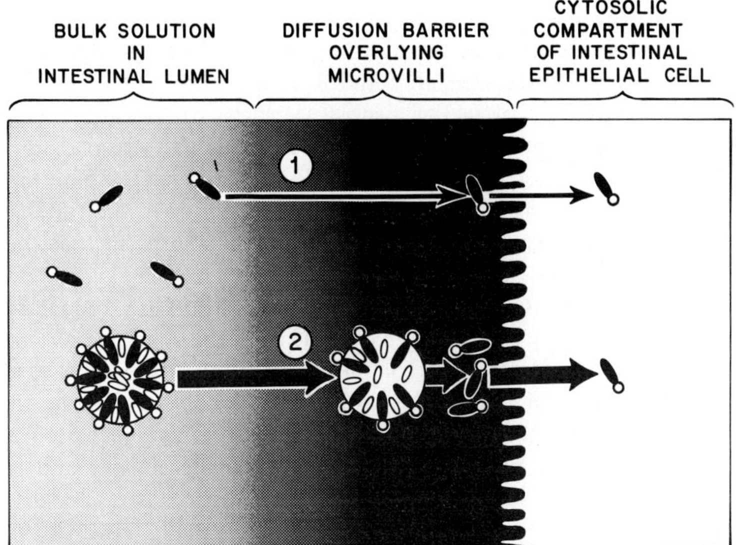

Fig. 3. Diagrammatical representation of the effect of bile acid micelles (or vesicles) in overcoming diffusion barrier resistance. In the absence of bile acids, individual lipid molecules must diffuse across the barriers overlying the microvillus border of the intestinal epithelial cell (arrow 1). Hence, uptake of these molecules is largely diffusion limited. In the presence of bile acids (arrow 2) large amounts of these lipid molecules are delivered directly to the aqueous–membrane interface so that the rate of uptake is facilitated [11].

may be absorbed daily by the normal human intestine under circumstances where sterol absorption equals only 0.5–1.0 g. Furthermore, the uptake of the very hydrophobic sterols is exquisitely sensitive to the diffusion barrier resistance. When bile acids are diverted from the intestinal lumen, cholesterol uptake is nearly abolished while the absorption of the longer-chain-length fatty acids is reduced by only 15–20% [15–17].

(III) Intestinal cholesterol synthesis

A second major source for cholesterol in the intestinal epithelial cell is de novo synthesis from acetyl-CoA. This section reviews the methods available for measuring such synthesis and discusses the localization and regulation of this process.

(1) Methodology

Older techniques used to measure the rates of cholesterol synthesis in the small bowel have led to errors with respect to the importance, localization and regulation of this process. For example, the specific activity of various ^{14}C-labeled precursors such as [^{14}C]acetate or [^{14}C]glucose undergoes considerable dilution inside the mucosal cell which leads to serious underestimation of the importance of the small intestine as a source of newly synthesized cholesterol in the body [18–21]. This problem can be largely circumvented by use of a substrate such as [^{3}H]water which rapidly enters cells and is not appreciably diluted by endogenously formed, unlabeled water [22]. Recent data obtained in vivo using this substrate suggest that the small intestine accounts for 24% of whole-body cholesterol synthesis in the rat [20] and may be quantitatively even more important in other animal species such as the rabbit, guinea pig and primate [21].

Similar problems have complicated the quantitation of HMG-CoA reductase activity as a measure of the rate of cholesterol synthesis. For example, it has not been established as firmly for the intestine as for the liver that this enzyme is rate limiting to the overall synthesis of the cholesterol molecule [23]. Furthermore, HMG-CoA reductase in both the intestine and liver is subject to a phosphorylation–dephosphorylation reaction that modifies enzyme activity and is involved in the activation of an inactive (phosphorylated) to an active (dephosphorylated) form during homogenization of the mucosa [24,25]. Finally, HMG-CoA reductase is incompletely recovered from the mucosa during preparation of microsomes [26,27] and is very sensitive to inactivation by proteases present in the intestine [28]. These various technical problems have led to considerable confusion with respect to various aspects of intestinal cholesterol synthesis and have made it difficult to interpret quantitatively some of the results presented below.

(2) Localization

Early studies established that the rate of cholesterol synthesis is not uniform down the length of the bowel [18,29]. Although there is detectable cholesterol synthesis all along the intestinal tract from the esophagus to the colon in the rat, the highest rates are found in the stomach, duodenum, terminal ileum and distal colon [18]. A detailed profile of 10 different levels of the small intestine of the rat is shown in Fig. 4 and illustrates the high synthetic activity in both the segments immediately proximal to the entry of the bile duct and in the terminal ileum. In contrast, rates of sterol synthesis are low in the mid-small bowel where most cholesterol absorption is thought to take place [30]. A similar profile has been found in the rabbit although there is no significant rise in synthetic activity in the terminal ileum of this species [31]. Both in the squirrel monkey [32] and man [33] high rates of cholesterol synthesis are also seen in the terminal ileum when the data are normalized to tissue weight. HMG-CoA reductase activity also is higher in the ileum than in the jejunum of the rat [34], whereas such a difference is not observed in the intestine of the rabbit [35]. While these rates were obtained mostly under in vitro conditions and with ^{14}C-labeled precursors, more recent in vivo studies using [^{3}H]water have essentially confirmed this distribution of synthetic activity in the rat and rabbit, and have also demonstrated that the rates of cholesterol synthetic activity are more uniform along the length of the small intestine in the hamster and guinea pig [21]. It should be

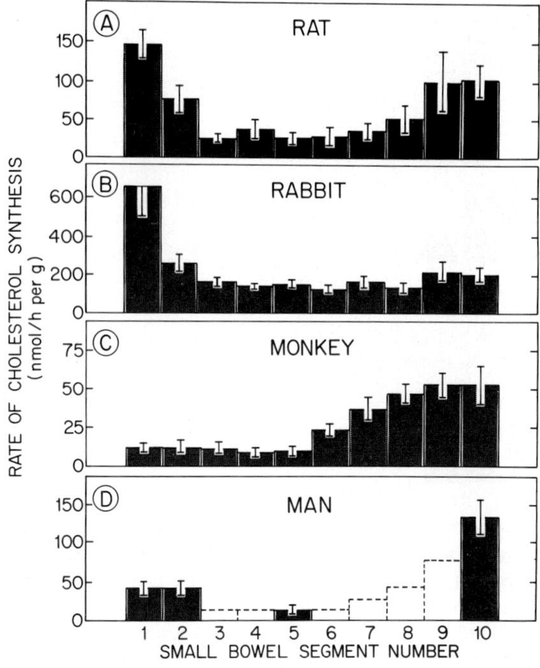

Fig. 4. Rate of cholesterol synthesis along the length of the intestine in 4 species. Cholesterol synthesis was determined in vitro in small intestinal slices obtained from segments 1 (proximal duodenum) through 10 (terminal ileum) using [^{14}C]octanoate (panels A and B) or [^{14}C]acetate (panels C and D). The data represent the flux of acetyl-CoA units to cholesterol from the two substrates in nmoles/h/g wet weight and are uncorrected for dilution by endogenous acetyl-CoA. Thus, the absolute numbers are not strictly comparable between the different species and substrates. The columns and bars represent the means ± 1 S.E.M.

pointed out that because of the greater mucosal thickness and weight in the proximal intestine, the absolute rate of cholesterol synthesis is actually greater in the jejunum than in the ileum of the rat, hamster, rabbit, and guinea pig. Thus, despite the higher rates of synthesis seen in the distal intestine when the data are expressed per gram of tissue, the jejunum is equal to or even of greater importance than the ileum as a potential source for newly synthesized cholesterol in the body. Very likely, this situation is also true in man when the mucosal weight of both portions of the intestine is taken into consideration.

In addition to these variations in rates of synthesis found longitudinally along the length of the intestine, there is also a gradient of synthetic activity found vertically along the villus–crypt axis. Although it was originally believed that virtually all cholesterol synthesis takes place in the crypt cells [18], this concept has been modified as more refined techniques for isolating individual cell fractions have become available [36]. For example, when the inhibitory effect of proteolytic enzymes on HMG-CoA reductase activity is circumvented (by use of trypsin

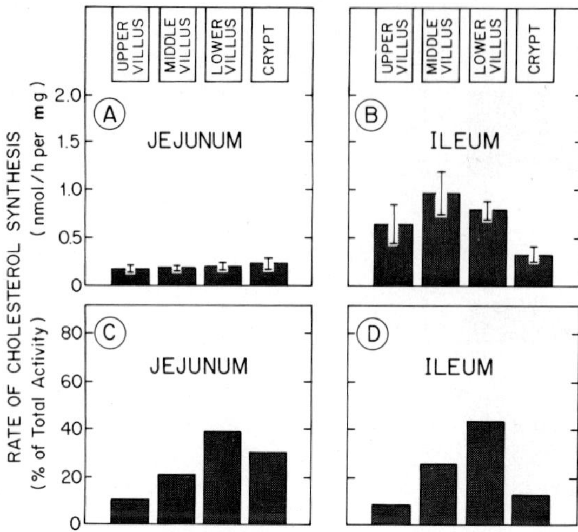

Fig. 5. Rate of cholesterol synthesis in the mucosa along the villus–crypt axis in the rat intestine. Enriched mucosal cell fractions were obtained from the mucosa by EDTA treatment and these viable cells were subsequently incubated in the presence of [^{3}H]water. Panels A and B represent the rate of cholesterol synthesis expressed as the nmoles of acetyl-CoA units incorporated into cholesterol/h/mg of cell protein in the jejunum and ileum, respectively. Panels C and D represent the total activity found in the isolated cell fractions taking into account the cell protein recovered in each fraction. The columns and bars represent means ± 1 S.E.M.

inhibitors or washed, isolated enterocytes) active sterol synthesis can be demonstrated in both crypt and villus cells, although there is little agreement on the relative specific activities found in these different cell fractions [28,36–40]. In a recent effort to more precisely identify the location of sterol synthesis along the villus–crypt axis in the rat, it has been found that, when normalized to a constant cell weight, rates of sterol synthesis in the jejunum are similar in villus and crypt cells while in the ileum, the villus cells manifest considerably more activity (Fig. 5). However, when these data are calculated in terms of the percentage of total recoverable mucosal activity, the great majority of sterol synthetic activity is found in the cells of the lower villus and crypt regions, and this is true regardless of whether the activity is measured under in vivo or in vitro conditions [36].

(3) Regulation

Just as there have been problems with localizing cholesterol synthetic activity, there has also been controversy as to the nature of the regulators, as well as the mechanism of action of such regulators, that control sterol synthesis in the intestine. Although less well established than in liver (Chapter 2), most evidence suggests that HMG-CoA reductase is the key enzyme in regulating the overall rate of cholesterol synthesis in mucosal cells [34,35,41]. In theory, the activity of this enzyme could be altered by changes in rates of enzyme synthesis or degradation, or by changes in the activity state of preformed enzyme as, for example, might occur through a phosphorylation–dephosphorylation reaction. However, there is little evidence to support the concept that a change in the activity level of the enzyme is important in long-term regulation of sterol synthesis in the intestine, although short-term regulation through alteration of the activity state of the enzyme has been described and is potentially important [25,42]. Most of the long-term effects of various regulators are mediated most likely through changes in the amount of enzyme protein, as has been described most extensively for the hepatic enzyme [23]. More recent work also indicates that there is little or no regulation of the enzymatic steps beyond that mediated by HMG-CoA reductase, although there is very little information on the characteristics of these enzymes in the intestinal mucosal cell [43,44].

Much of the early work in this area indicated that the rate of intestinal cholesterol synthesis is related to the size of the bile acid pool [18,32,33,45]. For example, mucosal cholesterol synthesis is high in rats with a biliary fistula or in animals fed cholestyramine. Furthermore, the infusion of whole bile or bile acid solutions suppresses the elevated rates seen in animals with biliary fistula, while cholestyramine-treated bile is ineffective in promoting such suppression [45]. In contrast, cholesterol feeding in the rat only marginally inhibits rates of sterol synthesis and even this inhibition is apparently related to an increase in luminal bile acid concentration [45]. However, since bile acids are required for the effective absorption of luminal cholesterol (see Section II), it was not possible in these studies to conclusively establish whether the regulator of sterol synthesis in the intestine was bile acids or whether the presence of bile acids merely facilitated the uptake of molecular cholesterol which, in turn, was the actual inhibitor of synthetic activity. More recent data, however, strongly suggest that this latter possibility is correct and that it is molecular cholesterol (or one of its oxygenated derivatives) that is actually responsible for regulation of intestinal cholesterol synthesis [35,42,46–50]. Thus, although cholesterol feeding is only marginally effective in the rat, both the guinea pig [51] and the rabbit [31,35] respond with more significant inhibition of mucosal sterol synthesis. The results in the rabbit are particularly relevant to this question since in this species bile acid synthesis is not increased by cholesterol feeding and, therefore, the lack of a secondary rise in the bile acid pool size suggests that cholesterol itself is the regulator of intestinal sterol synthesis [35]. While the limited data available in man show only a marginal effect of dietary cholesterol [33], other primates appear to be more responsive [32,52]. On the other hand, blocking cholesterol absorption with various agents such as surfomer [41,53], cholestyramine [41,53] and diosgenin [54] consistently enhances the rate of sterol synthesis at various locations along the length of the small intestine, as well as down the villus–crypt axis. An example of such experiments is shown in Fig. 6 which illustrates the effects of various dietary additions on cholesterol synthesis rates in the lower villus cells of the jejunum and ileum of the rat [41].

More direct evidence that cholesterol itself regulates sterol synthesis in the intestine has been obtained in studies using various in vitro techniques such as organ culture of intestinal mucosa. In such a system, cholesterol dissolved in ethanol

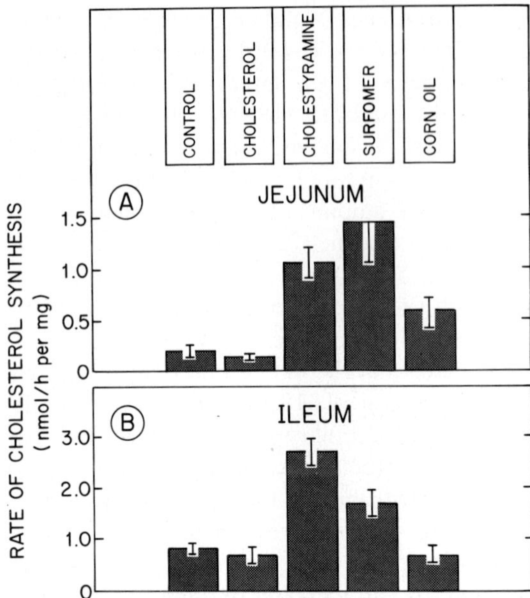

Fig. 6. Rate of cholesterol synthesis under conditions of varying cholesterol flux and demand in lower villus cells of rat intestine. The rats were fed for 2 weeks with normal rat chow (control) or with chow containing 0.5% (w/w) cholesterol, 2.0% cholestyramine, 2.0% surfomer, or 10% corn oil. The data are expressed as the nmoles of acetyl-CoA incorporated into cholesterol/h/mg of cell protein in the jejunum (panel A) and ileum (panel B). The columns and bars represent means ± 1 S.E.M.

inhibits the rise in HMG-CoA reductase activity seen during culture in cholesterol-free media of both canine and rabbit mucosa [46,48]. In long-term cultures of rabbit mucosa, bile acids at non-toxic concentrations not only do not inhibit rates of sterol synthesis but actually increase HMG-CoA reductase levels [42,48]. Concomitant with the increased rate of sterol synthesis there is a drop in the mucosal levels of cholesterol, suggesting that the rise in rates of synthesis are a compensatory response to a detergent-induced depletion of mucosal cholesterol. Both the depletion of tissue cholesterol and the rise in HMG-CoA reductase activity can be prevented by saturating the bile acid micelles with exogenous cholesterol. Such results, along with those described above in the intact animal, strongly suggest that changes in the size of the bile acid pool alter rates of intestinal cholesterol synthesis only secondarily by changing the flux of cholesterol into or out of the epithelial cells. This situation is analogous to that described in the liver where the conclusion has also been reached that bile acids have no direct regulatory role in altering hepatic cholesterol synthesis but act only indirectly by changing the rate of cholesterol flux across the liver cell [55].

In addition to cholesterol present in the lumen, the intestinal epithelial cells are also exposed on their basal-lateral surfaces to cholesterol carried in circulating lipoproteins. It is of interest, therefore, to determine if variations in this source of cholesterol also lead to alterations in rates of sterol synthesis. One approach to this question has been to treat rats with 4-aminopyrazolo[3,4-*d*]pyrimidine which inhibits the secretion of hepatic lipoproteins and leads to a precipitous fall in the plasma cholesterol to levels below 5 mg/dl [56,57]. Under these conditions the rate of cholesterol synthesis in the mucosa increases severalfold while the infusion of LDL intravenously prevents this rise [57]. Although the drug is toxic and alters intestinal morphology [38], these findings suggest a regulatory role for circulating LDL on intestinal cholesterol synthesis. Further support for this concept comes from experiments using long-term cultured mucosa where LDL has been found to be an effective suppressor of HMG-CoA reductase activity [24]. In contrast, both VLDL and HDL stimulate HMG-CoA reductase activity, presumably by inducing net sterol loss from the cells as cholesterol is partitioned from the cell membranes into the lipoprotein particles [49]. Finally, it has also been shown that when such cultured intestinal tissue is exposed to mevalonate there is marked suppression of HMG-CoA reductase, while inhibition of sterol synthesis by a drug like compactin stimulates the synthesis of the enzyme [49]. Thus, taken together these various observations indicate that the rate of cholesterol synthesis in the intestinal epithelial cell is under complex control by cholesterol reaching the regulatory sites from the intestinal lumen, from the plasma space and from local synthesis within the cell itself. Any experimental or physiological manipulation that alters the availability of cholesterol from any of these 3 sources is met by an appropriate, reciprocal increase in HMG-CoA reductase activity within the epithelial cells.

Even in the face of a constant supply of extracellular cholesterol, it is possible that a change in the demand for intracellular sterol, for either chylomicron synthesis or membrane differentiation, may also lead to alterations in the rate of cholesterol synthesis. Thus, for example, feeding fatty acids or triglycerides, with the accompanying need for chylomicron synthesis, is associated with an increased rate of cholesterol synthesis, as also shown in Fig. 6 [41,47]. This effect of fat feeding on intestinal sterol synthesis rates is dependent upon the type of fatty acid administered, but this dependency is not clearly related to either chain length or the degree of saturation [47,58]. Similarly glucocorticoids, which inhibit mucosal growth in vitro, suppress HMG-CoA reductase activity whereas thyroid hormone, which promotes mucosal growth, is associated with enhanced sterol synthetic activity [59].

Finally, both light cycling and fasting alter rates of cholesterol synthesis in the intestine although these effects are of much lower magnitude than seen in the liver [60,61]. Little is known of the response of mucosal sterol synthesis to diets varying in carbohydrate content; however, purified diets rich in sucrose, glucose or potato and corn starches eliminate the normal jejunal–ileal gradient of reductase activity [62]. Dietary fiber has also been recently reported to decrease cholesterol synthesis in the rat intestine, although this effect cannot be explained by the intraluminal physical–chemical properties of the fiber [63]. Thus, although it is clear that these various experimental diets do alter intestinal sterol synthesis, the mechanisms of action are presently unknown but may be related to the carbohydrate and other nutrient supply available to the intestinal mucosal cell.

(4) Function

From these considerations it is apparent that the localization and regulation of intestinal sterol synthesis are complex and subject to a variety of control mechanisms. The high rates of synthesis found in the differentiating cells of the crypt and lower villus region suggest that a major part of locally synthesized cholesterol may be incorporated into newly formed membranes and, thus, subserves the important functions of intestinal cell generation and maturation. This concept is compatible with the profound effect of various surgical and hormonal interventions that result in altered mucosal growth rates [59,64] and with other studies suggesting that microvillus membrane fluidity is influenced by locally synthesized cholesterol, rather than by absorbed luminal cholesterol [65]. Most of these data, therefore, point to an important function of locally synthesized cholesterol in membrane synthesis and differentiation. On the other hand, the fact that the relatively low rates of cholesterol synthesis found in the mature absorptive cells of the jejunal villi can be greatly increased by fat feeding indicates that newly synthesized cholesterol may also be utilized for synthesis of the surface coat of chylomicrons.

(IV) Intestinal lipoprotein uptake

As noted above, there is substantial evidence that the rate of cholesterol synthesis in the small intestinal mucosa can be regulated by changing the circulating levels of plasma cholesterol. Nevertheless, there is relatively little information on the importance of the intestine as a site for the uptake and degradation of lipoproteins and, particularly, of LDL.

(1) Methodology

The relative lack of quantitative data on these important transport processes is largely due to various methodological limitations. First, with the possible exception of a crypt cell line from rat mucosa [66] it has not been possible to maintain epithelial cells in culture for prolonged periods of time. Thus, receptor-binding studies such as those described in cultured fibroblasts, smooth muscle cells and hepatocytes have not been feasible with mucosal epithelial cells. Second, although some high-affinity binding of LDL and HDL to intestinal tissue has been described, it is not possible to extrapolate from these data to the quantitative importance of the intestine in lipoprotein degradation. Third, most of the work on lipoprotein uptake using labeled, non-metabolizable cholesterol esters in the particle core [67] or [^{14}C]sucrose attached to the apoprotein moiety [68,69] is difficult to interpret because of the use of human lipoproteins which do not bind well to the lipoprotein receptors of animals [70,71]. Finally, errors may also arise from the rapid cell turnover that takes place in the intestine and from biliary secretion of [^{14}C]sucrose with subsequent absorption of the radiolabeled metabolic products into the mucosal cells [69]. Some of these problems have been recently addressed using an improved technique for the quantitation of lipoprotein uptake in the intestine and other organs.

(2) Localization

From studies with freshly isolated rat intestinal epithelial cells, there do appear to be specific binding sites on the basal-lateral membranes for both rat and human LDL [72]. Furthermore, the lipoprotein particles appear to be taken up rapidly and degraded by lysosomal proteases [73]. In contrast, under in vivo conditions specific binding of only rat LDL is detectable [71]. On the other hand, radioactivity is found in the intestinal mucosa of the rat after the intravenous administration of human LDL labeled with [^{14}C]sucrose [69,74] or with [^{3}H]cholesterol ethers [67]. Comparable studies have also been performed in rabbits using human LDL labeled with radioactive iodine [75]. Thus, while these various studies suggest that intestine is capable of lipoprotein uptake, none provides quantitative information on the role of the bowel in lipoprotein degradation. Such data have been obtained more recently using a constant infusion technique that allows accurate in vivo measurements of receptor-dependent and receptor-independent uptake in the intestine and other organs of the body. With this technique it has been shown that the small intestine is the second most important site for LDL degradation in both the rat [2,10,76] and hamster [9] and accounts for approximately 10% of total LDL turnover. Although 50–60% of LDL uptake in the intestine is receptor dependent, the proportion of intestinal LDL uptake that is receptor independent is considerably higher than in other organs such as the liver and endocrine glands [2,9,77]. In contrast to the profile of cholesterol synthetic activity (Fig. 4), the uptake of LDL is relatively uniform along the length of the small intestine, as shown in Fig. 7. However, there is a gradient of LDL transport activity down the villus–crypt axis such that the rate of uptake increases approximately 3-fold in going from the cells of the upper villus to

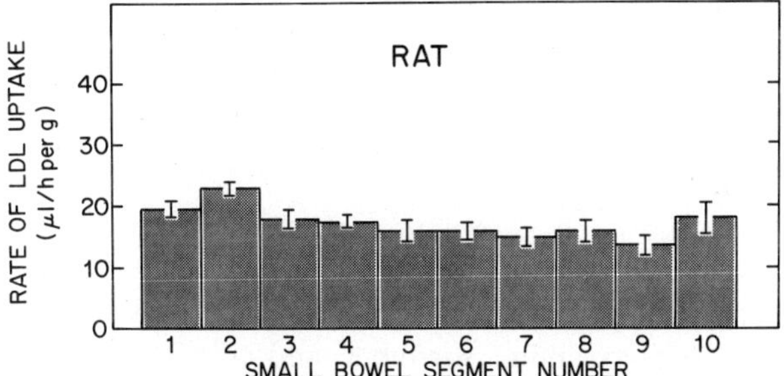

Fig. 7. Rate of LDL uptake along the length of the rat small intestine. The tissue clearance of rat LDL (LDL uptake) was determined in vivo using a constant infusion technique and [^{14}C]sucrose-labeled LDL. The data are expressed as the μl of plasma cleared of [^{14}C]sucrose–LDL/h/g wet weight. The columns and bars represent the means ± 1 S.E.M.

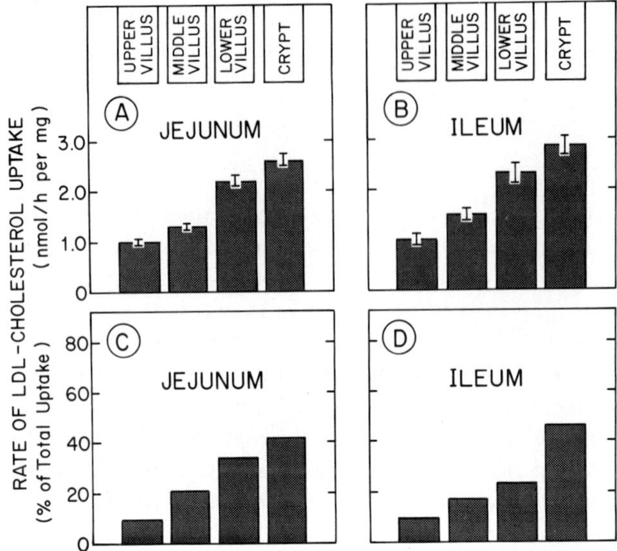

Fig. 8. Rate of LDL–cholesterol uptake in the mucosa along the villus–crypt axis in the rat intestine. The rates of LDL–cholesterol uptake were determined by measuring the tissue clearance of [^{14}C]sucrose-labeled LDL in vivo and then isolating different cell fractions from the mucosa. These clearance values were multiplied by the LDL–cholesterol concentration in plasma and expressed as the nmoles of LDL–cholesterol taken up per h/mg of cell protein (panels A and B) or as the percentage of total mucosal uptake found in each cell fraction (panels C and D). The columns and bars represent means ± 1 S.E.M.

those of the lower villus and crypt regions (Fig. 8) [77]. This is true regardless of whether the LDL transport data are expressed per mg of cell protein or as a percentage of total demonstrable transport activity. Unfortunately, comparable data are not available for other species. Thus, at least in the rat, the great majority of both cholesterol synthetic activity and LDL–cholesterol transport activity is found in the cells of the lower villus and crypt regions where active cell division and membrane differentiation take place.

(3) Regulation

In contrast to the extensive literature on the regulation of intestinal cholesterol synthesis, only a few studies are available on regulation of lipoprotein uptake in this organ. Notably, recent studies have compared the effect of various interventions such as the feeding of cholesterol, cholestyramine, surfomer, and corn oil on both rates of cholesterol synthesis and LDL transport in the rat intestine in vivo, as shown in Fig. 9. While these various manipulations all alter rates of cholesterol synthesis, there is no consistent effect upon LDL uptake at any location in the mucosa, with the possible exception of a slight increase in the jejunum after feeding

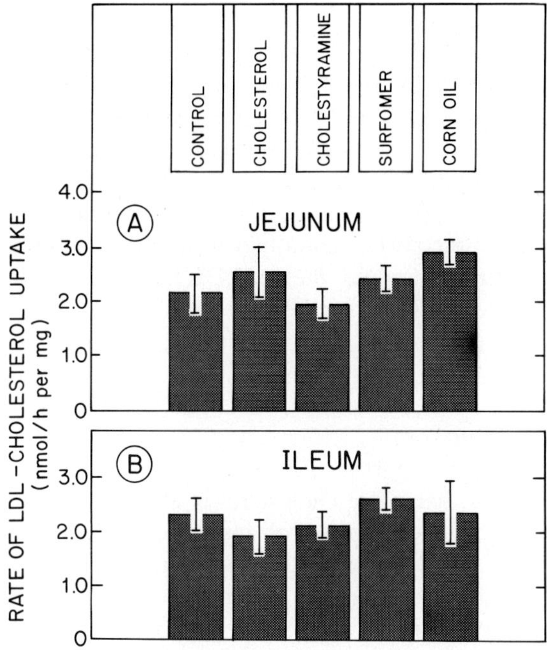

Fig. 9. Rate of LDL–cholesterol uptake under conditions of varying cholesterol flux and demand in lower villus cells of rat intestine. These data were obtained in animals treated as described in Fig. 6 for both jejunum (panel A) and ileum (panel B). The data are expressed as the nmoles of LDL–cholesterol taken up per h/mg of cell protein. The columns and bars represent means ± 1 S.E.M.

corn oil [77]. Thus, under conditions where the rate of cholesterol production varies over a 7-fold range, there is no consistent change in LDL uptake. This is true both longitudinally along the length of the intestine and vertically along the villus–crypt gradient. Thus, in the intestine the rate of cholesterol synthesis appears to be regulated independently of the rate of LDL transport. Comparable data are not available in other species although preliminary evidence suggests that LDL uptake in the hamster and rabbit intestine also is unresponsive to dietary manipulations (unpublished data).

(4) Function

The preferential localization of mucosal LDL uptake to the cells of the intestinal crypt and lower villus regions suggests that this lipoprotein supplies cholesterol for membrane formation and differentiation. However, two features of this system indicate that LDL uptake is not quantitatively important in this regard. First, dietary and drug interventions that dramatically alter the rate of cholesterol synthesis in these cells have little effect upon the rate of LDL transport. Second, it can be calculated that approximately 4 times more cholesterol is acquired by the intestinal epithelial cells through local synthesis than is taken up in the LDL particle. Thus, it seems likely that cholesterol that is locally synthesized and that is taken up from the intestinal lumen represents the major sources for sterol in meeting the needs of the intestinal epithelial cells, while receptor-dependent and receptor-independent uptake of LDL supplies only a minor amount of cholesterol to these cellular pools. Furthermore, any drug or dietary intervention that alters the availability of luminal cholesterol is rapidly adapted for by an appropriate change in the rate of cholesterol synthesis while the rate of LDL transport remains essentially constant. It should be emphasized, however, that at this time it is not known whether LDL transport would change if these adaptive responses in cholesterol synthesis were blocked by the administration of an inhibitor such as mevinolin.

(V) Intestinal cholesterol esterification

It has been recognized for many years that while cholesterol is absorbed exclusively in the unesterified form, the majority of cholesterol appearing in lymph is esterified to various long-chain unsaturated fatty acids [78]. The fraction of cholesterol in the esterified form varies with the load of dietary sterol so that the mass of cholesterol esters in lymph increases in proportion to the amount of cholesterol absorbed [79]. Such observations, therefore, suggest that absorbed cholesterol is a preferred substrate for the esterification reaction in the intestine. Since there is little detectable esterifying activity in intestinal lymph [80,81], the esterification process must be localized in the mucosa cell itself. The two enzymatic mechanisms proposed to mediate this esterification have very different origins and biochemical characteristics and will be described separately.

(1) Acyl-CoA : cholesterol acyltransferase (ACAT)

(a) Methodology

Acyl-CoA : cholesterol acyltransferase (ACAT) is the principal cholesterol esterifying enzyme in a variety of mammalian tissues [82, Chapter 4]. ACAT activity also has been detected in the intestine of the rat [83], guinea pig [84], rabbit [85], and man [86], and it has been suggested that this enzyme plays an important role in the mucosal esterification of cholesterol. The substrate for the microsome-bound ACAT is apparently free cholesterol on the membrane in the vicinity of the enzyme and fatty acid acyl-CoA [41,83]. In contrast to pancreatic esterase, ACAT has a more physiological pH optimum of 7.2, does not require high concentrations of bile acids for activity and does not utilize unactivated free fatty acids as substrate for the reaction [83]. In the original assay procedure radioactive cholesterol was equilibrated with microsomal cholesterol in vitro and used as the substrate. More recently, the rate of incorporation of [^{14}C]oleoyl-CoA into cholesterol esters has been used as a measure of ACAT activity, and the period of incubation has been shortened greatly to avoid hydrolysis of the substrate [86,87]. The apparent rate of esterification catalyzed by both the intestinal and hepatic enzymes can be markedly increased by incubating either microsomes or the partially purified enzyme with cholesterol-rich liposomes, suggesting that substrate supply is also an important determinant of the apparent rate of enzyme activity [41,88]. In addition, it has also been shown that the activity of the enzyme can be modulated by a phosphorylation–dephosphorylation reaction similar to that described for HMG-CoA reductase; however, phosphorylation activates ACAT but inactivates HMG-CoA reductase [88,89]. Thus, interpretation of ACAT activity is complex and, in some cases, ambiguous since the activity of the enzyme measured in vitro is influenced by both substrate (cholesterol) availability and the activity state of the enzyme itself. Hence, such activity may only indirectly reflect the actual rate of esterification occurring in the intact cell under in vivo conditions.

(b) Localization

Like cholesterol synthetic activity, ACAT activity also varies along the length of the intestine. In the rat, the highest specific activity is found in the jejunum with only slightly lower values being found in the ileum [41]. In contrast, in the guinea pig the specific activity of ACAT is approximately 3-fold higher in the proximal bowel than in the more distal intestine [84]. Similar findings have been reported in the

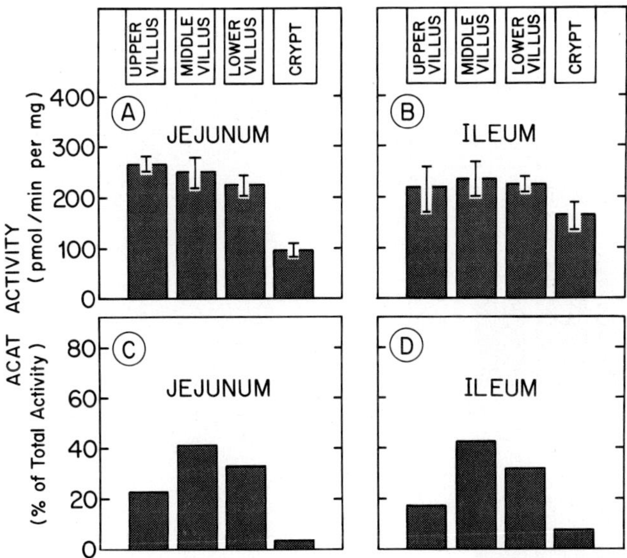

Fig. 10. ACAT activity in the mucosa along the villus–crypt axis in the rat intestine. Viable intestinal epithelial cells were isolated and ACAT activity was measured in whole cell homogenates using [^{14}C]oleoyl-CoA as a substrate. The data are expressed as the pmoles of [^{14}C]oleoyl-CoA incorporated into cholesterol esters/min/mg of cell protein (panels A and B) or as the percentage of total mucosal ACAT activity found in each cell fraction (panels C and D). The columns and bars represent means ± 1 S.E.M.

rabbit [85] and man [86]. Thus, the highest levels of ACAT in most species are found in the same region of the bowel where the majority of cholesterol absorption takes place [90]. Another indication that ACAT may be involved in cholesterol absorption is the distribution of enzyme activity vertically along the villus–crypt axis. Thus, as shown in Fig. 10, the highest specific activity of the enzyme is seen in the more mature cells of the villi so that more than 90% of total mucosal ACAT activity is recovered in these villus cells in both the jejunum and ileum of the rat [41,91]. Very little ACAT activity is detected in the immature cells of the intestinal crypts. A comparable villus–crypt gradient is found in the rabbit intestine only after feeding a diet rich in cholesterol and fat [85]. It is noteworthy that there seems to be a consistent inverse relationship between the distribution of cholesterol synthetic activity (low in mid-small bowel and the upper villus cells) and ACAT activity (high in the mid-small bowel and in the villus cells).

(c) Regulation

Intestinal ACAT activity can be increased by feeding a cholesterol-rich diet in species such as the rat (Fig. 11) [41,91], guinea pig [84] and rabbit [85]. However, it is possible that this increase in apparent enzyme activity is due solely to the fact that more substrate cholesterol is available on the microsomes harvested from the

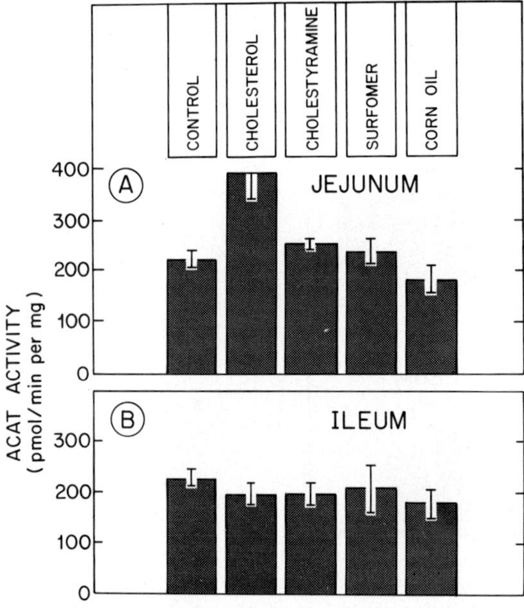

Fig. 11. ACAT activity in the intestine under conditions of varying cholesterol flux and demand in the villus cells of rat intestine. ACAT activity was measured in animals administered various dietary additions as described in Fig. 6. ACAT activity was then measured in villus cells obtained both from the jejunum (panel A) and ileum (panel B). The column and bars represent the means ±1 S.E.M.

cholesterol-fed animals. This possibility is supported by the recent demonstration that incubation of mucosal homogenates with cholesterol-rich liposomes increases apparent ACAT activity both in control animals and in cholesterol-fed animals to approximately the same level. Furthermore, in mucosal organ cultures, apparent ACAT activity can be increased by adding cholesterol to the medium, and this apparent induction of enzyme activity cannot be blocked by an inhibitor of protein synthesis such as cycloheximide [85]. Thus, taken together, these various observations suggest that the high levels of ACAT activity seen in the intestinal mucosa after cholesterol feeding merely represent an increase in the available supply of cholesterol on the microsomes and not a change in either the activity state of the enzyme or the amount of enzyme protein.

As also shown in Fig. 11, the administration of cholestyramine, surfomer or corn oil to experimental animals results in essentially no change in the level of ACAT activity even though all three of these dietary manipulations increase rates of sterol synthesis in the mucosal cells (Fig. 6). Presumably after treatment with these agents that either block the uptake of luminal cholesterol or increase the intracellular demand for sterol, the rate of synthesis increases and just compensates for the changing needs for intracellular sterol. If such compensation is nearly perfect, then the metabolically active pool of cholesterol on the microsomal membranes would remain constant, as would apparent ACAT activity measured in these membranes.

Finally, recent data in the rat intestine have shown an increase in ACAT activity with fasting. Since the microsomes harvested from these animals are also found to have a higher content of unesterified cholesterol, this result is also consistent with the view that assayable, microsomal ACAT activity primarily reflects substrate availability on the microsomal membranes [92].

(d) Function

Several lines of evidence strongly suggest that ACAT activity is of paramount importance for the mucosal esterification of absorbed cholesterol. First, the highest activities of this enzyme are found in the mature absorptive cells of the jejunum where most cholesterol absorption occurs. Second, all data on the regulation of ACAT activity also suggest that absorbed cholesterol is the predominant substrate for this enzyme. Third, it has been calculated that, as judged from the in vitro activity of ACAT, this enzyme is quantitatively sufficient to account for essentially all cholesterol esters secreted into mesenteric lymph [92]. Fourth, the regulation of ACAT activity through both substrate supply and phosphorylation–dephosphorylation suggests tight metabolic control and, therefore, an important physiological function for this enzyme within the intestine. Finally, the recent development of an inhibitor of intestinal ACAT has allowed direct examination of the role of this enzyme in cholesterol absorption. It has been demonstrated, for example, that both mucosal ACAT activity and the absorption of cholesterol can be suppressed in intact rats [93]. Taken together, these various arguments strongly point to a major role for intestinal ACAT in the esterification and, thus, the absorption of luminal cholesterol.

(2) Cholesterol esterase of pancreatic origin

This enzyme and its possible functions have been recently reviewed [78]. Cholesterol esterase is secreted by the pancreas into the intestinal lumen where it hydrolyzes dietary cholesterol esters. It has been suggested that the intact enzyme is subsequently bound to the brush border membrane, possibly to high-affinity binding sites, and taken up by the mucosal cell. Once inside the cell, the enzyme is supposed to re-esterify absorbed cholesterol with various free fatty acids [78].

(a) Methodology

The conditions for assaying this enzyme are considerably different from those described above for measuring ACAT activity. The pH optimum for cholesterol esterase in extracts of intestinal mucosa is approximately 6.2. The enzyme requires high concentrations of bile acids and does not, apparently, utilize the CoA derivatives of fatty acids as substrate. In contrast to ACAT, most of the enzymatic activity is found in the supernatant fraction of mucosal cell homogenates and, under varying conditions, both esterifying and hydrolyzing activities can be identified [94]. There is evidence suggesting that both the pancreatic and intestinal enzymes are immunologically identical [95]. Furthermore, there is a marked decrease in mucosal cholesterol esterase activity following diversion of pancreatic secretions from the intestinal lumen [96].

(b) Localization

Using immunocytochemical techniques with a specific antibody against the pancreatic enzyme, it has been shown that there is an immune reaction within the mature absorptive cells from the villus tips to approximately half-way down the length of the villus [97]. Sometimes, reaction products are also seen on the microvillus surface and, surprisingly, in the lamina propria and submucosal space [97]. Inside the mucosal cell most of the staining is localized to the smooth endoplasmic reticulum immediately below the terminal web. Unfortunately, there is little quantitative information on the distribution of mucosal esterase activity either longitudinally along the length of the intestine or vertically down the villus–crypt axis.

(c) Regulation

Apart from the fact that mucosal esterase activity can be reduced by diverting pancreatic secretions from the intestinal lumen, no studies are available on how dietary manipulations alter the activity of this enzyme. Thus, for example, there is no indication that esterase activity can be increased by increasing the load of dietary cholesterol [98], as is the case with ACAT activity [41,85].

(d) Function

Most of the evidence implicating the pancreatic cholesterol esterase as playing an important role physiologically in the intestinal mucosa during cholesterol absorption is based on the observation that the lymphatic secretion of cholesterol esters is decreased in animals deprived of pancreatic juice [78,96]. Other studies, however, have reported that pancreatic secretions are not absolutely required for cholesterol absorption since the proportion of cholesterol in the esterified form often is unaffected by pancreatic diversion [99]. Furthermore, other authors have calculated that mucosal esterase activity in pancreatectomized animals cannot account for the mass of cholesterol esters appearing in mesenteric lymph in such animals [98]. On the other hand, it has been demonstrated that purified cholesterol esterase increases the esterification rate, but not the rate of cholesterol uptake, in isolated intestinal cells [100]. Other work, however, has reported that porcine pancreatic cholesterol esterase increases both the absorption of free cholesterol and its esterification, and it has been suggested that cholesterol uptake is actually mediated through some sort of interaction with the esterase [101]. Thus, the role of this esterase derived from the pancreas in cholesterol absorption and esterification in the intestine is controversial, and there is no conclusive evidence that this enzyme actually plays a major physiological role in the mucosal cell to promote cholesterol esterification. Nevertheless, it cannot be excluded that two competing enzyme systems exist for mucosal esterification of cholesterol, and further work must be done to quantitate the contribution of both ACAT and the pancreatic esterase to this process.

(VI) Origin of the cholesterol in intestinal lymph

Cholesterol found in intestinal lymph may ultimately be derived from a number of different sources. These include sterol taken up from the lumen which, in turn, may come from the diet, bile or sloughed intestinal cells; cholesterol that is synthesized locally in the intestinal mucosa; and sterol that is carried in different plasma lipoprotein fractions and reaches the lymph within the core of the intestinal villus.

(1) Total cholesterol mass

Early work using the lymph fistula rat demonstrated that the amount of cholesterol appearing in intestinal lymph is directly proportional to the amount of dietary cholesterol present in the intestinal lumen [102]. Although less complete data are available in other species, this relationship also appears to be true in rabbit [103] and man [104]. Thus, in the post-absorptive state, after the intake of a diet containing substantial amounts of sterol, most cholesterol in intestinal lymph is probably derived from the diet [98].

It is less clear, however, what proportion of sterol reaching the lymph is derived from other luminal sources, particularly when the diet contains little or no cholesterol. This problem has been approached in several ways. One is to feed a newly available, non-absorbable polymer called surfomer that binds to the mucosal membrane of the intestine and reduces the passive permeability coefficient for hydrophobic molecules such as cholesterol. In animals fed this polymer and only trace quantities of cholesterol labeled with ^{14}C, the content of cholesterol mass and [^{14}C]cholesterol in the intestinal lymph is reduced approximately 65% and 75%, respectively. Such a result suggests that approximately three-fourths of the sterol present in intestinal lymph under these conditions are still derived from the intestinal lumen even when no dietary cholesterol is fed. When the bile is diverted from the intestinal lumen there is a similar decrease in the concentration of cholesterol in the lymph suggesting that biliary cholesterol is the major source of this luminal sterol [105]. Under these experimental conditions, the remaining cholesterol in lymph could have come either from sterol synthesized in the intestinal mucosal cells or from the movement of plasma lipoproteins from the blood into the lymph within the intestinal villus.

(2) Newly synthesized cholesterol

It is equally difficult to define in quantitative terms how much newly synthesized cholesterol is present in the intestinal lymph under different physiological circumstances and to determine where such sterol comes from. In theory, such newly synthesized cholesterol could be derived from the intestinal mucosal cells directly or from a more remote organ after either being secreted into the lumen of the bowel or after being delivered to the intestinal villi in plasma lipoproteins.

The results of recent experiments designed to elucidate this problem are shown in Fig. 12. In this study, rats were fitted with catheters in the mesenteric lymph vessel and were given a priming dose of [^{3}H]water followed by a continuous infusion to maintain the specific activity of body water constant. Under these circumstances, all organs in the body synthesize cholesterol at rates which are linear with respect to time. This results, as seen in the control group in Fig. 12, in an essentially linear increase in the amount of newly synthesized cholesterol appearing in the intestinal lymph. When large amounts of chylomicrons are infused into such animals there is selective inhibition of sterol synthesis only in the liver [106]; yet, surprisingly, there is a marked reduction in the amount of newly synthesized cholesterol appearing in the lymph (Fig. 12). This finding suggests that much of the newly synthesized sterol in intestinal lymph ultimately is synthesized in the liver and reaches the lymph only after being secreted into the intestinal lumen or after being delivered to the intestinal villi in plasma lipoproteins. The quantitative aspects of this relationship are further shown by the data in Fig. 13. As is apparent from these results, the amount of newly synthesized cholesterol appearing in intestinal lymph is a linear function of the rate of cholesterol synthesis in the liver and, of particular importance, when hepatic sterol synthesis is fully suppressed, no newly synthesized cholesterol appears in intestinal lymph even though the mucosal cells are actively synthesizing sterol under these experimental conditions [105]. Such a finding indicates that in the absence of active triglyceride absorption, essentially no sterol newly synthesized in the intestinal mucosal cells is delivered into the intestinal lymph; rather, the [^{3}H]cholesterol detected in lymph must ultimately have come from the liver. Since treatment of such animals with surfomer or with biliary diversion reduces the appearance of newly synthesized cholesterol in the lymph by about two-thirds, it is likely that about this

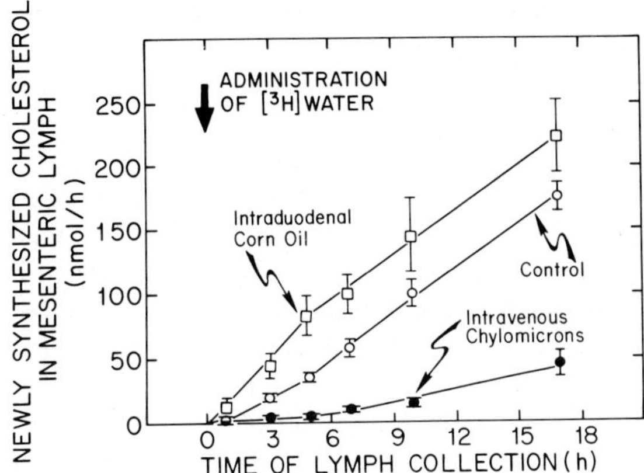

Fig. 12. Appearance of newly synthesized cholesterol in mesenteric lymph of the rat. The experimental animals had indwelling lymph fistulae and were infused intraintestinally with a glucose–amino acid–electrolyte solution. One group of these animals was also administered intravenously chylomicrons containing 105 mg of cholesterol, while another group was infused intraduodenally with corn oil. 24 h after the initial surgery, each animal was administered [^{3}H]water intravenously and the secretion of labeled cholesterol in intestinal lymph was followed for 18 h. The amount of [^{3}H]water incorporated into cholesterol was used to calculate the amount of newly synthesized cholesterol present in lymph. These values are expressed as the nmoles of newly synthesized cholesterol secreted into the lymph each hour. The data points represent means ± 1 S.E.M.

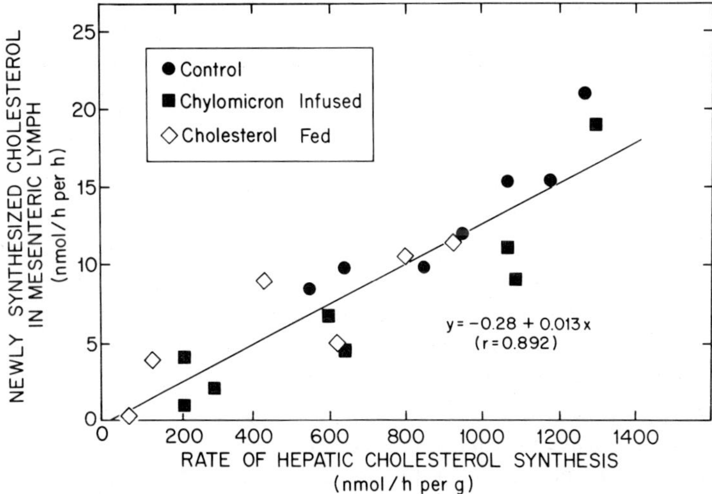

Fig. 13. The relationship between the appearance rate of newly synthesized cholesterol in mesenteric lymph and the rate of hepatic cholesterol synthesis in the same animal. These studies were carried out as described in the legend to Fig. 12 but contained an additional group of animals that were fed different amounts of cholesterol to alter rates of hepatic cholesterol synthesis.

fraction of the newly synthesized cholesterol reaches the lymph after being secreted into the bile and being absorbed across the intestinal mucosa. The remaining [^{3}H]cholesterol presumably is carried from the liver to the intestinal villi in plasma lipoproteins.

As also shown in Fig. 12, when active triglyceride absorption is induced by the infusion of corn oil into these animals, there is a significant increase in the appearance of newly synthesized cholesterol in intestinal lymph which, in this situation, is independent of any similar change in the rate of hepatic cholesterol synthesis. Thus, during triglyceride absorption and chylomicron formation there is an increase in the rate of cholesterol synthesis in the intestinal epithelial cells (Fig. 6), and a portion of this newly synthesized sterol becomes incorporated into the surface coat of chylomicrons and appears in the intestinal lymph. Under the conditions of this experiment it can be calculated that the mucosa contributes about 0.04 mg/h of newly synthesized cholesterol to the lymph which equals about one-fourth of the mass of cholesterol found in the lymphatic drainage. Nevertheless, this contribution is only a very small fraction of the cholesterol actually synthesized in the intestine during this same time period. This finding is consistent with the view that the intestine contributes little newly synthesized sterol to the body but, rather, most cholesterol that is synthesized goes into membrane maintenance and synthesis.

Thus, in summary, it may be concluded that much of the cholesterol synthesized in the intestine is apparently used for local purposes. Under circumstances where there is no triglyceride absorption taking place essentially no newly synthesized sterol of intestinal origin can be detected in the lymphatic outflow from the gut. During active triglyceride absorption, however, the rate of sterol synthesis increases markedly in the intestinal absorptive cells, and a portion of this newly synthesized cholesterol is incorporated into chylomicrons and other intestinal lipoproteins and delivered into the lymph. Thus, both the rate of sterol synthesis by the intestine and the rate of entry of this sterol into the body pools is partially dictated by the rate of triglyceride absorption.

(VII) Compartmentalization of cholesterol in the enterocyte

On the basis of the data reviewed in this chapter, it seems likely that there are functionally distinct pools of cholesterol in the intestinal epithelial cell that serve different metabolic functions. These pools are illustrated diagrammatically in the model of an epithelial cell shown in Fig. 14. Pool A is defined as having been derived largely from the uptake of luminal unesterified cholesterol (arrow 1) and serves as a major substrate for the CoA-dependent esterification reaction (arrow 2). The cholesterol esters that result from this reaction are incorporated into the hydrophobic core of the chylomicron particle. Following cholesterol feeding there is a marked increase in apparent ACAT activity in the intestinal epithelium that seems to be related to an increase in the amount of intracellular cholesterol available to the enzyme under the in vitro conditions of the assay rather than to an increase in the

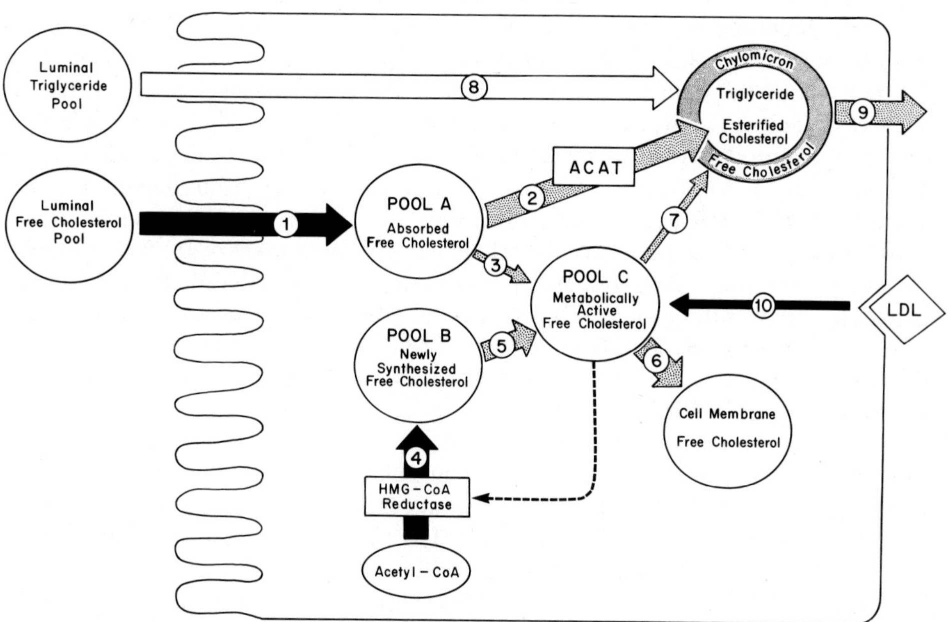

Fig. 14. Diagrammatic representation of the pools and fluxes of cholesterol within the intestinal mucosal cell. Based upon the experimental data presented in this review, it is likely that at least 3 distinct subpools of cholesterol exist within the cell; these include pool A, which is derived from sterol absorbed from the intestinal lumen (arrow 1) and serves principally as a substrate for acyl-CoA:cholesterol acyltransferase (ACAT) (arrow 2) while that in pool B is supplied primarily by de novo synthesis from acetyl-CoA (arrow 4). pool C presumably receives a major contribution of sterol from pool B (arrow 5) and a lesser contribution from pool A (arrow 3). The free sterol in this metabolically active pool is used for the synthesis of cell membranes (arrow 6) and for the surface coat of nascent chylomicrons (arrow 7). Triglycerides are also absorbed (arrow 8) and secreted in chylomicrons (arrow 9) into lymph. Finally, low-density lipoproteins (LDL) are taken up from the plasma and contribute to the metabolically active pool of cholesterol (arrow 10) [41].

absolute amount of ACAT protein. Increasing the rate of cholesterol synthesis and, therefore, the flux of cholesterol through pool B, by feeding surfomer, cholestyramine or corn oil, does not increase ACAT activity. Furthermore, in isolated intestinal epithelial cells newly synthesized sterol is esterified only to a limited extent if the rate of cholesterol synthesis is driven by incubating these cells with high concentrations of mevalonic acid [107,108]. Finally, newly synthesized cholesterol that is incorporated into the chylomicron is predominantly in the unesterified form. Thus, it may be concluded that newly synthesized cholesterol formed in the mucosa is normally not a major substrate for the ACAT reaction.

Pools A and B also appear to be functionally distinct with respect to the role of the sterol in these pools to effectively regulate the rate of cholesterol synthesis within the intestinal epithelial cell. For example, cholesterol feeding in the rat and in man exerts little inhibitory effect on the rate of cholesterol synthesis in the intestine. Such feedback inhibition may be seen, however, in species such as the guinea pig and rabbit. However, in all species there is an increase in the rate of mucosal cholesterol synthesis when the uptake of luminal cholesterol is blocked by feeding substances such as surfomer or cholestyramine. Thus, there must be a contribution of cholesterol (arrow 3) from pool A to the metabolically active, intracellular pool of sterol (pool C). Similarly, a contribution to pool C also must come from the uptake and degradation of low-density lipoproteins (arrow 10). Hence, when the contribution of cholesterol either from pool A (by blocking cholesterol uptake) or from lipoproteins (by treatment with 4-aminopyrazolo[3,4-*d*]pyrimidine) is reduced, there is an appropriate compensatory increase in the rate of cholesterol synthesis so that the size of pool C presumably remains constant, and the cell has adequate amounts of unesterified cholesterol for the synthesis of chylomicrons and for cell membrane maintenance and differentiation.

The relative importance of each of these contributions to pool C is likely to be different in epithelial cells located at different points along the villus–crypt axis. The fact that cholesterol derived from synthesis and from the uptake of LDL is critically important for membrane formation and differentiation is suggested by the finding that 70–80% of total mucosal sterol synthetic activity and LDL transport activity are localized to the immature cells of the lower villus and crypt regions in both the proximal and distal intestine. In the mature absorptive cells of the upper villus in the jejunum, where most sterol absorption takes place, the rate of cholesterol synthesis appears to be suppressed. In the absence of fat absorption, cholesterol newly synthesized in these cells apparently is sloughed into the lumen and not reabsorbed. However, with active triglyceride absorption cholesterol synthesis in these cells is increased and a portion of this sterol appears in the intestinal lymph. Only under this condition does pool B apparently supply sterol for lipoprotein formation.

Acknowledgements

A portion of the original research reviewed in this chapter was supported by United States Public Health Service Research Grants HL 09610 and AM 19329 and by a grant from the Moss Heart Foundation.

The authors would also like to acknowledge the help of Imogene Robison in the preparation of the manuscript.

References

1 Turley, S.D. and Dietschy, J.M. (1982) in: The Liver: Biology and Pathobiology (Arias, I., Popper, H., Schachter, D. and Shafritz, D.A., Eds.) pp. 467–492, Raven Press, New York.

2 Dietschy, J.M. (1984) Klin. Wochenschr. 62, 338–345.

3 Thomson, A.B.R. and Dietschy, J.M. (1981) in: Physiology of the Gastrointestinal Tract (Johnson, L.R., Ed.) pp. 1147–1220, Raven Press, New York.

4 Fielding, C.J. (1978) in: Disturbances in Lipid and Lipoprotein Metabolism (Dietschy, J.M., Gotto Jr., A.M. and Ontko, J.A., Eds.) pp. 83–98, Waverly Press, Baltimore, MD.
5 Sherrill, B.C. and Dietschy, J.M. (1978) J. Biol. Chem. 253, 1859–1867.
6 Cooper, A.D. and Yu, P.Y.S. (1978) J. Lipid Res. 19, 109–117.
7 Shelburne, F., Hanks, J., Meyers, W. and Quarfordt, S. (1980) J. Clin. Invest. 65, 652–658.
8 Kita, T., Brown, M.S., Bilheimer, D.W. and Goldstein, J.L. (1982) Proc. Natl. Acad. Sci. (U.S.A.) 79, 5693–5697.
9 Spady, D.K., Bilheimer, D.W. and Dietschy, J.M. (1983) Proc. Natl. Acad. Sci. (U.S.A.) 80, 3499–3503.
10 Dietschy, J.M., Spady, D.K. and Stange, E.F. (1983) Biochem. Soc. Trans. 11, 639–641.
11 Westergaard, H. and Dietschy, J.M. (1976) J. Clin. Invest. 58, 97–108.
12 Carey, M.C., Small, D.M. and Bliss, C.M. (1983) Annu. Rev. Physiol. 45, 651–677.
13 Dietschy, J.M. (1978) in: Disturbances in Lipid and Lipoprotein Metabolism (Dietschy, J.M., Gotto, A.M. and Ontko, J.A., Eds.) pp. 1–28, Waverly Press, Baltimore, MD.
14 Westergaard, H. and Dietschy, J.M. (1974) J. Clin. Invest. 54, 718–732.
15 Westergaard, H. and Dietschy, J.M. (1974) Med. Clin. N. Am. 58, 1413–1427.
16 Wilson, F.A. and Dietschy, J.M. (1971) Gastroenterology 61, 911–931.
17 Wilson, F.A. and Dietschy, J.M. (1972) Arch. Intern. Med. 130, 584–594.
18 Dietschy, J.M. and Siperstein, M.D. (1965) J. Clin. Invest. 44, 1311–1327.
19 Andersen, J.M. and Dietschy, J.M. (1979) J. Lipid Res. 20, 740–752.
20 Turley, S.D., Andersen, J.M. and Dietschy, J.M. (1981) J. Lipid Res. 22, 551–569.
21 Spady, D.K. and Dietschy, J.M. (1983) J. Lipid Res. 24, 303–315.
22 Jeske, D.J. and Dietschy, J.M. (1980) J. Lipid Res. 21, 364–376.
23 Brown, M.S., Goldstein, J.L. and Dietschy, J.M. (1979) J. Biol. Chem. 254, 5144–5249.
24 Stange, E.F., Alavi, M., Schneider, A., Preclik, G. and Ditschuneit, H. (1980) Biochim. Biophys. Acta 620, 520–527.
25 Panini, S.R. and Rudney, H. (1980) J. Biol. Chem. 255, 11633–11636.
26 Young, N.L., Saudek, C.D., Crawford, S.A. and Zuckerbrod, S.L. (1982) J. Lipid Res. 23, 257–265.
27 Field, F.J., Erickson, S.K., Shrewsburg, M.A. and Cooper, A.D. (1982) J. Lipid Res. 23, 105–113.
28 Sugano, M., Ide, T., Okamatsu, H. and Takahara, H. (1977) Biochem. Biophys. Res. Commun. 79, 1092–1097.
29 Dietschy, J.M. (1973) in: Nutrition and Metabolism in Medical Practice (Luhby, A.L., Ed.) pp. 37–48, Futura, Mount Kisco.
30 Sylvén, C. and Borgström, B. (1969) J. Lipid Res. 10, 179–182.
31 Andersen, J.M., Turley, S.D. and Dietschy, J.M. (1982) Biochim. Biophys. Acta 711, 421–430.
32 Dietschy, J.M. and Wilson, J.D. (1968) J. Clin. Invest. 47, 166–174.
33 Dietschy, J.M. and Gamel, W.G. (1971) J. Clin. Invest. 50, 872–880.
34 Shefer, S., Hauser, S., Lapar, V. and Mosbach, E.H. (1973) J. Lipid Res. 14, 400–405.
35 Stange, E.F., Alavi, M., Schneider, A., Ditschuneit, H. and Poley, J.R. (1981) J. Lipid Res. 22, 47–56.
36 Stange, E.F. and Dietschy, J.M. (1983) J. Lipid Res. 24, 72–82.
37 Shefer, S., Hauser, S., Lapar, V. and Mosbach, E.H. (1972) J. Lipid Res. 13, 402–412.
38 Panini, S.R., Lehrer, G., Rogers, D.H. and Rudney, H. (1979) J. Lipid Res. 20, 879–889.
39 Muroya, H.H., Sodhi, S. and Gould, R.G. (1977) J. Lipid Res. 18, 301–308.
40 Merchant, J.L. and Heller, R.A. (1977) J. Lipid Res. 18, 722–733.
41 Stange, E.F., Suckling, K.E. and Dietschy, J.M. (1983) J. Biol. Chem. 258, 12868–12875.
42 Stange, E.F., Schneider, A., Preclik, G. and Ditschuneit, H. (1981) Biochim. Biophys. Acta 666, 291–293.
43 Tabacik, C., Aliau, S., Astruc, M. and DePaulet, A.C. (1981) Biochim. Biophys. Acta 666, 433–441.
44 Sable-Amplis, R. and Sicart, R. (1982) Biochem. Biophys. Res. Commun. 108, 1093–1100.
45 Dietschy, J.M. (1968) J. Clin. Invest. 47, 286–300.
46 Gebhard, R.L and Cooper, A.D. (1978) J. Biol. Chem. 253, 2790–2796.
47 Gebhard, R.L. and Prigge, W.F. (1981) J. Lipid Res. 22, 1111–1118.

48 Stange, E.F., Schneider, A., Alavi, M., Ditschuneit, H. and Poley, J.R. (1981) in: Bile Acids and Lipids (Paumgartner, G., Stiehl, A. and Gerok, W., Eds.) pp. 57–66, MTP, Lancaster.
49 Stange, E.F., Preclik, G., Schneider, A., Alavi, M. and Ditschuneit, H. (1981) Biochim. Biophys. Acta 663, 613–620.
50 Stange, E.F., Schneider, A., Preclik, G., Alavi, M. and Ditschuneit, H. (1981) Lipids 16, 397–400.
51 Turley, S.D. and West, C.E. (1976) Lipids 11, 511–517.
52 Feingold, K.R., Wiley, M.H., Moser, A.H., Lau, D.T., Lear, S.R. and Siperstein, M.D. (1982) J. Lab. Clin. Med. 100, 405–410.
53 Turley, S.D. and Dietschy, J.M. (1980) J. Cardiovasc. Pharm. 2, 281–297.
54 Cayen, M.N. and Dvornik, D. (1979) J. Lipid Res. 20, 162–174.
55 Weis, H.J. and Dietschy, J.M. (1969) J. Clin. Invest. 48, 2398–2408.
56 Andersen, J.M. and Dietschy, J.M. (1976) Science 193, 903–905.
57 Andersen, J.M. and Dietschy, J.M. (1977) J. Biol. Chem. 252, 3652–3659.
58 Bochenek, W.J. and Rodgers, J.B. (1979) Biochim. Biophys. Acta 575, 57–62.
59 Stange, E.F., Preclik, G., Schneider, A., Seiffer, E. and Ditschuneit, H. (1981) Biochim. Biophys. Acta 678, 202–206.
60 Shefer, S., Hauser, S., Lapar, V. and Mosbach, E.H. (1972) J. Lipid Res. 13, 571–573.
61 Andersen, J.M. and Dietschy, J.M. (1977) J. Biol. Chem. 252, 3646–3651.
62 Sugano, M., Fujisaki, Y., Oku, H. and Ide, T. (1981) J. Nutr. 112, 51–59.
63 Schwartz, S.E., Starr, C., Bachman, S. and Holtzapple, P.G. (1983) J. Lipid Res. 24, 746–752.
64 Weis, H.J. and Dietschy, J.M. (1974) Eur. J. Clin. Invest. 4, 33–42.
65 Brasitus, T.A. and Schachter, D. (1982) Biochemistry 21, 2242–2246.
66 Quaroni, A.J., Wands, R.L., Trelstad, R.L. and Isselbacher, K.J. (1979) J. Cell. Biol. 80, 248–265.
67 Stein, Y., Halperin, G. and Stein, O. (1981) Biochim. Biophys. Acta 663, 569–574.
68 Pittman, R.C., Green, S.R., Attie, A.D. and Steinberg, D. (1979) J. Biol. Chem. 254, 6876–6879.
69 Pittman, R.C., Attie, D., Carew, T.E. and Steinberg, D. (1982) Biochim. Biophys. Acta 710, 7–14.
70 Innerarity, T.L., Pitas, R.E. and Mahley, R.W. (1980) J. Biol. Chem. 255, 11163–11172.
71 Koelz, H.R., Sherrill, B.C., Turley, S.D. and Dietschy, J.M. (1982) J. Biol. Chem. 257, 8061–8072.
72 Suzuki, N., Fidge, N., Nestel, P. and Yin, J. (1983) J. Lipid Res. 24, 253–264.
73 Suzuki, N., Fidge, N. and Nestel, P. (1983) Biochim. Biophys. Acta 750, 457–464.
74 Pittman, R.C., Carew, T.E., Attie, A.D., Witztum, J.L., Watanabe, Y. and Steinberg, D. (1982) J. Biol. Chem. 257, 7994–8000.
75 Slater, H.R., Packard, C.J., Bicker, S. and Shepherd, J. (1980) J. Biol. Chem. 255, 10210–10213.
76 Dietschy, J.M., Turley, S.D. and Spady, D.K. (1983) in: Liver in Metabolic Diseases (Bianchi, L., Gerok, W., Landmann, L., Sickinger, K. and Stalder, G.A., Eds.) pp. 25–39, MTP, Lancaster.
77 Stange, E.F. and Dietschy, J.M. (1983) Proc. Natl. Acad. Sci. (U.S.A.) 80, 5739–5743.
78 Treadwell, C.R. and Vahouny, G.V. (1968) in: Handbook of Physiology (Code, C.F., Ed.) pp. 1407–1438, Waverly Press, Baltimore, MD.
79 Vahouny, G., Falwal, V. and Treadwell, C.R. (1957) Am. J. Physiol. 188, 342–346.
80 Vahouny, G.V. and Treadwell, C.R. (1958) Proc. Soc. Exp. Biol. Med. 99, 293–295.
81 Bennett Clark, S.K. and Norum, R. (1977) J. Lipid Res. 18, 293–300.
82 Spector, A.A., Mathur, S.N. and Kaduce, T.L. (1979) Progr. Lipid Res. 18, 31–53.
83 Haugen, R.K. and Norum, R. (1976) Scand. J. Gasteroenterol. 11, 615–621.
84 Norum, K.R., Lilljeqvist, A.-C. and Drevon, C.A. (1977) Scand. J. Gastroenterol. 12, 281–288.
85 Field, F.J., Cooper, A.D. and Erickson, S.K. (1982) Gastroenterology 83, 873–880.
86 Helgerud, P., Saarem, K. and Norum, K.R. (1981) J. Lipid Res. 22, 271–277.
87 Norum, K.R., Helgerud, P. and Lilljeqvist, A.-C. (1981) Scand. J. Gastroenterol. 16, 402–410.
88 Suckling, K.E., Stange, E.F. and Dietschy, J.M. (1983) FEBS Lett. 151, 111–116.
89 Beg, F.H., Stonik, J.A. and Brewer, H.B. (1978) Proc. Natl. Acad. Sci. (U.S.A.) 75, 3678–3682.
90 Sylvén, C. and Nordstrom, C. (1970) Scand. J. Gastroenterol. 5, 57–63.
91 Norum, K.R., Helgerud, P., Peterson, L.B., Groot, P.H.E. and DeJonge, H.R. (1983) Biochim. Biophys. Acta 751, 153–161.
92 Helgerud, P., Haugen, R. and Norum, K.R. (1982) Eur. J. Clin. Invest. 12, 493–500.

93 Heider, J.G., Pickens, C.E. and Kelly, L.A. (1983) J. Lipid Res. 24, 1127–1134.
94 Gallo, L.L. and Treadwell, C.R. (1963) Proc. Soc. Exp. Biol. Med. 114, 69–72.
95 Gallo, L.L., Cheriathundam, E. and Vahouny, G.V. (1978) Arch. Biochem. Biophys. 191, 42–48.
96 Borja, C.R., Vahouny, G.V. and Treadwell, C.R. (1964) Am. J. Physiol. 206, 223–228.
97 Gallo, L.L., Chiang, Y., Vahouny, G.V. and Treadwell, C.R. (1980) J. Lipid Res. 21, 537–545.
98 Watt, S.M. and Simmonds, W.J. (1981) J. Lipid Res. 22, 157–165.
99 Lossow, W.J., Migliorini, R.H., Brot, N. and Chaikoff, I.L. (1964) J. Lipid Res. 5, 198–202.
100 Gallo, L. (1977) Proc. Soc. Exp. Biol. Med. 156, 277–281.
101 Bhat, S.G. and Brockman, H.L. (1982) Biochem. Biophys. Res. Commun. 109, 486–492.
102 Sylvén, C. and Borgström, B. (1968) J. Lipid Res. 9, 596–601.
103 Rudel, L.L., Morris, M.D. and Felts, J.M. (1972) J. Clin. Invest. 51, 2686–2692.
104 Quintao, E.C., Drewiacki, R.A., Stechhahn, K., de Faria, E.C. and Sipahi, A.M. (1979) J. Lipid Res. 20, 941–951.
105 Stange, E.F. and Dietschy, J.M. (1985) J. Lipid Res., 26, 175–184.
106 Nervi, F.O., Weis, H.J. and Dietschy, J.M. (1975) J. Biol. Chem. 250, 4145–4151.
107 Field, F.J. and Mathur, S.N. (1983) J. Lipid Res. 24, 1049–1059.
108 Herold, G., Schneider, A., Ditschuneit, H. and Stange, E.F. (1984) Biochim. Biophys. Acta, 796, 27–33.

H. Danielsson and J. Sjövall (Eds.), *Sterols and Bile Acids*

CHAPTER 6

Cholesterol and biomembrane structures

D. CHAPMAN, MARY T.C. KRAMERS and C.J. RESTALL

Department of Biochemistry and Chemistry, Royal Free Hospital School of Medicine (University of London), Rowland Hill Street, London NW3 2PF (Great Britain)

(I) Introduction

The modern view of biomembrane structure is that it consists of an asymmetric lipid bilayer having proteins, both intrinsic and extrinsic, associated with it. The intrinsic proteins are embedded within and can span the bilayer [1–5]. Associated with this view of biomembrane structure is the idea that in many cases the lipid matrix can be in a fluid condition where the lipids are essentially above their transition temperatures (T_c) and able to diffuse within the bilayer matrix. An additional feature of certain biomembrane systems is the presence of cholesterol.

The organisation and function of cholesterol in biological membranes and the possible interactions with other lipids and proteins need to be clarified in order to achieve an understanding of many cellular functions at the molecular level. Various disease conditions have been linked with abnormal cholesterol concentrations in cell membranes. Recently the evolutionary development of cholesterol and its role in membrane specialisation have become of some interest.

In the present review we attempt to relate the insights obtained from a variety of biophysical studies to consider the role of cholesterol in biomembranes.

(II) The occurrence of sterols

Sterols in biological membranes possess an alcoholic hydroxyl group at C-3 and a branched chain of 8 or more carbon atoms at C-17. In mammalian cells, cholesterol is the major sterol present. Cellular membranes such as liver plasma membranes [6], erythrocyte [7,8] and myelin [7,9] membranes contain high levels of cholesterol in the molar ratios cholesterol : phospholipid of 0.83, 0.90 and 1.32 respectively. Taking into account the high level of cerebrosides in the myelin membrane, the sterol : lipid ratio is about 0.83.

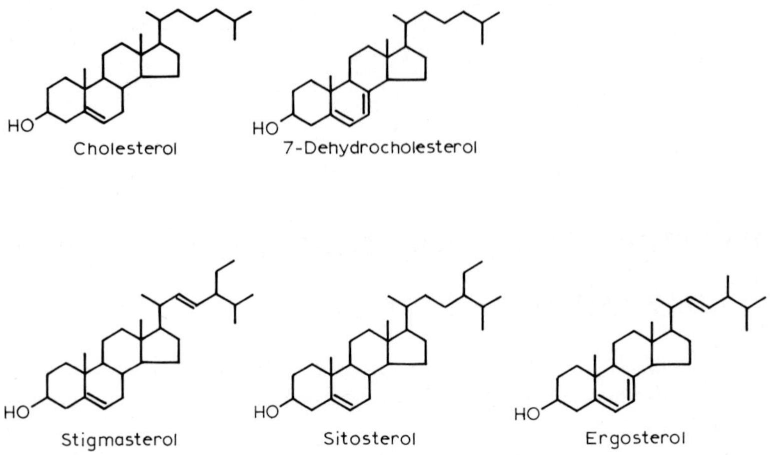

Fig. 1. Molecular structures of various sterols associated with membrane systems.

Relatively low cholesterol concentrations occur in membranes of nuclei, mitochondria and liver microsomes. The cholesterol : phospholipid ratio ranges from 0.11 to 0.33 [7,10]. However, mitochondria from brain and intestine are found to have cholesterol : phospholipid ratios of 0.51 and 0.60.

Although cholesterol is always the major sterol present, a few closely related sterols are detected in mammalian cells, namely 7-dehydrocholesterol (cholest-5,7-dien-3β-ol) [11], cholestanol (5α-cholestan-3β-ol) [12,13], lathosterol (5α-cholest-7-en-3β-ol) [14] and desmosterol (cholest-5,24-dien-3β-ol) [15]. 7-Dehydrocholesterol can make up 6–9% of the sterol content in subcellular membranes and in skin [11]. The structures of the most relevant mammalian and plant sterols are given in Fig. 1.

The sterols, with planar sterol nuclei and 3β-hydroxyl groups, are found in membranes in the free form, whereas the sterol esters are present only in trace amounts. Coprostanol, the A/B *cis* isomer of cholestanol, is excreted in faeces but formed by microbial action. In plants, sterols such as stigmasterol (24-ethyl-cholest-5,22-dien-3β-ol), sitosterol (24-ethyl-cholest-5-en-3β-ol) and campesterol (24-methyl-cholest-5-en-3β-ol) occur. Ergosterol (24-methyl-cholest-5,7,22-trien-3β-ol) is the predominant sterol in fungi and yeast. These sterols also possess a double bond in the side chain at C-22 and/or a methyl or ethyl group at C-24. Bacterial membranes are devoid of sterols. In a few membranes the sterol content can be varied. *Acholeplasma laidlawii* cells are of special interest. These organisms can grow in the absence of sterols, but are able to incorporate several sterols when present in the growth medium [16–18].

(III) Cholesterol–phospholipid interactions

The interactions between cholesterol and the other components of the biomembrane are important for understanding its biological function.

Monolayer studies were among the earliest techniques used to study cholesterol and to examine its role in biomembranes. Cholesterol itself forms a liquid condensed monomolecular film with very little compressibility [19]. This means that cholesterol is perpendicularly oriented at the surface at all surface pressures. The same behaviour is found for the other naturally occurring sterols in mammalian cells, such as 7-dehydrocholesterol, cholestanol and lathosterol [20]. The molecular area for these sterols ranges from 36.7 to 39.5 $Å^2$. The molecular area of the plant sterols is comparable with that of mammalian sterols [20]. The interaction forces between the sterol molecules seem to be little affected by the double bond in the ring system or modifications in the side chain. Also the change in orientation of the hydroxyl group from 3β to 3α does not alter significantly the cross-sectional area of the sterol at the surface. However, replacement of the hydroxyl group by an oxo group, or changes in the planar structure of the sterol nucleus, increase the molecular area.

Many monolayer studies have been made with phospholipids and sterols which have helped to clarify the details of the molecular properties of both types of molecule required to bring about the so-called "condensation effect" [21–23,27]. After various speculations and suggestions, it was shown that a *cis* double bond at the 9,10 position of the acyl chain was not necessary for condensation, and that *trans* isomers and even fully saturated phospholipid could bring about this "condensation" effect [24]. The condensation effects are not restricted to particular phospholipid classes but have been demonstrated to occur with phosphatidylcholines and phosphatidylethanolamines as well as with phosphatidic acid [25], sphingomyelin, phosphatidylglycerol and phospholipid derivatives [26].

Long-chain saturated phosphatidylcholines such as dipalmitoyl- and distearoylglycerophosphocholine which give a very condensed film do not show a reduction in cross-sectional area in the presence of cholesterol [27,28]. The shorter-chain saturated phosphatidylcholines which give a liquid expanded film such as dimyristoylglycerophosphocholine, dilauroylglycerophosphocholine, diundecanoylglycerophosphocholine and didecanoylglycerophosphocholine, show a reduction in mean molecular area in the presence of cholesterol [27]. Short-chain phosphatidylcholines such as dinonanoylglycerophosphocholine and dioctanoylglycerophosphocholine do not however show any "condensation effect" [29]. Phosphatidylcholines with one unsaturated chain containing up to 4 double bonds show a marked condensation effect, but little or no condensation is found for those with a fatty acid containing 6 double bonds or when both fatty acid chains are polyunsaturated [30].

The effects of cholesterol on phospholipid dispersions in water have been studied by a variety of biophysical techniques. These have created an understanding of the cholesterol condensation effect in molecular terms. Such studies have been made above and below the main phospholipid melting transition temperature (T_c) at which the phospholipid changes from the L-β gel phase to the L-α liquid-crystalline phase.

When cholesterol is present in dipalmitoylglycerophosphocholine dispersions in water, the transition temperature between the gel and fluid crystalline phase is lowered and the enthalpy of the transition is reduced [31]. The transition is

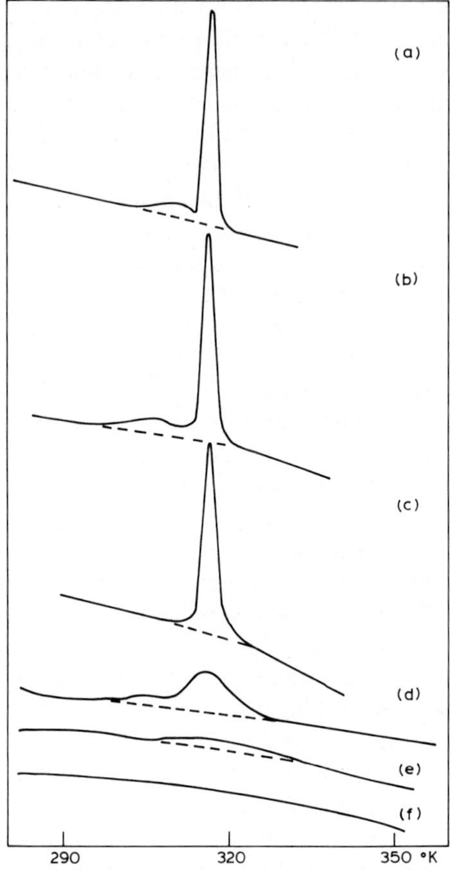

Fig. 2. Differential scanning calorimetry thermograms of 50 wt% dispersions in water of dipalmitoyl-glycerophosphocholine–cholesterol mixtures containing: (a) 0 mole%, (b) 5 mole%, (c) 12 mole%, (d) 20 mole%, (e) 32 mole%, (f) 50 mole% cholesterol [31].

completely removed at equimolar ratio of lipid to cholesterol (see Fig. 2). This ratio corresponds to the maximum amount of cholesterol which can be introduced into the lipid–water dispersions before cholesterol precipitation occurs.

These effects are not specific for dipalmitoyl glycerophosphocholine; thus, unsaturated phosphatidylcholines and the lipid extract of human erythrocyte ghosts exhibit similar behaviour. The explanation for this behaviour is that addition of cholesterol to the lipid–water system causes a reduction in the cohesive forces between adjacent ordered hydrocarbon chains of the lipid preventing chain crystallisation leading to an increase in fluidity of the lipid chains. The presence of water is also of prime importance in this interaction and cholesterol is precipitated when most of the water is removed.

The first calorimetric studies to show that the main phospholipid endotherm is removed with increasing amounts of cholesterol were the studies of Ladbrooke et al. [31]. They suggested that the enthalpy was totally removed at 50 mole%, whilst later studies by Hinz and Sturtevant [32] were interpreted to indicate that this occurred at 33 mole%. Later studies [33] using sensitive scanning calorimeters confirm the early conclusion of Ladbrooke et al. [31].

Both sonicated and unsonicated dispersions of dipalmitoylglycerophosphocholine and cholesterol in water have been studied by proton nmr spectroscopy. The observed line widths provide a useful indication of the mobility of the system. Analysis of the relative intensities of the observed signals locates the steroid between the phospholipid hydrocarbon chains of the bilayer with the steroid hydroxyl group adjacent to the phosphate groups of the phosphatidylcholines [34]. The number of hydrocarbon chain *gauche-trans* isomers of the phospholipid are reduced by the presence of the cholesterol molecules.

Deuterium magnetic resonance studies have also been carried out with phospholipid–cholesterol dispersions. The first experiments were done by Oldfield et al. [35] with perdeuterated phospholipids. Later, selectively deuterated phospholipids have been employed. The effect of cholesterol is to increase the deuterium quadrupole splittings, e.g. from 3.6 kHz to 7.8 kHz at an equimolar level, indicating an ordering of the lipid hydrocarbon chains. Other studies [36] have shown that different parts of the phospholipids are affected by the addition of cholesterol. The region of the lipid bilayer closer to the polar head group is more ordered than the terminal methyl region. Below the T_c phase transition a decrease in the deuterium quadrupole splitting occurs, consistent with an increase in fluidity [35]. More recently, deuterium nmr has been used to compare the molecular ordering of cholesterol in human erythrocyte membranes with results obtained in model systems [37]. [2,2,3,4,4,6-$^2H_6$]Cholesterol was incorporated into the erythrocyte membrane and measurements of the deuterium quadrupole splittings used to calculate the axis of motional averaging of cholesterol. The axis was found to make an angle of $81 \pm 2°$ with the C_3–^2H bond vector, very close to the $84 \pm 2°$ and $79 \pm 2°$ found for cholesterol in dimyristoylglycerophosphocholine and in egg phosphatidylcholine [37].

The interaction of cholesterol with dipalmitoylglycerophosphocholine and dipalmitoylglycerophosphoethanolamine has also been investigated using ^2H- and ^{31}P-nmr [38]. It was found that up to 50 mole% cholesterol could be incorporated without significantly changing the ^{31}P chemical shielding anisotropy. However, some of the deuterium quadrupole splittings were reduced by a factor of almost 2. These results were interpreted as showing that cholesterol has opposite effects on the hydrocarbon and polar head group regions of phospholipids; the ordering of the lipid chains by cholesterol is not accompanied by corresponding conformational changes in the polar region of the molecules. Instead the conformation of the head group is very similar to that observed in the liquid crystalline phase of pure phospholipids [38].

Later, more detailed studies of cholesterol–dipalmitoylglycerophosphoethanolamine (DPPE) interactions have been made using DPPE ^{13}C-labelled at the carbonyl group of the *sn*-2 chain and with ^{2}H introduced at the 4 position of the same chain or the 1 position of the ethanolamine head group [39,40]. The ^{13}C spectra show a characteristic change from an axially symmetric powder pattern in the L-β phase to an isotropic-like line in the L-α phase. This spectral change is due to an alteration in the conformation of the glycerol backbone as the bilayer expands. The presence of cholesterol can also induce this change and causes it to occur at progressively lower temperatures with increasing concentration. The ^{2}H spectra of acyl chain and head group labelled DPPE showed the presence of two components, one of these is very similar to gel-state lipid whilst the second has properties of both gel and liquid-crystalline lipid. These spectral changes are suggestive of the cholesterol molecule acting as a space that disrupts the lipid packing in pure DPPE bilayers.

A number of ESR experiments have been performed using spin label probes to investigate the effects of cholesterol. It is concluded that above T_c, a decrease in fluidity of the phospholipid bilayer occurs with increasing cholesterol content [41–43].

Studies have also been made using both steady-state and time-resolved fluorescence techniques. In some cases the effects of cholesterol have been interpreted in terms of an increase in the "microviscosity" [44]. In other cases the effects of cholesterol are discussed in terms of a change in the angle through which the fluorescent probe can reorient, and the wobbling diffusion coefficient (D_w), a measure of the dynamic friction. The cone angle is said to be decreased above T_c and increased below T_c by the presence of the cholesterol molecules [45]. However, the wobbling diffusion constant does not show the same effect. D_w increases below the phase transition but changes little above the transition in the presence of cholesterol.

Model studies have suggested that cholesterol is randomly arranged within the phospholipid bilayer [46]. This has led to a re-examination of the effect of cholesterol in phospholipid bilayers when studied by fluorescence spectroscopy [47] or deuterium nmr spectroscopy [36].

When the normalised change (polarisation and quadrupole splitting, respectively) is plotted against cholesterol concentration in the phospholipid bilayer, it is found that all the data can be fitted by the same exponential function. This applies over the whole concentration range. This is in contrast to the expected dependence which would be obtained if cholesterol formed a stoichiometric complex with the phospholipid molecules and is taken as evidence that random packing of cholesterol occurs.

IR analyses of phospholipid–water systems have shown that the main endothermic phase transition is accompanied by an abrupt change in the methylene band parameters [48]. The frequency of the band maximum has been used to monitor changes in lipid conformation. C–H and C–^{2}H stretching frequencies provide information on the static order (proportions of *trans* and *gauche* isomers) of the hydrocarbon chains. The temperature profiles of the band-maximum frequencies for the methylene stretching vibrations of dimyristoylglycerophosphocholine (DMPC) and dipalmitoylglycerophosphocholine (DPPC) are shown in Fig. 3. This method detects cooperative transitions at 23°C and 41°C, respectively, in agreement with the

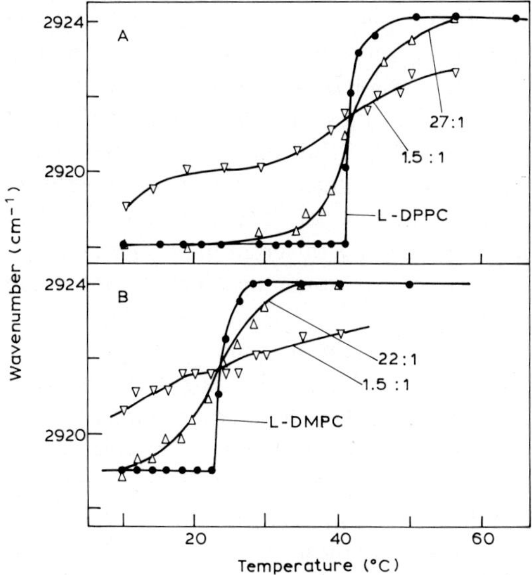

Fig. 3. Temperature dependence of the maximum wave number of the CH_2 asymmetric stretching vibrations in (a) DPPC–cholesterol and (b) DMPC–cholesterol dispersions at the molar ratios indicated. The temperature dependence for the pure lipids is also given [48].

results obtained by a variety of physical methods. The cholesterol effect may also be observed by the IR method. Elevation of the cholesterol content increases the number of *gauche* conformers (i.e. decreases the order) below the T_c, and decreases the number of *gauche* conformers (i.e. increases the order) above the T_c. The magnitude of this effect increases with cholesterol concentration. At very high cholesterol concentrations, there is almost no temperature-dependent change in the relative populations of *gauche* and *trans* conformers (i.e. the abrupt lipid phase transition is essentially smeared out and removed; Fig. 3).

A sophisticated theoretical treatment has been reported on cholesterol–phospholipid systems [49]. These calculations use statistical mechanics and cluster theory. In general it is agreed that cholesterol causes an ordering of the phospholipid hydrocarbon chain above the gel to liquid-crystalline phase transition temperature and a disordering of chain packing below this temperature.

The effect of cholesterol on lateral diffusion has also been studied. Rubenstein and co-workers [50] have found that the lateral diffusion of a fluorescent labelled phospholipid, phosphatidyl-*N*-(4-nitrobenzo-2-oxa-1,3-diazole)ethanolamine, exhibited an abrupt change in its lateral diffusion coefficient at 20 mole% cholesterol in a binary mixture of cholesterol and dimyristoylglycerophosphocholine. Two explanations for this behaviour have been proposed based on the existence of ordered microscopic domains characterised by ripples or strips of solid phase interspread with the more fluid domains of the phospholipid–cholesterol complex [51–53]. Such a structure would form barriers to free lateral diffusion. An alternative explanation put forward by Snyder and Freire [54] was based on mathematical modelling using Monte-Carlo methods. These authors proposed that at 20 mole% cholesterol, the microdomains of phospholipid–cholesterol complex were able to merge, thereby interrupting the pathway for diffusing molecules. Using monolayer studies, Muller-Landau and Cadenhead [55] suggested that the fitting of phospholipid molecules around the cholesterol molecules was altered at particular cholesterol levels. At certain molar ratios, a different number of layers of phospholipid surrounded the cholesterol molecule, thereby reaching a different molecular arrangement. A similar model has also been put forward by Martin and Yeagle [56] which also does not require the existence of phase boundaries.

In analysing the physical properties of bilayer membranes one must differentiate between (a) *the ordering* of the phospholipid molecules i.e. the time-averaged orientation and amplitude of the angular excursions of particular groups within the hydrocarbon chains and the head group region and (b) *the rate of motion* of the various segments. Further studies are necessary using relaxation measurements to establish the dynamic nature of the cholesterol–phospholipid interaction.

There have been various suggestions in the literature that cholesterol forms stoichiometric complexes with phospholipids. Based on line-width measurements of proton nmr a 1 : 1 complex between phospholipid and cholesterol was suggested [34]. Other workers have also proposed on the basis of X-ray diffraction [50] and differential scanning calorimetry measurements [33] a phospholipid : sterol ratio of 2 : 1. It was suggested that for a cholesterol concentration at or below 33 mole% each sterol molecule is surrounded by fatty acyl chains without cholesterol–cholesterol interaction. At higher concentrations, cholesterol–cholesterol interactions would occur. Some investigators have suggested that hydrogen bonding occurs between the cholesterol hydroxyl group and the phosphate ester oxygen atoms of the phospholipid [58–60]. A bonding of this type is probably unlikely because (a) the ester groups of the phospholipid must also be considered hydrated, (b) cholesterol incorporation does not affect the ^{31}P-nmr spectrum of various phosphatidylcholine liposomes [61] and (c) in a ^{31}P (^{1}H) nuclear Overhauser effect study on cholesterol–phosphatidylcholine vesicles it was shown that cholesterol does not interact with the phosphate group of phosphatidylcholine [62]. The possibility of an alignment of phospholipid carboxyl, cholesterol hydroxyl and water in a hydrogen belt has also been suggested by Brockerhoff [63]. However, there is no direct experimental evidence to support this concept. Structural analysis of egg phosphatidylcholine–cholesterol bilayers using X-ray diffraction and neutron diffraction [64,65] has indicated that the cholesterol molecule is immersed in the hydrocarbon region of the bilayer with its hydroxyl group (at 19.5 ± 1.5 Å from the bilayer centre) near the water interface. Epicholesterol (an isomer with a 3α-hydroxyl group) does not interact with phospholipids [66]. This is not necessarily due to an inability to form a hydrogen bond with the phospholipid, but could also be due to a difference in hydration water or interaction between the sterol molecules.

Phospholipids move remarkably quickly, having an estimated neighbour exchange rate of somewhat less that 10^{-6} sec. Such facile motion, which also exists in sarcoplasmic reticulum [67], is only slightly affected by addition of cholesterol to the bilayer [68]. There are few measurements of cholesterol diffusion in the plane of the bilayer. The question of transbilayer flip-flop of cholesterol and its transfer from one type of liposome or cell to another in a mixed suspension in water is discussed later.

Cholesterol causes a strong reduction in glucose, glycerol and Rb^+ permeability only of those liposome systems for which an interaction of the phospholipid with cholesterol is demonstrated [69]. The reduced permeability (which is proportional to the concentration of cholesterol) has been explained as being due to the increased packing and decreased mobility of the hydrocarbon chains. Studies with related sterols show that no effect is found for compounds lacking the side chain (5α-androstan-3β-ol) or with a non-planar sterol nucleus (5β-cholestan-3β-ol). However, when other derivatives are tested it is clear that the polar head group is an important requirement to ensure that the sterol penetrates the phospholipid bilayer and affects permeability. The 3α-hydroxysterols (epicholesterol) and several oxosterols were not able to reduce the membrane permeability [20,70,71].

Modulation of the cholesterol content of membranes affects passive permeability to water and other molecules. For example, permeability to Na^+ and K^+ is known to increase at the boundary between domains of rigid and fluid phospholipid within a bilayer which may result from cholesterol removal [72,73].

(IV) The effects of cholesterol upon membrane proteins

A question of some importance is whether cholesterol in biomembranes can affect the function of membrane proteins. Several systems have now been examined and a number of conflicting ideas have been put forward. Let us first consider what is known about "intrinsic" protein–cholesterol interactions.

Based upon studies of the sarcoplasmic reticulum Ca^{2+}-ATPase, it has been stated that the structure of membrane proteins is designed so as to exclude direct interaction with cholesterol [74]. This exclusion was said to be due to the presence of a single shell of phospholipids, termed an annulus, bound relatively tightly to the protein. The suggested mechanism was that the annular interactions of phospholipids were more rigid and immobilised than the phospholipid distant from the protein. The cholesterol was envisaged as preferring the more fluid phospholipid environment to the more rigid annular environment. This effect was extended and generalised to include a major class of membrane proteins having diverse biochemical functions [74].

The evidence to support the idea that many, if not all, membrane proteins possess a immobile, long-lived annulus was of two kinds: (a) biochemical and (b) spin-label studies. The first was based upon the fact that to maintain full enzyme activity, at least 30 lipid molecules per protein are required. The second was the presence of an immobile ESR signal at high protein to phospholipid content. Tanford has shown however that phospholipid is not essential for full enzymatic activity and that the hydrophobic fluid environment of a detergent is quite sufficient [75]. Furthermore, deuterium magnetic resonance studies on reconstituted ATPase systems have cast considerable doubt on the existence of a long-lived phospholipid annulus associated with the Ca^{2+}-ATPase [76], i.e. all the phospholipid appears to completely exchange within a lifetime of at least 10^{-4} sec. Of course, the lipids adjacent to a membrane protein may be perturbed on a shorter time scale, 10^{-8} sec.

Other experiments carried out with sarcoplasmic reticulum membranes gave results that do not support the idea that cholesterol is excluded by a lipid annulus. This work showed that as the cholesterol content of the biomembrane was raised, the enzyme activity decreased [77,78]. Spin-labelled cholesterol has also been used to study this problem with the conclusion that cholesterol does contact the surface of the protein, but with a lower probability than does the lipid [79].

Experiments with other membrane proteins also show effects due to the presence of cholesterol. Bacteriorhodopsin for example shows a reduction in protein mobility and a lateral segregation of the protein when cholesterol is present [80]. Cholesterol has been shown to have an inhibitory effect upon the Na^+/K^+-ATPase. It was suggested this is probably associated with the general effect of reducing phospholipid fluidity [81,82]. The incorporation of cholesterol into membranes of rat kidney fibroblasts caused two cell membrane enzymes, adenylate cyclase and Na^+/K^+-ATPase to exhibit decreased activity. The decrease in adenylate cyclase activity was directly proportional to the uptake of cholesterol [83].

Effects on the Na^+–K^+ pump of erythrocytes when the membrane cholesterol is depleted have been demonstrated. K^+ influx was reduced [84] whereas other workers have reported increased Na^+ efflux [85] and increased selectivity of the pump for internal Na^+ [86]. We have simultaneously measured Na^+ and K^+ transport via the Na^+–K^+ pump in thymocytes [87,88]. Cholesterol depletion activated pump-mediated Na^+ efflux but inhibited pump-mediated K^+ influx, whereas under normal physiological conditions these two fluxes are stoichiometrically linked [88–90]. Furthermore, the mode of functioning of the pump was altered, i.e. Na^+–Na^+ exchange instead of the normal Na^+–K^+ exchange occurred. It was suggested that in this case cholesterol depletion may cause molecular rearrangements of the multimeric enzyme protein within the phospholipid bilayer [89].

Some workers suggest that cholesterol may modulate the depth to which integral proteins are inserted within the bilayer, and the expression, for example, of membrane antigens on the cell surface. Borochov and Shinitzky [92] have labelled SH groups of erythrocyte membrane proteins covalently with fluorescent reagents. Tagged cells were enriched with or depleted of cholesterol. Upon increasing the cholesterol–phospholipid ratio the fluorescence spectra changed in a manner suggesting increased exposure of fluorophores to a hydrophilic environment. That is, the labelled membrane proteins were more exposed at the cell surface. Similar results were reported by Shinitzky and Rivnay [93] for the effects of cholesterol on the vertical mobility of integral proteins in sarcoplasmic reticulum and erythrocyte membranes.

Having considered the biophysical studies of cholesterol in phospholipid bilayers, it is now necessary to examine the biological role of cholesterol in the light of these conclusions.

(V) The effects of cholesterol on cellular functions

Studies of intact cells have shown that manipulation of cellular cholesterol alters cellular physiology and morphology. Many of these observations may be related to the effects of cholesterol on membrane fluidity and permeability, or protein rotation and enzyme activity. For example, cholesterol depletion or enrichment affects pump-mediated Na^+ and K^+ transport in erythrocytes [84–86,94] and thymocytes [87,88], K^+ transport in fibroblasts [95], and the intracellular concentration of these cations [94]. However, modulation of membrane fluidity by cholesterol does not modify binding to the α-adrenergic receptor or platelet adenylate cyclase activity [96]. The physiological processes of cell–cell adhesion and fusion are important in endo- and exocytosis, aggregation, growth regulation and the cytotoxic response of T lymphocytes. Although such processes are not fully understood, cholesterol is clearly an important regulatory agent, and such processes are probably linked to the fluidity of the cell membrane. Enrichment of cellular cholesterol increases fusion of erythrocytes [97]. In contrast, Papahadjopoulos and co-workers [98] found that incorporation of equimolar quantities of cholesterol into vesicles composed of phospholipids in a liquid-crystalline state reduced their ability to fuse with one another. Cholesterol enrichment inhibits macrophage phagocytosis [99] but cholesterol depletion inhibits endocytosis [100]. Furthermore, cholesterol enhances epinephrine-stimulated platelet aggregation and serotonin secretion [101].

Cholesterol depletion of T lymphocyte membranes also inhibits the immune response, i.e. cell-mediated cytotoxicity [102]. Cholesterol enrichment or depletion inhibits Con A-stimulated transformation of lymphocytes [87,103]. However, functions dependent on protein synthesis may be inhibited in cholesterol-depleted cells, not primarily because of the loss of cholesterol, but because of the secondary loss of K^+.

Increased amounts of membrane cholesterol have been associated with abnormalities of cell shapes: for example, the erythrocytes of patients with liver disease develop a characteristic 'spur cell' appearance which is associated with an increase in membrane cholesterol. These cells regain their normal shape on removal of the excess cholesterol [94]. Increased osmotic fragility has been observed with cholesterol depletion in both mycoplasma [104] and in erythrocytes [94]. There are few rheological studies on cells and the role of cholesterol in determining normal cell shape is not known. However, it is almost certainly linked to the fluidity and permeability of the cell membrane.

Cholesterol serves as the biosynthetic precursor for several vital compounds, including a variety of steroid hormones and bile acids. Many of these compounds, and many other polyisoprenoid compounds biosynthetically related to cholesterol, act biologically as important regulatory compounds [105]. In mammals such regulatory compounds include steroid hormones and vitamins A and D. Steroids and other isoprene derivatives also play important regulatory roles in other phyla. Several insect hormones, for example, are isoprenoid derivatives [106] (cf. Chapter 8). Many of the floral scents of plants are isoprene derivatives.

In mammals, some of these regulatory compounds may act at membranes, by affecting membrane structure or the transport of ions or molecules [107–109]. It is possible that the chemical relationship between these compounds and cholesterol may determine their effects on biological membranes. In a recent review, Bloch [110] has extensively described the relationships between the structure of sterols and their effects on membrane function.

(VI) Cholesterol exchange

In mammals, cholesterol is carried via the plasma in each of the major lipoprotein classes, namely chylomicrons, very-low-density lipoproteins (VLDL), low-density lipoproteins (LDL) and high-density lipoproteins (HDL) [111–120] (cf. Chapters 2 and 4). Cholesterol delivered to the liver in the chylomicron remnant is mainly derived from the diet or from the novo synthesis in the intestine and so represents a net increase in cholesterol entering into the body and results in an appropriate compensatory suppression of hepatic cholesterol synthesis.

LDL transports cholesterol to most extrahepatic parenchymal cells [121]. In contrast, the adrenal gland, ovary and testis utilise HDL cholesterol [122]. Studies in vitro show that LDL uptake is mediated by high-affinity receptor binding of the lipoprotein, subsequent endocytosis and catabolism [123]. However, other studies show that a significant portion of free cholesterol in serum lipoproteins can be transferred to the mycoplasma cell membrane by simple exchange [123,124]. A similar process may occur in eucaryotic cells [94].

How does cholesterol leave the cell? Since most cells do not secrete cholesterol esters (the known exceptions are hepatocytes and intestinal epithelial cells), free cholesterol must take its way to the outer bilayer of the cell membrane, where it may be removed by appropriate acceptors. It is likely that a net loss from the cell membrane involves movement of cholesterol from an area in the membrane with a high cholesterol–phospholipid ratio to an area with a lower ratio in the acceptor. The appropriate acceptors for cholesterol removal include any phospholipid bilayer system that contains little or no free cholesterol [125]. In vivo this is intact or nascent HDL [126,127]. Nascent HDL is a disc of phospholipid surrounded on its hydrophobic perimeter by detergent-like apoproteins, such as the arginine-rich apoprotein and the HDL apoproteins, apo AI and apo AII [128]. It is secreted from the liver and probably from the intestine (Chapter 5) into the plasma. Cholesterol enters nascent or intact HDL, and the lecithin–cholesterol acyltransferase (LCAT) reaction converts it to cholesterol ester [129,130] (Chapter 4). Since the ester is insoluble in the phospholipid bilayer it oils out into the centre of the particle. In this way, nascent discs are converted to spheres, and space for a new substrate, cholesterol, is created at the surface of the particle. Lipoproteins in lymph may also produce similar effects on the cell surfaces exposed to this fluid.

A further route for cholesterol loss from the cell surface is via the fluid flowing past the exposed epithelial surfaces lining secretory or excretory ducts, for example

(a) in the bile from the bile canalicular face of the hepatic cell, (b) in the urine from the brush border of the kidney proximal tubular cell, (c) in milk from secretory tracts of the mammary glands. Further studies are required in this area.

(VII) The experimental manipulation of cholesterol

Experimentally, the cholesterol content of cell surface membranes may be modified in vivo e.g. in the guinea pig by dietary means [131] or by modification of the culture media of micro-organisms [104]. In vitro, cholesterol modulation has also been achieved by the use of inhibitors of sterol synthesis [95] or liposomes [97,103,132–134].

Pagano and Weinstein [135] suggest that there are 4 possible types of liposome–cell interaction, namely stable adsorption, fusion, endocytosis and lipid transfer. These can all occur depending upon the experimental conditions and the lipid used for the construction of the liposomes.

Liposomes have been used to assess how much of the erythrocyte cholesterol is exchangeable. This is a matter of controversy, with several investigators allowing for only a single pool of cholesterol [136–139], while others have observed significant non-exchangeable portions, leading to the conclusion that membrane cholesterol may exist in two or more distinguishable pools [140,141].

A number of studies have also attempted to measure the transmembrane movement, or “flip-flop”, of cholesterol. Poznansky and Lange [142] and Lenard and Rothman [143] have shown that in sonicated dipalmitoylglycerophosphocholine–cholesterol liposomes and in influenza virus membranes, respectively, the half-time for flip-flop of cholesterol was in excess of 6 days, if it occurred at all. However, other workers have reported rapid transmembrane and intermembrane movement of cholesterol in small unilamellar liposomes [144–147].

To interpret these conflicting reports, Poznansky and Lange [148] examined the exchange of cholesterol between phospholipid–cholesterol liposomes and an excess of erythrocyte ghosts. Under conditions of simple cholesterol exchange and in the absence of any net movement of cholesterol, only the cholesterol from the outer half of the bilayer is available for exchange. The process of cholesterol exchange requires the two membranes to come into close contact and is dependent on the nature of the fatty acid chains with respect to chain length and degree of unsaturation. However, if cholesterol is removed from the outer half of the liposome then flip-flop of cholesterol can occur from the inner half in response to this perturbation.

It is concluded that under equilibrium conditions lipids do not easily undergo transbilayer movement in liposomes or membranes [149–151]. On the other hand, phospholipids and cholesterol have been shown to undergo transmembrane movement in erythrocytes under non-equilibrium conditions or following membrane perturbation such as ghost formation or phospholipase treatment [152–154]. More recently Lange and co-workers have made studies of the rate of transmembrane movement of cholesterol in the membranes of human erythrocytes. Normally, cholesterol in intact erythrocytes is not accessible to cholesterol oxidase [155].

However, following enrichment of the cells with exogenous cholesterol or incubation with 0.1 mM chlorpromazine [156], the whole of the cholesterol pool becomes available to the cholesterol oxidase. This means that the time-course of cholesterol oxidation can be determined and hence the rate of flip-flop. Based on such studies, a half-time of less than 3 sec at 37°C has been found for transposition of cholesterol across the bilayers [157]. These studies have also been extended to probe features of lipid–cholesterol organisation in the human erythrocyte membrane [158]. Clearly, such studies are relevant to our understanding of the mechanisms of cholesterol loss from cells in vivo by the methods outlined earlier.

(VIII) Cholesterol and disease

Abnormalities in cholesterol content or topology in the membrane, or its metabolism in vivo may contribute to the development of some pathological conditions (cf. Chapters 2 and 4).

(1) Liver disease

In both obstructive jaundice and parenchymal liver disease the amount of plasma free cholesterol is increased and the percentage of phosphatidylcholines among the total phospholipids is raised. Studies [159] have characterised the different lipoproteins that occur in both parenchymal liver disease and obstructive jaundice and have related many, but not all, of the changes to reduced plasma LCAT activity. Three separate LDL particles are present in obstructive jaundice (lipoprotein-X (LP-X), large particles rich in triglyceride and free cholesterol, and "normal-sized particles" with less cholesterol ester and more triglyceride than usual. In parenchymal liver disease only the "normal-sized particle" is found, although occasionally LP-X may occur. Abnormalities have been demonstrated in HDL and VLDL in patients with both types of liver disease when LCAT activity was low [160].

Net transfer of lipid occurs from the plasma to the erythrocyte membrane, presumably because of a shift in the equilibrium as the plasma lipoproteins become saturated with the excess cholesterol and phosphatidylcholine. This leads to membrane abnormalities and cholesterol–phospholipid ratios of up to 2 : 1. Changes in cellular physiology of the type referred to in section IV have also been reported [94,96,161]. These must reflect an alteration in lipid–protein interactions within the membranes. The molecular arrangement of the excessive amounts of cholesterol present in the cell membranes in diseased liver cells is not known. In model systems cholesterol is not present in molar amounts greater than 1 : 1. In liver disease a major change is in cellular morphology with the formation of abnormally shaped erythrocytes, as discussed earlier.

(2) Familial hypercholesterolaemia

Patients with familial hypercholesterolaemia have a mutation in the gene specifying the LDL receptor. In these patients, LDL degradation through the physiologic pathway is blocked, and each LDL particle survives in the circulation 2–3 times longer than it does in normal subjects [162–164]. As a result, the lipoprotein accumulates to abnormally high levels in plasma, and elevated levels of cholesterol are found in the tissues, leading to early demise from myocardial infarction. Eventually, the LDL is degraded through an alternate pathway [165–167].

(3) Ageing and atherosclerosis

The studies discussed earlier strongly indicate that cholesterol could regulate the permeability of biological membranes by affecting the internal viscosity and molecular motion of the phospholipids within the membrane. The degree of cohesion between the phospholipid molecules will in turn determine the motional freedom and localization of membrane enzymes, "carriers" and "gating" systems involved in transport and other membrane functions. The role of cholesterol can thus be considered as a stabilizing or a "dampening" mechanism, inhibiting structural changes in the membrane due to thermal, mechanical and other stresses.

Papahadjopoulos and co-workers suggest that while cholesterol is needed in order to provide a generally stable membrane framework, it is excluded from highly functional areas of membranes such as those containing Na^+/K^+-ATPase. These areas are likely to require greater structural fluctuations and molecular motion than more functionally inert areas. Following the same argument, it can also be suggested that an increased cholesterol to phospholipid ratio, along with decreased unsaturation (which would tend to enhance the cholesterol-condensing effect) could be detrimental to the function of the plasma membrane and indirectly to the cellular metabolism. Increased cholesterol content and also decreased unsaturation have been observed to correlate with ageing and the process of atherosclerosis [168–172]. Moreover, a rise in the free cholesterol content is one of the earlier events involving changes of aortic lipid composition in the preatherotic lesions, the fatty streaks [173–175].

The above evidence, combined with the studies on model membranes discussed earlier, and the well known "atherogenic" effect of cholesterol feeding in animals [176,177] suggests the possibility that increased cholesterol content in the membranes of aortic cells could be involved as an initiator of the process of atherogenesis. An hypothesis to this effect has been advanced, proposing that increased incorporation of cholesterol into the plasma membranes of arterial intima cells (induced by high levels of circulating plasma β-lipoproteins and/or endothelial injury) could have a critical inhibitory effect on several important membrane enzymes, with consequent alterations of the metabolic state of the cells [178]. There is also some evidence which describes the modulation of membrane-associated enzymes such as adenylate cyclase and acetylcholinesterase and an alteration of cellular morphology by interaction of plasma lipoproteins with erythrocytes [179–181].

Many of the early and subsequent events in the development of atherosclerosis could be accounted for by the initial effects of increased membrane cholesterol.

(4) Muscular dystrophy

Compared with normal muscle, dystrophic muscle exhibits delayed relaxation suggesting a disturbance of the excitation–contraction coupling mechanism. This process involves the release of calcium from the sarcoplasmic reticulum when the membrane becomes depolarised in response to a nerve impulse and the calcium ions in contact with the myofibrils cause them to contract. The muscle reverts to a relaxed condition when the calcium ions are removed by sequestration within the sarcoplasmic reticulum, a process that depends upon the active transport of calcium mediated by Ca^{2+}-activated ATPase in conjunction with a repolarisation of the membrane.

Biochemical alterations have been found in fragmented sarcoplasmic reticulum isolated from dystrophic human, mouse and chicken muscle. Alterations in calcium transport, ATP hydrolysis and phosphoenzyme formation have been reported. Some of these biochemical alterations in the dystrophic sarcoplasmic reticulum are suggested to be due to alterations of the lipid environment of these membranes; it has been suggested that the cholesterol content of dystrophic sarcoplasmic reticulum is elevated [182–187].

(5) Malaria

When multiplying, intracellular parasites do not synthesise their own membrane sterol, but must derive it from the host cell. It is interesting that the changes observed in erythrocytes infected with malaria merozoites are very similar to those brought about by depleting plasma membranes of cholesterol: increased permeability, changes in Na^+ and K^+ concentrations, increased acetylcholinesterase and adenylate cyclase activities [188–191].

(6) Cholesterol and cancer

Recent studies imply that sterol synthesis in proliferating cells is usually controlled by sterols that are produced intracellularly and is, therefore, independent of extracellular cholesterol [192]. Furthermore, a linkage between de novo cholesterol synthesis, cell proliferation, and DNA synthesis is indicated [87]. A discrete period of sterol synthesis is required for completion of the cell cycle. Studies with lymphocytes stimulated to blastogenesis by phytohaemagglutinin showed that a cycle of sterol synthesis preceded the cycle of DNA synthesis and cell division [193]. When sterol synthesis was blocked in L cell cultures by addition of an inhibitory sterol, two significant changes occurred: (a) the rate of DNA synthesis began to decline soon after addition of the inhibitory sterol and approached zero after about 80 h; (b) the concentration of sterol in the whole cells and in their plasma membranes declined, reaching a level about one half of the initial concentration by 24 h. Thereafter, the sterol concentration remained constant as the cells rounded-up, ceased to divide, and eventually were lost or died.

Other studies with rat thymocytes have also shown that extensive depletion of membrane cholesterol (via liposomes) virtually inhibits transformation [79]. Other concomitant marked changes in $Na^{+} + K^{+}$ transport were discussed earlier.

The need for an enhanced rate of sterol synthesis for a discrete period of time preceding DNA synthesis and cell proliferation can be explained in two ways: (a) the cells need an increment in cellular sterol for the production of the additional plasma membrane required to enclose two daughter cells. De novo synthesis may be the mode developed by cells to obtain the sterol increment, even if a steady-state exchange with extracellular cholesterol exists. (b) Modulation of membrane fluidity may be required during the cell cycle as a means for altering transport of nutrients and ions and other membrane functions. This modulation may be accomplished by varying the concentration of membrane sterol via changes in the rate of sterol synthesis. These two explanations are not mutually exclusive, and sterol synthesis in dividing cells may meet both a need for the production of new membrane and a requirement for changes in membrane fluidity. It should also be mentioned that mevalonate-derived compounds other than cholesterol are essential in the period preceding DNA synthesis (Chapter 2).

Thus, the regulation of sterol synthesis in hepatomas and leukaemias may be compared with that in proliferating normal tissues such as developing brain, crypt cells of the intestine, and phytohaemagglutinin-stimulated lymphocytes rather than with that in liver or in normal, unstimulated peripheral lymphocytes. It is possible that abnormal (unregulated) sterol synthesis may push resting into unregulated proliferation, i.e. into a malignant state.

The existence of such an abnormality would not necessarily imply that the sterol concentration of the cancer cells must be different from that of the normal cells of origin. However, a decrease in the cholesterol/phospholipid (C/PL) ratio of leukaemic cells as compared to normal cells has been reported [194–197]. Gottfried suggested that the altered lipid patterns found in leukaemic cells reflected cell immaturity [195]. All these lipid analyses were performed in whole cell extracts; it is uncertain whether the difference in C/PL ratio was due to alteration in the lipid composition of cell surface membranes or to differences in the relative content of various intracellular membranes between normal and leukaemic cells. Membranes from nuclei, mitochondria, endoplasmic reticulum, and other intracellular membranes contain phospholipid, but insignificant amounts of cholesterol, or none at all. Ideally, analysis of the lipids of isolated cell membranes from normal and tumour cells is necessary if firm conclusions concerning the nature of the changes in lipid composition are to be made.

No difference in the cholesterol–phospholipid ratio of the purified surface membranes of virally transformed and normal fibroblasts has been found [198–200]. However, an increase in the proportion of esterified cholesterol has been reported in virally transformed fibroblasts which appears to be caused by alterations in cholesterol metabolism [201].

Shinitzky and Inbar [202] found that lymphoma cells had a lower microviscosity (thus were more "fluid") than normal lymphocytes, a result consistent with the reported lower cholesterol content of these tumour cells. The same workers [203] also reported a lower microviscosity in human chronic lymphatic leukaemic cells as compared to normal lymphocytes. However, their studies have been contested. No difference was found in the microviscosity or C/PL ratio of leukaemic cells and normal lymphocytes [204,205]. The discrepancy is attributed to platelet contamination of the populations of normal but not leukaemic lymphocytes in the earlier studies.

The possibility of changes in the topology of membrane components cannot be excluded by the experimental technique used at present, and would contribute to alterations in cellular physiology.

(IX) Cholesterol evolution

The influence of plant sterols on the phase properties of phospholipid bilayers has been studied by differential scanning calorimetry and X-ray diffraction [206]. It is interesting that the phase transition of dipalmitoylglycerophosphocholine was eliminated by plant sterols at a concentration of about 33 mole%, as found for cholesterol in animal cell membranes. However, less effective modulation of lipid bilayer permeability by plant sterols as compared with cholesterol has been reported. The molecular evolution of biomembranes has received some consideration [207–209]. In his speculation on the evolution of sterols, Bloch [207] has suggested that in the prebiotic atmosphere "chemical evolution of the sterol pathway" if it did indeed occur, must have stopped at the stage of squalene "because of lack of molecular oxygen, an obligatory electron acceptor in the biosynthetic pathway of sterols". Thus, cholesterol is absent from anaerobic bacteria (procaryotes).

However, in procaryotes derivatives of one triterpene family, the hopanes, are widely distributed [207,208]. They may be localised in membranes, fulfilling there the same role as sterols play in eucaryotes, as a result of their similar size, rigidity and amphiphilic character. Their biosynthesis has many primitive features compared to that of sterols; it involves a hydration of squalene and does not require molecular oxygen, but could have evolved toward the latter once aerobic conditions had been established. Membrane reinforcement appears to be achieved in other procaryotes by other mechanisms, involving either 40-Å-long rigid hydrocarbon chains terminated by one polar group acting like a peg through the double layer or similar chains terminated by two polar groups acting like tie-bars across the membrane. These inserts can be tetraterpenes, e.g. carotenoids.

The triterpenes, e.g. tetrahymanol, are larger in cross-section than cholesterol. A better intermolecular fit is restored with acyclic lipids which have a larger cross-section than do the *n*-acyl chains found in eucaryotes. Increased effective cross-sections can be achieved by the introduction of *cis* double bonds; this is partly how *Tetrahymena pyriformis* adjusts the composition of its phospholipids in its sterol-free, tetrahymanol-containing state. Another way to obtain thicker lipids is to have branched chains. Whereas only *n*-acyl lipids have been reported in Tetrahymena and in cyanobacteria, branched-chain fatty acids are frequent in bacteria, and so are cyclopropyl or ω-cyclohexyl acids [209]. No data are available on whether triterpenes abolish lipid phase transitions and modify membrane permeability, features which are characteristic of cholesterol and other plant and animal sterols in model and eucaryotic cell surface membranes.

(X) Conclusions

(a) Cholesterol and related sterols are ubiquitous components of eucaryotic cell surfaces. The sterol molecule possesses certain unique features for incorporation into lipid bilayers and interdigitating among the hydrocarbon chains.

(b) Cholesterol–phospholipid interactions have been studied in monolayer and liposome systems using a variety of biophysical techniques. It is generally agreed that cholesterol modulates phospholipid fluidity and prevents or inhibits lipid chain crystallisation thereby removing the main melting phase transitions of the lipid matrix. The cholesterol molecules are probably randomly arranged in the plane of the lipid bilayer matrix. The possibilities of transmembrane movement of cholesterol, and whether cholesterol is symmetrically distributed within the membrane bilayer are still under debate.

(c) Cholesterol modifies membrane permeability e.g. to water molecules, and upon incorporation into a model or natural biomembrane has been shown to modify the function of some integral membrane proteins.

(d) Major changes in cell physiology may result from cell surface-cholesterol modulation. Furthermore, many biological regulatory compounds are derived from cholesterol. The chemical relationship between these compounds and cholesterol may determine their effects on biological membranes.

(e) Cholesterol exchange to and from cells in vivo is known to occur via the lipoproteins. In vitro, a variety of techniques is now available for the modulation of membrane cholesterol.

(f) Abnormalities in cellular cholesterol have been implicated in the development of several pathological conditions. An alteration in the content or topology of membrane cholesterol may lead to changes in membrane permeability and cellular physiology similar to those already investigated in model systems. Knowledge of the mechanisms of cholesterol transfer from cell surfaces via (a) lipoprotein–cell interaction, (b) cell–cell interaction and (c) from the membranes lining secretory tracts, may elucidate a variety of disease processes.

(g) Sterol synthesis requires an aerobic environment and sterols are absent from anaerobic bacteria. However, triterpenes are widely distributed in procaryotes; their biosynthesis has many primitive features compared to that of sterols. They may be localised in membranes fulfilling there the same role as sterols serve in eucaryotes as a result of their similar size, rigidity and amphiphilic character.

Acknowledgements

We wish to thank the Wellcome Trust and the Cancer Research Campaign for generous financial support, and Dr. Winfried Hoffmann and Dr. Richard Smallwood for helpful discussions.

References

1 Singer, S.J. and Nicholson, G.L. (1972) Science 175, 720–731.
2 Chapman, D. (1975) Quart. Rev. Biophys. 8, 185–235.
3 Oldfield, E. and Chapman, D. (1972) FEBS Lett. 23, 285–297.
4 Rothman, J.E. and Lenard, J. (1977) Science 195, 743–753.
5 Bretcher, M.S. (1973) Science 181, 622–629.
6 Dorling, P.R. and le Page, R.N. (1973) Biochim. Biophys. Acta 318, 33–40.
7 Ashworth, L.A.E. and Green, C. (1966) Science 151, 210–211.
8 Nelson, G.J. (1967) J. Lipid Res. 8, 374–379.
9 Demel, R.A., London, Y., Geurts van Kessel, W.S.M., Vossenberg, F.G.A. and van Deenen, L.L.M. (1973) Biochim. Biophys. Acta 311, 507–519.
10 Lee, T., Stephens, N., Moehl, A. and Snyder, F. (1973) Biochim. Biophys. Acta 291, 86–92.
11 Glover, J. and Green, C. (1957) Biochem. J. 67, 308–316.
12 Werbin, H., Chaikoff, J.L. and Imada, M.R. (1962) J. Biol. Chem. 237, 2072–2077.
13 Lasser, N.L. and Clayton, R.B. (1966) J. Lipid Res. 7, 413–421.
14 Miller, W.L. and Baumann, C.A. (1954) Proc. Soc. Exp. Biol. Med. 85, 561–564.
15 Smith, M.E., Fumagalli, R. and Paoletti, R. (1967) Life Sci. 6, 1085–1091.
16 Razin, S., Tourtellotte, M.E., McElhaney, R.N. and Pollack, J.D. (1966) J. Bacteriol. 91, 609–616.
17 de Kruijff, B., de Greef, W.J., van Eyk, R.V.W., Demel, R.A. and van Deenen, L.L.M. (1973) Biochim. Biophys. Acta 298, 479–499.
18 McElhaney, R.N. (1984) Biochim. Biophys. Acta 779, 1–142.
19 Pethica, B.A. (1955) Trans. Faraday Soc. 51, 1402–1411.
20 Demel, R.A. and de Kruijff, B. (1976) Biochim. Biophys. Acta 457, 109–132.
21 de Bernard, L. (1958) Bull. Soc. Chim. Biol. 40, 161–170.
22 Chapman, D. (1966) Ann. N.Y. Acad. Sci. 137, 745–754.
23 Phillips, M.C. and Chapman, D. (1968) Biochim. Biophys. Acta 163, 301–313.
24 Chapman, D., Owens, N.F. and Walker, D.A. (1966) Biochim. Biophys. Acta 120, 148–155.
25 Shah, D.O. and Schulman, J.H. (1967) J. Lipid Res. 8, 215–226.
26 de Kruijff, B., Demel, R.A., Stolboom, A.J., van Deenen, L.L.M. and Rosenthal, A.F. (1973) Biochim. Biophys. Acta 307, 1–19.
27 Demel, R.A., van Deenen, L.L.M. and Pethica, B.A. (1967) Biochim. Biophys. Acta 135, 11–19.
28 Ghosh, D., Williams, M.A. and Tinoco, J. (1973) Biochim. Biophys. Acta 291, 351–362.
29 Joos, P. and Demel, R.A. (1969) Biochim. Biophys. Acta 183, 447–457.
30 Demel, R.A., Geurts van Kessel, W.S.M. and van Deenen, L.L.M. (1972) Biochim. Biophys. Acta 266, 26–40.
31 Ladbrooke, B.D., Williams, R.M. and Chapman, D. (1968) Biochim. Biophys. Acta 150, 333–340.
32 Hinz, H.-J. and Sturtevant, J.M. (1972) J. Biol. Chem. 247, 3697–3700.
33 Mabrey, S., Mateo, P.L. and Sturtevant, J.M. (1978) Biochemistry 17, 2464–2468.
34 Phillips, M.C. and Finer, E.G. (1974) Biochim. Biophys. Acta 356, 199–206.
35 Oldfield, E., Chapman, D. and Derbyshire, W. (1971) FEBS Lett. 6, 102–104.
36 Jacobs, R. and Oldfield, E. (1979) Biochemistry 18, 5280–5285.
37 Kelusky, E.C., Duforc, E.J. and Smith, I.C.P. (1983) Biochim. Biophys. Acta 735, 302–304.

38 Brown, M.F. and Seelig, J. (1978) Biochemistry 17, 381–384.
39 Wittebort, R.J., Blume, A., Huang, T.-H., Das Gupta, S.K. and Griffin, R.G. (1982) Biochemistry 21, 3487–3502.
40 Blume, A. and Griffin, R.G. (1982) Biochemistry 21, 6230–6242.
41 Barratt, M.D., Green, D.K. and Chapman, D. (1969) Chem. Phys. Lipids 3, 140–144.
42 Hubbell, W.L. and McConnell, H. (1971) J. Am. Chem. Soc. 93, 314–326.
43 Oldfield, E. and Chapman, D. (1971) Biochem. Biophys. Res. Commun. 43, 610–616.
44 Shinitzky, M. and Barenholz, Y. (1978) Biochim. Biophys. Acta 515, 367–394.
45 Kawato, S., Kinosita, K. and Ikegami, A. (1977) Biochemistry 16, 2319–2324.
46 Cornell, B.A., Chapman, D. and Peel, W.E. (1974) Chem. Phys. Lipids 23, 223–237.
47 Hoffmann, W., Pink, D.A., Restall, C.J. and Chapman, D. (1981) Eur. J. Biochem. 114, 585–589.
48 Cortijo, M., Alonso, A., Gomez-Fernandez, J.C. and Chapman, D. (1982) J. Mol. Biol. 157, 597–618.
49 Pink, D.A. and Chapman, D. (1979) Proc. Nal. Acad. Sci. (U.S.A.) 76, 1542–1546.
50 Rubenstein, J.L.R., Smith, B.A. and McConnell, H.M. (1979) Proc. Natl. Acad. Sci. (U.S.A.) 76, 15–18.
51 Copeland, B.R. and McConnell, H.M. (1980) Biochim. Biophys. Acta 599, 95–109.
52 Presti, F.T. and Chan, S.I. (1982) Biochemistry 21, 3821–3830.
53 Presti, F.T., Pace, R.J. and Chan, S.I. (1982) Biochemistry 21, 3831–3835.
54 Snyder, B. and Freire, E. (1980) Proc. Natl. Acad. Sci. (U.S.A.) 77, 4055–4059.
55 Muller-Landau, F. and Cadenhead, D.A. (1979) Chem. Phys. Lipids 25, 315–328.
56 Martin, R.B. and Yeagle, P.L. (1978) Lipids 13, 594–597.
57 Engelman, D.E. and Rothman, J.E. (1972) J. Biol. Chem. 247, 3694–3697.
58 Darke, A., Finer, E.G., Flook, A.G. and Phillips, M.C. (1972) J. Mol. Biol. 63, 265–279.
59 Green, J.R., Edwards, P.A. and Green, C. (1973) Biochem. J. 135, 63–71.
60 Verma, S.P. and Wallach, D.F.H. (1973) Biochim. Biophys. Acta 330, 122–131.
61 Cullis, P.R., de Kruyff, B. and Richards, R.E. (1975) Biochim. Biophys. Acta 426, 433–446.
62 Yeagle, P.L., Hutton, W.C., Huang, C.-H. and Martin, R.B. (1975) Proc. Natl. Acad. Sci. (U.S.A.) 72, 3477–3481.
63 Brockerhoff, H. (1974) Lipids 9, 645–650.
64 Franks, N.P. (1976) J. Mol. Biol. 100, 345–358.
65 Worcester, D.L. and Franks, N.P. (1976) J. Mol. Biol. 100, 359–378.
66 Demel, R.A., Bruckdorfer, K.R. and van Deenen, L.L.M. (1972) Biochim. Biophys. Acta 255, 311–320.
67 Scandella, C.J., Devaux, P. and McConnell, H.M. (1972) Proc. Natl. Acad. Sci. (U.S.A.) 69, 2056–2060.
68 Devaux, P. and McConnell, H.M. (1972) J. Am. Chem. Soc. 94, 4475–4481.
69 Demel, R.A., Bruckdorfer, K.R. and van Deenen, L.L.M. (1972) Biochim. Biophys. Acta 255, 321–330.
70 de Gier, J., Mandersloot, J.G. and van Deenen, L.L.M. (1968) Biochim. Biophys. Acta 150, 666–675.
71 de Kruijff, B., Demel, R.A. and van Deenen, L.L.M. (1972) Biochim. Biophys. Acta 255, 331–347.
72 Papahadjopoulos, D., Jacobson, K., Nir, S. and Isac, T. (1973) Biochim. Biophys. Acta 311, 330–348.
73 Wu, S.H.-W. and McConnell, H.M. (1973) Biochem. Biophys. Res. Commun. 55, 484–491.
74 Warren, G.B., Houslay, M.D., Metcalfe, J.C. and Birdsall, N.J.M. (1975) Nature (London) 255, 684–687.
75 Dean, W.L. and Tanford, C. (1977) J. Biol. Chem. 252, 3551–3553.
76 Rice, D.M., Meadows, M.D., Scheinman, A.O., Goni, F.M., Gomez-Fernandez, J.C., Moscarello, M.A., Chapman, D. and Oldfield, E. (1979) Biochemistry 18, 5893–5903.
77 Madden, T., Chapman, D. and Quinn, P.J. (1979) Nature (London) 279, 538–541.
78 Ortega, A. and Mas-Oliva, J. (1984) Biochim. Biophys. Acta 773, 231–236.
79 Silvius, J.R., McMillen, D.A., Saley, N.D., Jost, P.C. and Griffiths, D.H. (1984) Biochemistry 23, 538–547.
80 Cherry, R.J., Muller, V., Holenstein, C. and Heyn, M.P. (1980) Biochim. Biophys. Acta 596, 145–151.

81 Kimelberg, H.K. and Papahadjopoulos, D. (1974) J. Biol. Chem. 249, 1071–1080.
82 Kimelberg, H.K. (1975) Biochim. Biophys. Acta 413, 143–156.
83 Klein, I., Moore, L. and Pastan, I. (1978) Biochim. Biophys. Acta 506, 42–53.
84 Poznansky, M., Kirkwood, D. and Solomon, A.K. (1973) Biochim. Biophys. Acta 330, 351–355.
85 Giraud, F., Claret, M. and Garay, R. (1976) Nature (London) 264, 646–648.
86 Claret, M., Garay, R. and Giraud, F. (1978) J. Physiol. 274, 247–263.
87 Bottomley, J.M., Kramers, M.T.C. and Chapman, D. (1980) FEBS Lett. 119, 261–264.
88 Kramers, M.T.C., Patrick, J., Bottomley, J.M., Quinn, P.J., and Chapman, D. (1980) Eur. J. Biochem. 110, 579–585.
89 Skou, J.C. (1964) Progr. Biophys. Mol. Biol. 14, 133–166.
90 Post, R.L., Merritt, C.R., Kinsolving, C.R. and Albright, C.D. (1960) J. Biol. Chem. 235, 1796–1802.
91 Glynn, I.M. (1956) J. Physiol. 134, 278–310.
92 Borochov, H. and Shinitzky, M. (1976) Proc. Natl. Acad. Sci. (U.S.A.) 73, 4526–4530.
93 Shinitzky, M. and Rivnay, B. (1977) Biochemistry 16, 982–986.
94 Cooper, R.A., Arner, E.C., Wiley, J.S. and Shattil, S.J. (1975) J. Clin. Invest. 55, 115–126.
95 Chen, H.W., Heiniger, H.-J. and Kandutsch, A.A. (1978) J. Biol. Chem. 253, 3180–3185.
96 Insel, P.A., Nirenberg, P., Turnbull, J. and Shattil, S.J. (1978) Biochemistry 17, 5269–5274.
97 Hope, M.J., Bruckdorfer, K.R., Hart, C.A. and Lucy, J.A. (1977) Biochem. J. 166, 255–263.
98 Papahadjopoulos, D., Poste, G., Schaeffer, B.E. and Vail, W.J. (1974) Biochim. Biophys. Acta 352, 10–28.
99 Dianzani, M.U., Torrielli, M.V., Canuto, R.A., Garcea, R. and Feo, F. (1976) J. Pathol. 118, 193–199.
100 Heiniger, H.J., Kandutsch, A.A. and Chen, H.W. (1976) Nature (London) 263, 515–517.
101 Shattil, S.J., Anaya-Galindo, R., Bennett, J., Colman, R.W. and Cooper, R.A. (1975) J. Clin. Invest. 55, 636–643.
102 Heiniger, H.-J., Brunner, K.T. and Cerottini, J.-C. (1978) Proc. Natl. Acad. Sci. (U.S.A.) 75, 5683–5687.
103 Alderson, J.C.E. and Green, C. (1975) FEBS Lett. 52, 208–211.
104 le Grimellec, C. and Leblanc, G. (1978) Biochim. Biophys. Acta 514, 152–163.
105 Shopf, W.J. (1978) Sci. Am. 239, 85–102.
106 Schneiderman, H.A. and Gilbert, L.I. (1964) Science 143, 325–333.
107 Schachter, D. (1963) in: Transfer of Calcium and Strontium Across Biological Membranes (Wasserman, R.H., Ed.) pp. 197–210, Academic Press, New York.
108 Fell, H.B. and Dingle, J.T. (1963) Biochem. J. 87, 403–408.
109 Lucy, J.A., Luscombe, M. and Dingle, J.T. (1963) Biochem. J. 89, 419–425.
110 Bloch, K. (1983) CRC Crit. Rev. Biochem. 14, 47–92.
111 Hotta, S. and Chaikoff, I.L. (1955) Arch. Biochem. Biophys. 56, 28–37.
112 Friedman, M., Byers, S.O. and Michaelis, F. (1951) Am. J. Physiol. 164, 789–791.
113 Lindsey Jr., C.A. and Wilson, J.D. (1965) J. Lipid Res. 6, 173–181.
114 Dietschy, J.M. and Wilson, J.D. (1970) New Engl. J. Med. 282, 1128–1138, 1179–1183, 1241–1249.
115 Dietschy, J.M. and Siperstein, M.D. (1967) J. Lipid Res. 8, 97–104.
116 Dietschy, J.M. and Wilson, J.D. (1968) J. Clin. Invest. 47, 166–174.
117 Carrella, M. and Dietschy, J.M. (1977) Am. J. Dig. Dis. 22, 318–326.
118 Nervi, F.O. and Dietschy, J.M. (1978) J. Clin. Invest. 61, 895–909.
119 Andersen, J.M. and Dietschy, J.M. (1977) J. Biol. Chem. 252, 3646–3651.
120 Weis, H.J. and Dietschy, J.M. (1975) Biochim. Biophys. Acta 398, 315–324.
121 Goldstein, J.L. and Brown, M.S. (1977) Annu. Rev. Biochem. 46, 897–930.
122 Anderson, J.M. and Dietschy, J.M. (1978) J. Biol. Chem. 253, 9024–9032.
123 Slutzky, G.M., Razin, S., Kahane, I. and Eisenberg, S. (1977) Biochemistry 16, 5158–5163.
124 Clejan, S., Bittman, R. and Rottem, S. (1978) Biochemistry 17, 4579–4583.
125 Sniderman, A.D., Carew, T.E., Chandler, J.G. and Steinberg, D. (1974) Science 183, 526–528.
126 Carew, T.E., Koschinsky, T., Hayes, S.B. and Steinberg, D. (1976) Lancet 1, 1315–1217.
127 Stein, Y., Glangeaud, M.C., Fainaru, M. and Stein, O. (1975) Biochim. Biophys. Acta 380, 106–118.

128 Hamilton, R.L., Williams, M.C., Fielding, C.J. and Havel, R.J. (1976) J. Clin. Invest. 58, 667–680.
129 Glomset, J.A. and Norum, K.R. (1973) Adv. Lipid Res. 11, 1–65.
130 Stein, O., Vanderhoeck, J. and Stein, Y. (1976) Biochim. Biophys. Acta 431, 347–358.
131 Kroes, J. and Ostwald, R. (1971) Biochim. Biophys. Acta 249, 647–650.
132 Bruckdorfer, K.R., Edwards, P.A. and Green, C. (1968) Eur. J. Biochem. 4, 506–511.
133 Bruckdorfer, K.R., Demel, R.A., de Gier, J. and van Deenen, L.L.M. (1969) Biochim. Biophys. Acta 183, 334–345.
134 Arbogast, L.Y., Rothblat, G.H., Leslie, M.H. and Cooper, R.A. (1976) Proc. Natl. Acad. Sci. (U.S.A.) 73, 3680–3684.
135 Pagano, R.E. and Weinstein, J.N. (1978) Annu. Rev. Biophys. Bioeng. 7, 435.
136 Hagerman, J.S. and Gould, R.G. (1951) Proc. Soc. Exp. Biol. Med. 78, 329–332.
137 Bruckdorfer, K.R. and Green, C. (1967) Biochem. J. 104, 270–277.
138 Basford, J.M., Glover, J. and Green, C. (1964) Biochim. Biophys. Acta 84, 764–766.
139 Quarfordt, S.H. and Hilderman, H.L. (1970) J. Lipid Res. 11, 528–535.
140 Bell, F.P. and Schwartz, C.J. (1971) Biochim. Biophys. Acta 231, 553–557.
141 d'Hollander, F. and Chevallier, F. (1972) J. Lipid Res. 13, 733–744.
142 Poznansky, M.J. and Lange, Y. (1976) Nature (London) 259, 420–421.
143 Lenard, J. and Rothman, J.E. (1976) Proc. Natl. Acad. Sci. (U.S.A.) 73, 391–395.
144 Patzer, E.J., Shaw, J.M., Moore, N.F., Thompson, T.E. and Wagner, R.E. (1978) Biochemistry 17, 4192–4200.
145 Sefton, B.M. and Gaffney, B.J. (1979) Biochemistry 18, 436–442.
146 Backer, J.M. and Dawidowicz, E.A. (1979) Biochim. Biophys. Acta 551, 260–270.
147 Smith, R.J.M. and Green, C. (1974) FEBS Lett. 42, 108–111.
148 Poznansky, M.J. and Lange, Y. (1978) Biochim. Biophys. Acta 506, 256–264.
149 Rothman, J.E. and Dawidowicz, E.A. (1975) Biochemistry 14, 2809–2816.
150 Johnson, L.W., Hughes, M.E. and Zilversmit, D.B. (1975) Biochim. Biophys. Acta 375, 176–185.
151 de Kruyff, B., van den Besselaar, A.M.H.P. and van Deenen, L.L.M. (1977) Biochim. Biophys. Acta 465, 443–453.
152 Bloj, B. and Zilversmit, D.B. (1976) Biochemistry 15, 1277–1283.
153 Renooij, W., van Golde, L.M.G., Zwaal, R.F.A. and van Deenen, L.L.M. (1976) Eur. J. Biochem. 61, 53–58.
154 Lange, Y., Cohen, C.M. and Poznansky, M.J. (1977) Proc. Natl. Acad. Sci. (U.S.A.) 74, 1538–1542.
155 Gottlieb, M.H. (1977) Biochim. Biophys. Acta 466, 422–428.
156 Lange, Y., Cutler, H.B. and Steck, T.L. (1980) J. Biol. Chem. 255, 9331–9337.
157 Lange, Y., Dolde, J. and Steck, T.L. (1981) J. Biol. Chem. 256, 5321–5323.
158 Lange, Y., Matthies, H. and Steck, T.L. (1984) Biochim. Biophys. Acta 769, 551–562.
159 Harry, D.S., Day, R.C., Owen, J.S., Agorastos, J., Foo, A.Y. and McIntyre, N. (1978) Scand. J. Clin. Lab. Invest. 38, Suppl. 150, 223.
160 Day, R.C., Harry, D.S., Owen, J.M., Foo, A.Y. and McIntyre, N. (1979) Clin. Sci. 56, 575–583.
161 Owen, J.S., Hutton, R.A., Hope, M.J., Harry, D.S., Bruckdorfer, K.R., Day, R.C., McIntyre, N. amd Lucy, J.A. (1978) Scand. J. Clin. Invest. 38, Suppl. 150, 228.
162 Simons, L.A., Reichl, D., Myant, N.B. and Mancini, M. (1975) Atherosclerosis 21, 283–298.
163 Bilheimer, D.W., Goldstein, J.L., Grundy, S.M. and Brown, M. (1975) J. Clin. Invest. 56, 1420–1430.
164 Goldstein, J.L. and Brown, M.S. (1977) Metabolism 26, 1257–1275.
165 Watanabe, T., Tanaka, K. and Yanai, N. (1968) Acta Pathol. Jpn. 18, 319–331.
166 Chomette, G., De Gennes, J.L., Delcourt, A., Hammou, J.C. and Perie, G. (1971) Ann. Anat. Pathol. 16, 233–250.
167 Goldstein, J.L., Ho, Y.K., Basu, S.K. and Brown, M.S. (1979) Proc. Natl. Acad. Sci. (U.S.A.) 76, 333–337.
168 Smith, E.B. (1965) J. Atheroscler. Res. 5, 224–240.
169 Rouser, G. and Solomon, R.D. (1969) Lipids 4, 232–234.
170 Bottcher, C.J.F. and Van Gent, C.M. (1961) J. Atheroscler. Res. 1, 36–46.
171 Small, D.M. (1977) Semin. Med. 297, 873.

172 Small, D.M. (1977) Semin. Med. 297, 924.
173 Insull, W. and Bartsch, G.E. (1966) J. Clin. Invest. 45, 513–523.
174 Portman, O.W., Alexander, M. and Maruffo, C.A. (1967) J. Nutr. 91, 35–46.
175 Portman, O.W. (1970) Adv. Lipid Res. 8, 41–114.
176 Kritchevsky, D. (1964) in: Lipid Pharmacology (Paoletti, R., Ed.) p. 63, Academic Press, New York.
177 Constantinides, P. (1965) in: Experimental Atherosclerosis, p. 49, Elsevier, Amsterdam.
178 Papahadjopoulos, D. (1974) J. Theoret. Biol. 43, 329–337.
179 Pairault, J., Levilliers, J. and Chapman, M.J. (1977) Nature (London) 269, 607–609.
180 Shore, V. and Shore, B. (1975) Biochem. Biophys. Res. Commun. 65, 1250–1256.
181 Shore, B. and Shore, V. (1975) Fed. Proc. 34, 1446–1448.
182 Samaha, F.J. and Gergely, J. (1969) New Engl. J. Med. 280, 184–188.
183 Martonosi, A. (1968) Proc. Soc. Exp. Biol. Med. 127, 824–828.
184 Hanna, S.D. and Baskin, R.J. (1977) Biochem. Med. 17, 300–309.
185 Hanna, S.D. and Baskin, R.J. (1978) Biochim. Biophys. Acta 540, 144–150.
186 Butterfield, D.A. and Leung, P.K. (1978) Life Sci. 22, 1783–1788.
187 Hidalgo, C., Thomas, D.D. and Ikemoto, N. (1978) J. Biol. Chem. 253, 6879–6887.
188 Sherman, I.W. (1977) Bull. Wld Health Org. 55, 211.
189 Homewood, C.A. (1977) Bull. Wld Health Org. 55, 227.
190 Anon. (1977) Bull. Wld Health Org. 55, 347.
191 Holz, G.G. (1977) Bull. Wld Health Org. 55, 237.
192 Chen, H.W., Kandutsch, A.A. and Heiniger, H.J. (1978) Progr. Exp. Tumour Res. 22, 275–316.
193 Chen, H.W., Heiniger, H.J. and Kandutsch, A.A. (1975) Proc. Natl. Acad. Sci. (U.S.A.) 72, 1950–1954.
194 Gottfried, E.L. (1967) J. Lipid Res. 8, 321–327.
195 Gottfried, E.L. (1971) J. Lipid Res. 12, 531–537.
196 Vlodavsky, I. and Sachs, L. (1974) Nature (London) 250, 67–68.
197 Montfoort, A., Boere, W.A.M. and van Griensven, L.J.L.D.V. (1976) Lipids 11, 798–801.
108 Perdue, J.F., Kletzien, R. and Miller, K. (1971) Biochim. Biophys. Acta 249, 419–434.
199 Perdue, J.F., Kletzien, R. and Wray, V.L. (1972) Biochim. Biophys. Acta 266, 505–510.
200 Perdue, J.F., Warner, D. and Miller, K. (1973) Biochim. Biophys. Acta 298, 817–826.
201 Mark-Malchoff, D., Marinetti, G.V., Hare, J.D. and Meisler, A. (1979) Exp. Cell Res. 118, 377–381.
202 Shinitzky, M. and Inbar, M. (1974) J. Mol. Biol. 85, 603–615.
203 Inbar, M. and Shinitzky, M. (1974) Proc. Natl. Acad. Sci. (U.S.A.) 71, 4229–4231.
204 Johnson, S.M. and Robinson, R. (1979) Biochim. Biophys. Acta 558, 282–295.
205 Johnson, S.M. and Kramers, M.T.C. (1978) Biochem. Biophys. Res. Commun. 80, 451–457.
206 McKersie, B.D. and Thompson, J.E. (1979) Pl. Physiol. 63, 802–805.
207 Bloch, K. (1976) in: Reflections in Biochemistry (Kornberg, A. et al., Eds.) p. 143, Pergamon Press, London.
208 Nes, W.R. (1976) Lipids 9, 596–612.
209 Rohmer, M., Bouvier, P. and Ourisson, G. (1979) Proc. Natl. Acad. Sci. (U.S.A.) 76, 847–851.

H. Danielsson and J. Sjövall (Eds.), *Sterols and Bile Acids*

CHAPTER 7

Biosynthesis of plant sterols

T.W. GOODWIN

Department of Biochemistry, University of Liverpool, P.O. Box 147, Liverpool, L69 3BX (Great Britain)

(I) Introduction

Animals confine their biosynthetic activity in the sterol field to producing cholesterol (4-A) *; in contrast plants produce a multiplicity of sterols of which cholesterol is generally a minor component. These are characterized by an additional alkyl group at C-24 with either α- or β-chirality, for example clionasterol (4-I) (β-chirality) and sitosterol (4-P) (α-chirality). Sterols with methylene and ethylidene substituents are also found, as for example 24-methylene cholesterol (4-F) and fucosterol (4-E). In the case of ethylidene derivatives both *E* and *Z* isomers are found; isofucosterol (4-C) (*Z*) exists as well as fucosterol (4-*E*). The other major characteristics of plant sterols is the presence of additional double bonds in the side chain, as exemplified by poriferasterol (4-*B*) (Δ^{22}), cyclosadol (2-*T*) (Δ^{23}), ergosta-5,24(25)-diene-3β-ol (4-O) ($\Delta^{24,25}$) and clerosterol (4-J) (Δ^{25}) [1–4].

Sterol esters, sterol glycosides and acylated sterol glycosides are also widespread in plants [5].

There is little doubt that the pathway from acetyl-CoA to squalene 2,3-oxide in plants is the same as that in animals and as it is detailed in the chapter on cholesterol biosynthesis it will not be reiterated here.

(II) Formation of cycloartenol

In animals (Chapter 1) squalene 2,3-oxide is first converted into lanosterol (1-A) and this reaction also occurs in yeasts. However, in higher plants and algae the first cyclic product is cycloartenol (2-A).

* In order to save space and repetition of structural formulae sterol structures are designated by a number (nucleus) and a letter (side chain). The keys are given in Figs. 1 and 2.

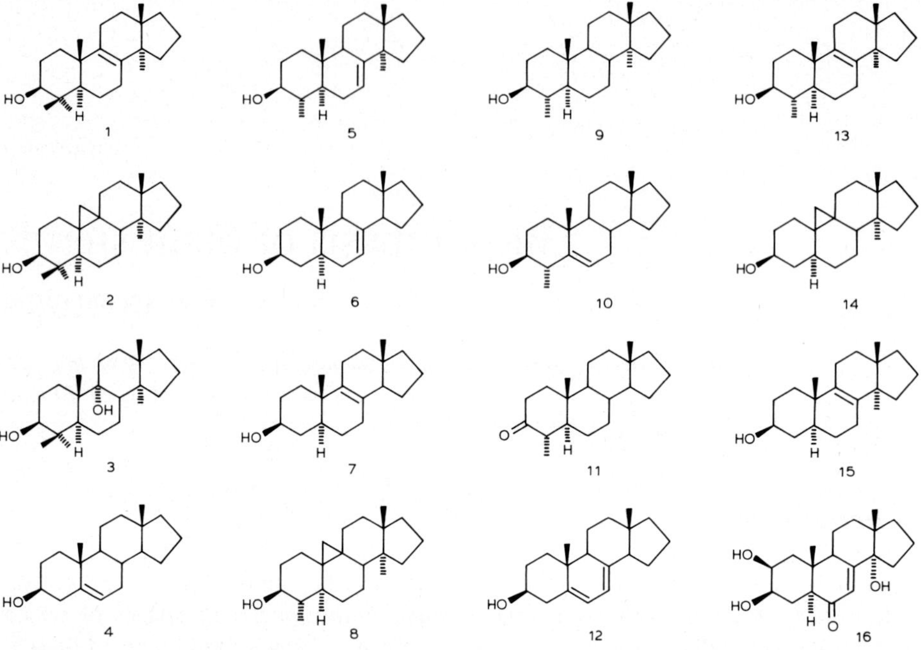

Fig. 1. Sterol nuclei discussed in text.

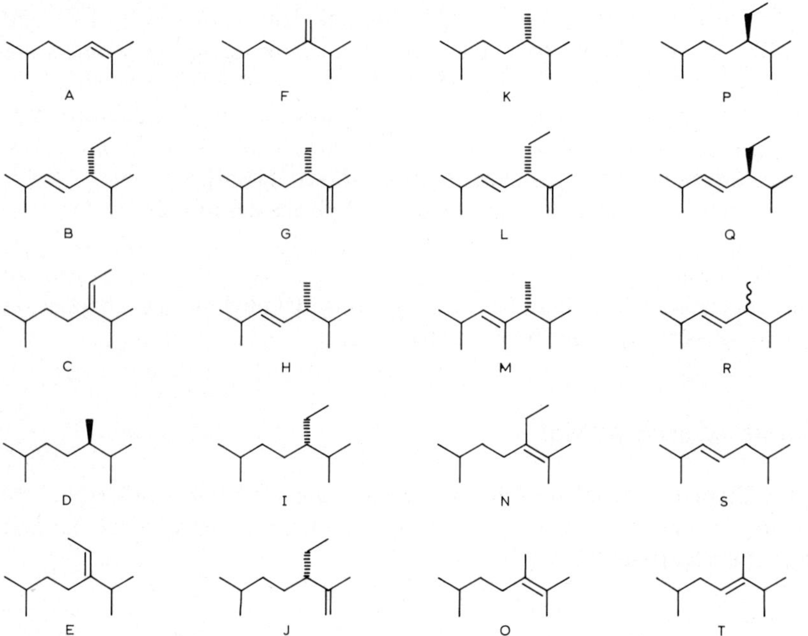

Fig. 2. Sterol side chains discussed in text.

The enzyme involved is squalene 2,3-oxide: cycloartenol cyclase and the substrate is the *S* enantiomer. The reaction is initiated by H^+ attack on the oxygen of the epoxy group of the substrate held in the chair, boat, chair, boat unfolded conforma-

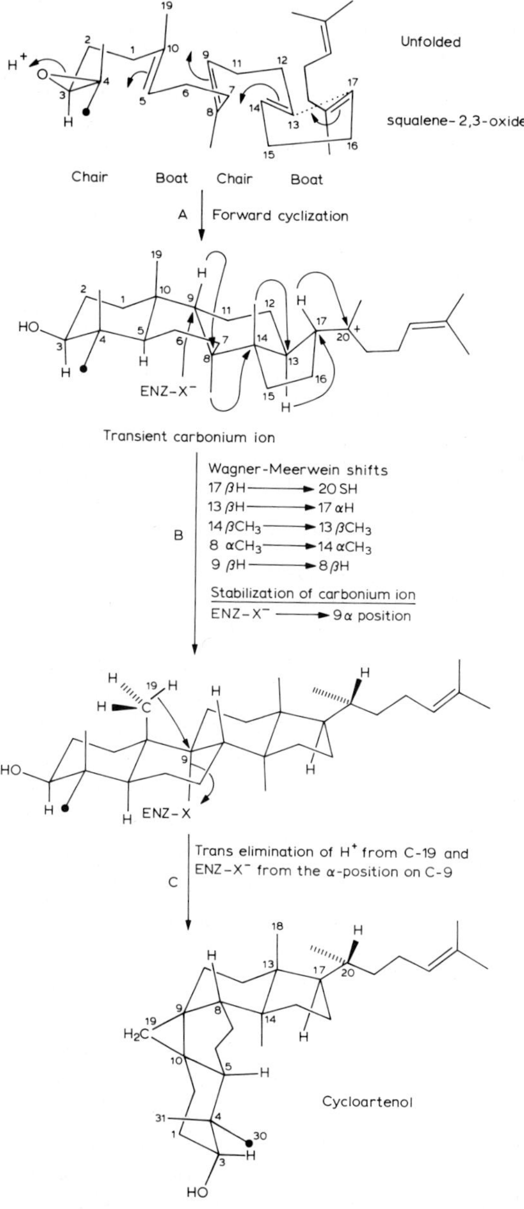

Fig. 3. Mechanism of cyclization of squalene 2,3-oxide to cycloartenol [9].

tion (Fig. 3). The resulting forward cyclization reaction (A, Fig. 3) stops at C-20 because of the unfolded conformation. The transient carbonium ion so produced undergoes a backward rearrangement (B, Fig. 3) involving a series of 1–2 (Wagner–Meerwein) shifts with stabilization at C-9 by the addition in the α-configuration of a nucleophilic group (enzyme $-X^-$). Finally a *trans* elimination of enzyme $-X^-$ and H^+ from C-19 with the concomitant formation of the 9,19-cyclopropane ring (C, Fig. 3) results in the formation of cycloartenol. The involvement of enzyme $-X^-$ is necessary to allow the final step to be a *trans* elimination according to the isoprene rule.

(III) Alkylation reactions

Alkylation in the formation of plant sterols involves methylation at C-24 with *S*-adenosyl methionine to produce C_{28} sterols. C-24 ethyl sterols are formed by the further methylation of a C-24 methylene substrate. The mechanism involved depends on the chirality of the product which is mainly but not exclusively β in algae and mainly but again not exclusively α in higher plants. The overall pattern of alkylation is outlined in Fig. 4. As the first methylation reaction in higher plants involves cycloartenol as substrate it is appropriate to consider it at this point. Furthermore, although as will be seen later, the second methylation does not involve the cycloartenol skeleton, it is convenient to consider it along with the first methylation because the two mechanisms are closely interrelated. Experiments which have led to our knowledge of the alkylation reactions involved the use of $[C^2H_3]$-methionine and stereospecifically labelled mevalonic acid, feeding experiment with labelled putative precursors and also, to some extent, enzyme studies. The approach can be demonstrated by considering the situation in some detail in the chrysophyte alga *Ochromonas malhamensis*. The pathways involved (1 and 2) are outlined in Fig. 4.

Experiments with $[C^2H_3]$methionine showed that only 2 and 4 deuteriums were present in brassicasterol (4-H) and poriferasterol (4-B), respectively. When $[2\text{-}^{14}C, 4R\text{-}^3H_1]$mevalonic acid is the substrate for sterol synthesis it was shown in the classical experiments of Cornforth and Popják that lanosterol, the precursor of cholesterol in animals, contained a tritium at C-24. This is also true for cycloartenol. In an alkylated derivative this tritium should, according to pathways 1 and 2 outlined in Fig. 4, be retained at C-25. This was shown to be so in the case of poriferasterol; in the case of brassicasterol tritium is retained but its location has not been experimentally determined. However this has been shown in the case of the 24β-methyl sterol, ergosterol (12-H) synthesized by yeasts. Furthermore studies with chiral acetate have indicated that the methyl group is transferred from *S*-adenosyl methionine with inversion, deprotonation and hydrogen addition at C-29. This is indicated in Fig. 5. In addition the proton lost in the formation of the methylene intermediate (A, Fig. 5) and that added on its reduction (B, Fig. 5) are under tight stereochemical control. This means that the protonation of the methylene group

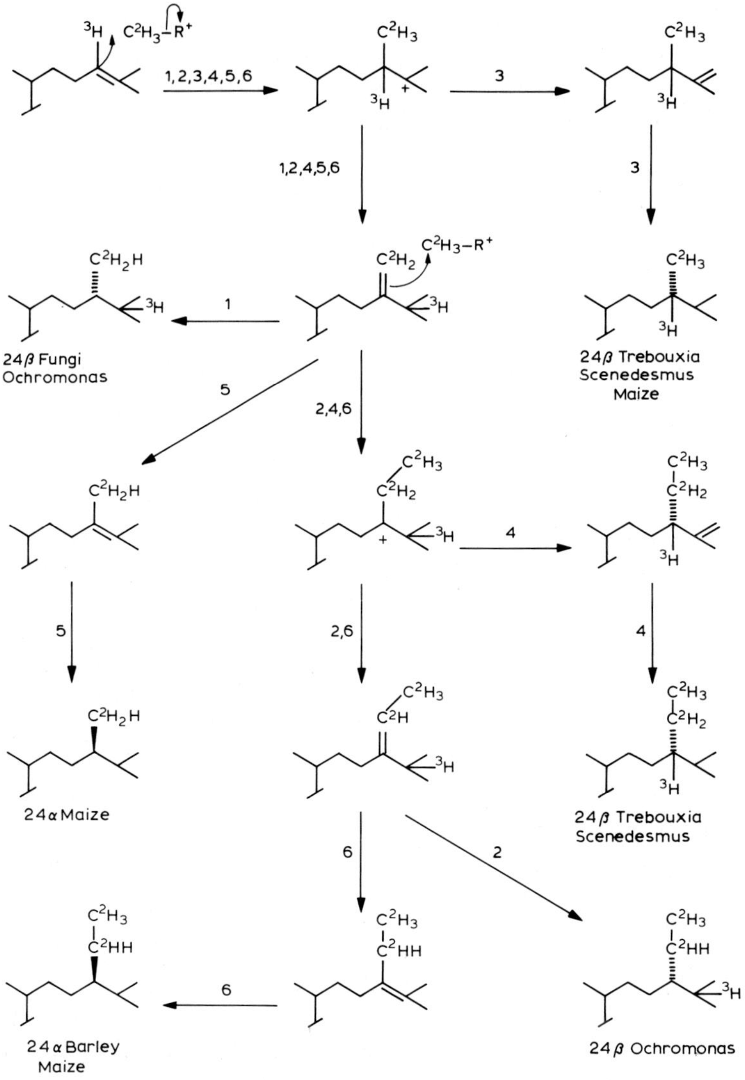

Fig. 4. Mechanisms involved in alkylating the sterol side chain.

must occur at the face of the double bond opposite to that from which the original proton was removed [6]. By using [2-^{13}C]mevalonic acid Arigoni also demonstrated that the methyl group transferred attacks the *si*-face of the C-24 double bond (see also ref. 7).

The presence of only 4 deuteriums in poriferasterol (4-B) formed from [C^2H_3]methionine in Ochromonas implies the formation of an intermediate ethylidene compound. Feeding experiments showed that the 28-*Z* isomers ethylidene lophenol (5-C) and isofucosterol (4-C) are both effectively incorporated into

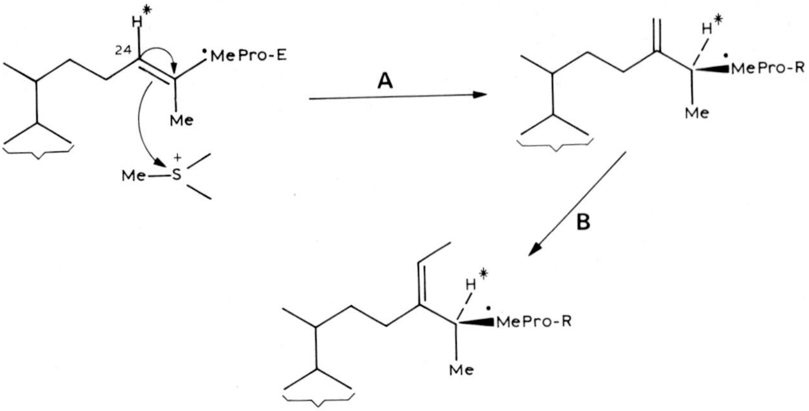

Fig. 5. The stereochemistry of methyl group transfer at C-28.

poriferasterol. On the other hand the 28-*E* isomer fucosterol (4-E) is less well incorporated. So it seems that the *Z* ethylidene derivatives are the true intermediates. The *E* isomers are probably active only in so far as the $\Delta^{24,28}$ reductase is not completely stereoselective. Furthermore isofucosterol is widely distributed in trace amounts, suggesting its intermediate role, whereas fucosterol is the major sterol in such algae as the giant kelps, which suggests an end product rather than a biosynthetic intermediate.

A similar mechanism for the formation of alkyl sterols functions in Euglena and the Xanthophyte *Monodus subterraneus.*

It eventually transpired that the mechanism involved in green algae for the formation of 24β-alkyl sterols was different from that in Ochromonas. Pathways 3 and 4 (Fig. 4) lead to the formation of 24β-methyl and 24β-ethyl sterols, respectively, in these organisms [8]. The evidence for these pathways include (i) 3 and 5 deuteriums from [C^2H_3]methionine are retained in the methyl and ethyl sterols respectively; (ii) the simultaneous formation of labelled 24-methylene cycloartanol (2-F) and cyclolaudenol (2-G) in the presence of [$^{14}CH_3$]methionine; (iii) the conversion of 31-norcyclolaudenol (8-G) only into 24β-methyl sterols (pathway 3, Fig. 4) and the conversion of nor-24β-methylene cycloartanol (cycloeucalenol, 8-F) only into 24β-ethyl sterols (pathway 4, Fig. 4); (iv) both 24β-methyl sterols (e.g. codisterol, 4-G) and 24β-ethyl sterols (e.g. clerosterol 4-J) with a double bond at C-25 occur naturally in green algae; (v) 22-dehydroclerosterol (4-L) is very effectively converted into poriferasterol (4-B). The fact that this substrate is not converted to any extent into clionasterol (4-I), combined with the observation that clerosterol (4-J) is converted into both clionasterol and poriferasterol rather ineffectively, points to the conclusion that desaturation at C-22 is not a terminal step in the biosynthesis of sterols in green algae (Fig. 6).

It has not yet been possible to show that the hydrogen originally at C-24 in cycloartenol is still present in the same position in the final alkylated products

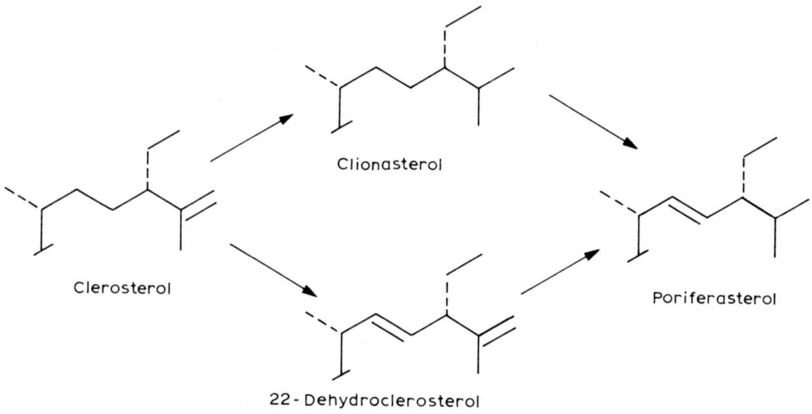

Clionasterol

Clerosterol

Poriferasterol

22-Dehydroclerosterol

Fig. 6. Pathways for the conversion of clerosterol into poriferasterol; only 22-dehydroclerosterol is effectively converted.

because green algae will not take up added mevalonic acid. However, in the higher plant *Clerodendron campbellii* 24β-ethyl sterols e.g. clerosterol (4-J) and 22-dehydroclerosterol (4-L) unexpectedly occur and it has been shown that in the latter case the original C-24 hydrogen in cycloartenol remains in the sterol in the same position.

The 24α-alkyl sterols which predominate in higher plants are formed by yet other mechanisms which are not yet completely understood. The most likely pathway for the biosynthesis of 24α-methyl sterols is route 5 (Fig. 4) and of 24α-ethyl sterols route 6 (Fig. 4). The evidence for route 5 includes (i) the retention of only 2 deuteriums from [C^2H_3]methionine in campesterol (4-D) formed by barley embryos; (ii) the formation of 24-methylene derivatives by plants, one of which, methylene lophenol (5-F), accumulates in place of campesterol when plant tissue cultures are grown in the presence of inhibitor the fenarimol; (iii) $\Delta^{24(25)}$-24-methyl sterols are occasionally found in nature, as, for example, (4-O) in *Withania somnifera.* The conversion of a $\Delta^{24(25)}$-24-methyl sterol into, for example, campesterol (4-D) has not yet been demonstrated. A number of observations point to pathway 6 for the synthesis of 24α-ethyl sterols, these include (i) only 4 deuteriums are incorporated into sitosterol (4-P) from [C^2H_3]methionine; (ii) isofucosterol is formed by barley embryos and retains its C-24 hydrogen at C-25; (iii) isofucosterol is rapidly transformed into sitosterol (4-P) by barley seedlings with the loss of its hydrogen at C-24; (iv) $\Delta^{24(25)}$-24-ethyl sterols have been reported in higher plants (e.g. 4α-methyl-24-ethylcholesta-7,24-dien-3β-ol, 10-N); (v) a $\Delta^{24(25)}$-24-ethyl sterol, stigmasta-5,24-dien-3β-ol (4-N) is converted into sitosterol in barley embryos but only to a very limited extent. However it has not yet been possible to trap 4-N as a biosynthetic intermediate. A possibility which has not yet been tested experimentally is that a $\Delta^{22,24(25)}$-diene is the natural intermediate as suggested for green algae.

24β-Methyl sterols are widespread in higher plants in traces whereas 24β-ethyl sterols are rather rare. Recent work has shown that higher plants utilize the 'green algal' pathway to produce these stereoisomers.

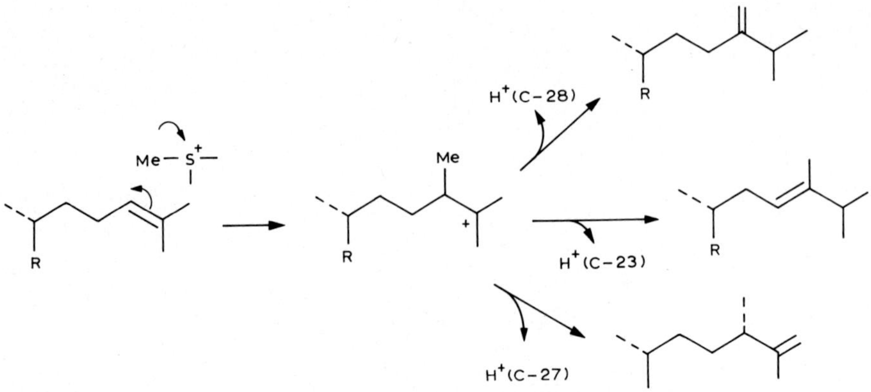

Fig. 7. The formation of 24-methylene cycloartanol, cyclolaudenol and cyclosadol by methylation of cycloartenol.

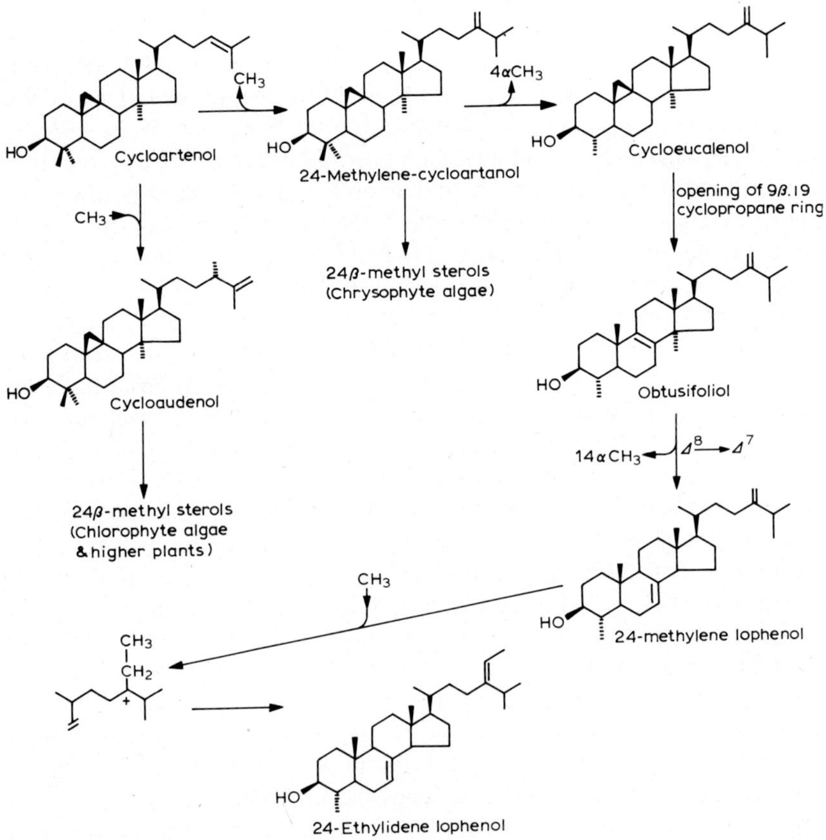

Fig. 8. Formation of 24-methylene lophenol and 24-ethylidene lophenol from 24-methylene cycloartanol [9].

Apart from 24-methylene cycloartanol (2-F) and cyclolaudenol (2-G), which in maize and barley embryos could give rise to 24α- and 24β-methyl sterols respectively, a further primary product of methylation, cyclosadol (2-T) has recently been found in maize and barley embryos. Its significance in the major pathway of sterol synthesis is still under investigation, but minor components such as 4-T and 8-T have also been reported in maize. The overall pattern of the type of compounds formed by the first attack of *S*-adenosyl methionine on cycloartenol is outlined in Fig. 7.

The next question is when in the biosynthetic pathway do the two methylations take place. As already indicated, experiments with enzyme preparations demonstrate that cycloartenol is the best substrate for the first methylation. However 24-methylene lophenol (5-F) and not 24-methylene cycloartanol (2-F), is the preferred substrate for the second methylation. This is formed by the pathway indicated in Fig. 8. 24-Methylene cycloartanol (2-F) is demethylated to cycloeucalenol (8-F) which is the substrate for cycloeucalenol: obtusifoliol isomerase which opens the 9,19-cyclopropane ring to form obtusifoliol (13-F); demethylation at C-14 and isomerization

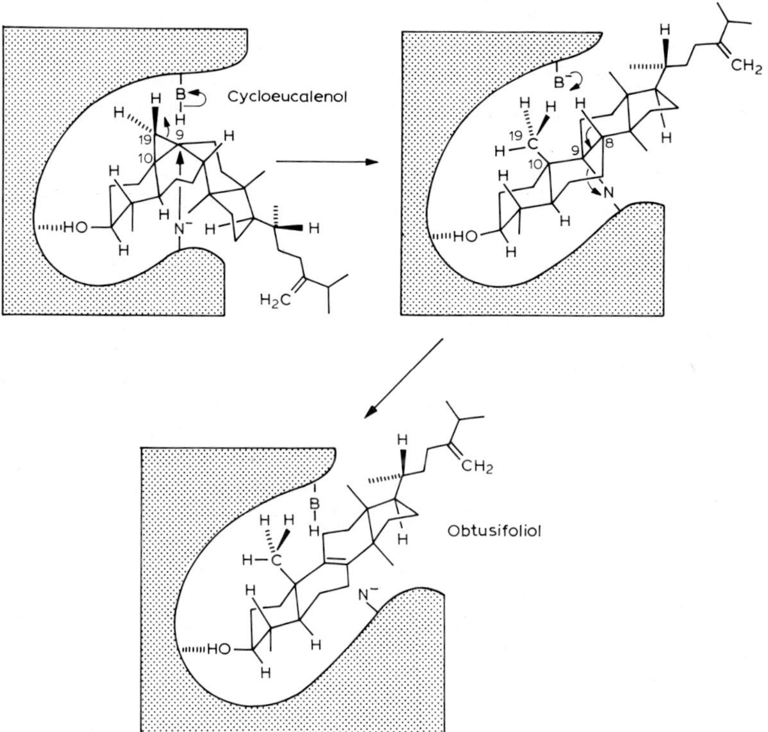

Fig. 9. Mechanism for the opening of the cyclopropane ring of cycloeucalenol; B and N are active groups at the active site of enzyme; the hydrogen which is transferred from B to C-19 can exchange with H^+ in the aqueous environment.

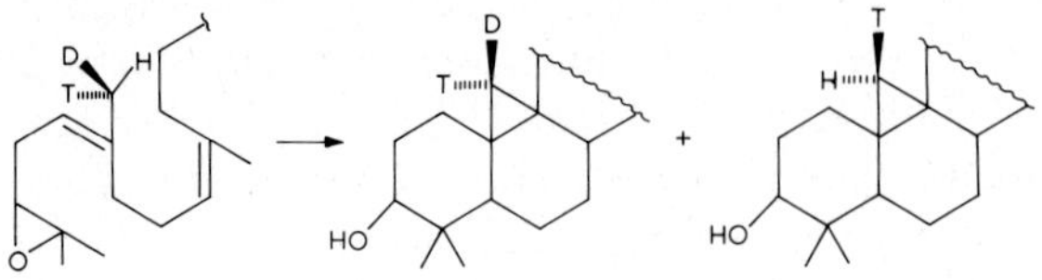

Fig. 10. Retention of configuration on formation of the cyclopropane ring of cycloartenol.

($\Delta^8 \rightarrow \Delta^7$) (details of these reactions are still obscure) yields 24-methylene lophenol which is then methylated to 24-ethylidene lophenol.

The mechanism proposed for the isomerase (Fig. 9) involves the stabilization of a carbonium ion generated at C-9 when the ring of cycloeucalenol is opened by proton attack by a suitable electrophilic group of the enzyme. A *trans* antiperiplanar elimination of the 8β-hydrogen and the enzyme results in the formation of obtusifoliol. This proposal is supported by the observation that when the reaction is carried out in ^2H_2O deuterium appears in the methyl group attached to C-9. Cycloartenol is formed from squalene 2,3-oxide carrying a chiral methyl group at C-6 with a methyl hydrogen replaced by C-9 with retention of configuration (Fig. 10). Experiments with 19*S*-[19-^{2}H, 19-^{3}H]-31-norcycloartenol have shown that the ring opening also occurs with retention of configuration; that is the reverse of the reaction indicated in Fig. 10.

The isomerase does not act on cycloartenol or 24-methylene cycloartanol which explains the absence of lanosterol (1-A) and 24-methylene lanosterol (1-F) from photosynthetic tissues.

It is important to note that in the methylation reaction in yeasts the best substrate for the methylase enzyme is zymosterol (7-A), a compound almost at the end of the line in the biosynthetic sequence. In contrast to the plant enzyme it is not active on the first product of cyclization of squalene 2,3-oxide, in this case lanosterol (1-A).

Some diatoms synthesize sterols with 2 methyl groups attached to different carbon atoms in the side chain, an example is dinosterol (9-M) which contains a methyl group at C-23 in addition to the usual C-24 substituent. Experiments with [C^2H_3]methionine have shown that the C-23 methyl group is introduced intact whereas the 24β-methyl group is introduced via a 24-methylene group.

(IV) Steps other than those involving methylation

(1) Demethylation

The steps immediately following the first methylation have already been indicated in Fig. 8 and the isomerization reaction discussed in the previous section. Demethyl-

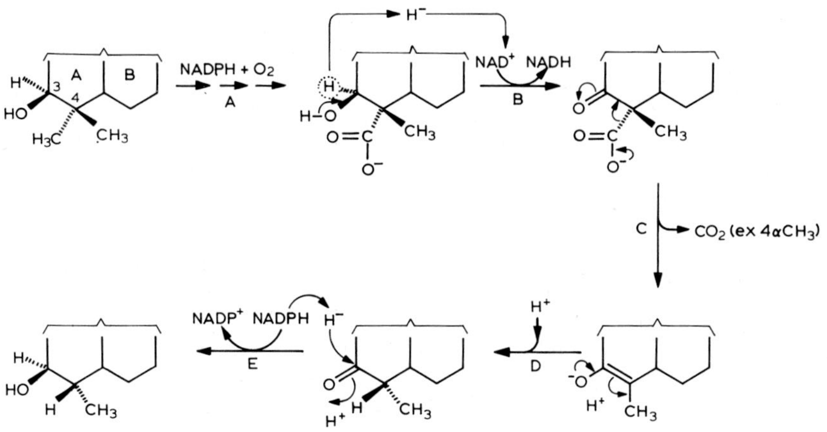

Fig. 11. Probable mechanism of demethylation at C-4 in the biosynthesis of plant sterols [9].

ation at C-4 has been examined in detail in *Polypodium vulgare.* The 4α-methyl group of cycloartenol arises from C-2 of mevalonic acid and is removed in the formation of 31-norcycloartenol (8-A) in which the 4β-methyl group takes up the 4α-position. During the reaction the 3α-hydrogen is exchanged so the reaction is clearly very similar to that which occurs in animals during cholesterol biosynthesis (Fig. 11) (see also Chapter 1). The first step in the reaction in animals (A, B) involves the stepwise oxidation of the methyl group to a carboxyl group under the influence of an NADPH/O_2-dependent oxidase. This is in contrast to the mechanism proposed for the removal of the 14α-methyl group which involves oxidation to a formyl derivative (see below). However the mechanism for the oxidation of the methyl group to a carboxyl group in plants has not been investigated, but it is highly likely to be very similar to that in animals. A clear difference between plant and animal systems is that in animals the methyl group at C-14 is removed before the first 4α-methyl group. In plants, except in rare cases, it is the other way round.

The question whether the Δ^8 bond of obtusifoliol is first isomerized to Δ^7 before demethylation at C-14 takes place to yield 24-methylene lophenol has not yet been answered, but it is clear that demethylation involves the formation and reduction of a double bond at C-14. During this reaction the 15α-hydrogen is exchanged with a proton and the 15β-hydrogen epimerized; simultaneously the hydrogen from NADPH appears in the 14α position (G, Fig. 12). The mechanism which has been worked out mainly in yeast and involves a cytochrome P-450 and NADPH-dependent decarboxylation is outlined in Fig. 12 (A $\rightarrow$ F). Sterols with a double bond at C-14 are present in traces in yeast and algae and are the major components of the sterols produced by *Methylococcus capsulatus,* one of the few procaryotes in which sterols have so far been clearly demonstrated. Obviously in this organism the Δ^{14} reductase is absent or only very weakly active.

The final demethylation step, the removal of the 4α group which was originally

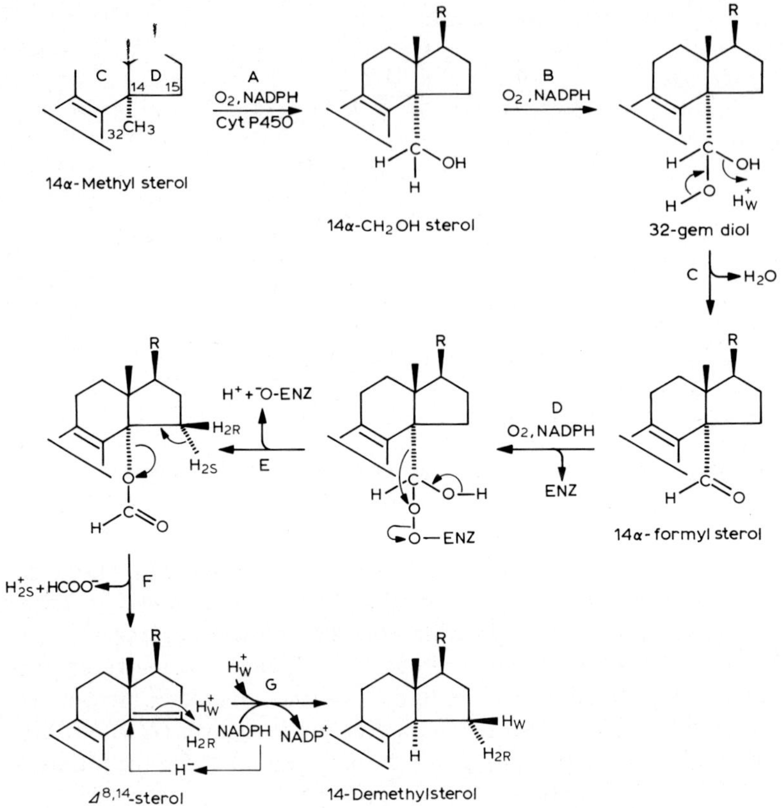

Fig. 12. Mechanism for the removal of the final 14α-methyl group in formation of plant sterols [9].

the 4β group in cycloartenol, was followed by observing the conversion of [2,2,4-$^3H_3$]obtusifoliol (13-F) into poriferasterol (4-B) in Ochromonas. It was found that the 4β-hydrogen (axial) was inverted to the 4α(equatorial) position during the demethylation. The mechanism outlined in Fig. 11 covers this observation; it is the same as that envisaged for the removal of the first 4α-methyl group from a 4,4-dimethyl derivative, but in this reaction the 4β-hydrogen takes the place of the 4β-methyl group. The exact substrate for this final demethylation is not known but is highly likely to be a Δ^7 compound because, as already indicated, ethylidene lophenol is effectively converted into poriferasterol in Ochromonas.

Although the major pathway of demethylation is 4,4,14α-trimethyl → 4α,14α-dimethyl → 4α-methyl, occasional deviations from the pattern can exist as for example 4,4-dimethyl sterols are major components in *Methylococcus capsulatus* and macdougallin (I), a 14α-methyl sterol, occurs in *Peniocerus macdougallii.*

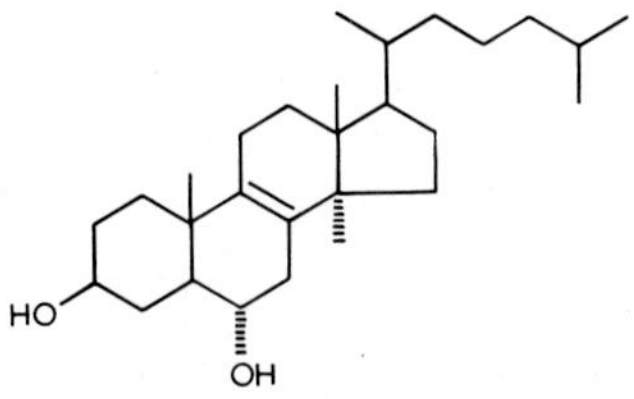

Formula I

(2) Isomerization of $\Delta^8 \rightarrow \Delta^5$

The isomerization in animals involves the pathway $\Delta^8 \rightarrow \Delta^7 \rightarrow \Delta^{5,7} \rightarrow \Delta^5$. The evidence for this pathway in plants is not as extensive as in animals but its existence, with one important variation of detail in yeast, is clear. The stereochemistry involved in the conversion in higher plants, Ochromonas and mammals is indicated in Fig. 13.

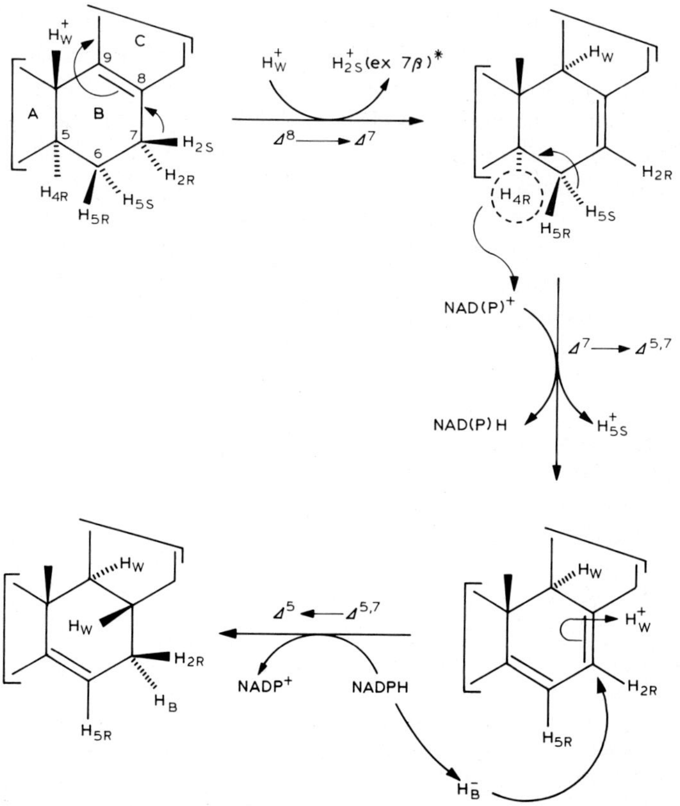

Fig. 13. Pathway for the conversion of Δ^8-sterols into Δ^5-sterols in Ochromonas and higher plants [9].

Formula II

In yeast, however, the 7α-hydrogen is lost in the $\Delta^8 \rightarrow \Delta^7$ step. This reaction is inhibited in bramble tissue cultures by the fungicide AY9944. The wide distribution in fungi of considerable amounts of $\Delta^{5,7}$-sterols such as ergosterol (12-H) may be due to the absence or low activity of the Δ^7 reductase in these organisms. The existence of lichesterol (II), a $\Delta^{5,8}$-sterol has not yet been rationalized biosynthetically.

(3) Insertion of the Δ^{22} double bond

Recent investigations now point to the insertion of the C-22 double bond, which has a *trans* configuration, at an early stage in the biosynthetic pathway rather than as the last step, which was previously thought to be the case. Some of the evidence for the present view has already been presented (Fig. 5); for example in Trebouxia clerosterol (4-J), although it can be converted into poriferasterol (4-B) to a slight extent, is a much less efficient precursor than 22-dehydroclerosterol (4-L). In the red alga *Porphyridium cruentum* Δ^{22} derivatives containing 4α- and 14α-methyl groups are the major sterols present. The fact that in *Ochromonas malhamensis* isofucosterol (4-C) is a better precursor of poriferastol (4-B) than is fucosterol (4-E) may be due to the fact that the C-29 methyl group of the latter could hinder attack of a dehydro-

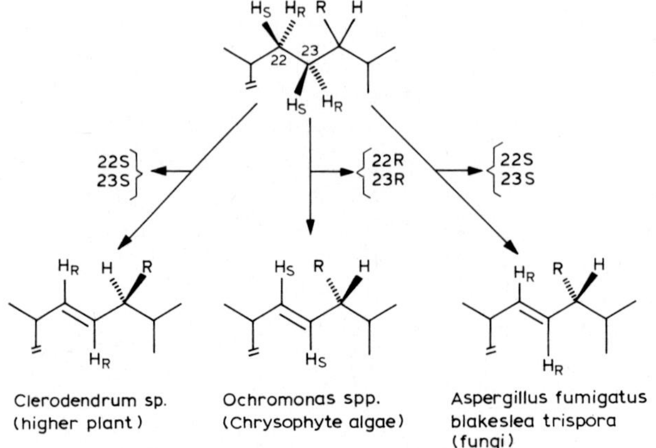

Fig. 14. The stereochemistry of desaturation of C-22,23 in higher plant, algal and fungal sterols [9].

genase at C-22,23 whereas that of isofucosterol would have no such effect. This is supported by the observation that in *Chlorella ellipsoidea,* fucosterol is reduced to clionasterol but not poriferasterol; unfortunately isofucosterol was not tested in this system. However, the protozoan *Tetrahymena pyriformis* can desaturate isofucosterol but not fucosterol at C-22.

The stereochemistry of the desaturation at C-22,23 varies with the organism under consideration, the 22pro-*S* and 23pro-*S* hydrogens are removed in higher plants and fungi whilst they are retained and the corresponding pro-*R* hydrogens lost in Ochromonas (Fig. 14).

(V) Cholesterol

Many plant tissues produce small amounts of free cholesterol whilst in some red algae it or the closely related desmosterol (4-A) are the major sterols. The pathway

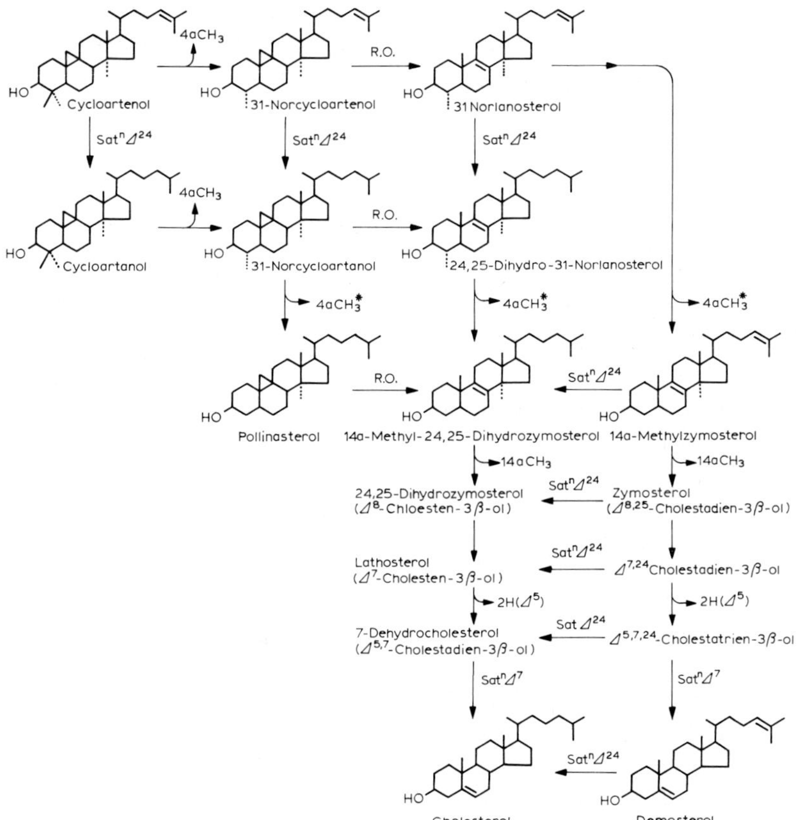

Fig. 15. The probable pathway of cholesterol biosynthesis in higher plants and algae [9].

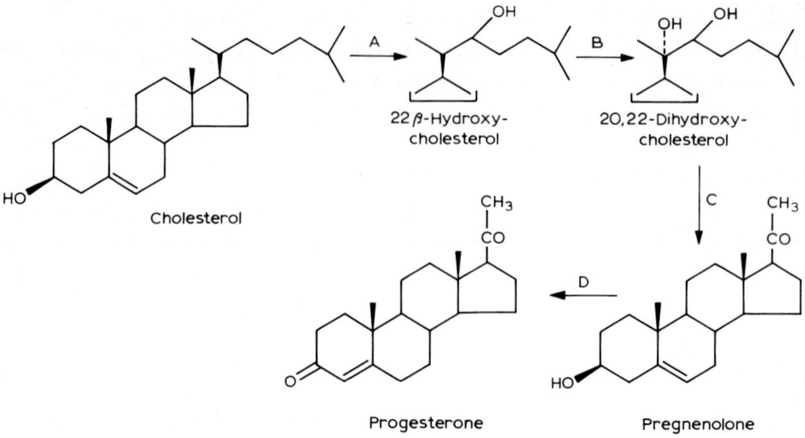

Cholesterol
A
22β-Hydroxy-cholesterol
B
20,22-Dihydroxy-cholesterol
C
Pregnenolone
D
Progesterone

Fig. 16. The pathway of progesterone synthesis in higher plants [9].

of synthesis of cholesterol in plants from cycloartenol has not been investigated in detail but the most likely possibility is outlined in Fig. 15. Most of the sterols in the scheme have been isolated from higher plants and the pattern which emerges fits well into the pathway for cholesterol synthesis in mammals.

(VI) Steroid hormones

In many plants the capacity for cholesterol synthesis may be greater than it may seem at first glance because of the marked synthesis of steroid hormones, cardenolides and ecdysones which are all derived from cholesterol.

Progesterone is synthesized from either cholesterol or alkylated plant sterols by a pathway similar to that in animals. Hydroxylation at C-20 and C-22 is a prerequisite for removal of the C-6 residue of the side chain (A, B, C, Fig. 16). The product pregnenolone is then reduced to progesterone (D, Fig. 16). Traces of oestrone, testosterone, deoxycorticosterone and closely related compounds have been found in plants but nothing is known of their biosynthesis.

(VII) Cardiac glycosides

Pregnenolone is also the precursor of cardenolides (C_{23} compounds) which are the aglycones of cardiac glycosides. The first steps in the biosynthetic sequence (A, Fig. 17) involve the oxidation of the hydroxyl at C-3 followed by the stereospecific reduction of the C-5 double bond to yield an A/B *cis* ring junction after reduction of the 3-keto group (B, Fig. 17). An interesting reaction involves the insertion of a hydroxyl group at C-14 with inversion of configuration (C, Fig. 17). A molecule of

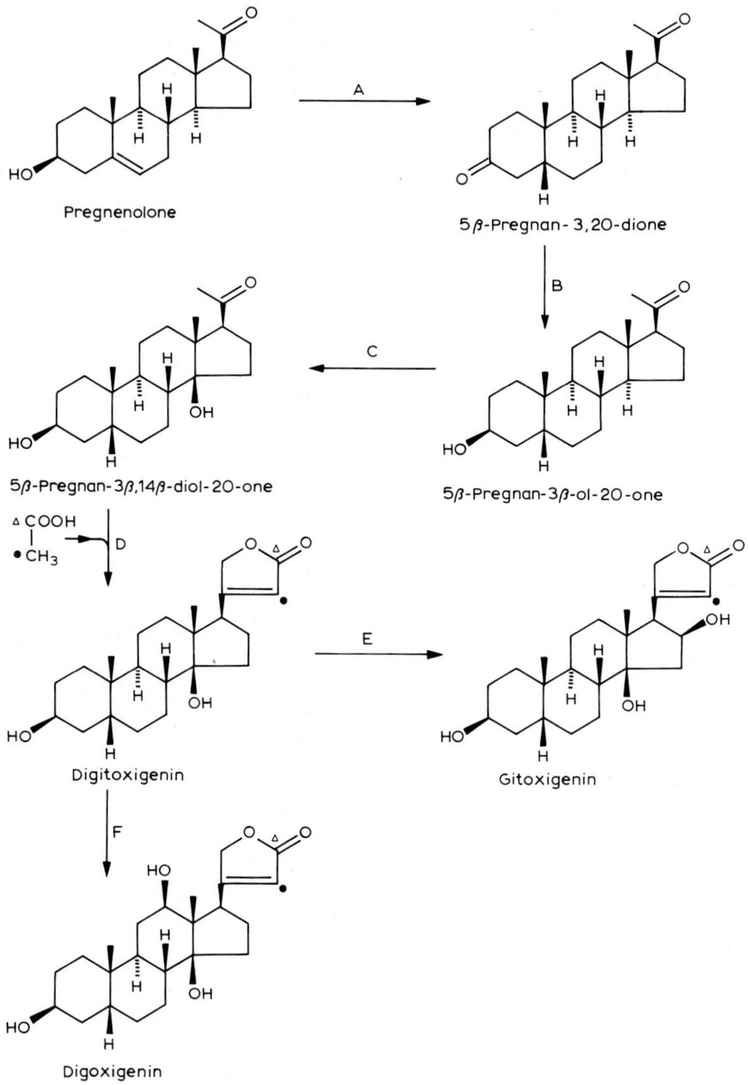
Pregnenolone
A
5β-Pregnan-3,20-dione
B
C
5β-Pregnan-3β,14β-diol-20-one
5β-Pregnan-3β-ol-20-one
△COOH
•CH3
D
E
Digitoxigenin
Gitoxigenin
F
Digoxigenin

Fig. 17. Biosynthesis of cardenolides from pregnenolone in higher plants [9].

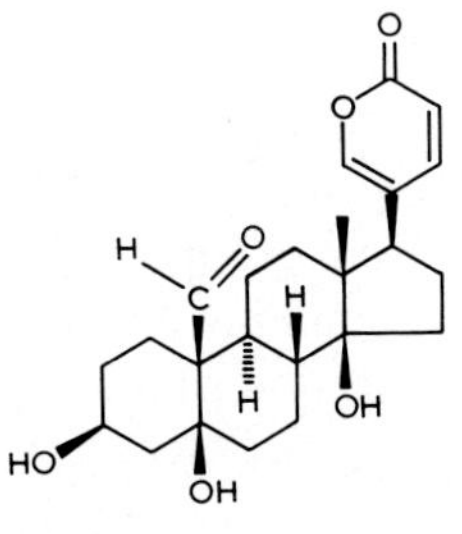

Formula III

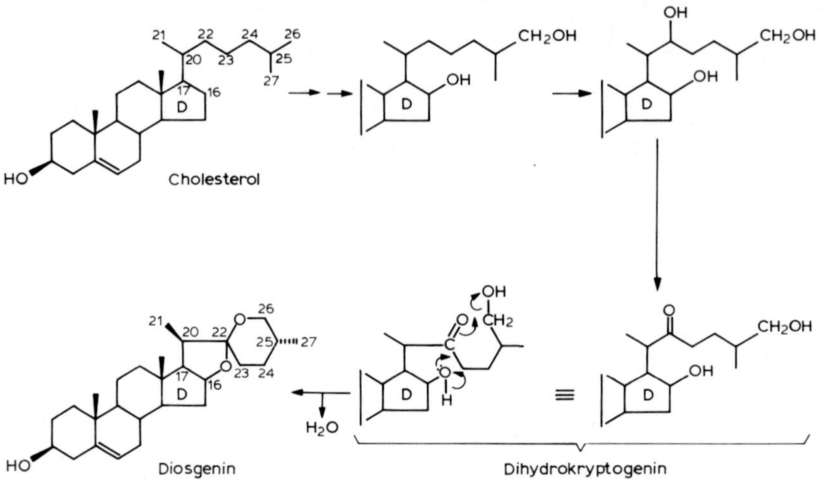

Fig. 18. Possible pathway for the conversion of cholesterol into sapogenins (diosgenin) [9].

acetate is then added to the side chain at this point (D, Fig. 17) and subsequent hydroxylations lead to the various known cardenolides (E, F, Fig. 17) (see ref. 9).

The biosynthesis of the C_{24}-bufadienolides, aglycones of the cardiac glycosides, e.g. hellibrigenin (III) is not known.

(VIII) Sapogenins

These are C_{27} sterols in which the side chain has been metabolized to a spiroketal. They are formed from cholesterol by a pathway illustrated for diosgenin in Fig. 18. Sapogenins are the aglycones of the naturally occurring saponins which are 3-*O*-glycosides.

(IX) Ecdysteroids

These compounds which are formed in insects from food sterols (Chapter 8) act as moulting hormones; a number of them, for example ecdysone (α-ecdysone) (Fig. 19) are also synthesized by plants such as Polypodium and Podocarpus. Labelling studies have revealed that they are formed from cholesterol and that formation of the *cis* A/B ring junction involves the migration of the 3α- and 4β-hydrogens of cholesterol to positions 4α and 5β, respectively. A possible mechanism involving the formation of a 5,6-epoxide and the subsequent formation of the keto group at C-6 has been suggested (B, C Fig. 19). The production of the Δ^7 double bond involves the stereospecific removal of the 7α- and 8β-hydrogens. This desaturation at C-7 is considered to occur before the formation of the saturated A/B ring junction at C-5.

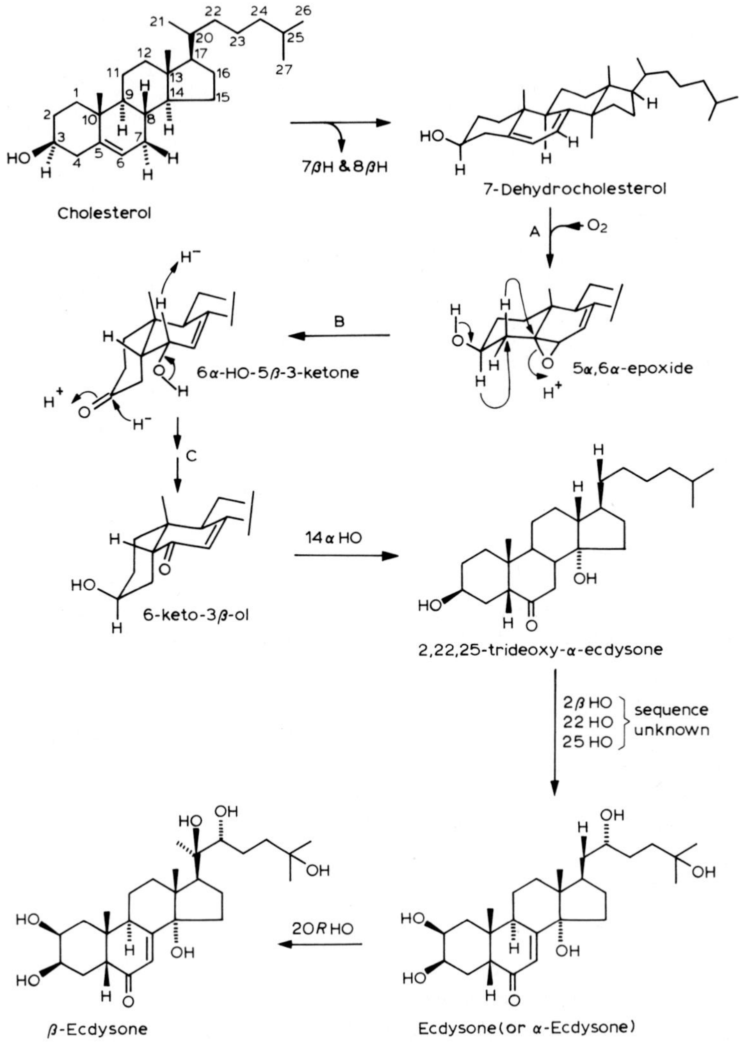

Fig. 19. Ecdysterone formation in higher plants [9].

Subsequent hydroxylation of α-ecdysone yields β-ecdysone (Fig. 19), the most oxidized ecdysone normally encountered in plants.

(X) Steroid alkaloids

Two main groups of steroid alkaloids are known: the C_{27} compounds such as solasodine (IV) and the C_{21} alkaloids such as holaphyllamine (V). The C_{27} com-

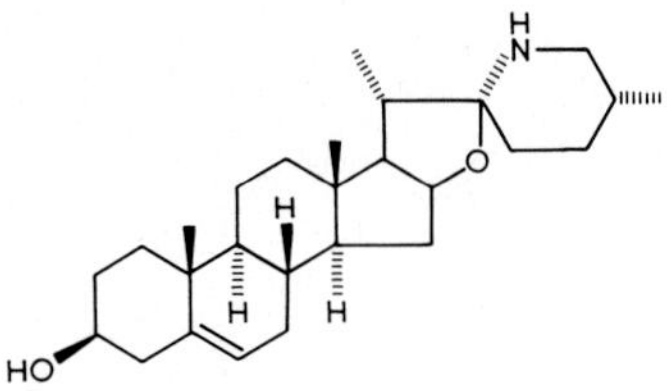

HO

Formula IV

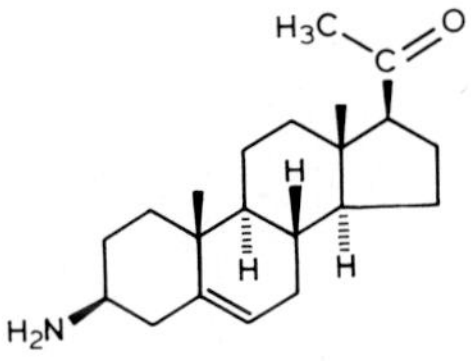

H_3C C O

H_2N

Formula V

pounds are nitrogen analogues of sapogenins (see Section VIII) and the basic pathways of formation are probably the same. The source of the nitrogen is not clearly known but L-arginine is possibly the donor in *Veratrum grandiflorum.* Holaphyllamine, the nitrogen analogue of pregnenolone (see Section VI) is, as would be expected, formed from it; however progesterone is apparently not a precursor.

Additional *N*-methyl and *O*-methyl groups frequently encountered in steroid alkaloids appear to arise conventionally from *S*-adenosyl methionine.

(XI) Withanolides

These are a group of ergostane steroids isolated from the family Solanaceae. They are characterized by highly oxygenated A and B rings and the presence of a side chain lactone. A typical example is withanolide E (1, Fig. 20) although compounds with the 14β configuration are also known as are compounds with the epoxide group in positions 6 and 7. 24-Methylcholesterol can act as a precursor of withanolides and a recently observed Δ^{16}-withanolide (4, Fig. 20) may be a precursor of withanolide E. This is indicated in Fig. 20 in which the way other naturally occurring withanolides may be converted into withanolide E is outlined [10].

(XII) Brassinosteroids

This is a relatively new group of naturally occurring steroids with remarkable biological activity (see Section XV.2). The first member isolated was brassinolide

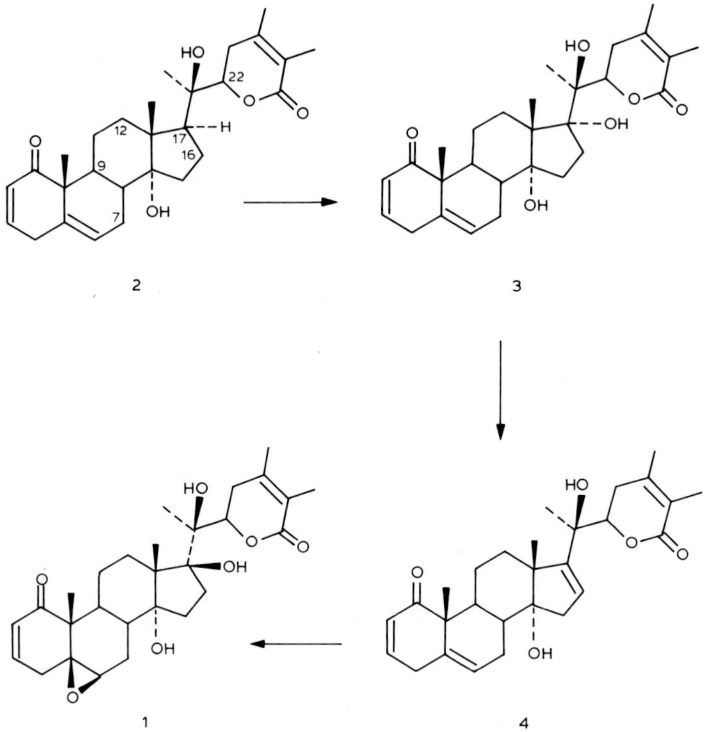

Fig. 20. Possible route for withanolide E(1) formation from withanolide G(2).

(VI) from the pollen of *Brassica napus* [11]. They have now been found in many other plant sources. The unique features of brassinolides are the 7-membered lactone B ring and a 22*R*-hydroxyl function. Brassinones, compounds with a normal B ring but with a 6-keto function and the same distribution of hydroxyls as in brassinolides, have been reported. One example is castasterone (VII) (24*S*-24-methylbrassinone) [12]; it also has the biological properties of the brassinolides. Nothing is known of the biosynthesis of these compounds but it has been suggested that castasterone is the precursor of brassinolide.

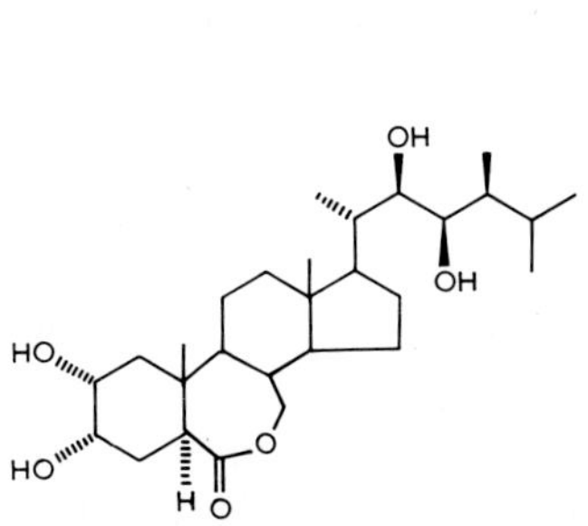

Formula VI

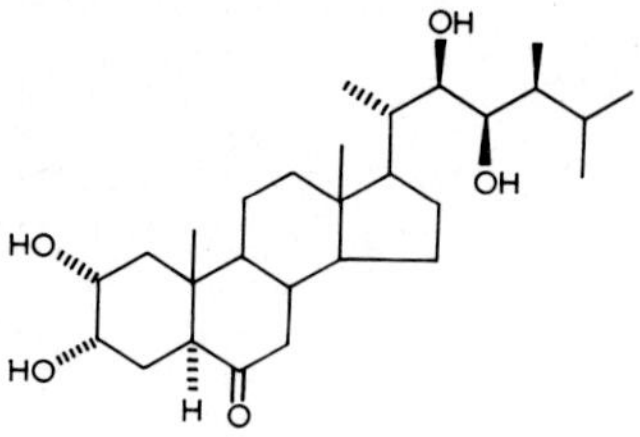

Formula VII

(XIII) Sterol esters

Particulate preparations from higher plants will esterify plant sterols; diacyl glycerols are the most effective acyl donors. However in *Phycomyces blakesleanus* the donor is phosphatidylcholine [5].

Sterol esterase activity is located in the cell membrane of white mustard (*Sinapsis alba*) seedlings; esters of C_{14}–C_{18} fatty acids are most rapidly attacked [13].

(XIV) Sterol glycosides and acylglycosides

Sterol glycosides are widely distributed in plants and are frequently accompanied by their 6-*O*-acyl derivatives. As might be expected, preparations have been obtained which glucosylate sterols with UDP-glucose as sugar donor:

UDP-glucose + sterol → sterol glucoside + UDP

Acylation of steroid glucosides is carried out by particulate preparations which catalyse the reaction:

Sterol glucoside + phosphatidylethanolamine

→ sterol-3-(6-acyl-D-)glucose + lysophosphatidylethanolamine

A soluble transacylase from carrot and radish roots used digalactosyldiglyceride as the most effective acyl donor [9,14].

(XV) Function of sterols

(1) In membranes

There is ample evidence that the sterols of plant cells are localized in the membranes of the intracellular organelles. Evidence for their function in the membranes is still only indirect. The polyene antibiotic filipin increases the cellular permeability to solutes by complexing with the membrane sterols. The degree of leakage is directly related to the sterol content of the membrane under question and the effect can be reversed by adding exogenous sterol to the membrane preparation. Ozone also increases membrane permeability whilst at the same time reducing the sterol content of the tissue; pretreatment with sterol protects again the effect [15,16].

(2) As hormones

Steroid hormones, particularly progestogens and the corticosteroid deoxycorticosterone, do exist in plants. The presence of androgens is more doubtful and oestrogens, if present, are probably there in much lower levels than originally reported. There is no doubt that exogenously applied androgens and oestrogens have physiological effects on plants so the debate, as Grunwald [15] remarks, "is whether or not these terpenes are naturally occurring products of plants". This is well exemplified by considering cortisone which enhances root growth, hypocotyl growth and lateral root formation. However it has not yet been unequivocally identified in higher plants. On the other hand deoxycorticosterone, which is a naturally occurring product, has no such stimulatory effects [17].

Steroid hormones control the sexual reproductive process in the saprophytic aquatic fungus Achlya. Antheridiol (VIII) is secreted by the vegetative female mycelium and stimulates both formation of the antheridial hyphae and the secretion of oogoniol (IX) in the male. Oogoniol then stimulates the formation of oogonia in the female. These in turn are stimulated to secrete more antheridiol which causes the chemotactic growth of the antheridial hyphae to the oogonia when mating takes place [18].

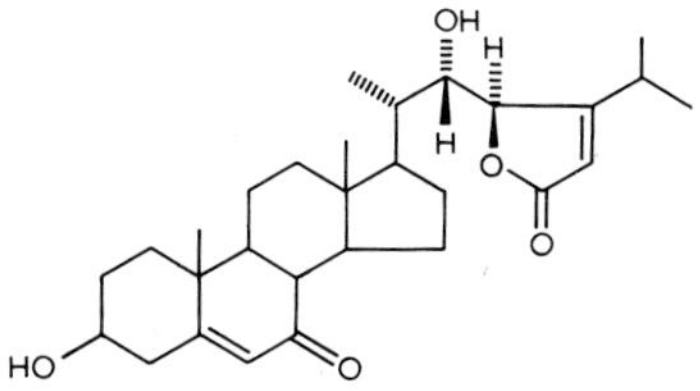

Formula VIII

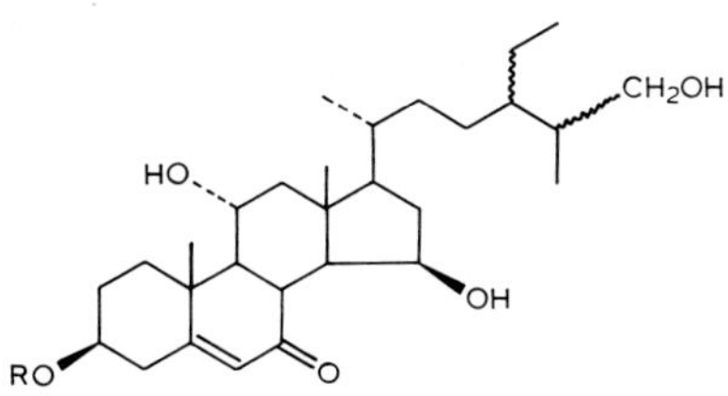

Formula IX

The brassinolides have been described as the most important discovery of plant physiologists and biochemists since the discovery of gibberellic acid. Be that as it may, their multiple biological effects are remarkable and include stimulation of cell elongation and cell division associated with splitting of the internode in the bean second-internode bioassay [11] and activity in the rice lamina inclination assay [12]. The structural requirements for activity are (i) a *trans* A/B ring system; (ii) a 6-oxo or 7-oxo system; (iii) *cis*-(α)hydroxyls at C-2 and C-3; (iv) *cis*-hydroxyls at C-22 and C-23); and (v) either a methyl or ethyl group at C-24 [19].

References

1 Nes, W.R. and McKean, M.L. (1977) Biochemistry of Steroids and other Isoprenoids, University Park Press, Baltimore, MD.
2 Goodwin, T.W. (1980) in: Biochemistry of Plants (Stumpf, P.K., Ed.) Vol. 4, Academic Press, New York.
3 Goodwin, T.W. (1981) in: Biosynthesis of Isoprenoid Compounds (Porter, J.W. and Spurgeon, S.L., Eds.) Wiley, New York.
4 Goodwin, T.W. (1985) in: The Enzymes of Biological Membranes (Martinelli, A., Ed.) Vol. 2, 2nd Edn., Plenum Press, New York.
5 Mudd, J.B. (1980) in: Biochemistry of Plants (Stumpf, P.K., Ed.) Vol. 4, Academic Press, New York.
6 Arigoni, D. (1978) Ciba Found. Symp. 60, 243.
7 Floss, H.G. and Tsai, M.-D. (1979) Adv. Enzymol. 50, 302.
8 Goad, L.J. and Goodwin, T.W. (1972) Progr. Phytochem. 3, 113–298.
9 Goodwin, T.W. and Mercer, E.I. (1983) Introduction to Plant Biochemistry, 2nd Edn., Pergamon, London.
10 Van der Velde, V. and Lavie, D. (1982) Phytochemistry 21, 731–733.
11 Grove, M.D., Spencer, G.F., Rohwedder, W.K., Mandava, N., Worley, J.F., Warthen Jr., J.D., Steffens, G.L., Flippen-Anderson, J.L. and Cook Jr., J.C. (1979) Nature (London) 281, 216–217.
12 Ikekawa, N., Takatsuto, S., Marumo, S., Abe, H., Morishita, T., Uchiyama, M., Ikeda, M., Sasa, T. and Kitsuwa, T. (1983) Proc. Jpn. Acad. 59B, 9–12.
13 Kalinowska, M. and Wojciechowski, A. (1983) Phytochemistry 22, 59.
14 Wojciechowski, Z.A. (1983) Biochem. Soc. Trans. 11, 565–568.
15 Grunwald, C. (1978) Phil. Trans. Roy. Soc. 284B, 541–558.
16 Grunwald, C. (1980) Encyclopaedia of Plant Physiology, Vol. 8, pp. 221–256, Springer, Heidelberg.
17 Geuns, J.M.C. (1972) Trends Biochem. Sci. 7, 7–9.
18 McMorris, T.C. (1978) Phil. Trans. Roy. Soc. 284B, 459–470.
19 Thompson, M.J., Meudt, W.J., Mandava, N.B., Dutky, S.R., Lusby, W.R. and Spandding, D.W. (1981) Steroids 39, 89–105.

H. Danielsson and J. Sjövall (Eds.), *Sterols and Bile Acids*

CHAPTER 8

Structures, biosynthesis and function of sterols in invertebrates

NOBUO IKEKAWA

Department of Chemistry, Tokyo Institute of Technology, Tokyo (Japan)

(I) Sterols in marine invertebrates

(1) Introduction

Recent progress on the analytical techniques of steroids by gas chromatography (GC) and high-performance liquid chromatography (HPLC) and their combination with mass spectrometry (MS) has opened a new field for studies on natural sterols. Thus, during the past decade, a great deal of information has become available on the structure and biosynthesis of sterols in invertebrates.

Sterols of marine invertebrates have been found to comprise most complex mixtures: more than 120 sterols have been isolated and their structures determined [1]. Analysis of these sterols has been performed largely by GC, GC/MS and HPLC. Stereochemical details were determined by NMR or by synthetic work. Fig. 1 demonstrates the effectivity of a capillary column; a and b showing the GC analysis of a sterol fraction obtained from the sponge, *Hymeniacidon perleve* using a packed and a capillary column, respectively [2].

Sterol patterns in marine invertebrates reflect the complexity of mixtures of sterols arising through food chains. Even in the same species, the sterol fractions show different patterns depending upon the location where the organisms have been collected. The capability of further biochemical modification of the dietary sterols makes the sterol mixtures even more complex. The symbiotic relationship between organisms also complicates the sterol compositions. These conditions are quite different from those affecting sterols of terrestrial organisms. Many sterols of unprecedented structures have now been isolated from marine sources.

Several excellent comprehensive reviews [1–11] on the structures and biosynthesis of marine sterols are available. This chapter focuses mainly on recent advances. Sterols widely distributed in marine invertebrates are shown in Fig. 2, which shows

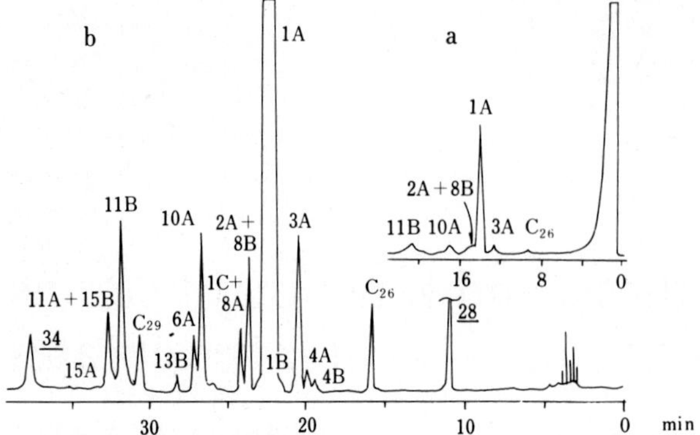

Fig. 1. GC separation of the trimethylsilyl derivatives of sterols from *Hymeniacidon perleve*. (a) Packed column, 1%OV-1, 3.6 m×3 mm i.d., 265°C. (b) Capillary column coated with OV-1, 50 m, 275°C.

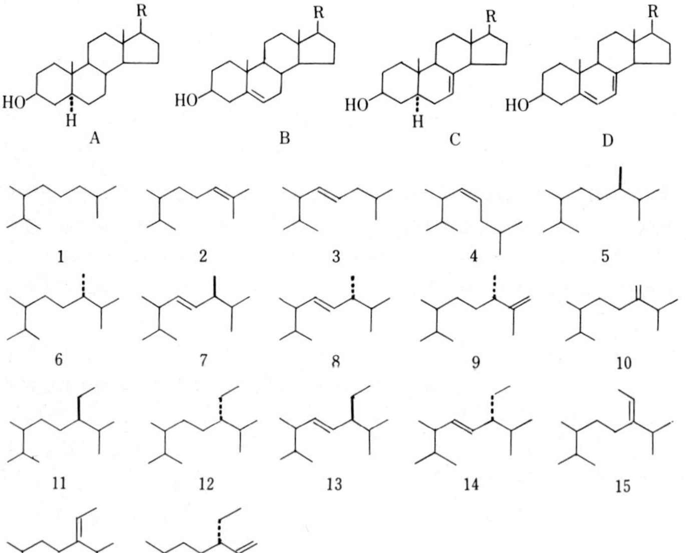

Fig. 2. Structures of conventional sterols. 1A: cholestanol, 1B: cholesterol, 1C: lathosterol, 1D: 7-dehydrocholesterol, 2B: desmosterol, 3B: 22-dehydrocholesterol, 5A: campestanol, 5B: campesterol, 5D: 7-dehydrocampesterol, 6A: ergostanol, 6B: dihydrobrassicasterol, 6C: fungisterol, 6D: 22-dihydroergosterol, 7B: pincasterol (crinosterol), 7C: stellasterol, 8B: brassicasterol, 8C: 5-dihydroergosterol, 8D: ergosterol, 9B: codisterol, 10A: 24-methylenecholestanol, 10B: 24-methylenecholesterol (chalinasterol), 10C: episterol, 11A: stigmastanol, 11B: sitosterol, 11C: stigmast-7-enol (scottenol), 11D: 7-dehydrositosterol, 12B: clionasterol, 12C: dihydrochondrillastenol, 12D: 7-dehydroclionasterol, 13B: stigmasterol, 13C: spinasterol, 13D: corbisterol (7-dehydrostigmasterol), 14B: poriferasterol, 14C: chondrillasterol, 15A: fucostanol, 15B: fucosterol, 16A: 28-isofucostanol, 16B: 28-isofucosterol (avenasterol), 16C: Δ^7-avenasterol, 17B: clerosterol.

common structures of the A/B ring system and side chain. The distribution of these sterols in marine organisms is given in the reviews of Goad [9,10].

(2) Sterols in Porifera (sponges)

Porifera (sponges) were the first invertebrates found to contain sterols other than cholesterol. Clionasterol (12B), poriferasterol (14B), chondrillasterol (14C), and chalinasterol (10B) were isolated by Bergmann. Minale et al. isolated sterols having an additional methyl group at C-26, aplysterol (18) and 24,28-dehydroaplysterol (19) as the principal sterols of *Aplysia aerophoba* [12]. They also found that the sterols of *Axinella polypoides* were a mixture of 19-nor-stanols (21) which have conventional side chains [13].

After the discovery of the C_{26}-sterols in marine planktons, all the marine C_{26}-sterols were suggested to have originated from a phytoplankton. The occurrence of 19-nor-C_{26}-sterol in *A. polypoides*, probably originating from C_{26}-sterol in the diet, suggests that one of the processes involved in the biosynthesis of these 19-nor-sterols could be the removal of the C_{10}-methyl group from the substrates [13]. The sterols in *Axinella verrucosa* were found to consist of a mixture of unique stanols containing a 3β-hydroxymethyl-A-nor-5α-cholestane (22) nucleus with conventional side chains [14]. Cholest-4-en-3-one was found to be an intermediate in the bioconversion of cholesterol into 3β-hydroxymethyl-A-nor-5α-cholestane [15].

One of the characteristic structures of the sponge sterol group is an extended and branched side chain. Two 26-methylated sterols, stelliferasterol (23) and isostelliferasterol (24) were isolated from the *Jaspis stellifera* [16]. Strongylosterol (25) was isolated as the sole sterol of *Strongylophora purissima* [17]. A 26,27-bismethylated sterol, verongulasterol (26) was isolated from the Belize sponge, *Verongula cauliformis* [18]. The major sterol in this sponge is aplysterol (18). The major sterol of the Caribbean sponge *Xestspongia muta* is xestosterol (27) which is the 25,26-dihydro-24(28)-dehydro analogue of verongulasterol [19]. Other major trimethylated sterols from Pseudaxinyssa sp. are 24-isopropylcholesterol (28) and 24-isopropyl-22-dehydrocholesterol [20]. The structurally related 24-isopropenylcholesterol (29) was isolated from *V. cauliformis*.

Recently, 24- and 25-methylated sterols were isolated from sponges by Djerassi's group. GC/MS analysis of *X. muta* from Barbados showed that at least 18 sterols were present, the main sterol being 24(28)-dehydroaplysterol (19). In addition, 24-isopropenylcholesterol (29), verongulasterol (26), and a new sterol named mutasterol (30) were identified [21] (Fig. 3).

Capillary GC analysis of the sterols of the Caribbean Xestospongia species, containing predominantly xestosterol (27), indicated a new sterol, xestospongesterol (31) which was separated by reversed-phase HPLC [22]. The structure was determined by mass spectrometry and NMR as a hitherto unprecedented quadruply biomethylated sterol. From the Indopacific sponge *Strongylophora durissima*, which has been reported to contain over 90% of strongylosterol, a new sterol named

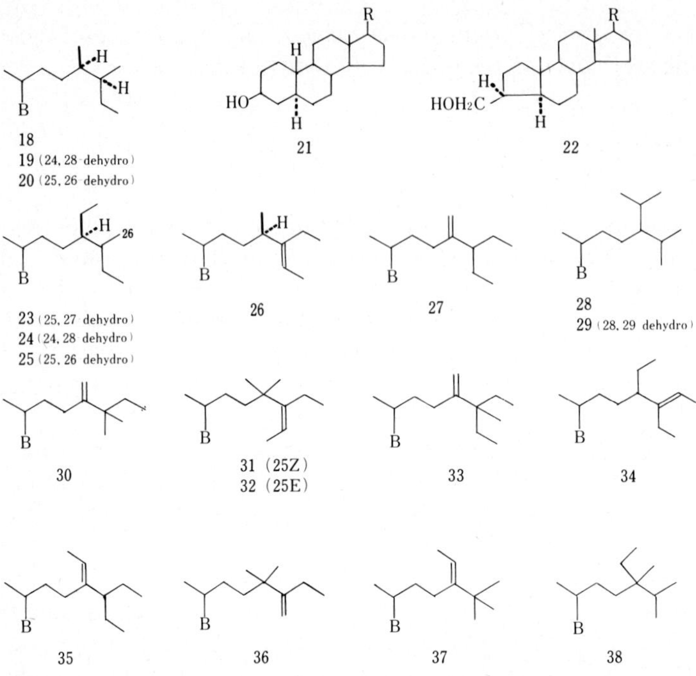

Fig. 3.

isoxestospongesterol (32) [22] was isolated and the structure was determined as the 25*E* isomer of xestospongesterol (31).

Several other quadruply methylated sterols were reported by Djerassi's group: 25-methylxestosterol (33) [23] from a Caribbean sponge Xestospongia sp.; 26-methylstrongylosterol (34), 28-methylxestosterol (35), and a new sterol named durissimasterol (36), from the Indopacific sponge *S. durissima* [24]. Other sterols with highly branched side chain, axinyssasterol (25-methylfucosterol) (37) and 24-ethyl-24-methylcholesterol (38), were isolated from Pseudoaxinyssa sp. collected in the region of the Australian Great Barrier Reef [25].

After identification of several sterols with a cyclopropane ring in the side chain from gorgonian species, modified cyclopropane sterols were also found in porifera. Calysterol (39) was isolated from the *Calyx niceaensis* by Sica et al. in 1975 [26]. Subsequent investigation led to the isolation of a new sterol, stigmasta-5,23-dien-3β-ol as the principal sterol of this sponge. Although the sponge has no capacity of sterol biosynthesis, conversion of [^{3}H]fucosterol to calysterol indicated an ability to modify dietary sterols [27]. In a reinvestigation of the same sponge, (23*R*)-23*H*-isocalysterol (40) [28], (24*S*)-24*H*-isocalysterol (41) [29] and 23,24-dihydrocalysterol [28] were identified in addition to two new Δ^{23}-sterols, (23*E*)- and (23*Z*)-stigmasta-5,23-dien-3β-ol [29].

Another cyclopropane sterol, petrosterol (42) was isolated as the major sterol from *Petrosia ficiformis* and Halichondria sp. The structure was determined as

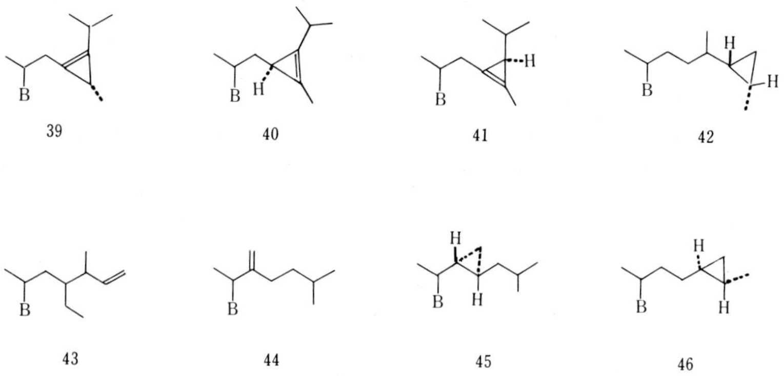

Fig. 4.

26,27-cycloaplysterol [30,31]. By careful analysis of the sterol fraction of *P. ficiformis* [26], a new C_{29}-sterol, ficisterol [32], was isolated and the structure determined as 23-ethyl-24-methyl-27-norcholesta-5,25-dien-3β-ol (43). 22-Methylenecholesterol (44) as the first example of a 22-monoalkylated cholesterol, was identified in the sterol fraction of *Halichondria panicea* [33] (Fig. 4). These two sterols are of interest in respect of the biosynthesis of marine sterols, indicating the occurrence of alkylation at C-22 and C-23 in contrast to the limitation of alkylation to C-24 in terrestrial plants.

In a continuing search by Djerassi's group, a new cyclopropane sterol was isolated from various sponges as a minor component and the structure was determined as (22*R*,23*R*)-methylenecholesterol (45) [34] which has the opposite configuration to naturally occurring demethylgorgosterol. This indicates that bioalkylation of the Δ^{22} double bond is possible even in the absence of a C-24 alkyl substituent. Another novel cyclopropyl sterol, 24,26-cyclocholesterol (46) [35] was isolated from the Spheciospongia sp.

Conventional marine sterols have Δ^5-, Δ^7- or $\Delta^{5,7}$-diene nuclei, but the occurrence of Δ^8-sterols was reported in *Axinella cannabina* [36]. Recently a complete analysis of sterols in the same species by Itoh et al. [37] showed the presence of 74 sterols with a variety of nuclei ($\Delta^{5,7,9(11)}$, $\Delta^{5,7}$, Δ^8, Δ^7, Δ^5, 5α-saturated and 5α-methoxy-$\Delta^{6,8(14)}$) and with different side chains. Sterols having $\Delta^{5,7,9(11)}$ and $\Delta^{7,9(11)}$ nuclei have also been reported [38].

A survey by Djerassi et al. indicated that sterols with different side chains exist in an A-nor form (22). Notably, they isolated an A-nor sterol with a gorgosterol side chain [39]. Since gorgosterol has so far been found in only coelenterate–zooxanthellae combinations (with the exception of Δ^7-gorgosterol, from a starfish and A-nor-sterols only in the sponge), the authors assumed that *Stylotella agminata* had converted gorgosterol or its 5,6-dihydro analogue of dietary origin into the A-nor form.

Teichaxinella morchella from the Gulf of Mexico has been shown to contain solely 3-hydroxymethyl-A-nor-sterols, two of which are the new 3-hydroxymethyl-A-nor-

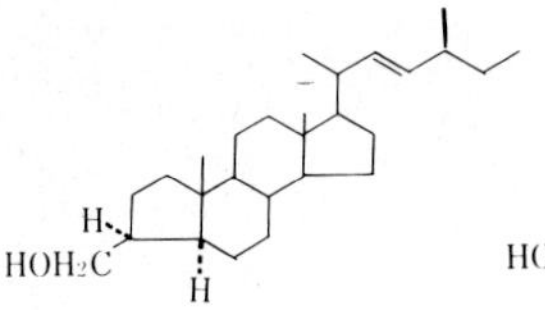

Fig. 5.

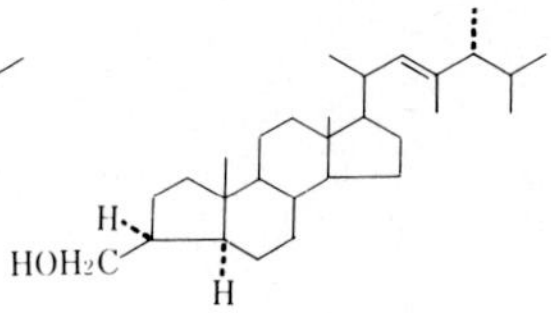

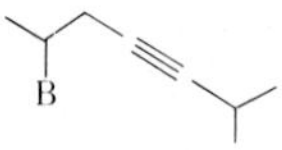

patinosterol (47) and 3-hydroxymethyl-A-nor-dinosterol analogue (48) isolated as acetate [40]. Sixteen 3-hydroxymethyl-A-nor sterols have been found in the Red Sea sponge *Acanthella aurantiaca,* which contains no sterols with conventional skeletons [41]. A new A-nor-sterol, 3-hydroxymethyl-A-nor-5α-cholest-15-ene, has been found in the Pacific sponge *Homaxinella tracys* together with 10 other A-nor-sterols [42]. The majority of the sponges containing A-nor-sterols lack sterols with conventional nuclei. This probably means that they have a very effective enzyme system for the transformation of dietary sterols into A-nor-sterols.

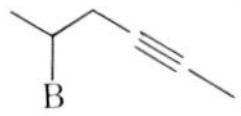

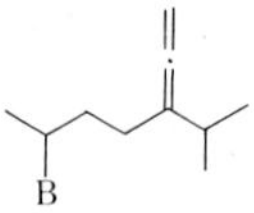

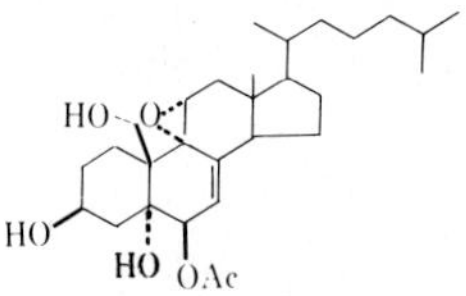

Several 5α,8α-epidioxysterols with Δ^6 or $\Delta^{6,9(11)}$ and conventional side chains have been isolated from sponges [43]. Two new unsaturated sterols having $\Delta^{8(14)}$ and 4-methylene nuclei, conicasterol and theonellasterol, were isolated as the principal sterols from the Red Sea sponges *Theonella conica* (Kieschnick) and *Theonella swinhoei* (Gray), respectively [44].

It is of interest to note that two acetylenic sterols, cholest-5-en-23-yn-3β-ol (49) and 26,27-dinorcholest-5-en-23-yn-3β-ol (50), were isolated from *Calyx nicaensis* as minor sterols [45], and 24-ethyl-$\Delta^{5,24(28),28}$-cholestatrien-3β-ol (51) from *Callyspongia diffusa* [46]. A new polyhydroxysterol (52) with a 19-hydroxyl group was reported by Schmitz in Dysidea sp. collected in Guam [47] (Fig. 5).

(3) Sterols in Coelenterata

Cholesterol is a major sterol in Coelenterata. The predominant sterol is gorgosterol

(53) whose occurrence was first reported in the gorgonian *Plaxaura flexuosa* by Bergmann in 1943. This sterol was later isolated from several gorgonians by Ciereszko, Gupta and Scheuer. Ciereszko also demonstrated that the occurrence of this sterol was associated with zooxanthellae, the symbiotic unicellular algae. The presence of the unprecedented cyclopropane side chain was indicated by mass spectrometry and NMR, and finally the structure of gorgosterol was determined by X-ray crystallography [48,49]. 23-Demethylgorgosterol (54) was isolated from *Gorgonia flabellum* and *G. ventilina* by Schmitz [50]. Recently, stereocontrolled synthesis of these cyclopropane sterols was achieved by our group [51,52].

9,11-Secogorgost-5-ene-3,11-diol-9-one (55) was isolated from *Pseudopterogorgia americana* [53]. Recently, the 9,11-secosteroids with conventional side chains (1, 6, 10 in Fig. 2), and their C-8 epimers were found in the soft coral, Sinularia sp. [54]. Minor and trace sterol analysis of *Pseudoplexaura porosa* and *Plexaura homomalla* has been reported by Djerassi, and 49 sterols, including 3-keto-4-ene and 5α analogues of gorgosterol, were identified [55].

A number of polyhydroxy sterols were isolated from coelenterata: 25-hydroxy-24-methylcholesterol [56] from Nephtea sp., 24-methylcholestane-3β,5α,6β,25-tetrol 25-acetate [57] and its 12-hydroxy analogue [58] from *Sarcophyton elegans*, 24-methylcholestane-1β,3β,5α,6β,25-pentol 25-acetate (56) and its 1β,3β,5α,6β-tetrahydroxy analogue from *Sarcophyton glaucum* [59]. 1β,3β,5α,6β-Tetrahydroxy-5α-androstan-17-one [60] and new $\Delta^{5,17(20)}$ sterols [61] were also isolated from the same soft coral.

The most notable sterol isolated by Kobayashi from the soft coral *S. glaucum* was a new C_{27}-sterol named glaucasterol (57) [62], shown to have the same structure as papakusterol isolated from deep sea gorgonians [63]. The 24*S*,25*S* stereochemistry of this sterol has been established by synthesis [64] and correlation with occelasterol [65].

Several polyhydroxy sterols were isolated from octocorals, alcyonaceans, gorgonians and other marine sources. Hippurin-I (58) [66], 3α-acetoxy-11β-hydroxy-24-methyl-22,25-epoxy-5α-furostan-18,20β-lactone (59), 3α-acetoxy-24-methyl-11β,18;18,20β;22,25-triepoxy-5α-furostane (60) and several of their analogues were isolated from *Isis hippuris* collected in Okinawa by Higa [67]. A polyhydroxy sterol (61) containing the gorgosterol side chain was also present [68] (Fig. 6).

24-Methylenecholest-5-ene-3β,7β,19-triol (62) [69] and 4α-methyl-3β,8β-dihydroxy-5α-ergost-24(28)-en-23-one (63) [70] were isolated from the soft coral *Litophyton viridis*. The former compound might be a biosynthetic precursor of 19-norsteroids. Other 4α-methylated sterols and 19-norcholesterol derivatives were also reported from several gorgonians. Higgs isolated new 3-ketopregnanes (64) and two 3α-acetoxypregnanes (65) from soft corals [71]. 23,24-Dimethylcholesta-5,22-dien-3β-ol (66) [72] and its Δ^{23} isomer [73] were obtained from *S. elegans* by Kanazawa et al. The 19-nor-5,6-dihydro analogue [74] of (66) was isolated from the sponge *Axinella polypoides*. The 4-methyl analogue of (66), dinosterol (67) [75], was also isolated from the plankton *Gonyaulax tamarensis*.

Unusual 20-epicholanic acid derivatives (68,69) were isolated from the sea pen, *Ptilosarcus gurneyi* [76]. A characteristic property of these compounds is the shorter

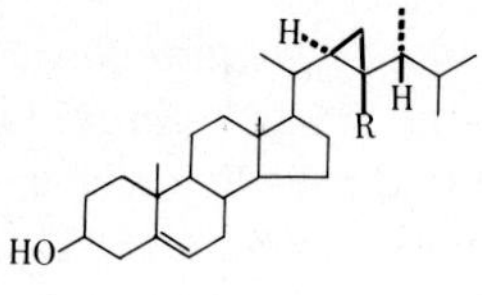

53 R=CH3
54 R=H

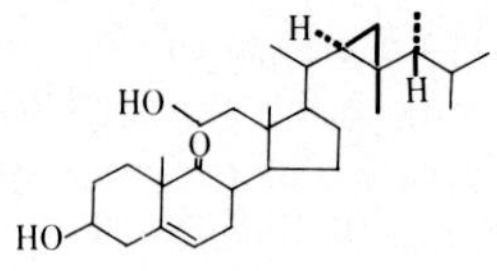

55

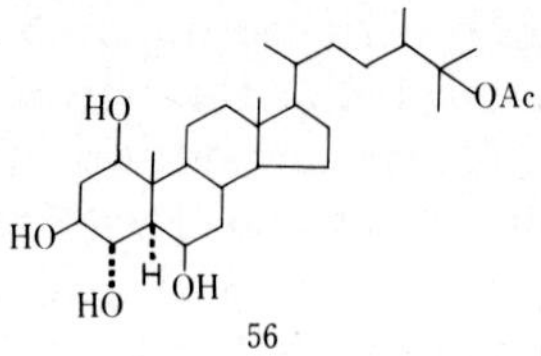

56

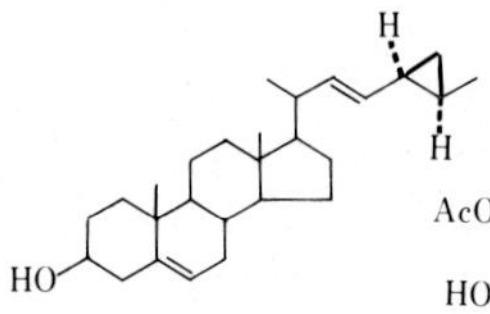

57

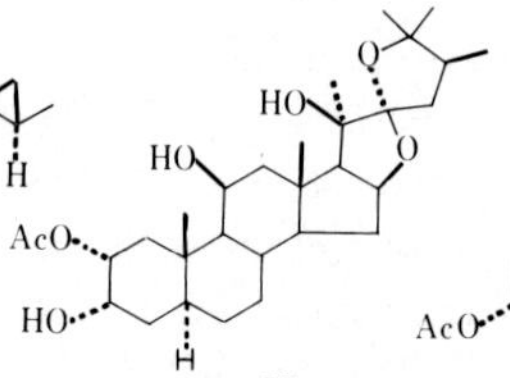

58

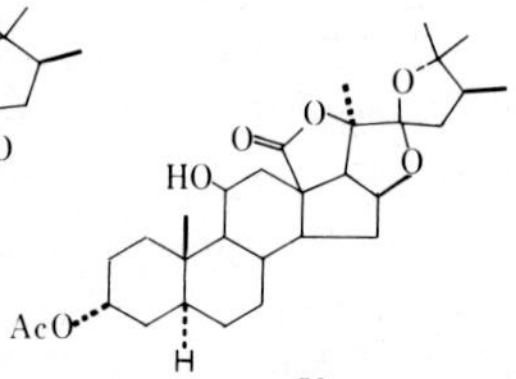

59

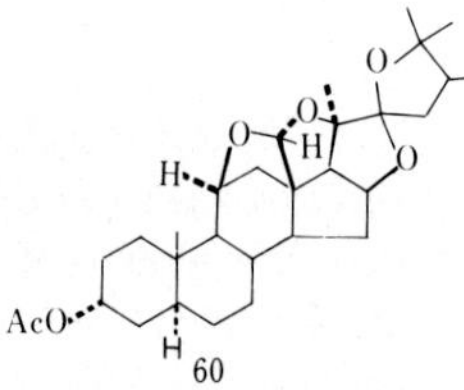

60

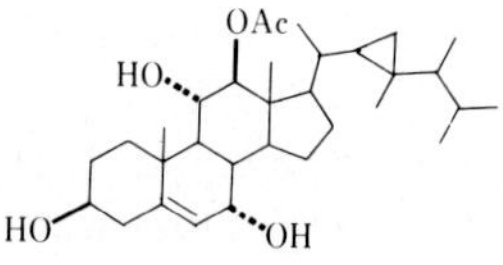

61

Fig. 6.

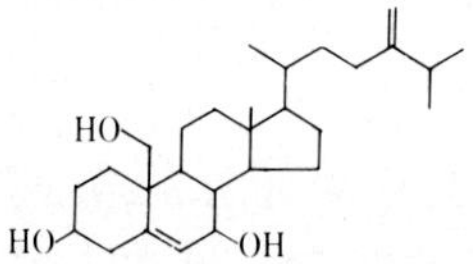

62

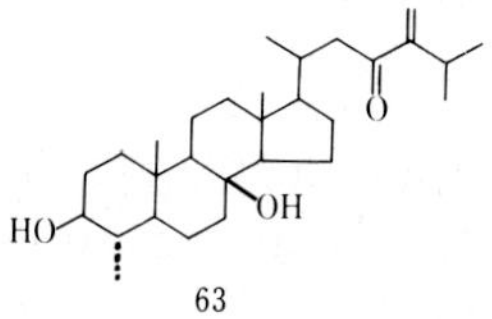

63

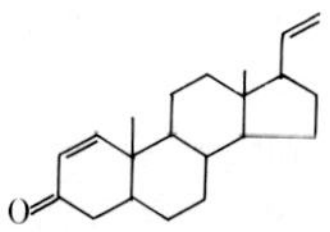

64 (5α-H & Δ1)

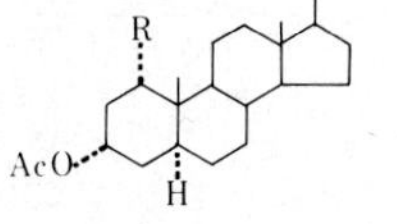

65 (R=H & OH)

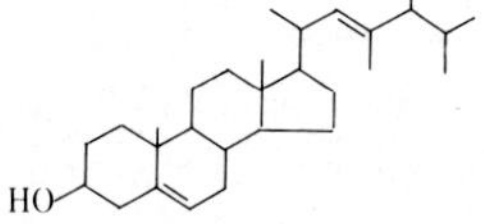

66

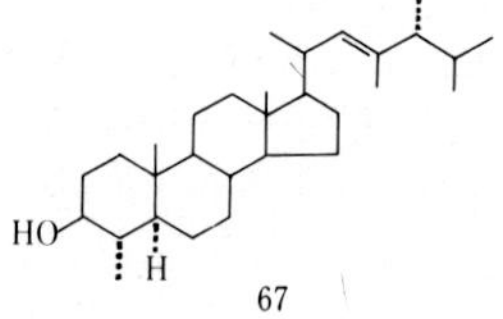

67

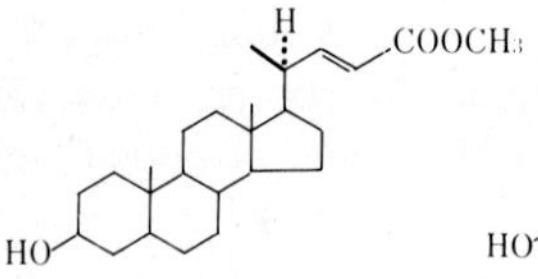

68 =Δ5 & 5α

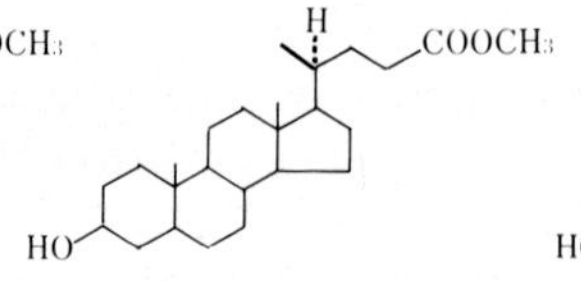

69 =Δ5 & 5α

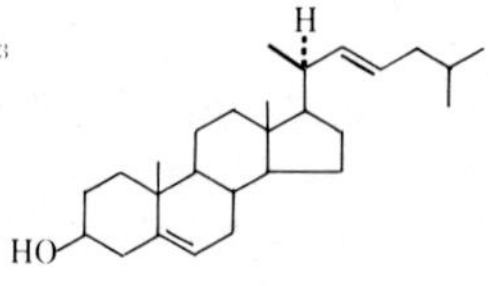

70

Fig. 7.

retention time than those of their natural C-20 isomers on GC analysis. The isolated steroids, as methyl esters, were identical with the synthetic 20-epicholenic acid methyl esters. Idler probably obtained the C-20 epimer of cholesta-5,22-dien-3β-ol (70) [77] from the scallop *Placopecten magellanicus* (Fig. 7). The structure is proposed from its short retention time on GC.

The incorporation of labelled acetate into cholesterol in coelenterata has not been demonstrated. Thus, it is likely that various sterols in coelenterata are of algal origin. They may be obtained either in the diet or by transfer from symbiotic zooxanthellae.

Djerassi et al. have found a group of characteristic sterols in marine organisms which have side chains ranging from 0 to 6 carbon atoms. They occur as minor components in various species of Porifera and Coelenterata [78] and may be formed by in vivo auto-oxidation, or be of dietary origin. Accumulation of auto-oxidation products may be more prevalent in marine invertebrates than in mammals, since many marine organisms are known to store excretion products. The side chains are apparently too short for the sterols to be functional membrane constituents, but if these sterols are shown to arise by in vivo or environmental auto-oxidation in the oceans, it will have important implications in marine biochemistry and ecology.

(4) Sterols in Echinodermata (starfish)

The major sterols of Echinodermata are C_{27}-sterols. Cholesterol is the principal sterol in echinoids (70–80%), ophiuroids, and crinoids. 5α-Cholest-7-en-3β-ol is the major sterol in asteroids and sea cucumbers. A C_{26}-sterol, 24-norcholesta-5,22-dien-3β-ol (83) is also a common sterol in Echinodermata: the content is especially high (6–10%) in ophiuroids and crinoids [79]. Asterosterol (70), a Δ^7-C_{26}-sterol, is common in asteroids and sea cucumbers [80], and amuresterol (71) was isolated from *Asterias amurensis* [81].

Acanthasterol [82] (acansterol) [83,84] (72), the Δ^7 isomer of gorgosterol, was isolated from *Acanthaster planci* by Scheuer. Gorgostanol [85] and demethylacanthasterol (73) [86] were also found in *A. planci* [86] (Fig. 8). Transformation from Δ^5- to Δ^7-sterol may be a common bioconversion in Echinodermata, because gorgonians are components of the diet of *A. planci* in which gorgosterol cannot be found.

In addition to cholesterol and 5α-cholest-7-en-3β-ol, many C_{28} and C_{29} conventional sterols are present in Echinodermata. These sterols are probably derived from the diet. However, echinoderms are able to synthesize sterols. Thus, [^{14}C]mevalonic acid was incorporated into squalene, lanosterol and desmosterol by the sea urchin, *Echinus esculentus* [87]. The ability of ophiuroids to synthesize sterol from [^{14}C]acetate has also been demonstrated [88]. Sterol biosynthesis by a holothuroid was first investigated by Numura [89], and sterol biosynthesis from [^{14}C]acetate in sea cucumbers has also been reported [90].

The ability of starfish to synthesize sterols was first demonstrated by Smith and Goad, who found a slow incorporation of [^{14}C]mevalonate into 4-desmethylsterols [91]. The main labelled sterol in *A. rubens* was 5α-cholest-7-en-3β-ol [92]. Evidence

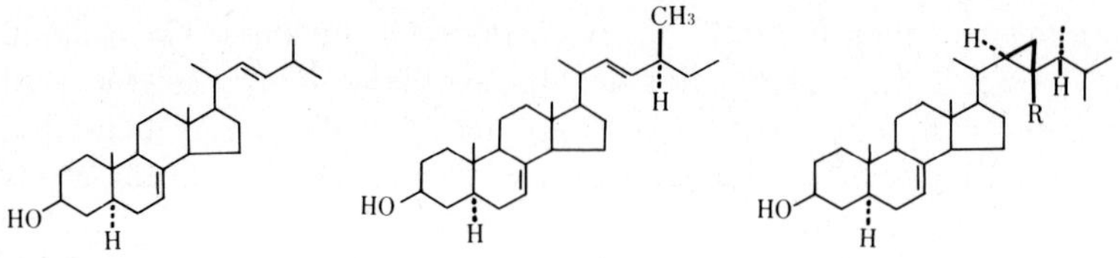

Fig. 8.

that cholesterol was converted into cholestanol and 5α-cholest-7-en-3β-ol, and that cholestanol was converted to 5α-cholest-7-en-3β-ol was also obtained.

Estradiol and progesterone have been tentatively identified in extracts of ovaries of the starfish *Pisaster ochraceus* [93] and the sea urchin *Stronglyocentrotus franciscanus* [94]. Progesterone was also identified in the ovaries of the starfish *Asterias amurensis* by Ikegami [95]. The physiological role of progesterone in starfish ovaries is unknown, but probably is connected with oocyte maturation.

In marine invertebrates, saponins have been found exclusively in the Echinodermata and particularly in Holothuroidea (sea cucumbers) and Asteroidea (starfishes) [96]. Saponins from sea cucumbers are triterpenoid glycosides, and those from starfishes are sulphated steroidal glycosides. The structure of the major saponin, thornasteroside A (74) in *Acanthaster planci* was determined by Kitagawa et al. [97]. The structure of glycoside B_2, an asterosaponin isolated from the ovaries of *Asterias amurensis* by Ikegami, is quite similar to that of thornasteroside A except that the terminal fucose is replaced by quinovose [98]. Ikegami et al. have also determined the structure of asterosaponin A (75) [99], one of the two major saponins from the sea starfish. This saponin was found to be the spawning inhibitor of the starfish, and also to inhibit the production of 1-methyladenine in the follicle cell. Several sapogenins having 20-ketone, $\Delta^{20(22)}$ or $\Delta^{17(20)}$ groupings may be artifacts produced during the purification of 20-hydroxy sapogenins. Structures of several "asterosaponins" from *Marthasterias glacialis* were also determined by Minale et al. [96].

A new type of saponin was discovered as toxic substances in starfishes of the genus Echinaster. The structure of steroidal cyclic glycosides, sepositoside A (76) from the Mediterranean starfish *Echinaster sepositus* [100] was determined. Three major saponins in the same starfish were isolated, and their structures were found to have 22,23-epoxide groups in the side chain [101].

Other new types of saponin which have a 24-*O*-glycoside group were isolated by Minale et al. and their complete structures were determined. Nodonside (77) [102] was isolated from the Pacific *Protoreaster nodosus*, while 5 related glycosides were isolated from the Mediterranean *Hacelia attenutata* (Fig. 9).

Three polyhydroxy steroids, 3β,6α,8β,15α,16β,26-hexa-, 3β,6α,7α,8β,15α,16β,26-hepta- and 3β,4β,6α,7α,8β,15α,16β,26-octahydroxy steroids were isolated from *P.*

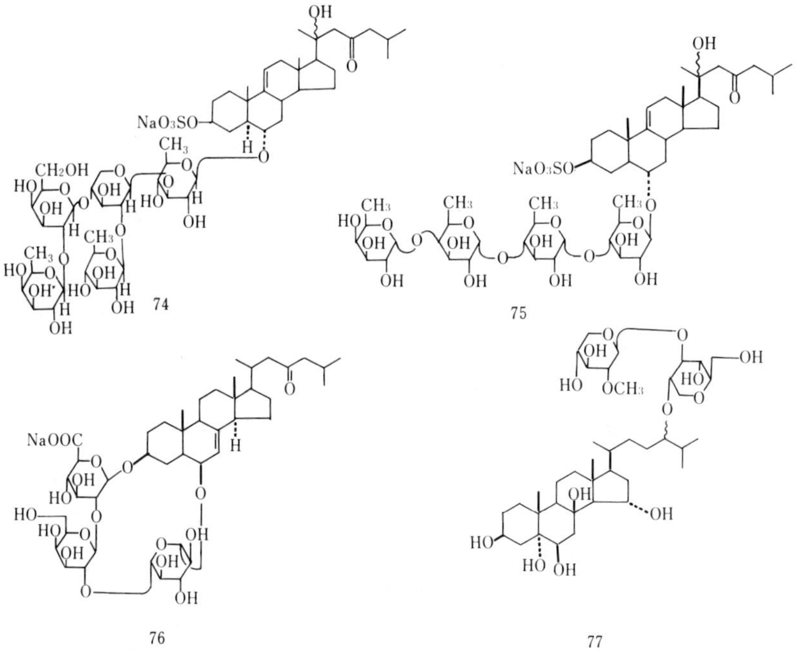

NaO$_3$SO CH$_3$ CH$_2$OH HO OH O H CH$_3$ OH HO OH 74

NaO$_3$SO CH$_3$ HO OH 75

NaOOC HO OH O H 76

HO OH OCH$_3$ 77

Fig. 9.

nodosus [103]. The octahydroxy steroids are the most highly hydroxylated sterols isolated from natural sources to date.

The toxicity of starfishes may be derived from the saponins. The biological activities of these compounds were reported, including haemolytic properties, and antitumour [104] and antibacterial activities [105]. Inhibition activities for influenza virus multiplication, and anti-inflammatory activity towards contraction of the rat phrenic nerve diaphragm preparation, were also reported [106]. Saponins are chemical defence agents in starfishes, and they also induce escape reactions in bivalve molluscs [107]. It is of interest to note that the sperm agglutination substance in the egg jelly of starfish is similar to asterosaponin A [108].

(5) Sterols in crustaceans

In crustaceans cholesterol is a predominant sterol, but considerable amounts of desmosterol and small amounts of C_{28}- and C_{29}-sterols are also present. It is now established that [^{14}C]acetate and [^{14}C]mevalonate are not incorporated into sterols, indicating incapability for the de novo synthesis of sterols. A nutritional requirement for sterol has been demonstrated for the prawn *Penaeus japonicus* [109]. After feeding prawns phytosterol, the sterol isolated was predominantly cholesterol [110]. Dealkylation of 24-methyl and 24-ethyl sterols to yield cholesterol has been demon-

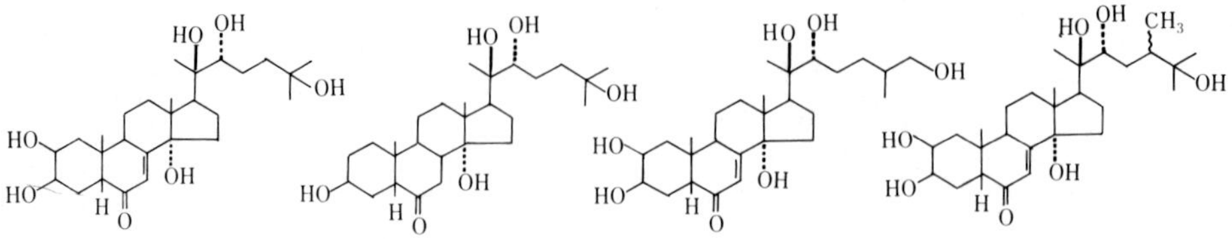

Fig. 10.

strated in several crustaceans, as in insects [111]. It is most likely that a similar mechanism to that described for insects is operating in crustaceans. The presence of high levels of desmosterol in some crustacean species supports this assumption.

Transformation of cholesterol into steroid hormones in crustaceans has been investigated [10]. Side chain cleavage of cholesterol affording C_{21}-steroids was reported in the lobster, *Panulirus japonica* [112]. Conversion of progesterone into corticosteroids was also demonstrated using homogenates of the androgenic gland of the male blue crab, *Callinectes sapidus* [113,114].

In 1960, the presence of a substance which showed ecdysone activity was detected in crabs by Karlson and Skinner [115]. Moulting in crustaceans is controlled by the Y-organ which is the organ analogous to the prothoracic gland in insects. In 1966, crustecdysone (20-hydroxyecdysone) (78) was first isolated from the crayfish, *Jasus lalandei*, by Horn et al. [116], and subsequently 2-deoxyecdysterone (79) [117] was isolated. 20-Hydroxyecdysteroids, callinecdysone A (inokosterone) (80) and callinecdysone B (makisterone A, possibly the 24-epimer) (81) were isolated from *Calinectes sapidus* [118].

Evidence that [^{14}C]cholesterol was converted into ecdysone in the lobster, *Homarus americanus*, was presented [119]. A detailed investigation of cholesterol uptake and turnover by the crab, *Hemigrapsus nudus*, was also reported [120,121]. Ecdysone was converted to 20-hydroxyecdysone by crustaceans. Moulting of crustaceans induced by administrated ecdysteroids was reported [122]. Changes of the moulting hormone concentration during the moulting cycle have been determined in the freshwater crayfish, *Orconectes limosus* [123] (Fig. 10).

(6) Sterols in Mollusca and others

Generally the sterols in Mollusca are a complex mixture of C_{26}-, C_{27}-, C_{28}- and C_{29}-sterols [124]. In the classes of Gastropoda, Bivalvia and Cephalopoda, Δ^5-sterols including cholesterol are the most abundant sterols. In the class Amphineura, Δ^7-sterols are predominant in all species, and 5α-cholest-7-en-3β-ol is the major sterol. Cephalopoda contain cholesterol as about 90% of the total sterols. Gastropoda and Bivalvia also contain cholesterol as the major sterol (50–60%). In some species of Bivalvia, the sterol fraction is a mixture of C_{27}-, C_{28}- and C_{29}-sterols, and in some species dihydrobrassicasterol is the major sterol (34–65%). The most significant feature in molluscs is the considerable amount of $\Delta^{5,7}$-diene sterols. Corbisterol, 7-dehydrostigmasterol (82), was first isolated [125]. The occurrence of these vitamin D precursors may be essential for calcium metabolism and shell formation.

In 1970, a new C_{26}-sterol was first isolated from *Placopecten magellanicus* by Idler [126], and its structure was determined as (22*E*)-24-norcholesta-5,22-dien-3β-ol (83). Subsequently C_{26}-sterols were found in many marine sources. These sterols may be of dietary origin from algae, but the mode of biosynthesis is still unknown. (22*Z*)-Cholesta-5,22-dien-3β-ol was reported from several molluscs [127].

A new C_{30}-sterol, (24*Z*)-24-propylidenecholest-5-en-3-β-ol (84) was isolated from the scallop, *P. magellanicus* [128]. Occelasterol (85), (22*E*,24*S*)-27-nor-24-methyl-cholesta-5,22-dien-3β-ol, and its 5,6-dihydro analogue, patinosterol, were isolated from the scallop, *Patinopecten yessoensis* [129] (Fig. 11).

Many investigations have been reported on the biosynthesis of sterols in molluscs [124]. Incorporation of acetate into sterol was not significant, but usually mevalonate was converted into sterol in high yield. Members of Amphineura, a primitive class of molluscs, contain mainly 5α-cholest-7-en-3β-ol, of which the biosynthesis has been investigated. Teshima and Kanazawa demonstrated that *Liolophura japonica* incorporated [^{14}C]mevalonate into 5α-cholest-7-en-3β-ol, but not into cholesterol [130]. Similar results were also observed in *Lepidochitona cinera* [131]. It is generally considered that molluscs can synthesize only C_{27}-sterols, and that their C_{28}- and C_{29}-sterols originate from their diet (algae). There is a report on the transmethylation of C_{27} to give C_{28}-sterol in molluscs [132]. However, [^{14}C]mevalonate was not incorporated into sterols in the oyster, *Ostrea gryphea* [133].

Dealkylation of phytosterols to cholesterol is now well known in insects and crustaceans. The transformation of [^{3}H]fucosterol into cholesterol and desmosterol was also observed in two species of molluscs [134]. Desmosterol is a widely distributed sterol in molluscs, and in some species the content is very high (30–35%) [127,135]. This sterol can be considered as the dealkylation product of 24-alkylsterols, and it is likely that desmosterol accumulates because of low activity of the Δ^{24}-sterol reductase. The capacity for both alkylation and dealkylation at the C-24 position in molluscs remains to be clarified.

The endocrinological system of steroid hormones in molluscs has been established, and many reports on the biosynthesis and metabolism of progesterone, estrogens and androgens have been published [10].

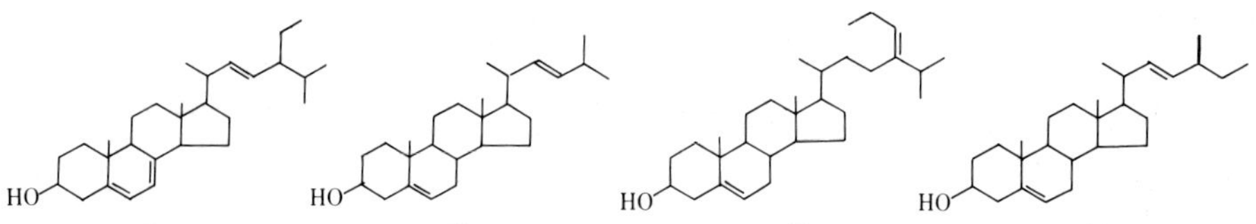

HO 82 HO 83 HO 84 HO 85

Fig. 11.

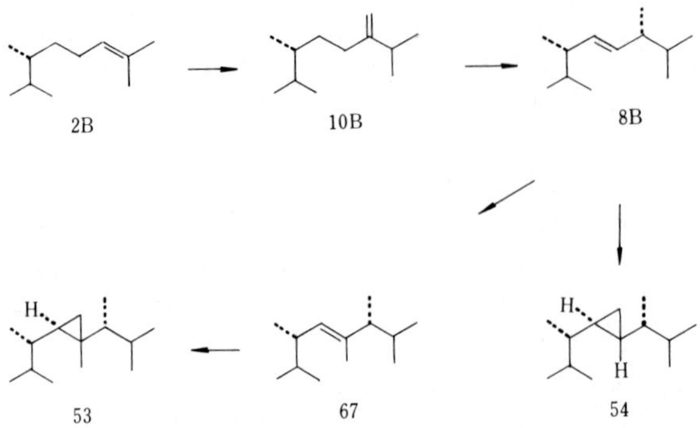

Fig. 12.

(7) Side chain modification of sterols in marine invertebrates

Biosynthesis of non-conventional sterols in marine invertebrates has not been much investigated, but the pathway can be postulated from consideration of the sterols isolated. The side chain of demethylgorgosterol may be constructed from brassicasterol (8B) which has been generated from desmosterol (2B) via 24-methylenecholesterol (10B) by transmethylation from *S*-adenosylmethionine (SAM). Bioalkylation of 8B would lead to demethylgorgosterol (54). Biosynthesis of gorgosterol (53) has not been investigated, but the isolation of dinosterol (67) from dinoflagellates, and of related sterols from the soft corals, suggests that gorgosterol may be of dinoflagellate origin and be biosynthesized from dinosterol. The transmethylation from [C^2H_3]methionine to dinosterol was demonstrated with a dinoflagellate by Withers et al. [215] (Fig. 12).

Biosynthesis of branched and highly alkylated sterols in marine invertebrates has been the subject of speculation. Tris- or quadruple-methylation would produce branched sterols in Porifera. Epi-codisterol (C-24-Epi-9B) can be assumed to be a precursor of 25(26)-dehydroaplysterol (20) which is biomethylated again to give

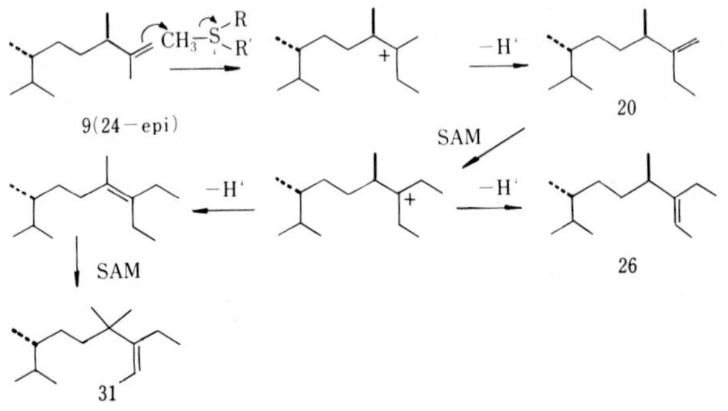

Fig. 13.

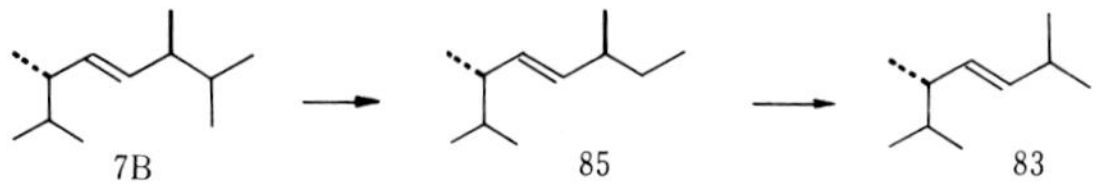

Fig. 14.

verongulasterol (26) or xestosterol (27). Transmethylation from SAM to the double-bond isomer of (26) would give xestospongesterol (31). Biosynthetic pathways of other non-conventional sterols can be postulated in the same way (Fig. 13).

The evidence that the C_{27}-nor-sterol, occelasterol (85), has the same 24α-configuration as 24α-methylcholesta-5,22-dien-3β-ol (7B) which was identified in a scallop, indicates the demethylation pathway from C_{27}-sterol to 27-nor-sterol. The C_{26}-sterol (83) may be formed from C_{27}-nor-sterol (85) (Fig. 14). Since C_{26}-sterol is widely distributed in marine invertebrates, it seems likely that this sterol may be produced in a rather early stage of the marine food chain.

(II) Sterol metabolism in insects

(1) Dealkylation of phytosterol

Insects, unlike most vertebrates and plants, lack the capacity for de novo sterol synthesis and require dietary sterol for their normal growth, development and reproduction. This sterol requirement is in most cases satisfied by cholesterol (86) which is one of the principal sterols in insects, serving as component of the cell membranes and as a precursor of ecdysone (107). The zoophagous species such as the house fly *Mucosa domestica* are unable to convert phytosterol to cholesterol. For this reason, cholesterol is an essential nutrient for these species. In phytophagous and omnivorous insects, sterols such as sitosterol (87), campesterol (88), and stigmasterol (89) are dealkylated to cholesterol. Thus, 24-dealkylation is one of the essential metabolic processes in phytophagous insects (Fig. 15).

Since the first rigorous demonstration of the dealkylative conversion of ergosterol into 22-dehydrocholesterol in the German cockroach *Blattela germanica,* several reports have appeared on the conversion of phytosterols into cholesterol in a variety of insects. The biochemical mechanism of the conversion has been investigated in

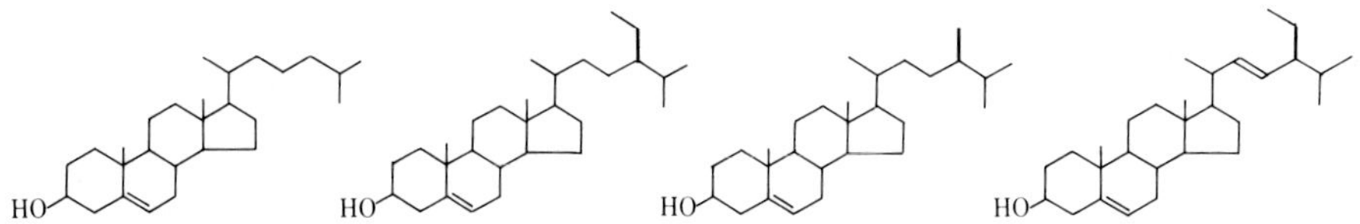

Fig. 15.

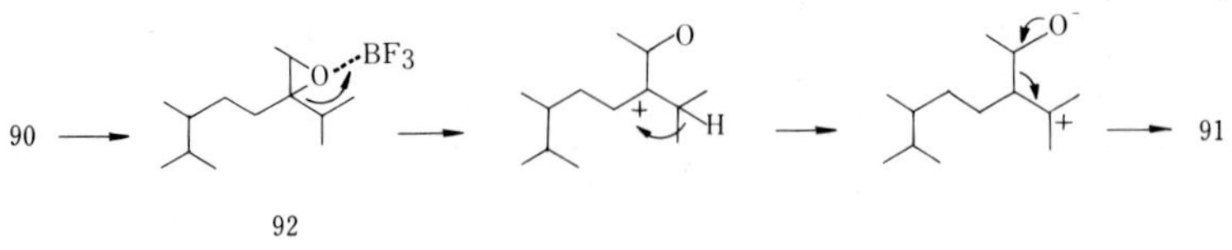

90 → 92 → → → 91

Fig. 16.

detail by the Beltsville group, using the tobacco hornworm [142–145]. They identified fucosterol (90) and desmosterol (91) as the intermediates in the conversion. The observation that fucosterol epoxide (92) yields desmosterol (91) [146] upon treatment with boron trifluoride-etherate, (Fig. 16) led us to propose that fucosterol epoxide is a key intermediate in the conversion of sitosterol to cholesterol [147]. This was subsequently verified in the silkworm *Bombyx mori*. When [^{3}H]fucosterol epoxide was ingested by silkworm larvae, it was converted to cholesterol in considerable yield, and the tritium of [^{3}H]fucosterol was trapped in fucosterol epoxide [148]. The tritium of [25-^{3}H]sitosterol migrated to the C-24 position during its conversion to desmosterol [149]. Fucosterol epoxide completely satisfied the silkworm sterol requirement.

Subsequently data from other insects support the biogenetic pathway show in Fig. 17. Goodwin's group found that the dealkylation of the synthetic [25-^{3}H, 26-^{14}C]clionasterol (C-24 epimer of sitosterol) to desmosterol by the insect, *Tenebrio molitor,* also involves migration of the C-25 hydrogen to the C-24 position [150–152]. The same mechanism was also proposed for the dealkylation of sitosterol in the locust *Locusta migratoria* L. [153].

For a detailed investigation of the mechanism of this dealkylation, it became necessary to determine the configuration of the epoxide (92). We developed a cell-free enzyme system prepared from the midguts of the silkworm *B. mori*. When samples of the supernatant obtained from a homogenate of silkworm guts were incubated separately with the [^{3}H](24*R*,28*R*)-epoxide (92a) and [^{3}H](24*S*,28*S*)-epoxide (92b), only the former was effectively converted to desmosterol (91) [154]. However, subsequent in vivo and in vitro studies demonstrated no absolute stereo-

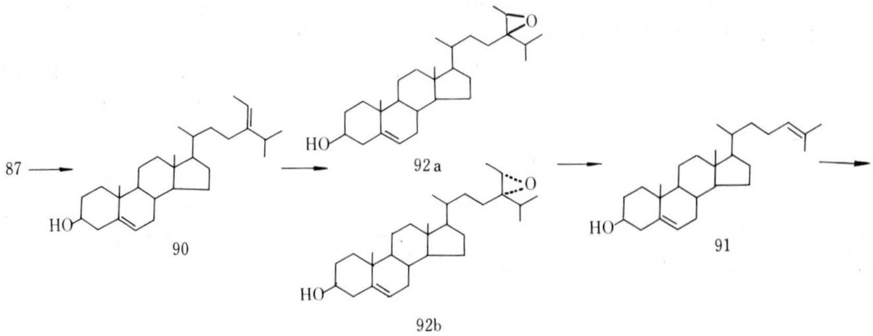

87 → 90 → 92a / 92b → 91 →

Fig. 17.

specificity, neither in the formation of the epoxide from fucosterol nor in the conversion to desmosterol, although the (24*R*,28*R*)-epoxide (92a) was a slightly better precursor than the (24*S*,28*S*)-epoxide (92b). These data suggested that both epoxides could be intermediates. This supposition was substantiated when the two epoxides were found to satisfy equally well the silkworm sterol requirement and the sterol profiles of the insects reared on them showed no significant difference. Moreover, both isomers of the epoxides (92a and b) were isolated from 5th instar larvae reared on mulberry leaves [155]. The low stereospecificity observed with fucosterol epoxide appears to be in line with the facts that both fucosterol (90) and isofucosterol (24(28)*Z* isomer of fucosterol) were identified in the silkworm [156], and that there is no difference in the nutritional effects of sitosterol and clionasterol. The intermediary role of isofucosterol epoxide is probably of less importance in *B. mori*, judging from its poor nutritional effect and its absence in the larvae. This, however, may not be the case in *T. molitor*, in which the (24*R*,28*S*)-isofucosterol epoxide was converted into cholesterol, but not the 24*S*,28*R* isomer. Both of the fucosterol epoxides were transformed into cholesterol to about the same extent [157,158].

In the dealkylation of campesterol (88), 24-methylenecholesterol has been identified as an intermediate. Recently, an intermediary role of the 24,28-epoxide of 24-methylenecholesterol has been demonstrated in the silkworm using [24-^{2}H]-, [25-^{2}H]- and [23,23,25-$^{2}H_3$]campesterols as well as [23,23,25-$^{2}H_3$]24-methylenecholesterol. The C-25 deuterium atom was shown to migrate to the 24 position of desmosterol during the dealkylation [159]. Similar results were also obtained in *T. molitor* using [23,23,25-$^{3}H_3$]24-methylenecholesterol [160,161,166].

In the case of stigmasterol (89), the proposed mechanism in Fig. 18 was evaluated as follows. [23-^{2}H]-, [24-^{2}H]- and [25-^{2}H]stigmasterols were synthesized and the fate of the deuterium atoms during the dealkylation was followed by mass spectrometry. The transfer of the deuterium atom from C-25 to C-24 was established in silkworm larvae [162]. Also, the chemically synthesized (24*E*)- and (24*Z*)-$\Delta^{22,24(28)}$-dienes (93 and 94) were found to satisfy the sterol requirement of the silkworm. The $\Delta^{22,24}$-diene (96) and desmosterol (91) were identified in significant amounts from the insects in accord with the previous observation by the Beltsville group. However, mass fragmentographic analysis of the sterols of insects fed on stigmasterol (89), the

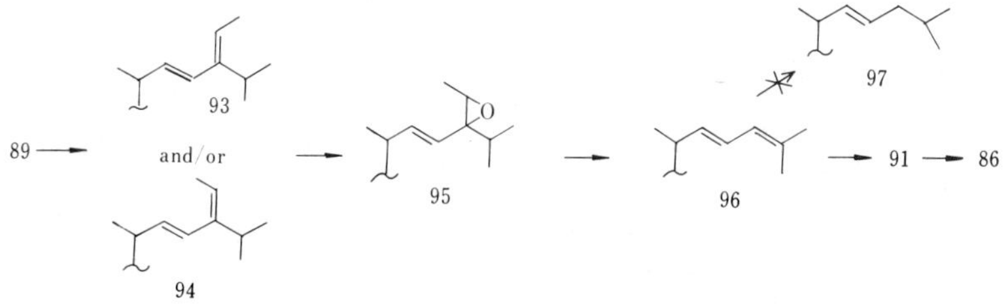

Fig. 18.

dienes (93) and (94), failed to detect 22-dehydrocholesterol (97), indicating that the saturation of the Δ^{24} double bond occurs at the last stage of the dealkylation. It is likely that a similar mechanism is operative for all phytosterols examined.

It is worthy of note that low stereospecificity in utilizing 24-stereoisomers of 24-methylcholesterol was demonstrated with *Manduca sexta*. However, it was reported that in *Dermestes maculatus* there was a preference for (24*R*)-alkylsterols (acetate) over 24*S* isomers, and *Drosophila melanogaster* utilizes both (24*R*)- and (24*S*)-methylcholesta-5,7-dien-3*β*-ol, while *Drosophila pachea* preferentially utilizes the 24*S* isomers and *Drosophila mojavensis* prefers the 24*R* isomers as reported by Kircher and Rosenstein [163]. Our studies revealed that 24-stereoisomers of 24-methyl- and 24-ethylcholesterols and their 22-dehydro analogues can sustain the growth of the silkworm *B. mori* and are all converted into cholesterol to a similar extent [164].

As discussed above, phytophagous insects generally are capable of converting dietary C_{28}- and C_{29}-phytosterols to cholesterol. However, several kinds of insects which show unusual variations in the utilization and metabolism of dietary phytosterols were found recently by Svoboda et al. [165–172].

In the Mexican bean beetle *Epilachna varivestis*, Δ^5-sterols were readily reduced to stanols, and the stanols produced were then dealkylated to cholesterol. Significant amounts of lathosterol (7-dehydrocholestan-3*β*-ol) are also produced from cholestanol in this insect [165–167].

The Milkweed bug, *Oncopeltus tasciatus* [168], is unable to dealkylate plant sterols into cholesterol before they are incorporated into the larval or adult tissues or into the egg, and is apparently able to utilize campesterol as a precursor for their C_{28} moulting hormone, makisterone A.

The Khapra beetle, *Trogoderma granrium* [169], cannot convert dietary phytosterols to C_{27}-sterol. However, there is an increase in the concentration of cholesterol and campesterol in its tissues relative to the dietary concentrations of these sterols, presumably as a result of selective uptake [170].

The honey bee, *Apis mellifera*, does not convert C_{28}- and C_{29}-sterols to cholesterol, but instead the workers and queens selectively transfer 24-methylenecholesterol, sitosterol, and isofucosterol from their endogenous sterol pools to the broad larvae regardless of the dietary sterols of the workers. The major portion of the sterols incorporated into the tissues of the broad larvae originated from the worker bees used to establish the colony [171,172].

Thus, it is evident that there is considerable diversification in the physiological and biochemical mechanisms concerned in the utilization of sterols as essential nutrients by insects.

The ability of crustaceans to biosynthesize sterols has been investigated by several groups and it is now established that they are incapable of de novo sterol synthesis. Dealkylation of 24-methyl and 24-ethyl sterols, giving cholesterol, was demonstrated in several crustaceans by Teshima and Kanazawa [111].

It is interesting to note that the protozoan, *Tetrahymena pyriformis*, lacks the capacity of sterol biosynthesis, but has the ability to dealkylate phytosterols [173].

(2) Inhibitors of phytosterol metabolism

The blocking effect of 22,25-diazacholesterol (98) and triparanol on a step of metabolism of phytosterols in *M. sexta* causing accumulation of desmosterol was discovered by the Beltsville group. Since then, more than 30 azasteroids were tested for their effects on moulting and metamorphosis. Certain of these inhibitors blocked development of insects when added to the diet or medium in less than ppm quantities. Among these steroids, 25-azacholesteryl methyl ether, 25-azacholestane (99) and 25-azacoprostane (100) (Fig. 19) [174] were the most active. The characteristic biological effects of minimal inhibitive concentrations that disrupt development in several test species, were related to the process of moulting and metamorphosis. Other studies have provided further evidence that certain of these azasteroids interfere with moulting hormone biosynthesis or deactivation.

By the modification of azasteroids, some of the nonsteroidal amines, such as bicyclic amines (e.g. 101) and straight-chain amines (e.g. 102 and 103) (Fig. 19) [175] were found to be strong inhibitors of moulting hormone metabolism. Strong inhibitory activities of these amines for pupation were observed in experiments in which they were fed to the hornworm larvae in combination with 22,25-dideoxyecdysone. Another interesting observation was made with the cultured cockroach leg

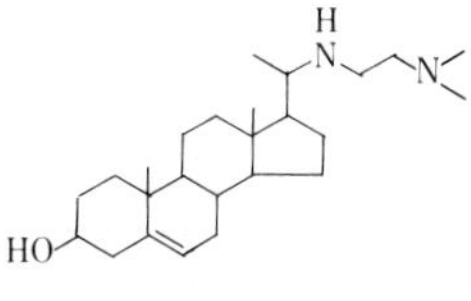

98 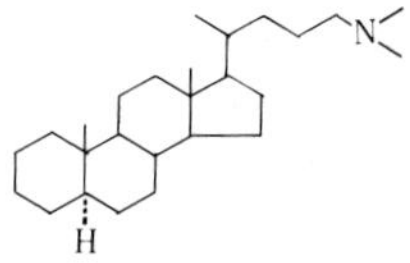 99 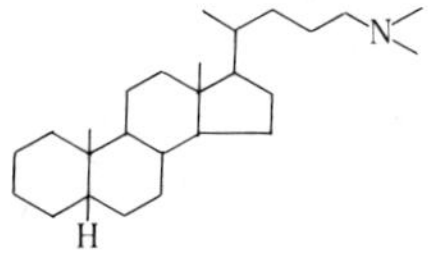 100

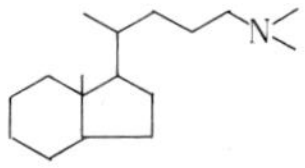

101 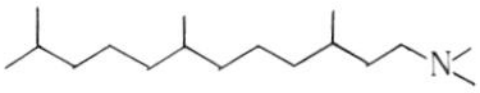 102 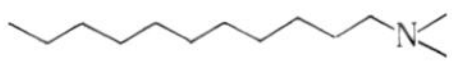 103

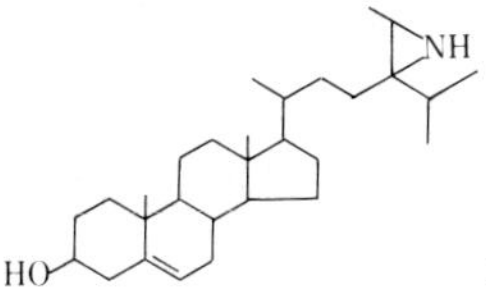

104 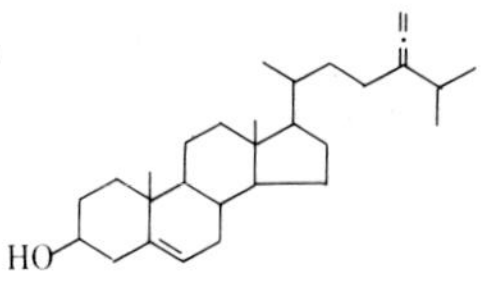 105 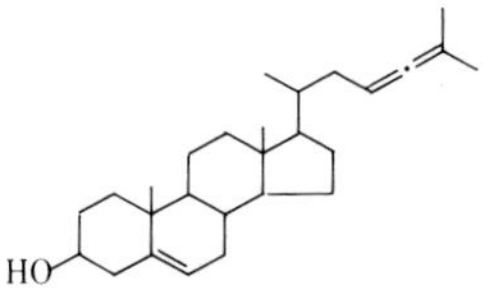 106

Fig. 19.

regenerate system. It was found that these amines interfered with hydroxylation of 22,25-dideoxyecdysone or formation of conjugate forms.

Another series of inhibitors of sterol metabolism in insects were synthesized by our group. These are 24,28-iminofucosterol (104) [176], stigmasta-5,24(28),28-trien-3β-ol (105) [177], and cholesta-5,23,24-trien-3β-ol (106) [177] (Fig. 19). When the imine (104) or the allene (105) was administered in the silkworm diet in combination with sitosterol or cholesterol, the growth and development of *B. mori* were markedly retarded. The imine was expected to inhibit the conversion of fucosterol epoxide to desmosterol, and this was verified by in vitro experiments where the imine, at the same level as the substrate [^{3}H]fucosterol epoxide (92), completely blocked the transformation into desmosterol. However, the imine may not exert its effect solely by limitation of desmosterol or cholesterol formation because cholesterol as the sole dietary sterol was unable to prevent the inhibitory effect. In contrast, the allene (106) seemed to exert little effect on sitosterol dealkylation because the sterols in silkworms fed on the allene (106) in combination with sitosterol were essentially the same as in controls.

The other allene (105) has more interesting properties. When *B. mori* was reared on fucosterol epoxide, desmosterol, or cholesterol, the addition of the allene (105) to the diets at the same concentration as those of nutritional sterol did not inhibit insect growth and development. In contrast, when the nutritional sterol was sitosterol or fucosterol, marked growth retardation was observed. In agreement with these results, the allene (105) induced accumulation of sitosterol or fucosterol when these were the dietary sterols. The results strongly suggest that the allene (105) is a highly specific inhibitor for the steps involving fucosterol; that is, for the conversion of sitosterol to fucosterol and/or fucosterol to the epoxide.

Prestwich has synthesized several sterols fluorinated in the side chain and tested their inhibitory action on the growth of tobacco hornworm, *M. sexta*. 29-Fluorinated compounds of sitosterol and stigmasterol and their 24 isomers gave significant impairment of growth and development of the larvae [178]. The Δ^{22}-sterols are more toxic and cause more severe stunting than 22-dihydro analogues. C-24 stereochemistry does not appear to be so important in determining relative toxicity. Abnormal development caused by the 29-fluorophytosterols is similar to that seen in the larvae fed sodium fluoroacetate or ω-fluoro fatty acids. Neither toxicity nor abnormal growth was found with 25- or 26-monofluorophytosterol or monofluorocholesterol, incorporated into diets fed to *M. sexta* [179]. These results suggested that 29-fluorinated sterol gave fluoroacetate by metabolism in the insect, causing the toxicity.

The effect of 22-dehydrocholesterols (97) on the growth of Drosophila was investigated by Kirchner et al. [180]. *cis*- and *trans*-22-dehydrocholesterols were added to media of diet for 10 species of Drosophila. The *cis* isomer prevented normal maturation of 4 species and the *trans* isomer was toxic to 9. These findings were corroborated by tests with 4 representative species on a sterol-deficient medium under axenic conditions. Addition of cholesterol to the latter overcame the toxicity of the *trans* isomer. *trans*-22-Dehydrocholesterol may be acting as a competitive inhibitor in the metabolism of phytosterols to cholesterol or ecdysone by the insects.

(3) Structure requirement of sterol for growth and development

We have synthesized several cholesterol analogues with modified side chains. These were added to the artificial diet of the silkworm, and growth and development were recorded [181]. Cholesterol was the best nutrient for silkworm and either lengthening or shortening of the side chain induced slight growth-retarding effects. All of the silkworms fed the compound with the longest side chain (20-undecyl-5-pregnen-3β-ol) during the first instar and those reared on the shortest (20-propyl-5-pregnen-3β-ol) failed to develop to the third instar. The branching pattern of the sterol side chain seemed to be another important factor for nutritional efficiency. Thus, comparing the three C_{27} congeners, the straight-chain compound (20-hexyl-5-pregnen-3β-ol), was less effective than cholesterol and all of the larvae fed the other isomer, 20-(3-methylpentyl)-5-pregnen-3β-ol, died during the first instar. The C_{27}-sterol is a cholesterol analogue but it can also be regarded as 27-norcampesterol or 26,27-dinorsitosterol. In view of the complete satisfication of the silkworm sterol requirement with cholesterol, campesterol and sitosterol, it is remarkable that such a slight modification as found in 20-(3-methylpentyl)-5-pregnen-3β-ol produced the dramatic deleterious effect. The terminally branched structures as in cholesterol and 20-(3-methylbutyl)-5-pregnen-3β-ol are superior to the straight-chain isomers as nutrients.

More than 20 analogues of cholesterol, cholesterol esters, cholestenols, and cholestadienols were tested for supporting the growth of the silkworm *B. mori* in our laboratory [182,183]. 5α-Cholest-7-en-3β-ol, cholesta-5,7-dien-3β-ol and 5α-cholest-6-en-3β-ol as well as cholesteryl acetate can replace cholesterol as sterol sources for *B. mori*. Good growth was also obtained with 5α-cholest-14-en-3β-ol, 5α-cholesta-6,8(14)-dien-3β-ol, (20*E*)-cholesta-5,20(22)-dien-3β-ol, (22*E*)-cholesta-5,22-dien-3β-ol, and cholesta-5,25-dien-3β-ol. Other cholestenols and cholestadienols such as 5α-cholest-14-en-3β-ol, 5α-cholest-8(14)-en-3β-ol, 5α-cholesta-7,14-dien-3β-ol and cholesta-5,23-dien-3β-ol were partially effective and the larvae fed on these sterols reached 2nd instars. 5α- and 5β-cholestan-3β-ols, cholest-4-en-3β-ol, and cholest-4-en-3-one are unable to support the growth of *B. mori*.

(III) Ecdysteroids in insects

(1) Introduction

The biosynthesis and metabolism of the insect moulting hormone, ecdysone have been the subject of recent reviews [184–186]. Ecdysone (107) was first isolated in a crystalline form from the silkworm, *Bombyx mori*, by Butenandt and Karlson in 1954, and the structure was determined in 1965. Soon after, the second moulting hormone was isolated and the structure was elucidated as 20-hydroxyecdysone (108). The same hormone was also isolated from the sea-water crayfish, *Jasus lalandei* by Horn in 1966. Many ecdysone analogues were isolated from arthropods and certain

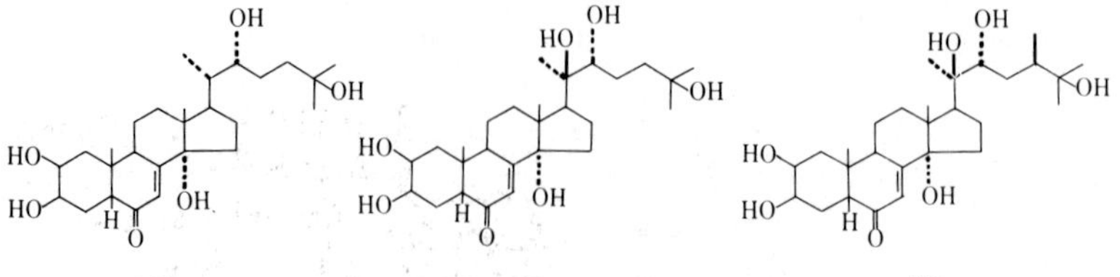

Fig. 20.

plant species, and they are named ecdysteroids. Ecdysone and 20-hydroxyecdysone are the most abundant ecdysteroids. They have been found in every arthropod species. Recently, an exceptional case was reported in that the milkweed bug has a C_{28}-ecdysteroid, makisterone A (109) as the moulting hormone [187] (Fig. 20).

Ecdysteroids are the most widespread and probably oldest steroidal hormone. Recent investigations suggest that the lower animals, namely Annelida, Nematoda and Mollusca might also use ecdysteroids to control certain vital processes in their life cycle. Ecdysteroids have been found in helminth parasites of humans and livestock (trematodes, filarial nematodes and cestodes [188].

In insects, ecdysone is secreted from the prothoracic glands (PG) at every moulting and pupal stage. Conversion of ecdysone to 20-hydroxyecdysone occurred in fat body, Malpighian tubules, gut and body wall tissues [189]. Although ecdysone may have direct hormonal effects, it is generally held that ecdysone serves as a prehormone that is converted to 20-hydroxyecdysone which functions as the active hormone. This is because in many bioassay systems, 20-hydroxyecdysone appears to be much more active than ecdysone.

(2) Ecdysteroids isolated from insects and their biosynthesis

Karlson and Hoffmeister first demonstrated the conversion of [^{3}H]cholesterol to ecdysone in *Calliphora erythrocephala*. Subsequently, the conversion was reported in other species. Direct evidence for the secretion of ecdysone from prothoracic glands has been provided by in vitro culture of such organs in appropriate media. The incorporation of radioactive cholesterol into ecdysone by such glands has been reported for *B. mori* [190], *Manduca sexta* [191], and *Leucophaea manderae* [192].

Since the elucidation of the structure of ecdysone, a number of synthetic cholesterol derivatives have been demonstrated as possible intermediates in the conversion of cholesterol into ecdysone. However, few attempts have been made to isolate the intermediates of ecdysone synthesis in the PG. Only 3β-hydroxy-5α-cholestan-6-one (111) was isolated from the organ culture medium of the silkworm PG as a possible intermediate [193]. The PG possesses a comparatively large percentage of 7-dehydrocholesterol (110) in several insects. Thus, 7-dehydrocholesterol may also be a possible early intermediate in the transformation of cholesterol into ecdysone [194].

The mode of formation of 7-dehydrocholesterol by larvae of *C. erythrocephala* was demonstrated by the Liverpool group. Recently the same group reported that

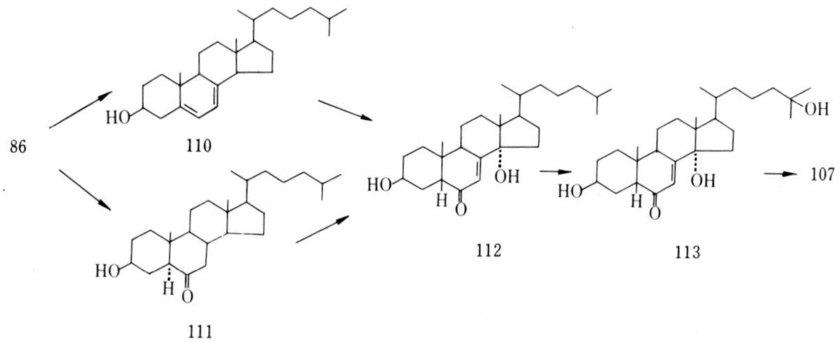

86 → 110 → 112 → 113 → 107; 86 → 111 → 112

Fig. 21.

the formation of the A/B *cis* ring junction of ecdysteroids apparently involves different mechanisms in plants and in insects. The 3-oxo-4-ene compound may be an intermediate in the formation of the A/B ring of ecdysteroids at least in the locust, *Schistocerca gregaria*. It is evident that the construction of the A/B ring occurs prior to the side chain hydroxylation, but the mechanism of the formation of the A/B *cis* ring junction is not clear. A tentative scheme for ecdysone biosynthesis is presented in Fig. 21. Biosynthesis of ecdysteroids in plants and insects [195], in the tobacco hornworm [196], and in the blowfly [197] was discussed in detail in reviews.

In 1971, high moulting hormone activity was found in the eggs of *B. mori* by Ohnishi et al. [198]. Kaplanis et al. found a high level of the active ecdysteroid, 26-hydroxyecdysone (117), in tobacco hornworm eggs [197]. The eggs of all insects investigated have been found to contain ecdysteroids. Eggs of several insect species contain high titres of ecdysteroids well before the embryonic prothoracic glands have differentiated. The ecdysteroids present in the newly laid eggs were predominantly in a conjugated form. These ecdysteroids are obviously of maternal origin, and indeed the ovary was shown to have the capacity of synthesizing ecdysteroids. Recently, a new ecdysiosynthetic tissue, the follicular cells of the developing ovary [199], has been detected and this finding has been used to explain the presence of ecdysteroids in the ovaries and eggs of many insect species. Garen et al. [200] isolated a temperature-sensitive mutant of *Drosophila melanogaster,* ecd^1, which has no capacity to synthesize ecdysone at elevated temperature. By use of this mutant, it was suggested that ecdysteroids might have significant roles not only at the post-embryonic stages but also at the embryonic stage as well as that of oogenesis.

In contrast to the rather simple pattern of ecdysteroids found at the post-embryonic stage, that found in ovaries or eggs is characterized by a variety of molecular species and a high proportion of conjugate forms. The term ‘oo-ecdysteroids’ was coined to distinguish them from ‘prothoraco-ecdysteroids’ which are found at post-embryonic stages. From the ovaries of *B. mori*, we have isolated and identified the following ecdysteroids; 2-deoxyecdysone (114) [201], ecdysone (107), 2-deoxy-20-hydroxyecdysone (116) [202], 2,22-dideoxy-20-hydroxyecdysone (115) [203], and 20-hydroxyecdysone (108). Our studies on the mode of accumulation of these

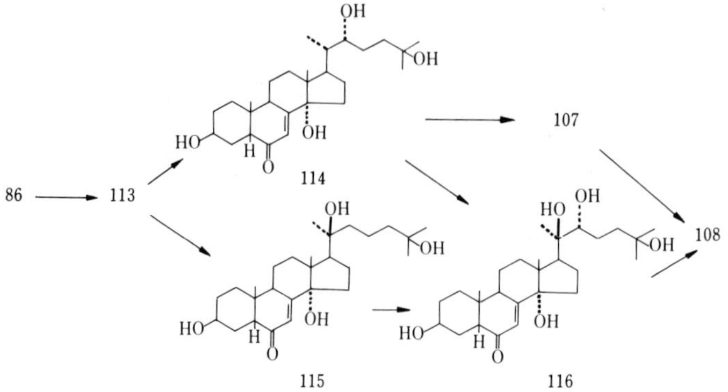

Fig. 22.

ecdysteroids during the ovarian development showed that the ecdysteroids that initially accumulated in the ovary were ecdysone and 20-hydroxyecdysone, and were followed by 2-deoxyecdysone, 2-deoxy-20-hydroxyecdysone and 2,22-dideoxy-20-hydroxyecdysone [215]. The last 3 ecdysteroids, together with a major part of ecdysone, were assumed to be synthesized de novo in the ovary. The most plausible biosynthetic pathway interrelating the ecdysteroids found in the ovary is shown in Fig. 22. Ecdysteroids in *B. mori* ovary differ from those of ovarian systems of *Galleria mellonella, S. gregaria* and macrotermes species, in which ecdysone and 20-hydroxyecdysone are predominant.

Many endogenous ecdysteroids which can be considered as the intermediates of ecdysone biosynthesis were isolated from the ovaries of *L. migratoria* by Hoffmann and Horn [204]. From the results of the bioconversion of labelled precursors, the following sequence in the biosynthetic pathway of ecdysteroids in vitellogenic ovaries of the insect was proposed: conversion of cholesterol to 3β-hydroxy-5β-cholest-7-en-6-one followed by 14α-hydroxylation to 3β,14-dihydroxy-5β-cholest-7-en-6-one (112); hydroxylation at C-25 and C-22 (in this order) to 2-deoxyecdysone (114); hydroxylation at C-2 to ecdysone (107).

(3) Ecdysone metabolism and biological activity

Only a few arthropod species have been examined for their ecdysteroid profiles. In addition to ecdysone and 20-hydroxyecdysone, 26-hydroxyecdysone (117), 20,26-dihydroxyecdysone (118), 3-epi-26-hydroxyecdysone and 3-epi-20,26-dihydroxyecdysone were isolated from the tobacco hornworm during pupal–adult development 5 days after the peak titre of moulting hormone activity [197]. 20-Hydroxyecdysone was the major moulting hormone present at peak titre during pupal–adult development. 26-Hydroxyecdysone is the major ecdysteroid present during embryonic development in this insect. 20,26-Dihydroxyecdysone, which has a lower biological activity and higher polarity, appears to be a deactivation product of 20-hydroxy-

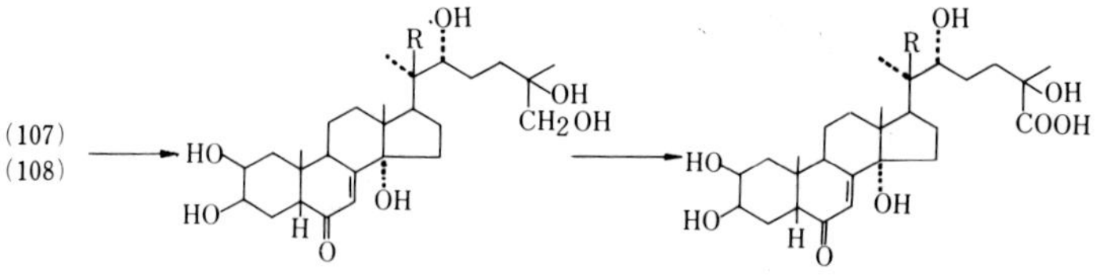

(107)
(108)

117(R=H)
118(R=OH)

119(R=H)
120(R=OH)

Fig. 23.

ecdysone. The configuration of 26-hydroxylated ecdysteroids at C-25 is not known.

The 26-hydroxyl group is further oxidized to ecdysonoic acid (119) and 20-hydroxyecdysonoic acid (120) [205] which have been identified in developing eggs of the desert locust, *S. gregaria* (Fig. 23). The occurrence of both compounds in *Spodoptera littoralis* pupae was also established. These oxidations are apparently inactivation steps. 26-Hydroxylation, 3-epimerization, 3-acetylation, and conjugation diminish the interaction with the steroid receptor and thus can be viewed as inactivation.

Recently, the first structure determination of the ecdysteroid conjugates was reported by Isaac et al. [206]. Ecdysone-22-phosphate (121) and 2-deoxyecdysone-22-phosphate were isolated from eggs of *S. gregaria,* and their structures were determined by fast atom bombardment mass spectrometry and NMR spectra. 22-Phosphates of ecdysteroids were also isolated from eggs of *L. migratoria* by Tsoupras et al. [207,208]. 22-Adenosine monophosphoric ester of 2-deoxyecdysone [209] was also identified in the eggs of the same species, but this might have been formed as an artifact during extraction [188]. A new ecdysone conjugate was recently isolated from newly laid eggs of *L. migratoria* and shown to be the 22-N^6-(isopentenyl)-adenosine monophosphoric ester of ecdysone [210].

Structure–function relationships among ecdysteroids have been reviewed by Bergamasco and Horn [211]. The 14α-hydroxy-7-en-6-one system is essential for activity. The 3β-hydroxyl group is essential but the 2-hydroxyl group is not. All active ecdysteroids have a *cis*-fused A/B ring. Ecdysteroids require a full side chain for activity, but a hydroxyl group on the side chain is not essential. The 22-hydroxyl group is essential for high activity, and the 22*R* configuration is also very important. The presence of a 5β-hydroxyl group in ecdysteroids enhances the activity. Recently an exceptional substance with high moulting hormone activity was reported: the phytoecdysone muristerone (122) was reported as a potent insect moulting hormone (Fig. 24). 14-Deoxymuristerone (123) [212], which was prepared from muristerone, was also found to show high activity. The biological activity of this compound was assayed by the morphological response of cultured Drosophila Kc-H cells. In this system various ecdysteroids have been shown to be active approximately in proportion to their reported affinities for the ecdysteroid receptor. Relative to 20-hydroxyecdysone, the activities of muristerone and 14-deoxymuristerone were approximately 10 and 80, respectively.

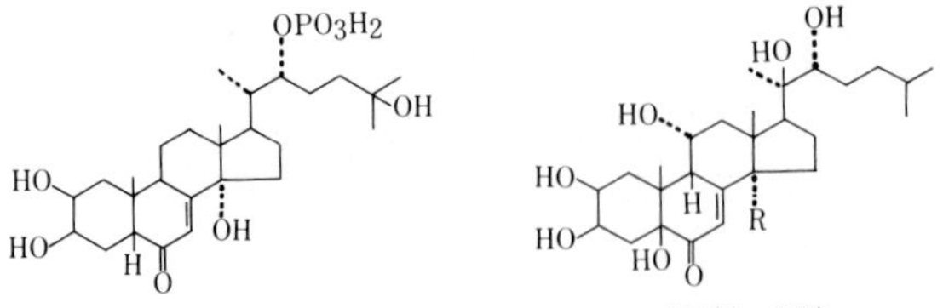

121

122(R=OH)
123(R=H)

Fig. 24.

Detoxication of exogenous phytoecdysteroids in *Bombyx mori* was investigated [213]. Some of the phytoecdysteroids show anti-feedant activity for insects [214].

The sterols in vertebrates have been studied for many years, while extensive research on the sterols in invertebrates started only about 20 years ago: the structure and biosynthesis of the latter sterols have become one of the most intensely investigated areas of chemistry and biochemistry. Recent studies have revealed the complexity of the sterols. Sterol, particularly cholesterol, plays a role as a precursor of ecdysone biosynthesis in Arthropoda [215,216]. Brassinolide (124) [217], recently identified plant growth hormones, are also phytosterol metabolites. 1,25-Dihydroxy-vitamin D (125) [218], hormonal metabolite produced in kidney, is derived from cholesterol. We can see the similarity in the structure and biosynthesis of those hormonally active steroids having hydroxylated side chains (Fig. 25). Also, we can imagine how animals and plants have utilized sterols for their growth and reproduction during evolution, since the appearance of sterol some 1.5 billion years ago. In addition to the role of sterols as precursors of hormones, the function of the constitutional sterols in invertebrates must await further investigation. Probably, the multifarious structures of the sterols may be important for invertebrate membrane physiology and biology. Functions of steroids in plants and animals are discussed in detail in a book of Nes and McKean [219], and recently Karlson [220] has discussed the relation between evolution and sterol metabolism.

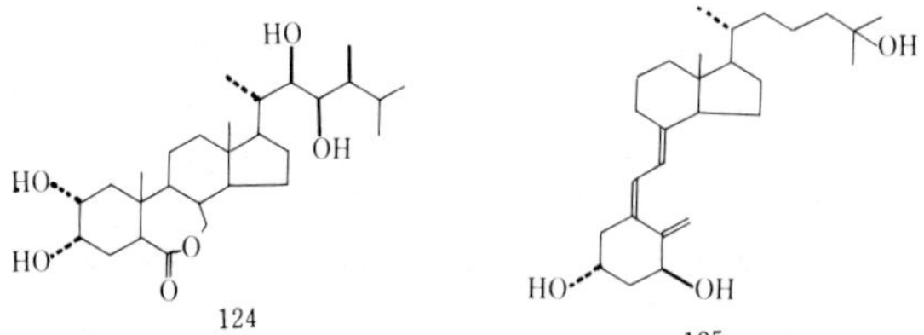

124

125

Fig. 25.

Acknowledgements

The author wishes to thank Prof. C.J.W. Brooks, University of Glasgow, and Prof. E. Ohnishi, Nagoya University, for their review of this manuscript.

References

1 Djerassi, C. (1981) Pure Appl. Chem. 53, 873–890.
2 Edmonds, C.G., Smith, A.G. and Brooks, C.J.W. (1977) J. Chromatogr. 133, 372–377.
3 Goad, L.J. (1981) Pure Appl. Chem. 51, 837–852.
4 Djerassi, C., Theobald, N., Kokke, W.C.M.C., Pak, C.S. and Carlson, R.M.K. (1979) Pure Appl. Chem. 51, 1815–1828.
5 Carlson, R.M.K., Tarchini, C. and Djerassi, C. (1980) in: Frontiers of Bio-Organic Chemistry and Molecular Biology (Ananchenko, S.N., Ed.) pp. 211–224, Pergamon Press, Oxford.
6 Minale, L. and Sodano, G. (1977) in: Marine Natural Products Chemistry (Faulkner, D.J. and Fenical, W.H., Eds.) pp. 87–109, Plenum Press, New York.
7 Teshima, S.I., Fleming, R., Gaffney, J. and Goad, L.J. (1977) in: Marine Natural Products Chemistry (Faulkner, D.J. and Fenical, W.H., Eds.) pp. 133–146, Plenum Press, New York.
8 Schmitz, F.J. (1978) in: Marine Natural Products (Scheuer, P.J., Ed.) Vol. I, pp. 241–297, Academic Press, New York.
9 Goad, L.J. (1978) in: Marine Natural Producs (Scheuer, P.J., Ed.) Vol. II, pp. 75–172, Academic Press, New York.
10 Goad, L.J. (1976) in: Biochemical and Biophysical Perspectives in Marine Biology (Malins, D.C. and Sargent, J.R., Eds.) Vol. 3, pp. 213–318, Academic Press, London.
11 Scheuer, P.J. (1973) Chemistry of Marine Natural Products, Academic Press, New York.
12 DeLuca, P., De Rosa, M., Minale, L. and Sodano, G. (1972) J. Chem. Soc., Perkin Trans. I, 2132–2135.
13 Minale, L. and Sodano, G. (1974) J. Chem. Soc., Perkin Trans. I, 1888–1892.
14 Minale, L. and Sodano, G. (1974) J. Chem. Soc., Perkin Trans. I, 2380–2384.
15 De Stefano, A. and Sodano, G. (1980) Experientia 36, 630–632.
16 Theobald, N., Wells, R.J. and Djerassi, C. (1978) J. Am. Chem. Soc. 100, 7677–7684.
17 Bortolotto, M., Braekman, J.C., Daloze, D. and Tursch, B. (1978) Bull. Soc. Chem. Belg. 87, 539.
18 Kokke, W.C.M.C., Fenical, W.H., Pak, C.S. and Djerassi, C. (1978) Tetrahedron Lett. 4373–4376.
19 Kokke, W.C.M.C., Tarchini, C., Stierle, D.B. and Djerassi, C. (1979) J. Org. Chem. 44, 3385–3388.
20 Kokke, W.C.M.C., Pak, C.S., Fenical, W. and Djerassi, C. (1979) Helv. Chim. Acta 62, 1310–1318.
21 Li, L.N., Sjöstrand, U. and Djerassi, C. (1981) J. Am. Chem. Soc. 103, 115–119.
22 Li, L.N. and Djerassi, C. (1981) J. Am. Chem. Soc. 103, 3606–3608.
23 Li, L.N., Sjöstrand, U. and Djerassi, C. (1981) J. Org. Chem. 46, 3867–3870.
24 Li, L.N. and Djerassi, C. (1981) Tetrahedron Lett. 22, 4639–4642.
25 Li, X. and Djerassi, C. (1983) Tetrahedron Lett. 24, 665–668.
26 Fattorusso, E., Magno, S., Mayol, L., Santacroce, C. and Sica, D. (1975) Tetrahedron 31, 1715–1716.
27 Minale, L., Riccio, R., Scalona, O., Sodano, G., Fattorusso, E., Magno, S., Mayol, L. and Santacroce, C. (1977) Experientia 33, 1550–1552.
28 Li, L.N., Li, H., Lang, R.W., Itoh, T., Sica, D. and Djerassi, C. (1982) J. Am. Chem. Soc. 104, 6726–6732.
29 Itoh, T., Sica, D. and Djerassi, C. (1983) J. Org. Chem. 48, 890–892.
30 Sica, D. and Zollo, F. (1978) Tetrahedron Lett. 837–838.
31 Ravi, B.N., Kokke, W.C.M.C., Delseth, C. and Djerassi, C. (1978) Tetrahedron Lett. 4379–4380.
32 Khalil, M.W., Durham, L.J., Djerassi, C. and Sica, D. (1980) J. Am. Chem. Soc. 102, 2133–2134.
33 Zielinski, J., Li, H., Milkova, T.S., Popov, S., Marekov, N.L. and Djerassi, C. (1981) Tetrahedron Lett. 22, 2345–2348.

34 Blanc, P.A. and Djerassi, C. (1980) J. Am. Chem. Soc. 102, 7113–7114.
35 Catalan, C.A.N., Lakshmi, V., Schmitz, F.J. and Djerassi, C. (1982) Steroids 40, 455–463.
36 Cafieri, F., Fattorusso, E., Frigerio, A., Santacroce, C. and Sica, D. (1975) Gazz. Chim. Ital. 105, 595–602.
37 Itoh, T., Sica, D. and Djerassi, C. (1983) J. Chem. Soc., Perkin Trans. I, 147–153.
38 Delseth, C., Kashman, Y. and Djerassi, C. (1979) Helv. Chim. Acta 62, 2037–2045.
39 Bohlin, L., Gehrken, H.P., Scheuer, P.J. and Djerassi, C. (1980) Steroids 35, 295–305.
40 Bohlin, L., Sjöstrand, U., Djerassi, C. and Sullivan, B.W. (1981) J. Chem. Soc., Perkin Trans. I, 1023–1028.
41 Bohlin, L., Sjöstrand, U., Sodano, G. and Djerassi, C. (1982) J. Org. Chem. 47, 5309–5314.
42 Eggersdorfer, M.L., Kokke, W.C.M.C., Crandell, C.W., Hochlowski, J.E. and Djerassi, C. (1982) J. Org. Chem. 47, 5304–5309.
43 Gunatilaka, A.A.L., Gopichand, Y., Schmitz, F.J. and Djerassi, C. (1981) J. Org. Chem. 46, 3860–3866.
44 Kho, E., Imagawa, D.K., Rohmer, M., Kashman, Y. and Djerassi, C. (1981) J. Org. Chem. 46, 1836–1839.
45 Steiner, E., Djerassi, C., Fattorusso, E., Magno, S., Mayol, L., Santacroce, C. and Sica, D. (1977) Helv. Chim. Acta 60, 475–481.
46 Theobald, N., Shoolery, J.N., Djerassi, C., Erdman, T.R. and Scheuer, P.J. (1978) J. Am. Chem. Soc. 100, 5574–5575.
47 Gunasekera, S.P. and Schmitz, F.J. (1983) J. Org. Chem. 48, 885–886.
48 Hale, R.L., Leclercq, J., Tursch, B., Djerassi, C., Gross Jr., R.A., Weinheimer, A.J., Gupta, K. and Scheuer, P.J. (1970) J. Am. Chem. Soc. 92, 2179–2180.
49 Ling, N.C., Hale, R.L. and Djerassi, C. (1970) J. Am. Chem. Soc. 92, 5281–5282.
50 Schmitz, F.J. and Pattabhiraman, T. (1979) J. Am. Chem. Soc. 92, 6073–6074.
51 Ishiguro, M., Akaiwa, A., Fujimoto, Y., Sato, S. and Ikekawa, N. (1979) Tetrahedron Lett. 763–766.
52 Terasawa, T., Hirano, Y., Fujimoto, Y. and Ikekawa, N. (1983) J. Chem. Soc., Chem. Commun. 1180–1182.
53 Enwall, E.L., van der Helm, D. Hsu, I.N., Pattabhiraman, T., Schmitz, F.J., Spraggins, R.L. and Weinheimer, A.J. (1972) J. Chem. Soc., Chem. Commun. 215–216.
54 Bonini, C., Cooper, C.B., Kazlauskas, R., Wells, R.L. and Djerassi, C. (1983) J. Org. Chem. 48, 2108–2111.
55 Popov, S., Carlson, R.M.K., Wegmann, A. and Djerassi, C. (1976) Steroids 28, 699–732.
56 Engelbrecht, J.P., Tursch, B. and Djerassi, C. (1972) Steroids 20, 121–126.
57 Moldowan, J.M., Tursch, B. and Djerassi, C. (1974) Steroids 24, 387–398.
58 Moldowan, J.M., Tan, W.L. and Djerassi, C. (1975) Steroids 26, 107–128.
59 Kobayashi, M., Hayashi, T., Nakajima, F. and Mitsuhashi, H. (1979) Steroids 34, 285–293.
60 Kobayashi, M. and Mitsuhashi, H. (1982) Steroids 40, 673–677.
61 Kobayashi, M., Tomioka, A. and Mitsuhashi, H. (1979) Steroids 34, 273–283.
62 Kobayashi, M. and Mitsuhashi, H. (1982) Steroids 40, 665–671.
63 Bonini, C., Kinnel, R.B., Li, M., Scheuer, P.J. and Djerassi, C. (1983) Tetrahedron Lett. 24, 277–280.
64 Fujimoto, Y., Kimura, M., Terasawa, T., Khalifa, F.A.M. and Ikekawa, N. (1984) Tetrahedron Lett., 1805–1808.
65 Catalan, C.A.N. and Djerassi, C. (1983) Tetrahedron Lett. 24, 3461–3464.
66 Higa, T., Tanaka, J., Tsukitani, Y. and Kikuchi, H. (1981) Chem. Lett. 1647–1650.
67 Higa, T., Tanaka, J. and Tachibana, K. (1981) Tetrahedron Lett. 22, 2777–2780.
68 Tanaka, J., Higa, T., Tachibana, K. and Iwashita, T. (1982) Chem. Lett. 1295–1296.
69 Bortolotto, M., Braekman, J.C., Daloze, D., Losman, D. and Tursch, B. (1976) Steroids 28, 461–466.
70 Bortolotto, M., Braekman, J.C., Daloze, D., Tursch, B. and Karlson, R. (1977) Steroids 30, 159–164.
71 Higgs, M.D. and Faulkner, D.J. (1977) Steroids 30, 379–383.
72 Kanazawa, A., Teshima, S., Ando, T. and Tomita, S. (1974) Bull. Jpn. Soc. Sci. Fish. 40, 729–730.
73 Kanazawa, A., Ando, T. and Teshima, S. (1977) Steroids 43, 83–88.
74 Minale, L. and Sodano, G. (1974) J. Chem. Soc., Perkin Trans. I, 1888–1892.

75 Shimizu, Y., Alain, M. and Kobayashi, A. (1976) J. Am. Chem. Soc., 98, 1059. Finer, J., Clardy, J., Kobayashi, A., Alain, M. and Shimizu, Y. (1978) J. Org. Chem. 43, 1990–1992.
76 Vanderah, D.J. and Djerassi, C. (1977) Tetrahedron Lett., 683–686.
77 Idler, D.R., Khall, M.W., Gilbert, J.D. and Brooks, C.J.W. (1976) Steroids 27, 155–166.
78 Carlson, R.M.K., Popov, S., Massay, I., Delseth, C., Ayanoglu, E., Varkony, T.H. and Djerassi, C. Bioorg. Chem. 7, 453–479.
79 Goad, L.J., Rubinstein, J. and Smith, A.G. (1972) Proc. Roy. Soc., Ser. B, 180, 223–246.
80 Kobayashi, M., Tsutu, R., Todo, K. and Mitsuhashi, H. (1972) Tetrahedron Lett. 2935–2938.
81 Kobayashi, M. and Mitsuhashi, H. (1974) Tetrahedron 30, 2147–2150.
82 Gupta, K.C. and Scheuer, P.J. (1978) Tetrahedron 24, 5831–5837.
83 Sheikh, Y.M., Djerassi, C. and Tursch, B. (1971) J. Chem. Soc., Chem. Commun. 217–218.
84 Sheikh, Y.M., Kaisin, M. and Djerassi, C. (1973) Steroids 22, 835–850.
85 Kanazawa, A., Teshima, S., Tomita, S. and Ando, T. (1974) Bull. Jpn. Soc. Sci. Fish. 40, 1077.
86 Sato, S., Ikekawa, N., Kanazawa, A. and Ando, T. (1980) Steroids 36, 65–71.
87 Goad, L.J., Lenton, J.R., Knapp, F.F. and Goodwin, T.W. (1974) Lipids 9, 582–595.
88 Voogt, P.A. (1973) Comp. Biochem. Physiol. 45B, 593–601.
89 Numura, T., Tsuchiya, Y., Andre, D. and Barbier, M. (1969) Bull. Jpn. Soc. Sci. Fish. 35, 299–302.
90 Voogt, P.A. and Over, J. (1973) Comp. Biochem. Physiol. 45B, 71–80.
91 Smith, A.C. and Goad, L.J. (1971) Biochem. J. 123, 671–673.
92 Smith, A.G. and Goad, L.J. (1975) Biochem. J. 146, 25–33.
93 Boticelli, C.-R., Hisaw, F.L. and Wotiz, H.H. (1960) Proc. Soc. Exp. Biol. Med. 103, 875–877.
94 Boticelli, C.-R., Hisaw, F.L. and Wotiz, H.H. (1961) Proc. Soc. Exp. Biol. Med. 106, 887–889.
95 Ikegami, S., Shirai, H. and Kamatani, H. (1971) Zool. Mag. 80, 26.
96 Minale, L., Pizza, C., Riccio, R. and Zollo, F. (1982) Pure Appl. Chem. 54, 1935–1950.
97 Kitagawa, I. and Kobayashi, M. (1978) Chem. Pharm. Bull. 26, 1864–1873.
98 Ikegami, S., Okano, K. and Muragaki, H. (1979) Tetrahedron Lett. 1769–1772.
99 Ikegami, S., Hirose, Y., Kamiya, Y. and Tamura, S. (1972) Agric. Biol. Chem. 36, 2453–2457.
100 De Simone, F., Dini, A., Finamore, E., Minale, L., Pizza, C., Riccio, R. and Zollo, F. (1981) J. Chem. Soc., Perkin Trans. I, 1855–1862.
101 De Simone, F., Dini, A., Minale, L., Pizza, C., Senatore, F. and Zollo, F. (1981) Tetrahedron Lett. 1557–1560.
102 Riccio, R., Minale, L., Pizza, C., Zollo, F. and Pusset, J. (1982) Tetrahedron Lett. 23, 2899–2902.
103 Riccio, R., Minale, L., Pagonis, S., Pizza, C., Zollo, F. and Pusset, J. (1982) Tetrahedron 38, 3615–3622.
104 Pettit, G.R., Day, J.F. Hartwell, J.L. and Wood, H.B. (1970) Nature (London) 227, 962–963.
105 Ruggieri, G.D. and Nigrelli, R.F. (1974) in: Bioactive Compounds From the Sea (Humm, H. and Lane, C., Eds.) pp. 183–195, Marcel Dekker, New York.
106 Shimizu, Y. (1971) Experientia 27, 1188–1189.
107 Mackie, A.M., Lasker, R. and Grant, P.T. (1968) Comp. Biochem. Physiol. 26, 415–428. Mackie, A.M. and Turner, A.B. (1970) Biochem. J. 117, 543–550.
108 Uno, Y. and Hoshi, M. (1978) Science 200, 58–59.
109 Kanazawa, A., Shimaya, M., Kawasaki, M. and Kashiwada, K.I. (1970) Bull. Jpn. Soc. Sci. Fish. 36, 949–954.
110 Teshima, S. and Kanazawa, A. (1971) Bull. Jpn. Soc. Sci. Fish. 37, 720–723.
111 Teshima, S. and Kanazawa, A. (1972) Bull. Jpn. Soc. Sci. Fish. 38, 1305–1310.
112 Kanazawa, A. and Teshima, S. (1971) Bull. Jpn. Soc. Sci. Fish. 37, 891–898.
113 Tcholakian, R.K. and Eik-Nes, K.B. (1969) Gen. Comp. Endocrinol. 12, 171–173.
114 Tcholakian, R.K. and Eik-Nes, K.B. (1971) Gen. Comp. Endocrinol. 17, 115–124.
115 Karlson, P. and Skinner, D.M. (1960) Nature (London) 185, 543–544.
116 Horn, D.H.S., Middelton, E.J. and Wunderlich, J.A. (1966) Chem. Commun. 339–341.
117 Gallbraith, M.N., Horn, D.H.S., Middleton, E.J. and Hackney, R.J. (1968) Chem. Commun. 83, 85.
118 Faux, A., Horn, D.H.S., Middleton, E.J., Fales, H.M. and Lowe, M.E. (1969) Chem. Commun. 175–176.

119 Gagosin, R.B., Bourbonnierre, R.A., Smith, W.B., Couch, E.F., Blanton, C. and Novak, W. (1974) Experientia 30, 723.
120 Kater, S.B. and Spaziani, E. (1971) Am. Zool. 11, 672.
121 Spaziani, E. and Kater, S.B. (1973) Gen. Comp. Endocrinol. 20, 534–549.
122 King, D.S. and Siddall, J.B. (1969) Nature (London) 221, 955–956.
123 Willig, A. and Keller, R. (1973) J. Comp. Physiol. 86, 377.
124 Voogt, P.A. (1972) in: Chemical Zoology (Florkin, M. and Scheer, B.T., Eds.) Vol. 4, p. 245, Academic Press, London.
125 Matsumoto, T. and Tamura, T. (1956) J. Chem. Soc. Jpn. 77, 376.
126 Idler, D.R. and Wiseman, P. (1970) Comp. Biochem. Physiol. 35, 678–687. Idler, D.R., Wiseman, P.M. and Safe, L.M. (1970) Steroids 16, 451–461.
127 Idler, D.R. and Wiseman, P. (1971) Int. J. Biochem. 2, 516.
128 Idler, D.R., Safe, L.M. and MacDonald, E.F. (1971) Steroids 18, 545–553.
129 Kobayashi, M., Minamizawa, T. and Mitsuhashi, H. (1977) Steroids 29, 823–826. Kobayashi, M. and Mitsuhashi, H. (1974) Steroids 24, 399–410; (1975) Steroids 26, 605–624.
130 Teshima, S. and Kanazawa, A. (1973) Comp. Biochem. Physiol. 44B, 881–887.
131 Voogt, P.A. and Van Rheenen, J.W.A. (1974) Comp. Biochem. Physiol. 47B, 131–137.
132 Teshima, S. and Kanazawa, A. (1973) Bull. Jpn. Soc. Sci. Fish. 39, 1309–1314.
133 Salaque, A., Barbier, M. and Lederer, E. (1966) Comp. Biochem. Physiol. 19, 45–51.
134 Saliot, A. and Barbier, M. (1973) J. Exp. Mar. Biol. Med. 144, 483.
135 Teshima, S. and Kanazawa, A. (1972) Bull. Jpn. Soc. Sci. Fish. 38, 1299–1304.
136 Voogt, P.A. (1974) Netherlands J. Zool. 24, 22.
137 Kobayashi, M. and Mitsuhashi, H. (1974) Steroids 24, 399–410.
138 Viala, J., Devys, M. and Barbier, M. (1972) Bull. Soc. Chim. Fr. 3626–3627.
139 Yasuda, S. (1975) Comp. Biochem. Physiol. 50B, 399–402.
140 Yasuda, S. (1976) Bull. Jpn. Soc. Fish. 42, 1307–1308.
141 Tam Ha, T.B., Kokke, W.C.M.C. and Djerassi, C. (1982) Steroids 40, 433–453.
142 Robbins, W.E., Kaplanis, J.N., Svoboda, J.A. and Thompson, M.J. (1971) Annu. Rev. Entomol. 16, 53–72.
143 Thompson, M.J., Kaplanis, J.N., Robbins, W.E. and Svoboda, J.A. (1973) Adv. Lipids Res. 11, 219–265.
144 Svoboda, J.N., Kaplanis, J.N., Robbins, W.E. and Thompson, M.J. (1975) Annu. Rev. Entomol. 20, 205–220.
145 Svoboda, J.A., Thompson, M.J., Robbins, W.E. and Kaplanis, J.N. (1978) Lipids 13, 742–753.
146 Ikekawa, N., Morisaki, M., Ohtaka, H. and Chiyoda, Y. (1971) Chem. Commun. 1498.
147 Ikekawa, N. (1983) Experientia 39, 466–472.
148 Morisaki, M., Ohtaka, H., Okubayashi, M., Ikekawa, N., Horie, Y. and Nakasone, S. (1972) J. Chem. Soc., Chem. Commun. 1272.
149 Fujimoto, Y., Awata, N., Morisaki, M. and Ikekawa, N. (1974) Tetrahedron Lett. 4335–4338.
150 Randall, P.J., Lloyd-Jones, J.G., Cook, I.F., Rees, H.H. and Goodwin, T.W. (1972) J. Chem. Soc., Chem. Commun. 1296–1298.
151 Pettler, P.J., Lockley, W.J.S., Rees, H.H. and Goodwin, T.W. (1974) J. Chem. Soc., Chem. Commun. 844–846.
152 Pettler, P.J., Lockley, W.J.S., Rees, H.H. and Goodwin, T.W. Biochem. J. 174, 397–404.
153 Allais, J.P., Alcaide, A. and Barbier, M. (1973) Experientia 29, 944–945.
154 Fujimoto, Y., Morisaki, M. and Ikekawa, N. (1980) Biochemistry 19, 1065–1069.
155 Ikekawa, N., Fujimoto, Y., Takasu, A. and Morisaki, M. (1980) J. Chem. Soc., Chem. Commun. 709–711.
156 Morisaki, M., Ying, B. and Ikekawa, N. (1981) Experientia 37, 336.
157 Nicotra, F., Ronchetti, F., Russo, G. and Toma, L. (1980) J. Chem. Soc., Chem. Commun. 479–480.
158 Nicotra, F., Pizzi, P., Ronchetti, F., Russo, G. and Toma, L. (1981) J. Chem. Soc., Perkin Trans. I, 480–483.
159 Maruyama, S., Fujimoto, Y., Morisaki, M. and Ikekawa, N. (1982) Tetrahedron Lett. 23, 1701–1704.

160 Nicotra, F., Ronchetti, F. and Russo, G. (1982) Lipids 17, 184–186.
161 Nicotra, F., Ronchetti, F., Russo, G. and Toma, L. (1983) J. Chem. Soc., Perkin Trans. I, 787–790.
162 Fujimoto, Y., Kimura, M., Takasu, A., Khalifa, F.A.M., Morisaki, M. and Ikekawa, N. (1984) Tetrahedron Lett., 1501–1504.
163 Kircher, H.W. and Rosenstein, F.Y. (1974) J. Am. Oil Chem. Soc. 51, 525A.
164 Fujimoto, Y., Kimura, M., Khalifa, F.A.M. and Ikekawa, N. (1984) Chem. Pharm. Bull., 32, 4373–4381.
165 Svoboda, J.A. and Thompson, M.J. (1974) Lipids 9, 752–755.
166 Nicotra, F., Ronchetti, F., Russo, G. and Toma, L. (1982) J. Chem. Soc., Chem. Commun. 922–923.
167 Svoboda, J.A., Thompson, M.J. and Robbins, W.E. (1975) Lipids 10, 524–527.
168 Svoboda, J.A., Dutky, S.R., Robbins, W.E. and Kaplanis, J.N. Lipids 12, 318–321.
169 Svoboda, J.A., Nair, A.M.G., Agarwal, N., Agarwal, H.C. and Robbins, W.E. (1979) Experientia 35, 1454–1455.
170 Svoboda, J.A., Nair, A.M.G., Agarwal, N. and Robbins, W.E. (1980) Experientia 36, 1029–1030.
171 Svoboda, J.A., Herbert Jr., E.W., Thomson, M.J. and Shimanuki, H. (1981) J. Insect Physiol. 27, 183–188.
172 Svoboda, J.A., Thompson, M.J., Herbert Jr., E.W., Shortino, T.J. and Szczepanik-Vanleeuwen, P.A. (1982) Lipids 17, 220–225.
173 Nes, W.R. and Alcaide, A. (1975) Lipids 10, 140–144.
174 Thompson, M.J., Serban, N.N., Robbins, W.E., Svoboda, J.A., Shortino, T.J., Dutky, S.R. and Cohen, C.F. (1975) Lipids 10, 615–622.
175 Robbins, W.E., Thompson, M.J., Svoboda, J.A., Shortino, T.J. and Cohen, C.F. (1975) Lipids 10, 353–359.
176 Fujimoto, Y., Morisaki, M., Ikekawa, N., Horie, Y. and Nakasone, S. (1974) Steroids 24, 367–375.
177 Awata, N., Morisaki, M., Fujimoto, Y. and Ikekawa, N. (1976) J. Insect. Physiol. 22, 403–408.
178 Prestwich, G.D. and Phirwa, S. (1983) Tetrahedron Lett. 24, 2461–2464.
179 Prestwich, G.D., Shieh, H.M. and Gayen, A.K. (1983) Steroids 41, 79–95.
180 Kircher, H.W., Phariss, R.L., Rosenstein, F.U., Baldwin, D. and Fogelman, J.C. (1982) Lipids 17, 209–214.
171 Isaka, Y., Morisaki, M. and Ikekawa, N. (1981) Steroids 38, 417–423.
182 Maruyama, S., Morisaki, M. and Ikekawa, N. (1982) Steroids 40, 341–346.
183 Kawakami, S., Morisaki, M. and Ikekawa, N. (1984) Chem. Pharm. Bull., 32, 1608–1611.
184 Rees, H.H., Greenwood, D.R., Dinan, L.N., Issac, R.E. and Goodwin, T.W. (1981) in: Regulation of Insect Development and Behavior (Sehnal, F., Zolza, A., Menn, J.J. and Gymboroski, B., Eds.) Part I, pp. 71–92, Wroclaw Technical University Press, Poland.
185 Koolman, J. (1982) Insect. Biochem. 12, 225–250.
186 Hoffmann, J.A. (Ed.) (1980) Progress in Ecdysone Research, Elsevier/North-Holland Biomedical Press, Amsterdam.
187 Aldrich, J.R., Kelly, T.J. and Woods, C.W. (1982) J. Insect. Physiol. 28, 857–861.
188 Whitehead, D.L. (1983) Nature (London) 306, 540.
189 King, D.S. (1972) Gen. Comp. Endocrinol Suppl. 3, 221.
190 Chino, H., Sakurai, S., Ohtaki, T., Ikekawa, N., Miyazaki, H., Ishibashi, M. and Abuki, H. (1973) Science 183, 529–530.
191 King, D.S., Bollenbacher, W.E., Borst, D.W., Vedeckis, W.V., O'Connor, J.D., Ittycheriah, P.I. and Gilbert, L.I. (1974) Proc. Natl. Acad. Sci. (U.S.A.) 71, 793–796.
192 King, D.S. and Marks, E.P. (1974) Life Sci. 15, 147.
193 Sakurai, S., Ikekawa, N., Ohtaki, T. and Chino, H. (1977) Science 198, 627–629.
194 Johnson, P., Cook, I.F., Rees, H.H. and Goodwin, T.W. (1975) Biochem. J. 152, 303–311.
195 Rees, H.H., Davies, T.G., Dinan, L.N., Lockley, W.J.S. and Goodwin, T.W. (1980) in: Progress in Ecdysone Research (Hoffman, J.A., Ed.) pp. 125–137, Elsevier/North-Holland Biomedical Press, Amsterdam.
196 Smith, S.L., Bollenbacher, W.E. and Gilbert, L.I. (1980) in: Progress in Ecdysone Research (Hoffmann, J.A., Ed.) pp. 139–161, Elsevier/North-Holland Biomedical Press, Amsterdam.

197 Kaplanis, J.N., Weirich, G.F., Svoboda, J.A., Thompson, M.J. and Robbins, W.E. (1980) in: Progress in Ecdysone Research (Hoffmann, J.A., Ed.) pp. 163–185, Elsevier/North-Holland Biomedical Press, Amsterdam.
198 Ohnishi, E., Ohtaki, T. and Fukuda, S. (1971) Proc. Jpn. Acad. 47, 413–415.
199 Goltzené, F., Lagueux, M., Charlet, M. and Hoffmann, J.A. (1978) Hoppe-Seyler's Z. Physiol. Chem. 259, 1427–1434.
200 Garen, A., Kauvar, L. and Lepesant, J.-A. Proc. Natl. Acad. Sci. (U.S.A.) 74, 5099–5103.
201 Ohnishi, E., Mizuno, T., Chatani, F., Ikekawa, N. and Sakurai, S. (1977) Science 197, 66–67.
202 Ohnishi, E., Mizuno, T., Ikekawa, N. and Ikeda, T. (1981) Insect Biochem. 11, 155–159.
203 Ikekawa, N., Fujimoto, Y., Takasu, A. and Morisaki, M. (1980) J. Chem. Soc., Chem. Commun. 709–711.
204 Hetru, C.C., Kappler, C., Hoffmann, J.A., Nearn, R., Bang, L. and Horn, D.H.S. (1982) Mol. Cell. Endocrinol. 26, 51–80.
205 Isaac, R.E., Milner, N.P. and Rees, H.H. (1983) Biochem. J. 213, 261–265.
206 Isaac, R.E., Rose, M.E., Rees, H.H. and Goodwin, T.W. (1982) J. Chem. Soc., Chem. Commun. 249–251.
207 Tsoupras, G., Hetru, C., Lagueux, L.M., Constantin, E. and Hoffmann, J.A. (1982) Tetrahedron Lett. 23, 2045–2048.
208 Tsoupras, G., Luu, B. and Hoffmann, J.A. (1982) Steroids 40, 551–558.
209 Tsoupras, G., Hetru, C., Luu, B., Constantin, E., Lagueux, M. and Hoffmann, J. (1983) Tetrahedron Lett. 39, 1789–1796.
210 Tsoupras, G., Luu, B. and Hoffmann, J.A. (1983) Science 220, 507–509.
211 Bergamasco, R. and Horn, D.H.S. (1980) in: Progress in Ecdysone Research (Hoffmann, J.A., Ed.) pp. 299–324, Elsevier/North-Holland Biomedical Press, Amsterdam.
212 Cherbas, P., Trainor, D.A., Stonard, R.J. and Nakanishi, K. (1982) J. Chem. Soc., Chem. Commun. 1307–1308.
213 Hikino, H., Ohizumi, Y. and Takemoto, T. (1975) J. Insect Physiol. 21, 1953–1963.
214 Kubo, I., Klocke, J.A. and Asano, S. (1981) Agric. Biol. Chem. 45, 1925–1927.
215 Withers, N.W., Tuttle, R.C., Goad, L.J. and Goodwin, T.W. (1979) Phytochemistry 18, 71–73.
216 Mizuno, T., Watanabe, K. and Ohnishi, E. (1981) Develop. Growth Differ. 23, 543–552.
217 Ikekawa, N., Takatsuto, S., Kitsuwa, T., Saito, H., Morishita, T. and Abe, H. (1984) J. Chromatogr., 290, 289–302.
218 DeLuca, H.F. and Schnoes, H.K. (1976) Annu. Rev. Biochem. 45, 631–666; (1983) Annu. Rev. Biochem. 52, 411–439.
219 Nes, W.R. and McKean, M.L. (1977) Biochemistry of Steroids and Other Isopentenoids, University Park Press, Baltimore, MD.
220 Karlson, P. (1983) Hoppe-Seyler's Z. Physiol. Chem. 364, 1067–1087.

H. Danielsson and J. Sjövall (Eds.), *Sterols and Bile Acids*

CHAPTER 9

Mechanism of bile acid biosynthesis in mammalian liver

INGEMAR BJÖRKHEM

Department of Clinical Chemistry, Huddinge Hospital, Karolinska Institutet, Stockholm (Sweden)

(I) Introduction

Generally the most important pathway for the metabolism and excretion of cholesterol in mammals is the formation of bile acids. The major primary bile acids, cholic and chenodeoxycholic acid, are formed from cholesterol in the liver and secreted with bile to the intestine. The reactions involved are saturation of the double bond, epimerization of the 3β-hydroxyl group, introduction of hydroxyl groups into the 7α and 12α positions, oxidation of the C_{27} side chain to a C_{24}-carboxylic acid, and conjugation with taurine or glycine (Fig. 1). The sequence of these reactions has been studied extensively and the major pathways have been defined with a high degree of certainty in rat and man. After secretion of the primary bile acids with bile to the intestine, microorganisms may transform them into secondary bile acids such as deoxycholic and lithocholic acid (Chapter 12). The major part of all bile acids in the intestine is absorbed and returns to the liver via the portal blood. Only a small fraction is excreted in the faeces. The bile acids returning to the liver in the enterohepatic circulation may be further metabolized before they are reconjugated and re-excreted into the bile.

The conversion of cholesterol into bile acids represents the most obvious example of the high capacity of the liver to convert lipid-soluble material into excretable water-soluble products. In principle, the reactions in the formation of bile acids are very similar to those generally involved in the metabolism and detoxication of various lipids and drugs: hydroxylations, oxidations, and conjugations. In contrast to detoxication reactions, however, some of the reactions are highly specific and at least one of the hydroxylations is subject to metabolic control. In view of the importance of the rate of elimination of cholesterol in diseases such as atherosclero-

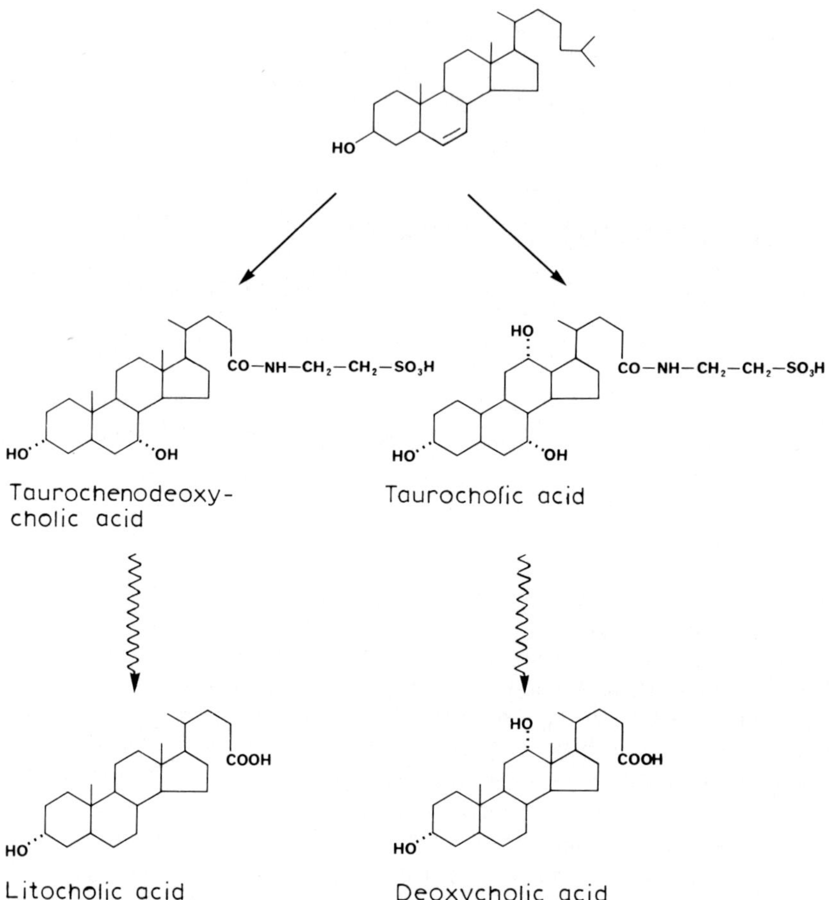

Fig. 1. Conversion of cholesterol into the major primary and secondary bile acids.

sis, hyperlipidaemia, gallstone disease and some lipid storage diseases, it is not surprising that the recently increasing interest in bile acid synthesis is focussed on its mechanism of regulation.

The scope of the present review is a detailed description of our knowledge of the biosynthesis of the primary bile acids in the mammalian liver and its regulation. In view of the vast literature, the survey cannot be regarded as complete, and it is inevitable that the specific interests of the author have influenced the selection of material. Emphasis will thus be put on mechanistic aspects. The literature has been followed up to June 1983. It should be mentioned that several excellent reviews have been published [1–9] which cover the literature up to about 1975.

(II) *Formulation of the sequence of reactions in the biosynthesis of bile acids*

In 1943, Bloch et al. [10] showed that randomly deuterated cholesterol was converted into labelled cholic acid in a dog with cholecystonephrostomy. When ^{14}C-labelled cholesterol became available in the beginning of the 1950's, several groups began to study the quantitative aspects of the conversion of cholesterol into bile acids, mainly with use of bile fistula rats. Chaikoff and co-workers [11,12] showed that 80–90% of intravenously injected labelled cholesterol was ultimately metabolized to bile acids in the rat, the remainder being excreted as neutral steroid in faeces. From the distribution of label in cholic acid after administration of labelled acetate, Zabin and Barker concluded that the cholic acid side chain was derived from cholesterol by a direct removal of the 3 terminal carbon atoms [13]. During the following years, the most important information came from studies in which the conversion of labelled hypothetical intermediates into bile acids was studied in bile fistula rats. In some classical experiments by Bergström et al., it was shown that 5β-cholestane-3α,7α,12α-triol was efficiently converted into cholic acid, whereas 3β-hydroxy-Δ^5-cholenic acid was not [14,15]. It was concluded that the changes in the nucleus are completed before the oxidation of the side chain. The nuclear changes in the degradation of cholesterol to bile acids include an epimerization of the hydroxyl group in position 3β, saturation of the Δ^5 double bond, and introduction of hydroxyl groups at positions 7α and 12α. If the first two reactions occur initially, one of the following compounds would be expected to be an intermediate: 5-cholesten-3α-ol, 5β-cholestan-3α-ol, 5β-cholestan-3β-ol, 4-cholesten-3-one, 5-cholesten-3-one. None of these steroids was converted into cholic acid in a bile fistula rat. In contrast, 7α-hydroxycholesterol (5-cholestene-3β,7α-diol) was rapidly converted into cholic and chenodeoxycholic acid, indicating that 7α-hydroxylation may be an early step [16]. It was also shown that chenodeoxycholic acid as well as 3α,7α-dihydroxy-5β-cholestanoic acid were not converted into cholic acid, indicating that at least in the rat, 12α-hydroxylation does not occur once the side chain has been oxidized [16,17]. This was also supported by the finding that 25- and 26-hydroxycholesterol did not give rise to cholic acid [18].

From the above investigations, summarized in Fig. 2, it was concluded that 7α-hydroxylation of cholesterol may be the first step in the conversion of cholesterol into bile acids, and that 5β-cholestane-3α,7α,12α-triol probably is an intermediate in cholic acid formation. Since 5β-cholestane-3α,7α-diol was rapidly converted into chenodeoxycholic acid and only to a small part into cholic acid [19], it was concluded that 5β-cholestane-3α,7α-diol is a corresponding intermediate in the formation of chenodeoxycholic acid. Samuelsson showed that the conversion of cholesterol into bile acids most probably involves a ketonic intermediate, since [3α-^3H]cholesterol lost its tritium when converted into cholic acid [1,20]. Since 4-cholesten-3-one appeared excluded, 7α-hydroxy-4-cholesten-3-one could be a possible intermediate. This steroid was synthesized by Danielsson [21], and it was shown

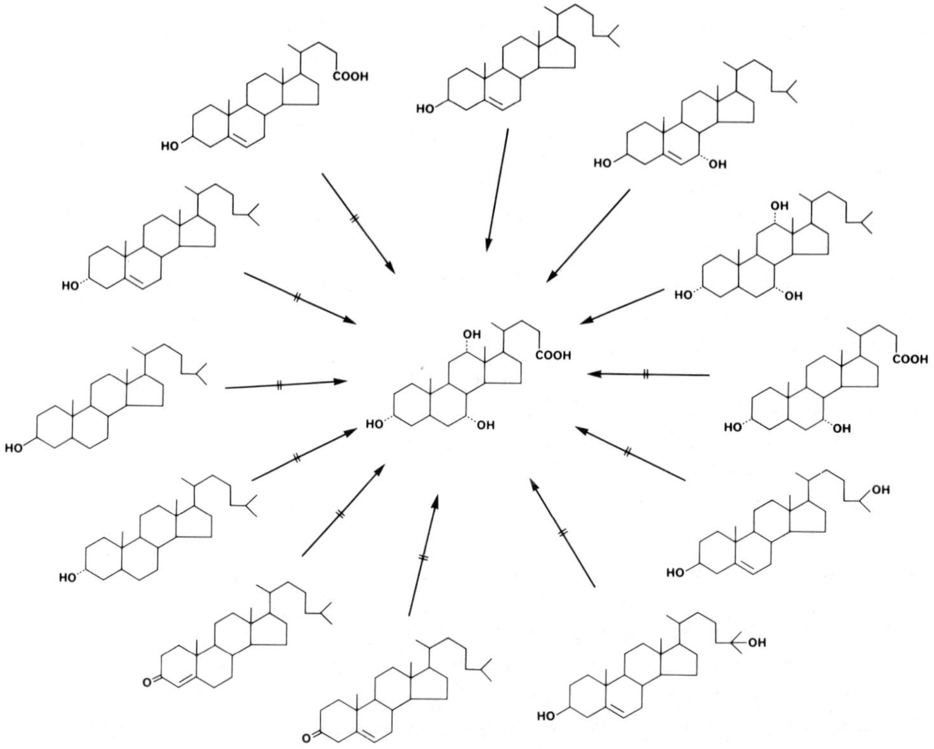

Fig. 2. Results of experiments with labelled hypothetical intermediates with use of bile fistula rats.

to be converted into cholic and chenodeoxycholic acid in a bile fistula rat. Several unidentified bile acids were formed in these experiments. In later studies, it was shown that cholic and chenodeoxycholic acids were the major products of 7α-hydroxy-4-cholesten-3-one in bile fistula rats, provided only trace amounts of the labelled precursor were injected [22].

During the 1960's, the above sequence of reactions was confirmed by different in vitro studies. Mendelsohn and Staple showed that labelled cholesterol could be converted into 5β-cholestane-3α,7α,12α-triol by $20\,000 \times g$ supernatant fluid of rat liver homogenates [23]. The enzymatic conversion of cholesterol into 7α-hydroxycholesterol was first shown by Danielsson and Einarsson using the microsomal fraction fortified with NADPH [24]. The conversion of 7α-hydroxycholesterol into 7α-hydroxy-4-cholesten-3-one was found to be catalysed by the microsomal fraction fortified with NAD^+ [25]. The latter steroid was converted into 7α,12α-dihydroxy-4-cholesten-3-one by the microsomal fraction and NADPH [26]. The conversion of 7α-hydroxy-4-cholesten-3-one and 7α,12α-dihydroxy-4-cholesten-3-one into the corresponding 3α-hydroxy-5β-saturated steroids was catalysed by soluble NADPH-dependent enzymes [25,27,28]. Since Hutton and Boyd found that 4-cholestene-3α,7α-diol was a product of 7α-hydroxy-4-cholesten-3-one in vitro [25], it was first suggested that 4-cholestene-3α,7α-diol could be an intermediate. It was later shown by direct as well as by indirect methods that the conversion of 7α-hydroxy-4-cholesten-3-one into 5β-cholestane-3α,7α-diol involves intermediary formation of 7α-hydroxy-5β-cholestan-3-one [28–30].

The above investigations led to the formulation of the sequence of reactions shown in Fig. 3 for the nuclear changes in the conversion of cholesterol into cholic acid and chenodeoxycholic acid. In this scheme, the 12α-hydroxyl group is introduced at the stage of 7α-hydroxy-4-cholesten-3-one. It was shown that also 7α-hydroxycholesterol could be 12α-hydroxylated by the microsomal fraction of a liver homogenate [31]. Since that hydroxylation occurred at a much lower rate, it was believed to represent a minor pathway [32]. The conversions shown in Fig. 3 were later also demonstrated in human liver [33].

It should be pointed out that the above investigations do not exclude the possibility that a 26-hydroxyl group is introduced in the side chain prior to completion of the nuclear changes. In particular, this may be the case in the biosynthesis of chenodeoxycholic acid. There is strong evidence that in human as well as rat liver, the 26-hydroxyl group normally may be introduced already at the stage of 7α-hydroxy-4-cholesten-3-one. In view of the high capacity of bile fistula rat to convert a number of different side-chain-modulated C_{27}-steroids into chenodeoxycholic acid, there might be several alternative pathways to chenodeoxycholic acid, even if the pathway involving 5β-cholestane-3α,7α-diol or 7α,26-dihydroxy-4-cholesten-3-one as intermediate appears to be the major one under normal conditions.

The mechanism of degradation of the C_{27}-steroid side chain is less well understood. According to the most accepted concept, this degradation starts with a hydroxylation in 26 position followed by oxidation to yield 3α,7α,12α-trihydroxy-5β-cholestanoic acid which is then transformed into cholic acid by reactions similar to those involved in β-oxidation of fatty acids (Fig. 4). 3α,7α-Dihydroxy-5β-cholestanoic acid is the corresponding intermediate in the biosynthesis of chenodeoxycholic acid. Supporting this pathway was the early finding that 3α,7α,12α-trihydroxy-5β-cholestanoic acid is a major bile acid in the bile of alligators [34], and that this acid is also present in trace amounts in human bile [35]. In addition, labelled 3α,7α,12α-trihydroxy-5β-cholestanoic acid was found to be a minor product of labelled cholesterol when administered to humans [36,37]. Labelled 3α,7α,12α-trihydroxy-5β-cholestanoic acid was rapidly converted into cholic acid in rat and man [37,38]. The results of various in vitro work were also consistent with the above pathway. Danielsson identified 5β-cholestane-3α,7α,12α,26-tetrol as well as 3α,7α,12α-trihydroxy-5β-cholestanoic acid as products of labelled 5β-cholestane-3α,7α,12α-triol in mouse liver homogenates [39]. The 26-hydroxylation step was catalysed by the mitochondrial fraction. The microsomal fraction of rat liver [40] but not human liver [41], was also able to catalyse 26-hydroxylation of some specific steroids such as 5β-cholestane-3α,7α,12α-triol. Staple and collaborators showed that NAD^+ was a necessary cofactor for conversion of the triol into the acid in the presence of a dehydrogenase from the soluble fraction [42].

Masui and Staple showed that a mitochondrial fraction supplemented with

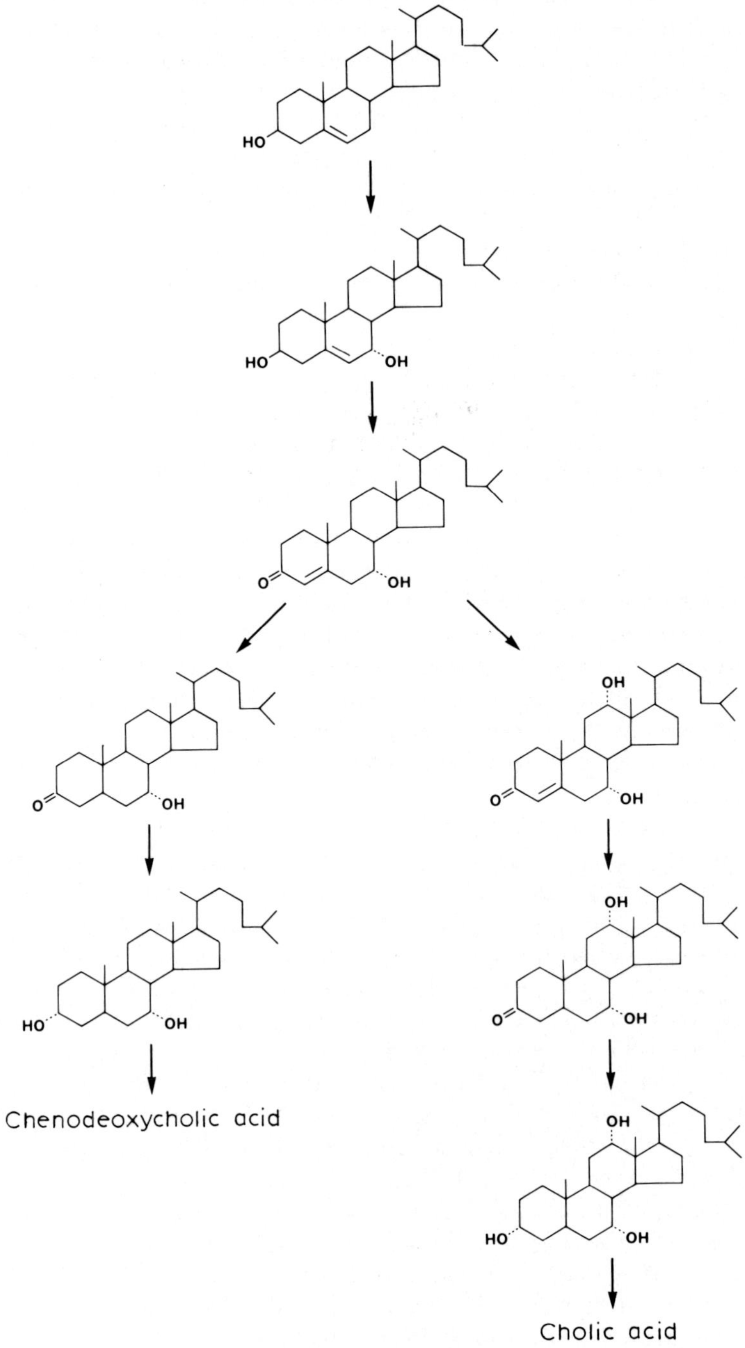

HO
HO
OH
O
OH
O
OH
OH
O
OH
HO
OH
OH
O
OH
Chenodeoxycholic acid
OH
HO
OH
Cholic acid

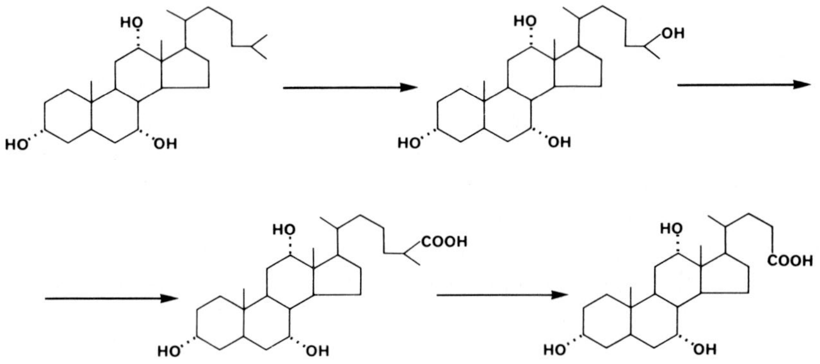

Fig. 4. Sequence of reactions in the degradation of the steroid side chain.

cytosol converted $3\alpha,7\alpha,12\alpha$-trihydroxy-5β-cholanoic acid into the corresponding 24-hydroxylated derivative [43], which in turn was converted into cholic acid by a cytosolic fraction fortified with NAD^+ or $NADP^+$. The cleavage of the side chain involved formation of propionic acid [42]. In similarity with β-oxidation of fatty acids it seems probable that the last reactions in the sequence involve CoA esters of the intermediates.

(III) Cholesterol 7α-hydroxylase

7α-Hydroxylation of cholesterol is the first step in the major pathway to bile acids (cf. Fig. 2). On the basis of their finding that the rate of this hydroxylation increased severalfold in rats after biliary drainage, Danielsson et al. suggested that this step is rate limiting in the biosynthesis of both cholic and chenodeoxycholic acid [44]. The cholesterol 7α-hydroxylase would thus be subjected to a negative feedback regulation by the bile acids returning to the liver. Biliary drainage also led to a small increase in the 12α-hydroxylase activity, but all other reactions studied were unaffected. The regulatory aspects of cholesterol 7α-hydroxylase activity will be reviewed in Section XV. The molecular basis for the regulation will be discussed here.

(1) Assay of cholesterol 7α-hydroxylase in liver microsomes

Assay of the enzyme activity is complicated by the fact that 7α-hydroxylation of cholesterol also may occur due to auto-oxidation or secondary to lipid preoxidation. In addition it is difficult to equilibrate exogenous cholesterol with endogenous microsomal cholesterol.

In the first studies on 7α-hydroxylation, the microsomal fraction together with the

---

Fig. 3. Sequence of nuclear changes in the conversion of cholesterol into bile acids.

cytosol was used as source of enzyme [23,24]. Under such conditions 7α-hydroxycholesterol and its metabolites were the major products, and only very small amounts of 7β-hydroxy- and 7-oxocholesterol were formed. When using the microsomal fraction with or without NADPH, considerable amounts of 7β-hydroxy- and 7-oxocholesterol were formed in addition to 7α-hydroxycholesterol [45,46]. Addition of EDTA or β-mercaptoethylamine reduced the formation of 7β-hydroxy- and 7-oxocholesterol and increased the formation of 7α-hydroxycholesterol due to inhibition of lipid peroxidation [47–49]. In most subsequent studies, the microsomal fraction prepared in EDTA-containing medium has been used as source of enzyme.

In most studies on 7α-hydroxylation, labelled cholesterol was added to the microsomal fraction dissolved in acetone, or as emulsion stabilized with serum albumin or detergents. The degree of equilibration of this added cholesterol with endogenous cholesterol may differ with experimental conditions, resulting in differences in rate of conversion of labelled substrate. Björkhem and Danielsson showed that the rate was much higher when the labelled cholesterol was added in Tween than in acetone [50]. On the other hand, the degree of stimulation or inhibition of enzyme activity was about the same with both types of assays. Cholesterol 7α-hydroxylase activity has also been measured by incubation of [7α-^{3}H]cholesterol followed by determination of the release of $^{3}H_2O$ to the medium [51]. This method gives values in close agreement with those obtained by incubation with [4-^{14}C]cholesterol. One way to overcome difficulties associated with use of exogenous substrate would be to label the microsomal cholesterol in liver by administration in vivo of labelled cholesterol or a precursor of cholesterol, and then measure the rate of production of labelled 7α-hydroxycholesterol in vitro. Such experiments in rats have shown that the metabolic fate of the labelled cholesterol present in the isolated microsomal fraction is the same as that of exogenously added cholesterol [52,53]. Another approach is to measure the rate of formation of 7α-hydroxycholesterol from endogenous microsomal cholesterol by use of [^{3}H]acetic anhydride [54] or by isotope dilution–mass spectrometry [50,55,56]. Still another possibility to eliminate the problem with endogenous microsomal cholesterol is to remove most of this cholesterol by preparation of an acetone powder from the microsome [57].

Since it appears impossible to saturate the 7α-hydroxylase system with cholesterol, all the above assays are deficient, and the maximal capacity of the system cannot be defined with certainty. Since all the different assays seem to give about the same answer with respect to degree of stimulation or inhibition under most conditions, all the assays may be used for studies of effects of different factors on the enzyme system. However, the best assays are those based on measurement of formation of products from endogenous cholesterol. Shefer et al. showed that the double isotope derivative method gave results in agreement with those obtained with the acetone powder method in studies on the effect of treatment with cholestyramine and cholic acid [57]. In contrast to the double isotope derivative assay, the acetone powder assay did not show any change in cholesterol 7α-hydroxylase activity during cholesterol feeding.

Balasubramaniam and co-workers have proposed the term "substrate pool" for the fraction of endogenous cholesterol that acts as substrate [58,59]. The size of this pool was estimated on the assumption that it equilibrates instantaneously and completely with all radioactive cholesterol added to the incubation mixture. Since the degree of equilibration differs with the method of addition the absolute size of the substrate pool cannot be determined. Nevertheless, the concept of a substrate pool appears to be useful since the apparent size of the pool measured under standardized conditions seems to change in response to e.g. cholesterol feeding.

(2) Substrate specificity and physiological substrate for cholesterol 7α-hydroxylase

Most studies on substrate specificity of cholesterol 7α-hydroxylase have been performed with intact microsomes. Results of such studies may be difficult to interpret since the enzyme system is embedded in a lipoprotein membrane, and may not be directly accessible to potential substrates [59]. Thus, differences in the rate of 7α-hydroxylation of various steroids could be due to differences in the rate at which the substrate reaches the active site of the enzyme rather than to differences in the intrinsic ability of the enzyme to interact catalytically with the substrate [59]. Further, occurrence of 7α-hydroxylation of a certain steroid may not reflect the substrate specificity of cholesterol 7α-hydroxylase activity since different species of cytochrome P-450 are present in the microsomes.

Esters of cholesterol cannot be directly attacked by the enzyme [60,61]. Rat liver microsomes catalyse 7α-hydroxylation of cholestanol at a rate comparable to that of cholesterol [62]. Since 7α-hydroxylation of cholestanol is stimulated after treatment with cholestyramine, it appears likely that the same enzyme is involved as in hydroxylation of cholesterol. Slight changes in the side chain lead to marked loss of activity [63,64]. Loss of a terminal methyl group reduces the rate to about 50% and addition of an ethyl group at C-24 (sitosterol) leads to almost complete loss of the activity. From a study with a great number of structurally closely related steroids, Aringer concluded that cholesterol 7α-hydroxylase requires a rather flat steroid (Δ^4, Δ^5 or 5α) and an equatorial or quasi-equatorial hydroxyl group at C-3 [65].

A coupling appears to exist between the rate-limiting enzyme in the biosynthesis of cholesterol, HMG-CoA reductase, and cholesterol 7α-hydroxylase. The two enzymes seem to be located close to each other on the endoplasmic reticulum membrane [66], and the two activities covariate under most conditions. Results from both in vivo and in vitro experiments show that newly synthesized cholesterol is the preferred substrate for cholesterol 7α-hydroxylase. In an early study by Staple and Gurin, it was shown that the bile acids in bile had a higher radioactivity than cholesterol after administration of labelled acetate to rats [67]. Björkhem and Danielsson found that the specific radioactivity of 7α-hydroxycholesterol was higher than that of cholesterol after incubation of labelled mevalonate with the $10\,000 \times g$ supernatant fluid of a rat liver homogenate [50]. Balasubramaniam et al. showed that 7α-hydroxycholesterol isolated from the livers of rats after intravenous administration of labelled cholesterol had a lower specific radioactivity than cholesterol [58]. Cronholm and collaborators measured the incorporation of isotope from [1-$^2H_2$]-,

[2-$^2H_3$]- and [1-^{13}C]ethanol into cholesterol and bile acids and concluded that the biliary cholesterol was derived from a pool of cholesterol with a turnover considerably slower than that of the pool of cholesterol used for bile acid biosynthesis [68]. From the incorporation of ^{18}O in 3 position of cholic and chenodeoxycholic acid isolated from the bile of a bile fistula rat which has inhaled $^{18}O_2$, Björkhem and Lewenhaupt calculated that at least 50% of the biosynthesized bile acids were derived from newly synthesized cholesterol [69]. It was assumed that all the ^{18}O in the 3 position had been introduced during the synthesis of cholesterol. Using an inhibitor of cholesterol synthesis, Long et al. obtained data suggesting that the bulk of bile acid is synthesized from equilibrated cholesterol when the determination is made within 2 h after fistulation of a rat [70]. With prolonged fistula times more of the bile acid originates from newly synthesized cholesterol.

An elegant demonstration of the relation between the activity of HMG-CoA reductase and cholesterol 7α-hydroxylase was performed by Mitropoulos et al. It was shown that administration of mevalonic acid to rats resulted in an increase of the size of the intracellular pool of cholesterol that is in the environment of the rate-limiting enzyme in cholesterol biosynthesis [71]. Since this enzyme seems to be located close to the cholesterol 7α-hydroxylase [66,72], and the activity of the latter enzyme was stimulated, it was suggested that the increased amount of free cholesterol available was the actual stimulating factor for cholesterol 7α-hydroxylase.

Some evidence indicates that among the different forms of preformed and equilibrated cholesterol reaching the liver, free cholesterol in HDL may be preferentially used as substrate for cholesterol 7α-hydroxylase [73,74].

(3) Mechanism of 7α-hydroxylation of cholesterol and experiments with purified enzyme components

The requirement of NADPH and O_2 in the microsomal 7α-hydroxylation of cholesterol indicates that the hydroxylase is a mixed function oxidase. Since the activity was found to be inhibited by carbon monoxide and an antibody against NADPH–cytochrome P-450 reductase [47,75,76], it was early suggested that a cytochrome P-450 species is involved. The mechanism of hydroxylation should thus be similar to that for hydroxylation of various drugs (Fig. 5). According to current concepts, in the presence of NADPH as the only source of reducing equivalents, the first step in the hydroxylation sequence starts with combination of the substrate with the oxidized form of cytochrome P-450 (Fe^{3+}). The substrate–cytochrome P-450 complex is then reduced by an electron from NADPH–cytochrome P-450 reductase. The substrate–cytochrome P-450 complex seems to be reduced at a faster rate than cytochrome P-450 alone. The reduced cytochrome P-450–substrate complex is then attacked by molecular oxygen to yield a ternary complex of cytochrome P-450, substrate and oxygen. This complex is reduced by transfer of a second electron to the ternary complex. After this event, there is a rearrangement in the ternary complex, resulting in introduction of one atom of oxygen into the substrate, expulsion of water and release of hydroxylated substrate and cytochrome P-450 in

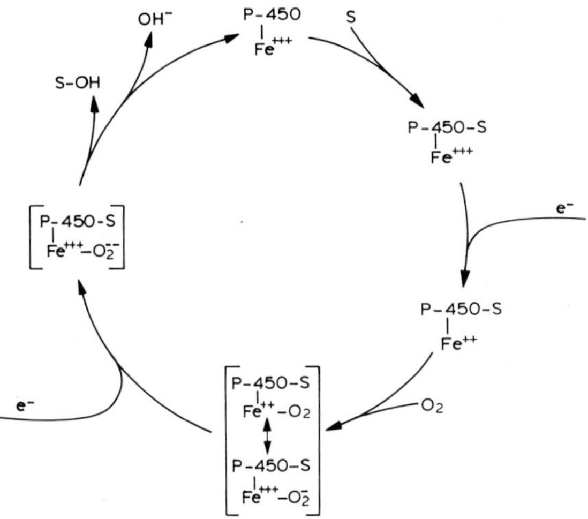

Fig. 5. Mechanism of hydroxylation by cytochrome-P-450-containing systems in liver microsomes.

the oxidized form. The second electron may come from NADPH–cytochrome P-450 reductase or from cytochrome b_5. If NADH is added to the incubation medium in addition to NADPH, there is a stimulation of the rate of reaction for certain substrates, presumably due to an increase in the rate of donation of the second electron by cytochrome b_5. A stimulatory effect of NADH has been shown also in the case of microsomal 7α-hydroxylation of cholesterol [77].

Kinetic data have been obtained for hydroxylation of some drugs that are consistent with the sequence of reactions shown in Fig. 6 [78]. In this scheme, the ternary cytochrome P-450–substrate–oxygen complex is formed after addition of the second electron. Such a mechanism explains better the presence of an isotope effect in the hydroxylation of some substrates labelled with ^{2}H or ^{3}H in the position which is hydroxylated [79]. However, there is no isotope effect in the enzymatic hydroxylation of [7α-^{3}H]- or [7α-^{2}H]cholesterol [80].

Björkhem et al. were the first to demonstrate 7α-hydroxylation of cholesterol in a reconstituted system consisting of partially purified cytochrome P-450, NADPH–cytochrome P-450 reductase, NADPH and a synthetic phosphatidylcholine [81]. The latter component is known to facilitate transfer of electrons from NADPH–cytochrome P-450 reductase. In later experiments with highly purified components there was no need for addition of lipids [82]. The specificity of the hydroxylation was found to be dependent mainly upon the cytochrome P-450 fraction [81]. It was further concluded that the cytochrome P-450 component must be different from the bulk of cytochrome P-450 in the liver. This is in accord with the finding that biliary drainage, which increases the rate of 7α-hydroxylation of cholesterol severalfold, has no effect on other hydroxylations [44] and results in no change or a slight reduction in the total cytochrome P-450 content. Treatment with phenobarbital which increases the rate of hydroxylation of a number of drugs and also increases the content

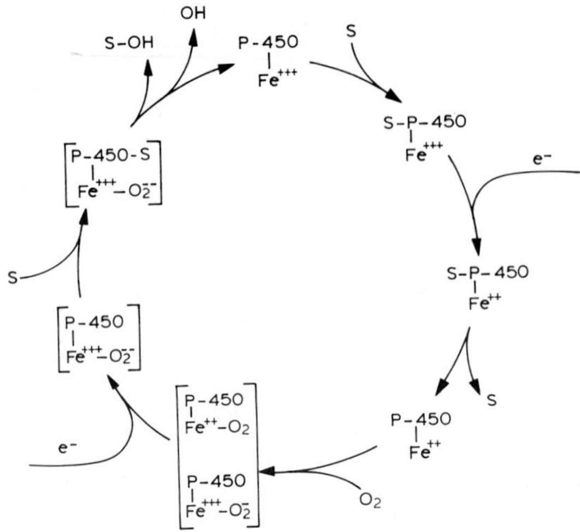

Fig. 6. Possible mechanism of hydroxylation by cytochrome-P-450-containing systems in liver microsomes according to Holtzman et al.

of cytochrome P-450 in the liver, leads to a decrease of the rate of 7α-hydroxylation in the rat [83].

The studies referred to were performed with crude preparations of cytochrome P-450. In a series of papers Wikvall, Hansson and collaborators have reported studies on 7α-hydroxylation of cholesterol in highly purified preparations of cytochrome P-450 from rats and rabbits [82,84,85]. They showed that electrophoretically homogenous cytochrome P-450 LM_4 isolated from cholestyramine-treated rabbits catalyses 7α-hydroxylation of cholesterol as well as some other hydroxylations. Chromatography of a cytochrome P-450 LM_4 fraction on octylamine–Sepharose resulted in 2 subfractions, cytochrome P-450 LM_4 I and cytochrome P-450 LM_4 II, with different catalytic properties. Cytochrome P-450 LM_4 I was unable to catalyse 7α-hydroxylation of cholesterol, but catalysed 12α- and 25-hydroxylations. Cytochrome P-450 LM_4 II efficiently catalysed cholesterol 7α-hydroxylation. It also catalysed the other hydroxylations, although at lower rates than the original cytochrome P-450 LM_4.

Cytochrome P-450 LM_4 I and cytochrome P-450 LM_4 II showed the same apparent molecular weight and spectral properties as the original cytochrome P-450 LM_4 fraction. However, the two subfractions differed in amino acid composition.

If the cholesterol 7α-hydroxylating system is of regulatory importance, a short half-life of the enzyme can be expected. Already in 1968 Einarsson and Johansson obtained evidence that this is the case [87]. It was calculated that the half-life for the breakdown of the 7α-hydroxylase was only 2–3 h. Other enzyme activities involved in the biosynthesis of bile acids from cholesterol, such as the 12α-hydroxylase, had a considerably longer half-life time. It seems likely that a cytochrome P-450 species with short half-life time is the component of the cholesterol 7α-hydroxylase. This was recently confirmed in some elegant experiments by Danielsson and Wikvall [88]. Newly synthesized cytochrome P-450 was labelled by administration of radioactive δ-aminolevulinic acid to rats 6 h prior to killing. Cytochrome P-450 fractions were isolated by solubilization of the microsomes with sodium cholate followed by chromatography on octylamine–Sepharose and hydroxylapatite. The cholesterol 7α-hydroxylase activity was separated from the other hydroxylase activities involved in bile acid biosynthesis (12α-, 25- and 26-hydroxylases). The cholesterol 7α-hydroxylase activity was found in a minor cytochrome P-450 fraction with low specific radioactivity whereas the 12α-, 25- and 26-hydroxylase activities were found in a major cytochrome P-450 fraction with higher specific radioactivity.

There seem to be distinct differences in the physical properties of the specific species of cytochrome P-450 involved in 7α-hydroxylation of cholesterol and most other species of cytochrome P-450. 7α-Hydroxylation is more sensitive to increasing concentrations of phosphate buffer and potassium thiocyanate than any other hydroxylation studied [77]. The 7α-hydroxylation is more dependent on reduced sulphydryl groups than the other C_{27}-steroid hydroxylations [89].

Many rate-limiting enzymes are modulated by reversible phosphorylation–dephosphorylation. Recently, it was suggested that cholesterol 7α-hydroxylase is subject to such modulation. Sanghvi et al. reported that the activity of cholesterol 7α-hydroxylase in crude microsomes was increased after inclusion of ATP, Mg^{2+} and a cytosolic protein fraction in the incubation [90]. There was a loss of enzyme activity in the presence of *E. coli* alkaline phosphatase which was proportional to the amount of phosphatase. Much of this loss was recovered upon addition of ATP, Mg^{2+} and the cytosolic protein fraction. Similar results were reported in a later publication by Goodwin et al. [91]. In contrast, Kwok et al. reported that ATP as well as ADP had an inhibitory effect on 7α-hydroxylation of cholesterol. AMP and cyclic AMP were found to be stimulatory [92]. The inactivation by ATP was dependent on Mg^{2+} and a cytosolic factor [92].

Whether or not phosphorylation–dephosphorylation is of importance, there is evidence that cytosolic proteins may modulate microsomal 7α-hydroxylase activity. It was early shown that the $20\,000 \times g$ supernatant fluid of rat liver homogenate catalyses 7α-hydroxylation of cholesterol more efficiently than the microsomal fraction fortified with NADPH [24]. Spence and Gaylor [93] and Craig et al. [94] have reported that cytosol as well as ammonium sulphate-fractionated cytosol has a stimulatory effect on 7α-hydroxylation in microsomes. Danielsson et al. have isolated two protein fractions from rat liver cytosol [95]. One fraction stimulated cholesterol 7α-hydroxylation of cholesterol 2–3 times in a reconstituted system containing highly purified cytochrome P-450. The other fraction inhibited the reaction markedly. Addition of ATP, $MgCl_2$ or NaF had no effect on the activities of the two protein fractions, indicating that phosphorylation–dephosphorylation was not important under the conditions employed. The dependence upon protein concentration and time suggested that the two protein fractions did not act through carrier effects or substrate solubilization (cf. also Chapter 3).

(IV) Conversion of 7α-hydroxycholesterol into 7α-hydroxy-4-cholesten-3-one

The conversion of 7α-hydroxycholesterol into 7α-hydroxy-4-cholesten-3-one (Fig. 3) is catalysed by the microsomal fraction of liver homogenate and NAD^+ is the preferred cofactor. In an early study on the transformation of [4β-^{3}H]cholesterol into bile acids in a bile fistula rat, Green and Samuelsson found that the main part of the 4β-hydrogen was lost and that a small part was transferred to the 6β position [20]. The 4β-hydrogen was probably lost during the formation of 7α-hydroxy-4-cholesten-3-one from 7α-hydroxycholesterol. The mechanism of this reaction has also been studied in vitro by Björkhem [96]. Conversion of [4β-^{3}H]7α-hydroxycholesterol into 7α-hydroxy-4-cholesten-3-one occurred with loss of most of the ^{3}H and only 3% was transferred to the 6β position. When the reaction was carried out with [4β-^{2}H]7α-hydroxycholesterol, the loss of isotope was about the same, but the extent of transfer was significantly higher, about 12%. The marked isotope effect in the transfer of the 4β-hydrogen to the 6β position was interpreted to mean that the extent of transfer observed with [4β-^{2}H]7α-hydroxycholesterol represents a minimum figure. Experiments in ^2H_2O and ^3H_2O showed only negligible incorporation into the product, indicating an almost complete intramolecular transfer of hydrogen. It should be borne in mind that the enzyme may not have been fully equilibrated with the labelled medium. In any case, it was concluded that the mechanism of isomerization of the Δ^5 double bond in 7α-hydroxycholesterol is different from that in the metabolism of steroid hormones in mammalian tissues.

There was a significant isotope effect in the conversion of [3α-^{3}H]7α-hydroxycholesterol into 7α-hydroxy-4-cholesten-3-one, indicating that abstraction of a hydride ion from the 3α position may be rate limiting in the reaction.

If oxidation of the 3β-hydroxyl group is rate limiting, 7α-hydroxy-5-cholesten-3-one could be an intermediate. Attempts to demonstrate this compound as an intermediate failed, however, possibly due to a rapid rate of isomerization as compared to the slow rate of oxidation of the 3β-hydroxyl group. Since chemical synthesis of 7α-hydroxy-5-cholesten-3-one failed due to the lability of the 7α-hydroxyl group, it was suggested that if 7α-hydroxy-5-cholesten-3-one is an intermediate in the reaction, the 7α-hydroxyl group must be protected from elimination by association to a suitable group on the enzyme. In view of this, the hypothesis of a single enzyme, catalysing both the oxidoreduction and the isomerization seemed attractive.

The idea that only one enzyme is involved in the conversion of 7α-hydroxycholesterol into 7α-hydroxy-4-cholesten-3-one was recently supported by an investigation by Wikvall [97]. He solubilized the enzyme activity from rabbit liver microsomes by treatment with a mixture of sodium cholate and the non-ionic detergent Renex 690. The enzyme was purified about 200-fold by different chromatographic steps. The purified enzyme showed only one protein band with an apparent molecular weight of 46 000. Whereas the microsomal fraction had a broad substrate specificity, NAD^+-supported oxidation with the purified oxidoreductase only occurred with 7α-hydroxycholesterol as substrate. $NADP^+$ could not replace NAD^+ in the reaction. The high specificity is also evident from studies with the 3β-hydroxy-Δ^5-steroid oxidoreductase inhibitor 2α-cyano-4,4,17-trimethyl-17β-hydroxy-5-androsten-3-one which does not influence the formation of 7α-hydroxy-4-cholesten-3-one [98].

(V) 12α-Hydroxylation

Also the microsomal 12α-hydroxylase is dependent upon cytochrome P-450. In early work, the involvement of cytochrome P-450 was questioned, due to the relatively low sensitivity towards carbon monoxide of this hydroxylation [32,99]. Conclusive evidence that the 12α-hydroxylation involves participation of cytochrome P-450 was obtained by Bernhardsson et al., who showed that the hydroxylation could occur in a reconstituted system consisting of a crude fraction of cytochrome P-450 from rat liver, NADPH–cytochrome P-450 reductase and a phospholipid [100]. The specificity depended upon the cytochrome P-450 component. Starvation is known to stimulate 12α-hydroxylation, and use of cytochrome P-450 from starved rats led to increased rate of 12α-hydroxylation.

Recently Hansson and Wikvall studied 12α-hydroxylation in a reconstituted system consisting of highly purified cytochrome P-450 LM_4 from rabbits [101]. The cytochrome P-450 fractions used were electrophoretically homogenous, but the cytochrome P-450 from starved rabbits had up to 4 times higher capacity to catalyse 12α-hydroxylation than had cytochrome P-450 from untreated, phenobarbital-treated, or β-naphthoflavone-treated rabbits. It should be mentioned that treatment with β-naphthoflavone increases the amount of cytochrome P-450 LM_4 in the liver. Amino acid analyses, peptide-mapping experiments as well as absorption spectral and circular dichroism spectral analyses revealed physical differences between cytochrome P-450 LM_4 preparations from starved and phenobarbital-treated animals. It was concluded that the cytochrome P-450 LM_4 fraction was heterogenous and contained a species of cytochrome P-450 specific for 12α-hydroxylation.

The cytochrome P-450 component in the 12α-hydroxylase is more sensitive to high ionic strength than most other species of cytochrome P-450 [77]. There is no isotope effect in the 12α-hydroxylation of a 12α-^{2}H-labelled substrate [102], showing that cleavage of the C–H bond in the ternary complex is not rate limiting.

Recently, Danielsson et al. reported that the activity of a purified 12α-hydroxylating system from rabbit liver microsomes could be modulated by protein fractions from rabbit liver microsomes and cytosol [103]. The microsomal protein fraction had a stimulatory effect whereas the cytosolic protein was inhibitory. Addition of ATP and $MgCl_2$ or NaF had no effect on the activities of the two protein fractions, indicating that phosphorylation–dephosphorylation was of little or no importance. The microsomal 12α-hydroxylase stimulator also stimulated cholesterol 7α-hydroxylase activity.

In most studies on 12α-hydroxylation, labelled 7α-hydroxy-4-cholesten-3-one has been used as the substrate [32], and it is believed to be the most important substrate also in vivo. It cannot be excluded that 5β-cholestane-3α,7α-diol as well as 7α-hydroxycholesterol are substrates for the 12α-hydroxylase in minor pathways in vivo.

In a study by Ali and Elliott it was shown that 5α-cholestane-3α,7α-diol was an even better substrate for the 12α-hydroxylase in rabbit liver microsomes than 7α-hydroxy-4-cholesten-3-one (156%) [104]. This reaction is probably of importance in the formation of allocholic acid. The high specificity of the 12α-hydroxylase towards the coplanar 5α-sterol nucleus is also evident from the finding that allochenodeoxycholic acid can be converted into allocholic acid in rats, both in vivo and in vitro [105,106, Chapter 11]. Based on the known structural requirements of the 12α-hydroxylase, Shaw and Elliott prepared competitive inhibitors with different substitutions in the C_{12} position [107]. The best inhibitor of those tested was found to be 5α-cholest-11-ene-3α,7α,26-triol. Theoretically, such inhibitors may be used to increase the endogenous formation of chenodeoxycholic acid in connection with dissolution of gallstones.

The activity of the 12α-hydroxylase in rat liver is decreased by treatment with thyroid hormone and increased after thyroidectomy [108,109]. The activity also seems to be inhibited by feeding bile acids [110,111].

(VI) Saturation of the Δ^4 double bond

In the presence of $100\,000 \times g$ supernatant fraction of liver homogenate, 7α-hydroxy-4-cholesten-3-one as well as 7α,12α-dihydroxy-4-cholesten-3-one are efficiently converted into the corresponding 3α-hydroxy-5β-steroids via the 3-oxo-5β-steriods [27,28] (cf. Fig. 3). The NADPH-dependent Δ^4-3-oxosteroid 5β-reductase active on 7α-hydroxy-4-cholesten-3-one and 7α,12α-dihydroxy-4-cholesten-3-one has been partially purified by Berséus [112,113]. The preparation was also active towards 3-oxo-Δ^4-steroids of the C_{19}, C_{21} and C_{24} series. The results of some inhibition experiments indicated that there were different Δ^4-3-oxosteroid 5β-reductases with different substrate specificities in the preparation.

The mechanism of saturation of the Δ^4 double bond has been investigated by Berséus and Björkhem [114]. The conversion of [4-^{14}C]7α,12α-dihydroxy-4-cholesten-3-one into 7α,12α-dihydroxy-5β-cholestan-3-one in the presence of partially purified Δ^4-3-oxosteroid 5β-reductase was found to occur with incorporation of ^{3}H from [4A-^{3}H]NADPH but not from [4B-^{3}H]NADPH. The ^{3}H was incorporated in the 5β position. The source of the hydrogen at the 4 position was studied with ^3H_2O and unlabelled NADPH. ^{3}H was incorporated in the 4 but not in the 5β position. The mechanism thus seems to be a polarization of the 3-oxo group making C-5 electrophilic and C-4 nucleophilic. C-4 could then be protonated and C-5 subjected to an attack of a hydride ion from NADPH (Fig. 7). In later experiments with ^2H_2O and [4A-^{2}H]NADPH, Björkhem and Holmberg found that the addition of hydride

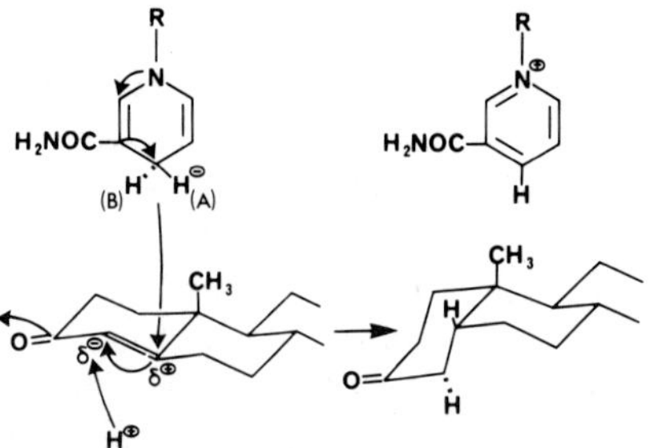

Fig. 7. Mechanism of 5β-saturation of the Δ^4 double bond.

ion from NADPH was rate limiting in the saturation of the double bond in progesterone catalysed by the same Δ^4-3-oxosteroid 5β-reductase preparation [115].

The stereochemistry in the addition of the proton to C-4 was also studied in vivo by Björkhem [116]. A mixture of [4-^{3}H]- and [4-^{14}C]7α-hydroxy-4-cholesten-3-one was converted into cholic acid in a bile fistula rat without loss of ^{3}H. By stereoselective dehydrogenation it was shown that the ^{3}H in the cholic acid isolated was located mainly in the 4β position. This means that the addition of the proton must occur in the 4α position. The enzymatic reduction of the Δ^4 double bond thus involves a *trans* diaxal addition of hydrogen (Fig. 7).

(VII) Reduction of the 3-oxo group

A 3α-hydroxysteroid dehydrogenase active on 7α-hydroxy-5β-cholestan-3-one and 7α,12α-dihydroxy-5β-cholestan-3-one (cf. Fig. 3), was partially purified (about 300-fold) from rat liver cytosol by Berséus [112,113]. NADPH was required as cofactor and hardly any activity was observed with NADH. The preparation was also active towards 3-oxo steroids of the C_{19}, C_{21} and C_{24} series, and in these cases appreciable activity was obtained also with NADH. The mechanism of reduction involves a stereospecific transfer of a hydride ion from the 4A position of NADPH to the 3β position of the steroid [114].

(VIII) 26-Hydroxylation

26-Hydroxylation (cf. Fig. 4) is catalysed both by the microsomal and the mitochondrial fraction of a rat liver homogenate [39,40]. In a human liver homogenate, however, there is only very small or insignificant 26-hydroxylation in the microsomal fraction [41]. Both the microsomal and the mitochondrial hydroxylation will be discussed here.

26-Hydroxylation corresponds to hydroxylation of one of the two terminal methyl groups in the steroid side chain. Since such a substitution creates an asymmetric carbon atom at C-25, 26-hydroxylation may be stereospecific. Berséus found that mitochondrial 26-hydroxylation of [1,7,15,22,27-$^{14}C_5$]cholesterol, synthesized from [2-^{14}C]mevalonate, was stereospecific [117]. This was confirmed by Mitropoulos and Myant who studied the release of propionic acid from [1,7,15,22,27-$^{14}C_5$]cholesterol [118]. It was later established that the methyl group of the side chain derived from C-2 of mevalonate corresponds to 25-pro-*R* and that derived from C-3 of mevalonate to 25-pro-*S* [119]. It may be concluded that it was the 25-pro-*S* methyl group that had been hydroxylated in the above experiments. Since hydroxylation of the 25-pro-*S* methyl group would give the 25*R* configuration in the product, it may be concluded that the 26-hydroxycholesterol isolated by Berséus had the 25*R* configuration. If this mitochondrial 26-hydroxylating system is of major importance under in vivo conditions and has the same stereospecificity towards the natural substrate (believed to be 5β-cholestane-3α,7α,12α-triol) as it has towards cholesterol, one could expect the naturally formed 3α,7α,12α-trihydroxy-5β-cholestanoic acid to be the 25*R* isomer. Batta et al. [120] as well as Hanson et al. [121] have shown that 3α,7α,12α-trihydroxy-5β-cholestanoic acid isolated from human bile in fact has the 25*R* configuration. A problem in the determination of configuration at C-25 in 3α,7α,12α-trihydroxy-5β-cholestanoic acid is that the alkaline hydrolysis commonly used in the isolation of this compound may cause some isomerization [122]. This problem was avoided in the work by Batta et al. by use of enzymatic hydrolysis.

That the mitochondrial system almost exclusively hydroxylates the 25-pro-*S* methyl group was later confirmed in vitro with 5β-cholestane-3α,7α,12α-triol and 5β-cholestane-3α,7α-diol as substrates [123,124]. Gustafsson and Sjöstedt showed that the microsomal fraction of rat liver mainly hydroxylates the 25-pro-*R* methyl group of 5β-cholestane-3α,7α,12α-triol [125].

In accordance with this, Shefer et al. found that the 25*S* isomer of 5β-cholestane-3α,7α-26-triol was the major product after incubation of 5β-cholestane-3α,7α-diol with the microsomal fraction of liver from several species [124].

It is evident that the microsomal and mitochondrial systems have opposite specificities. Since Popják et al. have suggested that the 25-pro-*R* methyl group should be denoted C-26 and the 25-pro-*S* methyl group C-27 [119], the mitochondrial ω-hydroxylation may be regarded as a 27- and the microsomal as a 26-hydroxylation. In this review, hydroxylation of any of the two methyl groups will be referred to as a 26-hydroxylation.

(1) Microsomal 26-hydroxylation

The microsomal 26-hydroxylase in rat liver has a higher substrate specificity than the mitochondrial. Of a number of C_{27}-steroids, only 5β-cholestane-3α,7α,12α-triol, 5β-cholestane-3α,7α-diol, 7α-hydroxy-4-cholesten-3-one and 7α,12α-dihydroxy-4-cholesten-3-one were 26-hydroxylated to a significant extent [126]. In addition to hydroxylation in the 26 position, 5β-cholestane-3α,7α,12α-triol was hydroxylated by the microsomal fraction of rat liver in the 23, 24α, 24β and 25 positions [40]. The hydroxylation in the 25 position was about as efficient as that in the 26 position.

The properties of the microsomal 26-hydroxylase seem to differ from those of the other microsomal side-chain hydroxylations. Treatment with phenobarbital had little or no influence on 26-hydroxylation of 5β-cholestane-3α,7α,12α-triol but stimulated the other hydroxylations up to 8-fold [126]. Thyroid hormone stimulated the microsomal 26-hydroxylase, which might be of importance for the regulation of the ratio between cholic and chenodeoxycholic acid in the rat (cf. below). Biliary obstruction inhibited [127] whereas biliary drainage and starvation have little or no effect [126].

Microsomal 26-hydroxylation is dependent upon cytochrome P-450, and the reaction can be studied in a reconstituted system consisting of microsomal cytochrome P-450 and NADPH–cytochrome P-450 reductase [128]. Björkhem et al. were able to obtain a partial separation of the 25-hydroxylase from the 26-hydroxylase activity [128]. Hansson et al. showed that there was a specific loss of 26-hydroxylase activity in the purification of some different cytochrome P-450 fractions [129].

(2) Mitochondrial 26-hydroxylation

The mitochondrial enzyme has a broad substrate specificity and catalyses 26-hydroxylation of a number of C_{27}-steroids. The most important substrates in vivo are believed to be 5β-cholestane-3α,7α-diol, 7α-hydroxy-4-cholesten-3-one and 5β-cholestane-3α,7α,12α-triol. Björkhem and Gustafsson found that 5β-cholestane-3α,7α,12α-triol and 7α-hydroxy-4-cholesten-3-one were the best substrates in rat liver mitochondria and that the least efficient 26-hydroxylation occurred with cholesterol as substrate [126,130]. There was also a small extent of 25-hydroxylation of cholesterol in the mitochondrial fraction [130]. The major part of the 26-hydroxylase is bound to the inner mitochondrial membranes [130,131]. Thus the hydroxylase activity is low with intact mitochondria and NADPH as cofactor. Under such conditions citric acid and isocitric acid, which are able to penetrate the inner mitochondrial membrane, stimulate 26-hydroxylation much more efficiently than NADPH [130,131]. It is evident that citric acid and isocitric acid generate NADPH inside the mitochondrial membrane. When using leaking mitochondria, NADPH stimulates the reaction about as efficiently as isocitrate [130,131].

Gustafsson has reported that Ca^{2+} and Mg^{2+} have different effects on mitochondrial 26-hydroxylation of endogenous cholesterol, exogenous cholesterol and 5β-cholestane-3α,7α,12α-triol [132]. He concluded that there might be different transport mechanisms for the two substrates through the mitochondrial membranes. This was later supported by studies by Pedersen et al., showing that the stimulatory effect of Mg^{2+} was similar for hydroxylation of several substrates catalysed by a partially purified system [133].

The mitochondrial 26-hydroxylase is inhibited by biliary drainage and is not influenced by starvation or treatment with phenobarbital [126]. Gustafsson reported that the mitochondrial 26-hydroxylation of cholesterol, 7α-hydroxycholesterol and 7α-hydroxy-4-cholesten-3-one was stimulated whereas 26-hydroxylation of 5β-cholestane-3α,7α,12α-triol was inhibited by biliary obstruction [127]. Whether the

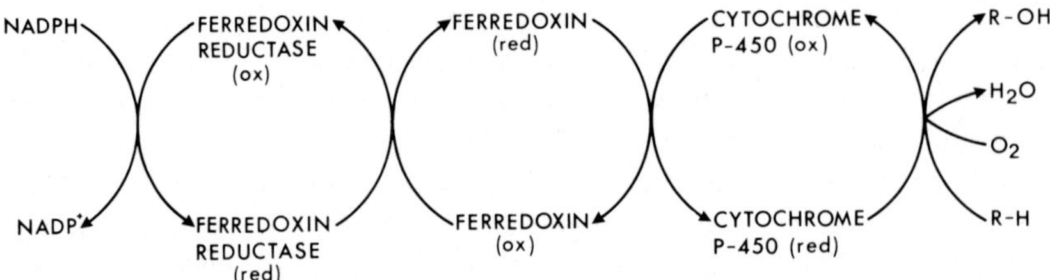

Fig. 8. Mechanism of 26-hydroxylation by the cytochrome P-450 system in liver mitochondria.

observed effects were due to effects on the 26-hydroxylase(s) per se or due to effects on the transfer of steroids to the site of the enzyme(s) could not be evaluated.

It was early suggested that a species of cytochrome P-450 could be involved in the 26-hydroxylation [126,130,131]. Björkhem and Gustafsson showed that the hydroxylase was a mixed-function oxidase by demonstrating incorporation of ^{18}O into 26-hydroxycholesterol when the reaction was performed in an $^{18}O_2$ atmosphere [130]. Conclusive evidence that a species of cytochrome P-450 was involved in the hydroxylation was presented by Okuda et al., who showed that the photochemical action spectrum for reversal of the carbon monoxide inhibition of 26-hydroxylation of 5β-cholestane-3α,7α,12α-triol in rat liver exhibited a maximum at 450 nm [134]. Pedersen et al. [135] and Sato et al. [136] reported simultaneously that small amounts of cytochrome P-450 could be solubilized from the inner membranes of rat liver mitochondria that was active towards cholesterol as well as 5β-cholestane-3α,7α,12α-triol in the presence of ferredoxin, ferredoxin reductase and NADPH. The mechanism of hydroxylation is thus the same as that operative in the biosynthesis of steroid hormones in the adrenals and in the 1α-hydroxylation of 25-hydroxyvitamin D in the kidney (Fig. 8). The liver mitochondrial cytochrome P-450 was not active in the presence of microsomal NADPH–cytochrome P-450 reductase [135,136]. Ferredoxin reductase as well as ferredoxin were active regardless of whether they were isolated from rat liver mitochondria or bovine adrenal mitochondria [133]. The partially purified cytochrome P-450 had a carbon monoxide difference spectrum similar to that of microsomal cytochrome P-450 from liver microsomes and adrenal mitochondria. In the work by Pedersen et al. [133], the concentration of mitochondrial cytochrome P-450 in rat liver mitochondria from untreated rats was calculated to be only about 0.1 nmole/mg protein. Treatment of rats with phenobarbital increased the specific content of cytochrome P-450 in the mitochondria more than 2-fold, without significant increase in the 26-hydroxylase activity. The carbon monoxide spectrum of the reduced cytochrome P-450 solubilized from liver mitochondria of phenobarbital-treated rats exhibited a spectral shift of about 2 nm as compared to the corresponding spectrum obtained in analysis of preparations from untreated rats. This was taken as evidence that more than one species of cytochrome P-450 was present in the preparation. It was later shown by Pedersen et al. [137] and Björkhem et al. [138] that the preparation was also able to catalyse 25-hydroxylation of vitamin D_3 and that different enzymes are involved in the 25- and the 26-hydroxylations. Pedersen et al. showed that the substrate specificity of a reconstituted system from rat liver mitochondria was similar to that in intact mitochondria but the rate of 26-hydroxylation was about 10-fold higher in the reconstituted system [133].

The turnover numbers found for 26-hydroxylation in the reconstituted system were 50–200 times higher than those reported for reconstituted systems from microsomes and it was concluded that the mitochondrial cytochrome P-450 has a much higher potential for 26-hydroxylation than the microsomal cytochrome P-450 [133].

All the above studies were carried out with preparations purified only 2–7-fold with respect to cytochrome P-450. In recent work by Atsuta and Okuda, up to 22-fold purification was reported [139]. The preparation was not homogenous as judged from sodium dodecyl sulphate polyacrylamide gel electrophoresis. It was shown by thermal inactivation as well as use of different inhibitors and activators that the same enzyme is involved in the 26-hydroxylation of 5β-cholestane-3α,7α-diol and 5β-cholestane-3α,7α,12α-triol.

(IX) Conversion of 5β-cholestane-3α,7α,12α,26-tetrol into 3α,7α,12α-trihydroxy-5β-cholestanoic acid

5β-Cholestane-3α,7α,12α,26-tetrol is rapidly oxidized to 3α,7α,12α-trihydroxy-5β-cholestanoic acid by the soluble fraction of a liver homogenate fortified with NAD^+ (Fig. 9). In general, the oxidation of the aldehyde is more efficient than that of the triol and the aldehyde is difficult to isolate as an intermediate. Using partially purified enzyme, Masui et al. were able to demonstrate accumulation of 3α,7α,12α-trihydroxy-5β-cholestan-26-al [141]. Okuda and Danielsson synthesized the aldehyde, which was reduced to 5β-cholestane-3α,7α,12α,26-tetrol by a cytosolic enzyme in the presence of NADH [140]. Okuda and Takigawa purified the 3α,7α,12α-trihydroxy-5β-cholestan-26-al reductase from rat and horse liver cytosol and showed that the reductase was identical with ethanol dehydrogenase (liver alcohol dehydrogenase) [142–144]. It was concluded that oxidation of 5β-cholestane-3α,7α,12α,26-tetrol is one of the important physiological functions of liver alcohol dehydrogenase. Alcohol dehydrogenase from horse liver contains 3 major isoenzymes, $LADH_{EE}$, $LADH_{ES}$ and $LADH_{SS}$. Björkhem et al. showed that the ω-hydroxysteroid dehydrogenase activity of $LADH_{SS}$ was much higher than that of

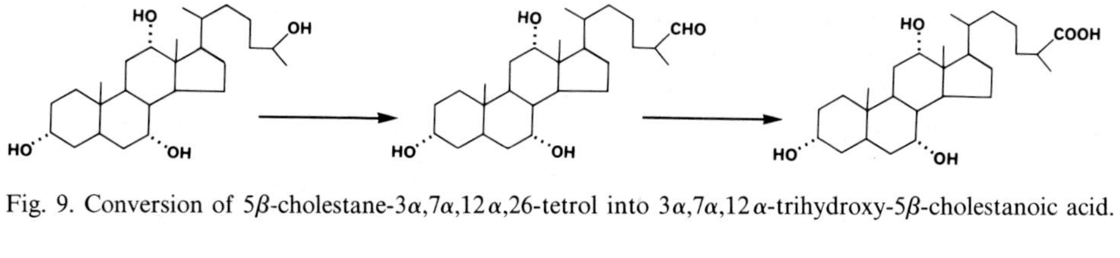

HO OH HO OH HO CHO HO OH HO COOH HO OH

Fig. 9. Conversion of 5β-cholestane-3α,7α,12α,26-tetrol into 3α,7α,12α-trihydroxy-5β-cholestanoic acid.

$LADH_{EE}$ and that the activity disappeared after carboxymethylation of a cysteine residue at the active site of $LADH_{SS}$ [145]. In a recent study by Okuda and Okuda it was demonstrated that the ω-hydroxysteroid dehydrogenase activity in human liver was associated with a major isoenzyme of liver alcohol dehydrogenase (β_2, β_2) and that the activity was inhibited by a chelating agent for Zn^{2+}, which resides in the active site of the enzyme [146]. Kinetic studies with the highly purified isoenzyme showed that neither a Theorell–Chance mechanism nor a simple ordered BiBi mechanism applied to the reaction. Evidence was obtained that the reaction was asymmetric in both directions. It has been established by Fukuba that the 4A-hydrogen in NADH is involved [147].

Okuda et al. have presented evidence that the aldehyde dehydrogenase of horse liver catalysing oxidation of 3α,7α,12α-trihydroxy-5β-cholestan-26-al is identical with the liver aldehyde dehydrogenase active on acetaldehyde [148]. Both acetaldehyde dehydrogenase activity and 3α,7α,12α-trihydroxy-5β-cholestan-26-al dehydrogenase activity were associated with one single protein and the two activities were reduced to a similar extent on inactivation with *p*-chloromercuribenzoate. The K_m value for NAD^+ of the 3α,7α,12α-trihydroxy-5β-cholestan-26-al dehydrogenase was roughly equal to that of liver acetaldehyde dehydrogenase. The stereochemistry in the transfer of hydrogen to NAD^+ was the same in both reactions [147]. It should be mentioned that a mitochondrial aldehyde dehydrogenase plays the predominant role in the oxidation of acetaldehyde formed during ethanol metabolism.

(X) Conversion of 3α,7α,12α-trihydroxy-5β-cholestanoic acid into cholic acid

The early work by Staple et al. showed that a mitochondrial fraction fortified with cytosol converted 3α,7α,12α-trihydroxy-5β-cholestanoic acid into 3α,7α,12α,24-tetrahydroxy-5β-cholestanoic acid [43] (cf. Fig. 3). It was suggested that this reaction was analogous to the formation of β-hydroxy fatty acids in the mitochondrial β-oxidation of fatty acids and would involve the CoA derivatives of the bile acids. No direct evidence for the intermediary formation of a Δ^{24}-unsaturated steroid was obtained. Gustafsson showed that a microsomal system from rat liver fortified with cytosol and ATP had a higher capacity to convert 3α,7α,12α-trihydroxy-5β-cholestanoic acid into the corresponding 24-hydroxylated acid than had the mitochondrial system fortified with ATP [149]. The system used by Gustafsson was less active towards the CoA ester of 3α,7α,12α-trihydroxy-5β-cholestanoic acid than towards the free acid. It was not possible to detect the intermediary formation of a Δ^{24}-unsaturated steroid, but evidence was presented that a desaturase and a hydratase were involved in the reaction. Thus, there was no incorporation of ^{18}O into the product when the reaction was performed in $^{18}O_2$ atmosphere. After incubation in a buffer containing ^2H_2O, there was significant incorporation ^2H into the product. The main product was the 24α isomer.

In spite of the high activity of the microsomal system, its physiological importance may be questioned in view of the very high concentrations of ATP needed for optimal conversion (2.5 mmoles/l) and the lack of need of activation of 3α,7α,12α-trihydroxy-5β-cholestanoic acid.

Staple et al. showed that the conversion of 3α,7α,12α,24-tetrahydroxy-5β-cholestanoic acid into cholic acid (cf. Fig. 3) can occur in rat liver microsomes or in cytosolic fractions fortified with NAD^+ or $NADP^+$ and that propionic acid is released [42,43]. Pedersen and Gustafsson showed recently that the peroxisomal fraction had a high capacity to convert 3α,7α,12α-trihydroxy-5β-cholestanoic acid into cholic acid [150]. Later, Kase et al. found that the peroxisomal fraction was more active than the microsomal and the mitochondrial fractions and that 3α,7α,12α-24-tetrahydroxy-5β-cholestanoic acid was an intermediate in the conversion [151]. Thus, some of the previous contradictory results may be explained by varying degrees of contamination of the microsomal and mitochondrial fractions with peroxisomes. In the work by Kase et al. it was shown that the over-all conversion of 3α,7α,12α-trihydroxy-5β-cholestanoic acid into cholic acid in the peroxisomes was absolutely dependent upon the presence of Mg^{2+}, CoA, ATP and NAD^+. The reaction was stimulated by FAD, by cytosolic protein, by microsomal protein and by bovine serum albumin. It is possible that the stimulatory effect of the microsomes and cytosol was unspecific and due to the increased protein concentration per se. The stimulatory effect of FAD was taken as evidence that 3α,7α,12α-trihydroxy-5β-cholestanoyl-CoA oxidase is a FAD-containing protein. There was a lag phase in the reaction, possibly due to the activation step, and it was suggested that the activation was rate limiting. Also in this case, it was not possible to isolate a Δ^{24}-unsaturated intermediate in the reaction. The participation of a desaturase and a hydratase was proved by the incorporation of ^2H from ^2H_2O into 3α,7α,12α,24-tetrahydroxy-5β-cholestanoic acid (Björkhem, Kase and Pedersen, unpublished study).

The specificity of the enzymes involved in the conversion of 3α,7α,12α-trihydroxy-5β-cholestanoic acid into cholic acid is not known. It is probable that the same or a similar system is involved in the conversion of 3α,7α-dihydroxy-5β-cholanoic acid into chenodeoxycholic acid. Cass et al. showed that there was a competitive inhibition of side-chain oxidation of 3α,7α-dihydroxy-5β-cholestanoic acid by 3α,7α,12α-trihydroxy-5β-cholestanoic acid in vivo in hamsters [152].

(XI) Conjugation of the carboxylic group

Conjugation of the carboxylic group in cholic acid involves participation of a cholic acid CoA ligase and a cholyl-CoA : glycine (taurine) acyltransferase [153–158]. Since the primary product of the thiolytic cleavage of the CoA ester of 3α,7α,12α-trihydroxy-24-oxo-5β-cholestanoic acid is the CoA ester of cholic acid, it is probable that only the transferase may be involved in the primary formation of cholic acid in the liver. A description of the properties of the CoA synthetase and the transferase is given in Chapter 11.

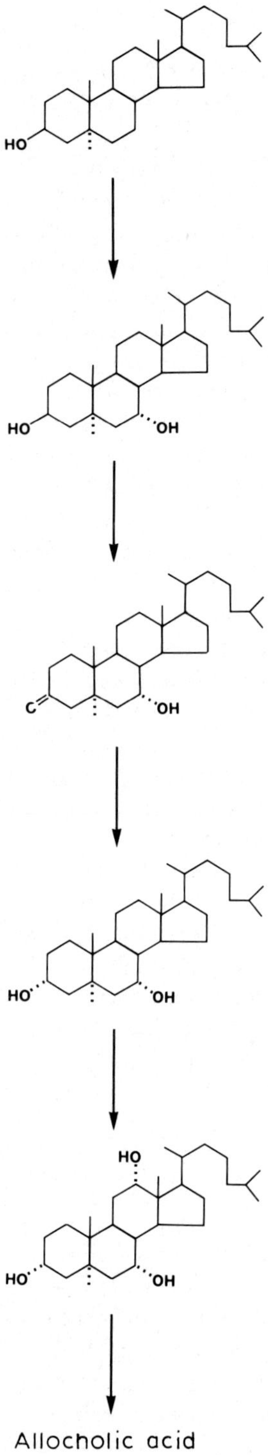

HO

HO OH

O OH

HO OH

HO

HO OH

Allocholic acid

Fig. 10. Sequence of reactions in the conversion of cholestanol into allocholic acid.

(XII) Formation of allo bile acids in the liver

5α-Bile acids (allo bile acids) are minor constituents in mammalian bile, ranging from 1% or less in man to more than 5% in rabbits. In several lower vertebrates, allo bile acids are the major bile acids (Chapter 10). Three different pathways have been described for formation of allo bile acids.

(1) Conversion of 5β-bile acids to allo bile acids

Deoxycholic acid can be converted into allodeoxycholic acid in rabbits and rats [159,160]. Kallner has shown that this conversion probably occurs by intermediate formation of the corresponding 3-oxo-5β-, 3-oxo-Δ^4- and 3-oxo-5α-bile acids [161,162]. Most or all of these reactions are catalysed by intestinal microorganisms. The reactions are reversible and it has been shown that allocholic, allochenodeoxycholic, allodeoxycholic and allolithocholic acid can be converted into the corresponding 5β-bile acids.

(2) Conversion of cholestanol into allo bile acids

Karavolas et al. [163] and Hofmann and Mosbach [164] found that the formation of 5α-bile acids can be induced by administration of cholestanol to rats and rabbits. From the results of in vitro work, it may be concluded that the sequence of reactions in the conversion of cholestanol into allo bile acids involves reactions analogous to those in the conversion of cholesterol into 5β-bile acids (Fig. 10). Shefer et al. have shown that cholestanol is 7α-hydroxylated in the microsomal fraction of rat liver about as efficiently as cholesterol [62]. Björkhem and Gustafsson have shown that 5α-cholestane-3β,7α-diol is efficiently oxidized to 7α-hydroxy-5α-cholestan-3-one by the microsomal fraction of rat liver fortified with NAD^+ [165]. The latter compound is reduced by the NADPH-dependent 3α-hydroxysteroid dehydrogenase in the cytosol to yield 5α-cholestane-3α,7α-diol [165]. This steroid is efficiently 12α-hydroxylated by the microsomal fraction fortified with NADPH to yield 5α-cholestane-3α,7α,12α-triol. 5α-Cholestane-3β,7α-diol as well as 5α-cholestane-3α,7α-diol are converted into allo bile acids, mainly allocholic acid in a bile fistula rat [165]. Noll et al. have shown that in addition to allocholic and allochenodeoxycholic acid, the corresponding 3β isomers are products of cholestanol in bile fistula rats [166]. The very high conversion of the 5α-steroids lacking a 12α-hydroxyl group into allocholic acid, can be explained by the high specificity of the 12α-hydroxylase towards 5α-steroids [104–106]. In the biosynthesis of cholic acid in the rat, introduction of a 26-hydroxyl group practically prevents 12α-hydroxylation. In contrast, Elliott and coworkers found 5α-cholestane-3α,7α,26-triol to be a very efficient precursor of allocholic acid [167] and allochenodeoxycholic acid is converted into allocholic acid both in vivo and in vitro [105,106].

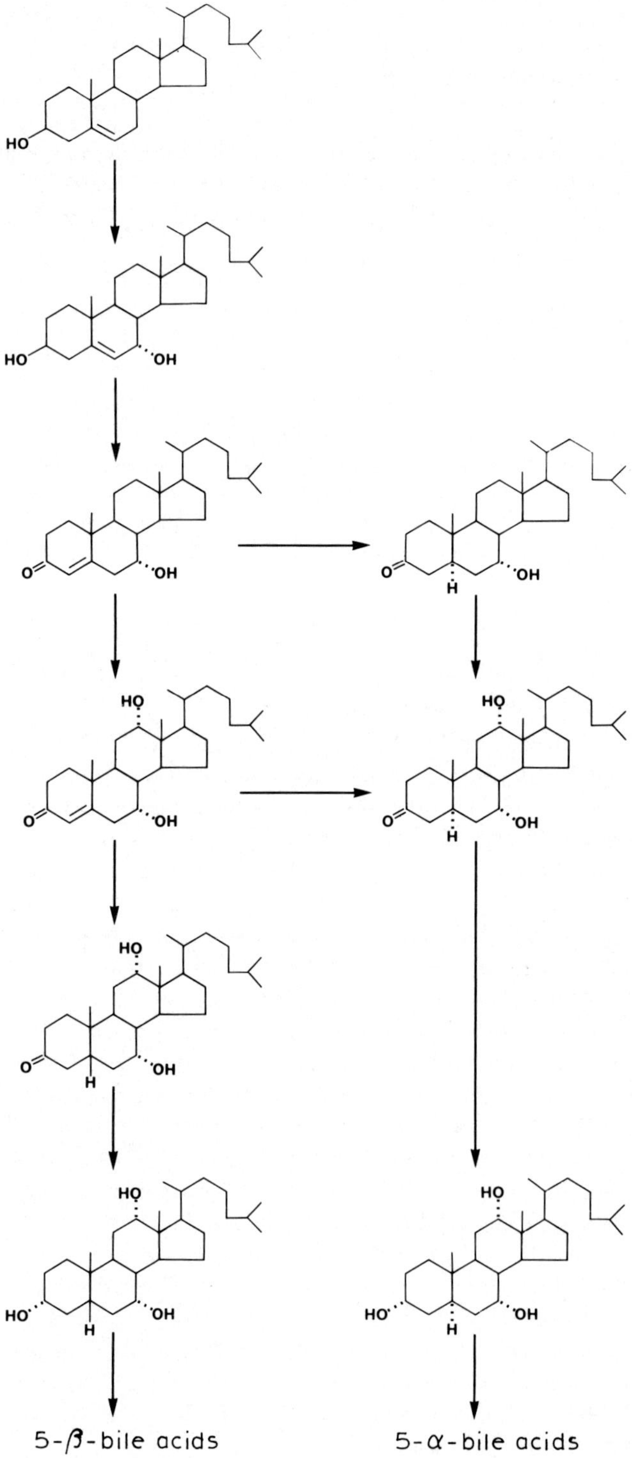

HO

HO OH

O OH

O OH
H

HO
O OH

HO
O OH
H

HO
O OH
H

HO
HO OH
H

HO
HO OH
H

5-β-bile acids

5-α-bile acids

(3) Conversion of 7α-hydroxy-4-cholesten-3-one into allo bile acids

Björkhem and Einarsson showed that rat liver microsomes in the presence of NADPH are able to convert 7α-hydroxy-4-cholesten-3-one and 7α,12α-dihydroxy-4-cholesten-3-one into the corresponding 3-oxo-5α-steroids (Fig. 11) [168]. Liver microsomes from female rats were 3–4 times more active than those from male rats. A similar sex difference was not found in human liver microsomes. The 3-oxo-5α-steroids were efficiently converted into allo bile acids in bile fistula rats. In the presence of both NADPH and NADH, the 3-oxo-5α-steroids were converted into the corresponding 3β-hydroxy-5α-steroids. As mentioned above, the 3-oxo-5α-steroids are efficiently converted into the corresponding 3α-hydroxy-5α-steroids in the cytosol.

In the microsomal 5α saturation of the double bond in 7α-hydroxy-4-cholesten-3-one there is a stereospecific transfer of a hydride ion from the 4B position of NADPH to the 5α position of the steroid [169]. From the results of experiments on the stereochemistry of the addition of the proton to the 4 position, it was concluded that the reduction of the double bond is likely to involve a non-stereospecific addition of hydrogens or a *cis* addition rather than a *trans* addition.

The quantitative importance of the pathway involving 7α-hydroxy-4-cholesten-3-one and 7α,12α-dihydroxy-4-cholesten-3-one as intermediates in formation of allo bile acids is not known. At least in the rat, the capacity of the microsomal Δ^4-3-oxosteroid 5α-reductase is high, and thus it is surprising that such small amounts of allo bile acids are formed under normal conditions in mammals. It seems probable that this enzyme is inhibited under in vivo conditions. Hoshita et al. found an efficient conversion of 7α,12α-dihydroxy-4-cholesten-3-one into 7α,12α-dihydroxy-5α-cholestan-3-one in the microsomal fraction of liver from *Iguana iguana* [170]. Allo bile acids are predominant in this species of iguana and it was suggested that the microsomal Δ^4-3-oxosteroid 5α-reductase is of major importance for their formation.

(XIII) Species differences and alternative pathways in the biosynthesis of bile acids

Most of the studies referred to above have been performed on rats. In vitro and in vivo studies have shown that the major pathways in man are similar to although not necessarily identical to those in the rat.

From in vitro experiments it may be concluded that there are several possible pathways for formation of chenodeoxycholic acid in rat liver. A number of different 26-hydroxylated steroids are converted into chenodeoxycholic acid in bile fistula

---

Fig. 11. Sequence of reactions in the conversion of cholesterol into allo bile acids with 7α-hydroxy-4-cholesten-3-one and 7α,12α-dihydroxy-4-cholesten-3-one as intermediates.

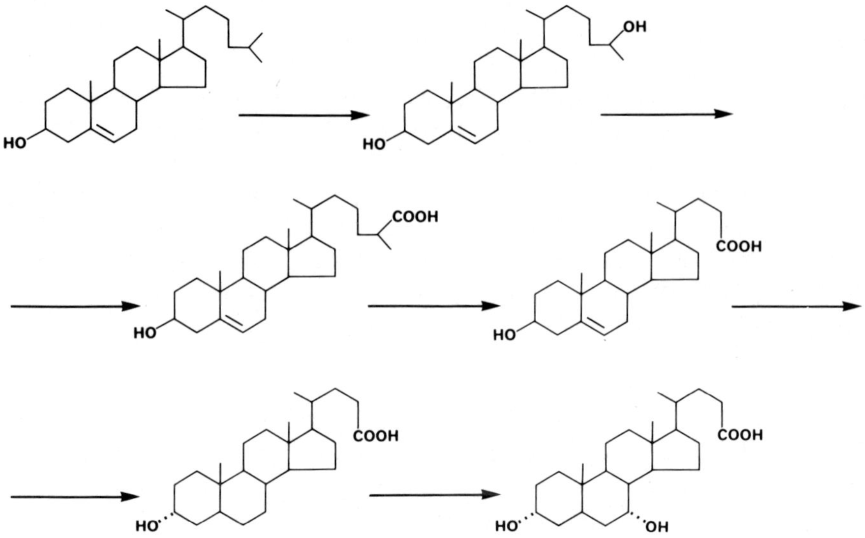

Fig. 12. Mitochondrial conversion of cholesterol into chenodeoxycholic acid.

rats, indicating that the side chain can be partially oxidized prior to the completion of the changes in the steroid nucleus. Such pathways are possible also in man, and Javitt and collaborators showed that labelled 26-hydroxycholesterol was efficiently converted into chenodeoxycholic acid in vivo [171]. In the extreme case, all the changes in the side chain would precede the changes in the nucleus. In such a pathway the sequence of reactions would be that shown in Fig. 12. Mitropoulos and Myant obtained a small conversion of labelled cholesterol into 3β-hydroxy-5-cholenoic acid, lithocholic acid and chenodeoxycholic acid in rat liver mitochondria supplemented with cytosol [172,173]. 26-Hydroxycholesterol was an intermediate [173]. Lithocholic acid is a less efficient precursor of chenodeoxycholic acid, and all available evidence suggests that this pathway is of little or no importance under normal conditions. Biliary drainage leads to an increased synthesis of both cholic acid and chenodeoxycholic acid. If a pathway involving initial 26-hydroxylation of cholesterol is of importance, the 26-hydroxylase would be expected to increase after biliary drainage. However, this is not the case [126]. This does not exclude the possibility that the pathway is of importance under some pathological conditions. Thus, it has been shown that urine from infants with biliary atresia and patients with liver disease contains elevated concentrations of 3β-hydroxy-5-cholenoic acid [174,175].

Yamasaki et al. have studied a pathway for formation of chenodeoxycholic acid in the rat involving intermediate formation of 7α-hydroxycholesterol, 3β-hydroxy-5-cholenoic acid and 7α-hydroxy-3-oxo-4-cholenoic acid [176–179]. In this pathway, changes in the side chain occur after the rate-limiting step. From the data available, it is not possible to evaluate the quantitative importance of this pathway.

Introduction of a 26-hydroxyl group almost completely prevents introduction of a 12α-hydroxyl group in rat liver. In contrast, there is an efficient conversion of 5β-cholestane-3α,7α,26-triol and 7α,26-dihydroxy-4-cholesten-3-one into both cholic and chenodeoxycholic acid in human liver [180–182]. From these findings it is possible to formulate a number of different pathways in the biosynthesis of cholic acid in human liver, with introduction of the 26- and the 12α-hydroxyl groups at different stages.

Studies on patients with the rare inborn disease cerebrotendinous xanthomatosis provide unique possibilities to evaluate the relative importance of different intermediates as substrates for the mitochondrial 26-hydroxylase. These patients appear to have a complete lack of mitochondrial 26-hydroxylase activity and may thus be expected to accumulate the normal substrates for the 26-hydroxylase in their livers. According to an investigation by Björkhem et al., in which the level of different intermediates in a liver biopsy was determined by isotope dilution–mass spectrometry, 7α-hydroxy-4-cholesten-3-one and 5β-cholestane-3α,7α,12α-triol seem to be the most important normal substrates for the 26-hydroxylase also in man [183].

5β-Cholestane-3α,7α,12α-triol is efficiently 25-hydroxylated in the microsomal fraction of liver from both rat and man [40,41]. Shefer et al. [184] and Salen et al. [185] have shown that 5β-cholestane-3α,7α,12α,25-tetrol is converted to 5β-cholestane-3α,7α,12α,24α,25-pentol, 5β-cholestane-3α,7α,12α,24β,25-pentol, 5β-cholestane-3α,7α,12α,23,25-pentol and 5β-cholestane-3α,7α,12α,25,26-pentol in the presence of microsomes fortified with NADPH. In the presence of NAD^+, 5β-cholestane-3α,7α,12α,24β,25-pentol, but not the other 5β-cholestanepentols formed, is efficiently converted to cholic acid by soluble enzymes (Fig. 13). The latter conversion must be assumed to involve formation of acetone. These experiments demonstrate the existence of a new pathway for side-chain degradation in cholic acid synthesis which does not involve hydroxylation at C-26 or the participation of mitochondria. The relative importance of this pathway is a matter of controversy. Salen et al. suggested that this may be the major pathway for biosynthesis of cholic acid in man [185]. The finding that 5β-cholestane-3α,7α,12α,25-tetrol is converted into cholic acid in vivo in rat and man considerably less efficiently than 5β-cholestane-3α,7α,12α,26-tetrol does not support this contention [40,186].

The possibility of multiple pathways in bile acid biosynthesis in man has been discussed by Vlahcevic et al. [180–182]. A number of labelled 7α-hydroxylated intermediates in bile acid biosynthesis were administered to bile fistula patients as well as patients with an intact enterohepatic circulation. In accordance with previous work with bile fistula rats, the specific activity of the isolated cholic acid was in general considerably lower than that of chenodeoxycholic acid. On the basis of this finding, it was suggested that a portion of cholic acid was synthesized via a route not involving initial 7α-hydroxylation of cholesterol. It must then be assumed that the administered intermediate mixes with the endogenous pool of the same steroid. However, due to compartmentation, the metabolic fate of a precursor reaching the hepatocyte might be different from that of the the same compound formed within the cell. Normally, the different precursors are present in the cells in trace amounts

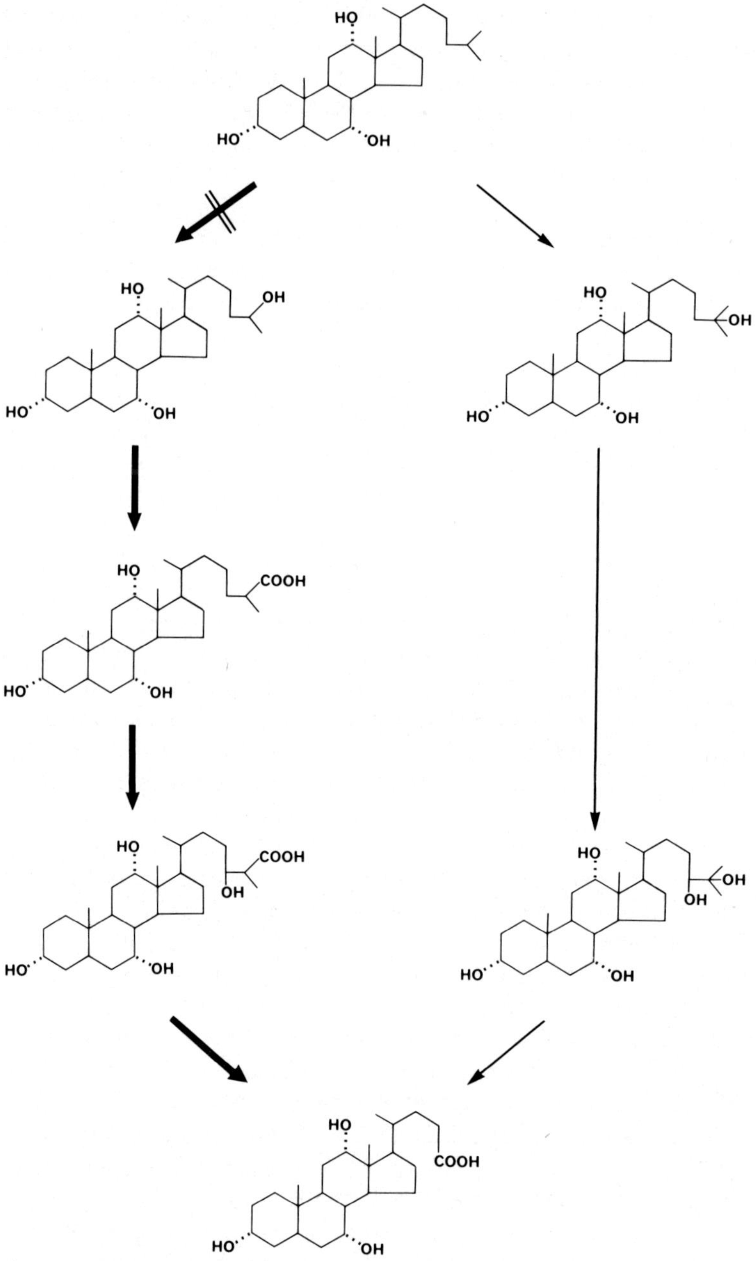

Fig. 13. Possible mechanism for accumulation of 5β-cholestane-3α,7α,12α,25-tetrol in patients with CTX.

only and a sudden expansion of the pool of a specific precursor may lead to an abnormal metabolism. In an early work by Björkhem et al., it was shown that the pattern of products formed from labelled 7α-hydroxy-4-cholesten-3-one in bile fistula rats varied with the amounts of labelled steroid administered [22]. In view of all this, it seems difficult to evaluate the relative importance of different possible pathways by determination of the relative conversion into cholic and chenodeoxycholic acid after intravenous administration of labelled precursors.

(XIV) Inborn errors of metabolism in bile acid biosynthesis

Information concerning the relative importance of metabolic pathways may be obtained from studies on inborn errors of metabolism. Two such disorders affecting bile acid biosynthesis have been described, cerebrotendinous xanthomatosis (CTX) and Zellweger's disease (cerebro-hepato-renal syndrome). The primary defect in cerebrotendinous xanthomatosis seems to be the absence of one enzyme involved in bile acid biosynthesis. The basic defect in Zellweger's disease has not yet been defined with certainty.

(1) Cerebrotendinous xanthomatosis

This rare inherited lipid storage disease is characterized by xanthomas, progressive neurological dysfunction, cataracts and the development of xanthomatous lesions in the brain and lung. In contrast to other diseases with tendon xanthomatosis, plasma cholesterol levels are remarkably low. Large deposits of cholesterol and cholestanol are present in most tissues, and the concentration of cholestanol is 10–100 times higher than normal. Salen and collaborators have made extensive and elegant studies on the various metabolic aspects of this disease [184,185,187–192]. They have conclusively shown that there is a subnormal synthesis of bile acids and that the metabolic defect is an impaired oxidation of the cholesterol side chain. The synthesis of chenodeoxycholic acid is reduced more than that of cholic acid. These patients excrete considerable amounts of bile alcohol in bile and faeces. The bile alcohols have been identified as 5β-cholestane-3α,7α,12α,25-tetrol, 5β-cholestane-3α,7α,12α,24,25-pentol and 5β-cholestane-3α,7α,12α,23,25-pentol. Two different explanations for the accumulation of these bile alcohols have been presented.

(1) Salen et al. reported that liver microsomes from 2 patients with CTX had a decreased capacity to 24β-hydroxylate 5β-cholestane-3α,7α,12α,25-tetrol [185]. It was suggested that the basic metabolic defect is a relative deficiency of the 24β-hydroxylase. To explain the severe metabolic consequences of such a defect, it must be assumed that the 25-hydroxylase pathway is the major pathway in the biosynthesis of cholic acid. This hypothesis does not explain the marked reduction in the biosynthesis of chenodeoxycholic acid. In view of the very low activity of the microsomal 25-hydroxylase towards 5β-cholestane-3α,7α-diol in human liver [41] it is evident that a 25-hydroxylase pathway cannot be of importance in the normal

biosynthesis of chenodeoxycholic acid. Part of the explanation for the reduced 24β-hydroxylase activity in the microsomal preparations from livers of CTX patients may be dilution of the exogenous labelled substrate with endogenous 5β-cholestane-3α,7α,12α,25-tetrol (cf. ref. 193).

(2) Oftebro et al. reported that the mitochondrial fraction of a liver homogenate from a biopsy of a CTX patient was completely devoid of 26-hydroxylase activity [193]. The possibility that there had been a general inactivation of the mitochondrial fraction seems excluded since there was a significant 25-hydroxylase activity towards vitamin D_3. There was a substantial accumulation of 5β-cholestane-3α,7α,12α-triol, the immediate substrate for the 26-hydroxylase in cholic acid biosynthesis. It was suggested that the accumulation of 5β-cholestane-3α,7α,12α-triol would lead to increased exposure to the action of the microsomal 23-, 24- and 25-hydroxylases. The alternative 25-hydroxylase pathway would then be of importance for the formation of cholic acid in patients with CTX (Fig. 13). If the 25-hydroxylase pathway has an insufficient capacity, this would explain the accumulation of the different 25-hydroxylated intermediates in patients with CTX. A lack of the mitochondrial 26-hydroxylase would also lead to accumulation of intermediates in chenodeoxycholic acid biosynthesis such as 5β-cholestane-3α,7α-diol and 7α-hydroxy-4-cholesten-3-one. Such accumulation would lead to increased exposure to the microsomal 12α-hydroxylase which would yield a relatively higher biosynthesis of cholic acid. This would explain the marked reduction in the biosynthesis of chenodeoxycholic acid in patients with CTX.

The contention that there is a lack of 26-hydroxylase activity in the liver of patients with CTX was recently supported by an investigation by Javitt et al. [194]. 26-Hydroxycholesterol in serum was quantitated by isotope dilution–mass spectrometry in normal subjects and in 5 subjects with CTX. The CTX patients had no detectable or markedly reduced levels of 26-hydroxycholesterol in their serum.

Results of various in vivo experiments with labelled bile acid precursors in patients with CTX have been published [185,190,195]. All these experiments show that there is a defect in the oxidation of the steroid side chain in the biosynthesis of cholic acid but are not fully conclusive with respect to the site of defect. Björkhem et al. administered a mixture of [^{3}H]7α,26-dihydroxy-4-cholesten-3-one and [^{14}C]7α-hydroxy-4-cholesten-3-one to a patient with CTX [195]. The ratio between ^{3}H and ^{14}C in the cholic acid and the chenodeoxycholic acid isolated was 40 and 60 times higher, respectively, than normal. Similar results were obtained after simultaneous administration of ^{3}H-labelled 5β-cholestane-3α,7α,26-triol and 4-^{14}C-labelled 5β-cholestane-3α,7α-diol. The results of these experiments are in consonance with the contention that the basic defect in CTX is the lack of the 26-hydroxylase, but do not per se completely exclude other defects in the oxidation of the side chain.

A specific finding in patients with CTX is the accumulation of cholestanol. The major pathway in the formation of cholestanol from cholesterol seems to involve intermediary formation of 4-cholesten-3-one and 5α-cholesten-3-one. The rate-limiting step in this conversion is probably the formation of 4-cholesten-3-one from cholesterol [196–198]. It is difficult to understand, however, how the oxidation of cholesterol to 4-cholesten-3-one can be accelerated due to a specific defect in the oxidation of the side chain of cholesterol in the biosynthesis of bile acids. Recently, Björkhem and Skrede showed that the bile of patients with CTX contains significant amounts of 7α-hydroxy-4-cholesten-3-one, presumably due to lack of the mitochondrial 26-hydroxylase [199]. After oral administration of labelled 7α-hydroxy-4-cholesten-3-one to rabbits, there was a significant conversion into cholestanol. This was shown to involve cholesta-4,6-dien-3-one and 4-cholesten-3-one as intermediates. It was suggested that this pathway may explain part of the accumulation of cholestanol in patients with CTX. The contention that the accumulation of cholestanol is secondary to the accumulation of 7α-hydroxylated intermediates in bile acid biosynthesis is further supported by results from a study in which a mixture of [7α-^{3}H]- and [4-^{14}C]cholesterol was administered to a patient with CTX (Skrede and Björkhem, unpublished experiments). Since the cholestanol isolated from bile and serum from this patient was almost devoid of ^{3}H, it was concluded that the conversion from cholesterol to cholestanol had involved 7α-hydroxylated intermediates.

(2) Zellweger's disease

This rare congenital disease is characterized by multiple craniofacial abnormalities, severe generalized hypotonia, central nervous system abnormalities, hepatomegaly, and renal cortical cysts. Most often the afflicted infants die within 6 months. Goldfischer et al. did not find any peroxisomes in the hepatocytes from such patients [200]. Histochemical studies of mitochondrial oxidation in the liver pointed to a defect between the succinate dehydrogenase flavoprotein and coenzyme Q, possibly in the region of the non-haeme iron protein. One important function of the peroxisomes seems to be oxidation of very-long-chain fatty acids, and such acids are in fact accumulated in tissues from patients with Zellweger's disease [201]. Another function of the peroxisomes seems to be the conversion of 3α,7α,12α-trihydroxy-5β-cholestanoic acid into cholic acid. Infants with Zellweger's disease accumulate 3α,7α,12α-trihydroxy-5β-cholestanoic acid and also some 3α,7α,12α,24-tetrahydroxy-5β-cholestanoic acid in bile and serum [202–204]. The metabolic block is not complete, since there is also some cholic acid. A similar accumulation has also been described in siblings with cholestasis due to intrahepatic bile duct anomalies [205]. In a recent work (Kase, Björkhem and Pedersen, unpublished study) it was shown that a patient with Zellweger's disease rapidly converted labelled 5β-cholestane-3α,7α,12α-triol into 3α,7α,12α-trihydroxy-5β-cholestanoic acid followed by a very slow conversion into cholic acid. A liver biopsy from this patient had no significant ability to convert 3α,7α,12α-trihydroxy-5β-cholestanoic acid into cholic acid. There was some conversion of 3α,7α-dihydroxy-5β-cholestanoic acid into chenodeoxycholic acid, which may explain the fact that in most cases there is little or no accumulation of 3α,7α-dihydroxy-5β-cholestanoic acid in this disease. The accumulation of 3α,7α,12α-trihydroxy-5β-cholestanoic acid may reflect the importance of the peroxisomes for the last steps in the biosynthesis of cholic acid from cholesterol. In addition, the accumulation of 3α,7α,12α-trihydroxy-5β-cholestanoic acid supports the contention that the major pathway in the biosynthesis of bile acids involves 3α,7α,12α-trihydroxy-5β-cholestanoic acid as an intermediate. Thus, it is difficult to understand the accumulation of this acid if it is believed that the 25-hydroxylase pathway is most important in the normal biosynthesis of cholic acid.

(XV) Regulation of the overall biosynthesis of bile acids

The regulation of the overall biosynthesis of bile acids has been studied intensively during the last decade, and only a small fraction of all the publications can be reviewed here. Cholesterol 7α-hydroxylase is the rate-limiting enzyme in the biosynthesis of both cholic acid and chenodeoxycholic acid. The publications in which a correlation has been demonstrated between bile acid biosynthesis and 7α-hydroxylation of cholesterol have been reviewed by Myant and Mitropoulos [59]. In the present review, emphasis will be put on the feedback regulation of the cholesterol 7α-hydroxylase by the bile-acid flux through the liver, the relation between HMG-CoA reductase and cholesterol 7α-hydroxylase and possible mechanisms for the regulation.

(1) Feedback regulation of bile acid biosynthesis

The possibility that the biosynthesis of bile acids is regulated by a negative feedback mechanism was supported by early experiments by Thompson and Vars [206] and Eriksson [207], who showed that the rate of bile acid synthesis in rats increased about 10-fold when a bile fistula is made. Bergström and Danielsson demonstrated that duodenal infusion of taurochenodeoxycholic acid in bile fistula rats restored the increased synthesis to a normal rate [208]. Danielsson et al. [44] showed that the cholesterol 7α-hydroxylase activity increased in parallel with the bile acid synthesis after cannulation of the bile duct in rats. In a subsequent work by Mosbach et al., it was reported that the incorporation of isotope from labelled acetate, mevalonate and cholesterol but not from labelled 7α-hydroxycholesterol into bile acids was inhibited by duodenal infusion of taurocholate to bile fistula rats [209]. The incorporation of isotope from labelled acetate, mevalonate and cholesterol but not from labelled 7α-hydroxycholesterol was stimulated in perfused livers of cholestyramine-treated rabbits [210]. It was concluded that there are essentially no rate-limiting steps beyond 7α-hydroxycholesterol in the biosynthesis of bile acids from acetate. Since both cholesterol and bile acid biosynthesis was subjected to negative feedback inhibition by bile acids, it cannot be excluded that inhibition of cholesterol biosynthesis precedes inhibition of the bile acid biosynthesis, and that the latter inhibition is secondary to the former.

The specificity of the inhibitory effect of bile acids on bile acid formation has been studied by Danielsson [110]. Taurocholic acid, taurochenodeoxycholic acid and taurodeoxycholic acid, fed at the 1% level in the diet for 3–7 days, were found to inhibit cholesterol 7α-hydroxylase activity. Feeding taurohyodeoxycholic acid and taurolithocholic acid had no effect on the activity. Shefer et al. showed that feeding taurocholate inhibited the biosynthesis of both taurochenodeoxycholic acid and taurocholic acid in rsts [211], and that taurochenodeoxycholic acid inhibited biosynthesis of taurocholic acid [212]. In man, chenodeoxycholic acid inhibits cholic acid synthesis and cholic acid inhibits chenodeoxycholic acid synthesis [213,214].

The possibility that cholesterol 7α-hydroxylase is directly inhibited by bile acids was studied by Mosbach et al. by addition of bile acids or bile salts to microsomal suspension [62]. An inhibition was observed, but this was probably due to non-specific detergent effects. From the time lag observed in the stimulation of bile acid biosynthesis after introduction of a bile fistula, it may be concluded that the effects of the bile acids most probably are mediated by effects on protein synthesis or protein catabolism.

The foregoing leads to the conclusion that there should be a relation between the concentration of bile acids in portal blood and the activity of the cholesterol 7α-hydroxylase as well as the overall biosynthesis of bile acids. Studies designed to directly correlate the concentration of bile acids in portal blood to the activity of the cholesterol 7α-hydroxylase have not appeared yet. Boyd and Lawson showed that the activity of the cholesterol 7α-hydroxylase in rats was increased after introduction of a portacaval anastomosis [215]. It was possible to further increase the activity in the operated animals by feeding them with a diet containing a bile-salt-sequestering agent. Thus, also the bile acids reaching the liver from the hepatic artery seem to be of some regulatory importance.

Dowling et al. and Small et al. have studied the effects of controlled interruption of the enterohepatic circulation in monkeys [216–218]. It was shown that the regulation of the bile acid biosynthesis was of "all or none" type. It was established that the increased bile acid biosynthesis in response to interruption of the enterohepatic circulation was limited and reached a maximum rate at only 20% interruption. Up to this level, the increased bile salt loss was compensated for by increased synthesis loss so that bile salt secretion and pool size were maintained at normal levels. With diversion of 37% or more, there was no further increase in hepatic bile salt synthesis to compensate for external loss, and a reduction in bile acid pool size and steathorrhoea were observed.

Angelin et al. reported recently that treatment with a bile-salt-sequestering agent reduced the postprandial but not the fasting serum bile acid levels in human [219]. It was concluded that the postprandial bile acid inflow to the liver may be more important as a regulator of bile acid biosynthesis than the fasting level of bile acids, supporting the contention that a certain concentration of bile acids must be reached in the portal blood to obtain an efficient inhibition of the cholesterol 7α-hydroxylase.

The effect of bile acid on bile acid biosynthesis has been studied also with isolated cells. Davis et al. reported that different bile acids added at concentrations up to 2.5 mmoles/l did not have a direct inhibitory effect on bile acid biosynthesis and secretion by cultured hepatocytes from rat liver [220]. It cannot be excluded that the cultured hepatocytes had lost an original ability to respond to bile acids.

(2) Relation between cholesterol 7α-hydroxylase and HMG-CoA reductase

There is a close relation between cholesterol 7α-hydroxylase and HMG-CoA reductase. The two enzymes are located near each other on the endoplasmic reticulum and newly synthesized cholesterol seems to be the preferred substrate for the cholesterol 7α-hydroxylase.

Table 1 summarizes studies in which a correlation between the two enzymes has been demonstrated.

In an early work by Myant and Eder, a time lag was observed between the increase in synthesis of cholesterol and synthesis of bile acids [221]. Such a time lag has not been reported in later studies, and it seems likely that the two rate-limiting enzymes respond to the same signal. The possibility that an increase of available cholesterol is responsible for the increase of cholesterol 7α-hydroxylation seems excluded by the work by Mitropoulos et al. in which attempts were made to measure the substrate of the enzyme under different condition [59,222]. In view of the time lag between introduction of a bile fistula and rise of enzyme activities, it is likely that protein synthesis is involved in the increase of both enzyme activities.

Since very little bile acids are transported via the lymph [224], the increased cholesterol 7α-hydroxylase activity observed after lymphatic drainage [225] is not due to depletion of bile acids. In view of the fact that the synthesis of cholesterol increases after lymphatic drainage, it is possible that the increased 7α-hydroxylation in this case may be due to increased supply of newly synthesized cholesterol.

The diurnal rhythm in both cholesterol 7α-hydroxylase and HMG-CoA reductase

TABLE 1

Effect of various modifying factors on cholesterol 7α-hydroxylase and HMG-CoA reductase

Modification	HMG-CoA reductase	Cholesterol 7α-hydroxylase	References
Bile fistula and treatment with cholestyramine	+	+	44, 49, 62, 221
Portacaval anastomosis	+	+	215, 223
Lymphatic drainage	+	+	225
Diurnal rhythm (dark period)	+	+	226–230, 234, 236
Glucocorticoids	+	+	234–236
Adrenalectomy	−	−	234–236
Thyroid hormone	+	+	75, 234, 235
Thyroidectomy	−	−	75, 234, 235
Glucose after starvation	+	+	237
Fasting	−	−	232, 245
Cholesterol feeding	−	+ or ±	49, 50, 222, 238, 239
Tomatine feeding	+	±	240
Sitosterol feeding	+	±	240, 241
Scurvy	+ or ±	−	242–244

activity has been studied by several groups [231–233]. There is no time lag between the nocturnal rise of the two activities in the rat, and it seems likely that both enzymes respond to the same signal. Since the rise in nocturnal activity of cholesterol 7α-cholesterase can be prevented by actinomycin D, it is evident that protein synthesis is involved [231]. The amplitude of the variations in the enzyme activity as well as the timing are influenced by the time for taking food and that of darkness and light. However, even in rats fasted for several days [231,232] and in genetically blind mice [233] there is some rhythmicity of cholesterol 7α-hydroxylase. Most likely, the diurnal rhythm in the cholesterol 7α-hydroxylase and HMG-CoA reductase is secondary to the diurnal rhythm in the secretion of glucocorticoids from the adrenal cortex. Administration of glucocorticoids to rats increases the activity of cholesterol 7α-hydroxylase after a lag period of 3 h or more [234–236], and this increase is prevented by pretreatment with actinomycin D [236]. Most or all of the diurnal rhythm is lost after bilateral adrenalectomy or hypophysectomy [226,234,236].

Treatment with thyroid hormone increases and thyroidectomy decreases cholesterol 7α-hydroxylase activity as well as HMG-CoA reductase activity [75,234,235]. As shown by Balasubramaniam et al. treatment with thyroid hormone increases first the cholesterol 7α-hydroxylase activity and then, after a time lag of several hours, HMG-CoA reductase [234]. Thus, it is likely that the rise in HMG-CoA reductase activity in this case is secondary to the depletion of cholesterol by cholesterol 7α-hydroxylase.

Takeuchi et al. measured cholesterol 7α-hydroxylase and HMG-CoA reductase activity in fasted rats refed glucose [237]. The administration of glucose to these rats resulted in increased cholesterol synthesis after 1 h and increased cholesterol 7α-hydroxylase activity after 2 h. These effects were not noted in rats pretreated with an inhibitor of cholesterol biosynthesis, suggesting that the effects on the cholesterol 7α-hydroxylase were secondary to those on cholesterologenesis. It was suggested that the stimulatory effect of glucose was due to increased availability of cholesterol for the cholesterol 7α-hydroxylase.

A dissociation between HMG-CoA reductase and the cholesterol 7α-hydroxylase has been reported in connection with feeding of cholesterol, tomatidine, sitosterol as well as in scurvy. Feeding cholesterol inhibits HMG-CoA reductase and in most [99,222,238,239] but not all [50] studies a stimulatory effect has been found on cholesterol 7α-hydroxylase. The stimulatory effect may be due to an expansion of the pool of cholesterol available for cholesterol 7α-hydroxylase. Feeding with tomatidine and sitosterol interferes with absorption of cholesterol from the intestine, and the increased HMG-CoA reductase activity is probably due to decreased inhibition by lymph cholesterol [240,241]. The cholesterol 7α-hydroxylase activity is only slightly increased or unaffected under these conditions [240,241].

Cholesterol 7α-hydroxylase activity is markedly reduced in scorbutic guinea pigs, probably due to decreased amount of the specific cytochrome P-450 [242]. HMG-CoA reductase is unaffected [243]. In another study, an increased incorporation of [^{14}C]acetate into cholesterol in liver of scorbutic guinea pigs was reported [244].

To summarize, it seems that HMG-CoA reductase and cholesterol 7α-hydroxylase respond in the same direction to the same signal in some cases (bile acids, glucocorticoids), that the rise in the activity of cholesterol 7α-hydroxylase is secondary to the rise in the activity of the HMG-CoA reductase activity in some cases (feeding with glucose or administration of mevalonate) and that the increase in HMG-CoA reductase activity is secondary to the rise in cholesterol 7α-hydroxylase activity in the case of treatment with thyroid hormone.

(3) Possible mechanisms for regulation of cholesterol 7α-hydroxylase activity

The regulation of cholesterol 7α-hydroxylase may involve some of the following mechanisms:

(1) Changes in the rate of synthesis or breakdown of a specific species of cytochrome P-450 with short half-life.

(2) Modulation by specific proteins in the cytosol.

(3) Short-term modulation by phosphorylation–dephosphorylation.

(4) Changes in the size of the substrate pool of cholesterol available to enzyme. The activity of HMGH-CoA reductase may be of importance for the size of this pool.

Myant and Mitropoulos have discussed the possibility of a yet unidentified component that regulates the activity of the enzyme, and whose induction and repression are responsible for the different effects on the enzyme activity [59]. The unidentified component could be an inducible protein carrier that facilitates access of cholesterol to the catalytic site of the enzyme (cf. Chapter 3).

The most important information concerning mechanisms of regulation of cholesterol 7α-hydroxylase is summarized in the model shown in Fig. 14. In view of the importance of HMG-CoA reductase for cholesterol 7α-hydroxylase activity, some important modulators of HMG-CoA reductase activity have also been included (cf. Chapter 2). It should be pointed out that the regulation of biosynthesis of cholesterol shown in Fig. 14 is oversimplified. For a discussion of the regulation of HMG-CoA reductase, the reader is referred to Chapter 2 and a recent review by Brown and Goldstein [246].

The bile acids returning to the liver in the portal blood inhibit both cholesterol 7α-hydroxylase and HMG-CoA reductase. Size, circulation rate and composition of the bile acid pool are of importance. The inhibitory effect of bile acids on cholesterol 7α-hydroxylase is mediated by an effect on synthesis or breakdown of proteins, most likely the specific species of cytochrome P-450 involved in the hydroxylation. Evidence that the rate of synthesis of the specific species of cytochrome P-450 is of major importance can be obtained only when it is possible to measure accurately the amount of specific cytochrome P-450 by means other than enzyme activity. Although less likely from the data available, it cannot be excluded at the present state of knowledge that the inhibitory effect of bile acids on cholesterol 7α-hydroxylase is mediated by the effect of bile acids on HMG-CoA reductase. Since the substrate pool for cholesterol 7α-hydroxylase does not seem to be affected [59,222], a hitherto unknown mechanism must then be responsible for the coupling between the two rate-limiting enzymes.

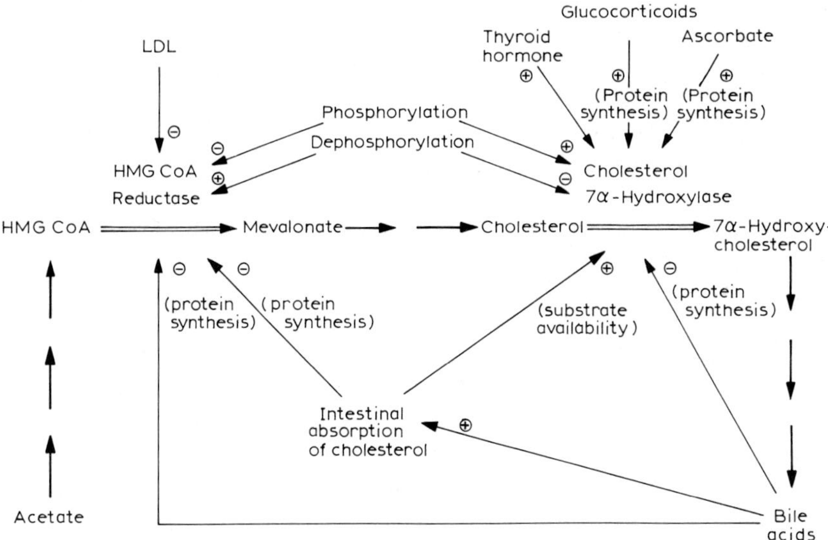

Fig. 14. Mechanisms for regulation of cholesterol 7α-hydroxylase.

The mechanism of the inhibition of the HMG-CoA reductase by bile acids shown in Fig. 14 is a matter of controversy. Weis and Dietschy did not observe any influence of taurocholate on cholesterol synthesis in bile fistula rats fed a cholesterol-free diet, and concluded that the inhibitory effect of bile acids on cholesterol synthesis may be related to the increased absorption of cholesterol by the presence of bile acids in the intestine [247]. However, Hamprecht et al. were able to demonstrate a reduction of HMG-CoA reductase activity in lymph fistula rats infused with cholate [248]. Results by Shefer et al. also indicate that bile acids inhibit HMG-CoA reductase directly [212]. It seems likely that the inhibitory effect of the bile acids on HMG-CoA reductase may involve both direct and indirect effects. It was recently established that the stimulation of HMG-CoA reductase activity in response to treatment with cholestyramine is associated with an increase of the specific mRNA [258].

It is well established that the size of the substrate pool may influence the activity of the substrate-unsaturated cholesterol 7α-hydroxylase under different conditions such as feeding with cholesterol or glucose. As shown also by the experiments by Mitropoulos et al. in which the synthesis of cholesterol was stimulated by mevalonate infusion [71], the activity of HMG-CoA reductase is of some importance for the pool of substrate available for the cholesterol 7α-hydroxylase.

According to the regulatory model in Fig. 14, the inhibitory effects of bile acids on cholesterol 7α-hydroxylase may be counteracted to some extent by the stimulatory effect of some bile acids on intestinal absorption of cholesterol which may increase the substrate pool for the cholesterol 7α-hydroxylase. The difficulties in different laboratories to get concordant results in studies of the effects of feeding different bile acids may be explained by such a mechanism. The concentration of cholesterol in the diet may be one factor influencing the results.

The importance of phosphorylation–dephosphorylation for modulation of cholesterol 7α-hydroxylase and HMG-CoA reductase activity is difficult to evaluate. Scallen and Sanghvi have suggested that this mechanism may be important for coordination of cholesterol 7α-hydroxylase, HMG-CoA reductase and acyl-CoA : cholesterol acyltransferase [249]. Phosphorylation decreases HMG-CoA reductase activity and probably increases acyl-CoA : cholesterol acyltransferase activity. According to Sanghvi et al. phosphorylation also increases the activity of cholesterol 7α-hydroxylase [90]. If so, such coordinated changes are suitable for removal of an excess of cholesterol. Dephosphorylation increases HMG-CoA reductase activity and possibly also decreases acyl-CoA : cholesterol acyltransferase activity. According to Sanghvi et al., dephosphorylation also decreases cholesterol 7α-hydroxylase activity [90]. If so, these changes are suitable under conditions of cholesterol deprivation. However, there is no experimental evidence yet that such coordinated changes of the 3 enzyme activities due to phosphorylation–dephosphorylation are of importance under in vivo conditions.

Since plasma lipoprotein cholesterol must be the major substrate for bile acid biosynthesis under conditions when the rate of hepatic synthesis of cholesterol is low, regulation of the uptake of lipoprotein cholesterol by the hepatocytes should be of importance not only for the rate of cholesterol synthesis but also for the activity of cholesterol 7α-hydroxylase. It should be mentioned that bile acids are included among the different factors known to be able to modulate the receptor-mediated uptake of cholesterol by the apo-B, E or LDL receptor. The apo-B, E receptor can thus be induced to high levels by treatment with a bile acid sequestrant]259]. Angelin et al. have shown that preparation of a bile fistula in adult dogs markedly induced the expression of the apo-B, E receptor and that the binding of this receptor could be almost totally abolished by reinfusion of taurocholate [260].

(XVI) Regulation of the ratio between cholic acid and chenodeoxycholic acid

Microsomal 12α-hydroxylation is the only unique step in the formation of cholic acid and is likely to be of regulatory importance for the ratio between newly synthesized cholic and chenodeoxycholic acid. Introduction of a 26-hydroxyl group seems to prevent subsequent 12α-hydroxylation in rat liver and the 26-hydroxylase could thus also have a regulatory role. It is possible that there are different precursor pools for the synthesis of cholic acid and chenodeoxycholic acid in rats. If so, the relative size of the two pools could be of importance for the relative rate of formation of the two bile acids.

Treatment with thyroid hormone leads to a marked depression in the ratio between cholic and chenodeoxycholic acid in rats, whereas treatment with propylthiouracil leads to an increase in this ratio [206,250,251]. Treatment of rats with thyroid hormone inhibits 12α-hydroxylase activity and stimulates microsomal 26-hydroxylase activity [108,109]. The mitochondrial 26-hydroxylase is not affected [109]. Thyroidectomy depresses the activity of the microsomal 26-hydroxylase [109]. Since thyroid hormone affects the ratio between microsomal 12α- and 26-hydroxylase activity in the same direction as it affects the ratio between cholic and chenodeoxycholic acid, it has been suggested that both activities are of regulatory importance in rat liver [109]. The 26-hydroxylase activity has probably no regulatory importance in human liver. Introduction of a 26-hydroxyl group does not seem to prevent subsequent 12α-hydroxylation in man. In addition, there is little or no 26-hydroxylase activity in the microsomal fraction of human liver, and thyroid hormone has only a small effect on the ratio between newly synthesized cholic acid and chenodeoxycholic acid in man [3,4].

The microsomal 12α-hydroxylase seems to be influenced by the flux of bile acids through the liver in a similar way as cholesterol 7α-hydroxylase. Biliary drainage in rats leads to a 2-fold stimulation of 12α-hydroxylase [44] perhaps due to reduced intake of food [252]. However, it was shown later that 12α-hydroxylation of 7α-hydroxy-4-cholesten-3-one was inhibited by feeding rats different taurine-conjugated bile acids at the 1% level [110]. Ahlberg et al. showed that the microsomal 12α-hydroxylase in human liver was inhibited by about 50% after treatment for 8 weeks with chenodeoxycholic acid, 15 mg/kg body weight [111]. The increased ratio between cholic acid and chenodeoxycholic acid observed after treatment with cholestyramine is also consistent with an inhibitory effect of reabsorbed bile acids on the 12α-hydroxylase [219].

The final ratio between cholic acid and chenodeoxycholic acid in bile is influenced also by factors other than the activity of the hepatic 12α-hydroxylase. Thus, the differential rates of enterohepatic cycling, intestinal absorption and degradation are of importance. Ahlberg et al. did not find a correlation between microsomal 12α-hydroxylase activity and the ratio between cholic acid and chenodeoxycholic acid in the bile of some normo- and hyperlipidaemic patients [253]. In a recent in vivo study, Björkhem et al. failed to show a correlation between the apparent 12α-hydroxylase activity and the ratio between biliary cholic and chenodeoxycholic acid in healthy subjects and a patient with liver cirrhosis [254]. In this study, a mixture of [^{3}H]7α,12α-dihydroxy-4-cholesten-3-one and [^{14}C]7α-hydroxy-4-cholesten-3-one was administered intravenously and the relative 12α-hydroxylase activity was calculated from the ratio between ^{3}H and ^{14}C in cholic acid.

Mitropoulos et al. have measured the rate of excretion and the specific activities of cholic acid and chenodeoxycholic acid in bile fistula rats fed [^{3}H]cholesterol and infused with [^{14}C]mevalonate or [^{14}C]7α-hydroxycholesterol [255]. It was concluded that newly synthesized hepatic cholesterol was the preferred substrate for the formation of cholic acid. It could not be excluded, however, that part of the chenodeoxycholic acid had been formed from a pool of cholesterol different from that utilized in cholic acid biosynthesis. The mitochondrial pathway, starting with a 26-hydroxylation, could have accounted for a significant fraction of the chenodeoxycholic acid formed. The cholesterol used for this pathway should then be derived from a pool which equilibrates more slowly with newly synthesized cholesterol than does the pool from which cholic acid is derived. However, such a mechanism would leave unexplained the diurnal rhythm in the biliary excretion of chenodeoxycholic acid observed in the above experiments. Schwartz et al. administered labelled cholesterol and mevalonate to bile fistula patients [256]. The specific activities of the newly synthesized cholic acid and chenodeoxycholic acid were virtually identical at all time periods. It was concluded that there is a common cholesterol substrate pool for both primary bile acids in man. On the other hand, Einarsson et al. reported small differences in specific activity between cholic and chenodeoxycholic acid isolated from bile fistula patients receiving a constant infusion of [^{3}H]mevalonate [257]. From the experiments by Schwartz et al. and Einarsson et al. it may be concluded that if there is a specific pool of cholesterol available for the synthesis of chenodeoxycholic acid, which is different from that available for the synthesis of cholic acid, the former should be of minor importance in man. To summarize, it seems less likely that distribution of cholesterol in different substrate pools is of major importance for the regulation of the ratio between synthesis of cholic acid and chenodeoxycholic acid.

Acknowledgements

The author is grateful to Maud Lindblad for typing the manuscipt and to Olle Falk and Anita Lövgren for drawing the figures.

The work performed in the author's laboratory referred to here has been supported by the Swedish Medical Research Council (Project 03x-3141).

References

1 Bergström, S., Danielsson, H. and Samuelsson, B. (1960) in: Lipid Metabolism (Bloch, K., Ed.) pp. 291–336, Wiley, New York.
2 Danielsson, H. (1960) Adv. Lipid Res. 1, 335–385.
3 Danielsson, H. and Tchen, T.T. (1968) Metab. Pathways 2, 117–168.
4 Danielsson, H. and Einarsson, K. (1969) Biol. Basis Med. 5, 279–315.
5 Elliott, W.H. and Hyde, P.M. (1971) A,. J. Med. 51, 568–579.
6 Boyd, G.S. and Percy-Robb, I.W. (1971) Am. J. Med. 51, 580–587.
7 Tyor, M.P., Garbutt, J.T. and Lack, L. (1971) Am. J. Med. 51, 614–626.
8 Nair, P.P. and Kritchevsky, D. (Eds.) (1973) The Bile Acids, Vol. 2, Plenum Press, New York.
9 Danielsson, H. and Sjövall, J. (1975) Annu. Rev. Biochem. 44, 233–253.
10 Bloch, K., Berg, B.N. and Rittenberg, D. (1943) J. Biol. Chem. 149, 511–517.
11 Chaikoff, I.M., Siperstein, M.D. and Dauben, W.G. (1952) J. Biol. Chem. 194, 413–416.
12 Siperstein, M.D. and Chaikoff, I.M. (1952) J. Biol. Chem. 198, 93–104.
13 Zabin, F. and Barker, W.F. (1953) J. Biol. Chem. 205, 633–636.
14 Bergström, S. (1955) Rec. Chem. Progr. (Kresge-Hooker Sci Lib) 16, 63–83.
15 Bergström, S., Pääbo, K. and Rumpf, J.A. (1954) Acta Chem. Scand. 8, 1109.

16 Lindstedt, S. (1957) Acta Chem. Scand. 11, 417–420.
17 Bergström, S. and Sjövall, J. (1954) Acta Chem. Scand. 8, 611–616.
18 Fredrickson, D.S. and Ono, K. (1956) Biochim. Biophys. Acta 22, 183–184.
19 Bergström, S. and Lindstedt, S. (1956) Biochim. Biophys. Acta 19, 556–557.
20 Green, K. and Samuelsson, B. (1964) J. Biol. Chem. 239, 2804–2808.
21 Danielsson, H. (1961) Acta Chem. Scand. 15, 242–248.
22 Björkhem, I., Danielsson, H., Issidorides, C. and Kallner, A. (1965) Acta Chem. Scand. 19, 2151–2154.
23 Mendelsohn, D. and Staple, E. (1963) Biochemistry 2, 577–579.
24 Danielsson, H. and Einarsson, K. (1964) Acta Chem. Scand. 18, 831–832.
25 Hutton, H.R.B. and Boyd, G.S. (1966) Biochim. Biophys. Acta 116, 336–361.
26 Danielsson, H. and Einarsson, K. (1966) J. Biol. Chem. 241, 1449–1454.
27 Berséus, O., Danielsson, H. and Kallner, A. (1965) J. Biol. Chem. 240, 2396–2401.
28 Björkhem, I., Danielsson, H. and Einarsson, K. (1968) Eur. J. Biochem. 2, 294–302.
29 Björkhem, I. and Danielsson, H. (1965) Acta Chem. Scand. 19, 2298–2302.
30 Björkhem, I. and Danielsson, H. (1967) Eur. J. Biochem. 2, 403–413.
31 Berséus, O., Danielsson, H. and Einarsson, K. (1967) J. Biol. Chem. 242, 1211–1219.
32 Einarsson, K. (1968) Eur. J. Biochem. 5, 101–108.
33 Björkhem, I., Danielsson, H., Einarsson, K. and Johansson, G. (1968) J. Clin. Invest. 47, 1573–1582.
34 Haslewood, G.A.D. (1952) Biochem. J. 52, 483–587.
35 Carey Jr., J.B. and Haslewood, G.A.D. (1963) J. Biol. Chem. 238, PC 855–PC 856.
36 Staple, E. and Rabinowitz, J.L. (1962) Biochim. Biophys. Acta 59, 735–736.
37 Carey Jr,. J.B. (1964) J. Clin. Invest. 43, 1443–1448.
38 Bridgewater, R.J. and Lindstedt, S. (1957) Acta Chem. Scand. 11, 409–413.
39 Danielsson, H. (1960) Acta Chem. Scand. 14, 348–352.
40 Cronholm, T. and Johansson, G. (1970) Eur. J. Biochem. 16, 373–381.
41 Björkhem, I., Gustafsson, J., Johansson, G. and Persson, P. (1975) J. Clin. Invest. 55, 478–486.
42 Suld, H.M., Staple, E. and Gurin, S. (1962) J. Biol. Chem. 237, 338–344.
43 Masui, T. and Staple, E. (1966) J. Biol. Chem. 241, 3889–3898.
44 Danielsson, H., Einarsson, K. and Johansson, G. (1967) Eur. J. Biochem. 2, 44–49.
45 Mitton, J.R. and Boyd, G.S. (1965) Biochem. J. 96, 60 pp.
46 Björkhem, I., Einarsson, K. and Johansson, K. (1968) Acta Chem. Scand. 22, 1595–1605.
47 Johansson, G. (1971) Eur. J. Biochem. 21, 68–79.
48 Johansson, G. (1971) Thesis, Opusc. Med. Suppl. XVII.
49 Boyd, G.S., Scholan, N.A. and Mitton, J.R. (1969) Adv. Exp. Med. Biol. 4, 443–456.
50 Björkhem, I. and Danielsson, H. (1975) Eur. J. Biochem. 53, 63–70.
51 Gielen, J., Van Cantfort, J. and Renson, J. (1968) Arch. Int. Physiol. Biochim. 76, 930–932.
52 Björkhem, I., Danielsson, H. and Einarsson, K. (1968) Eur. J. Biochem. 4, 458–463.
53 Balasubramanian, S., Mitropoulos, K.A. and Myant, N.B. (1973) Eur. J. Biochem. 34, 77–83.
54 Mitropoulos, K.A. and Balasubramaniam, S. (1972) Biochem. J. 128, 1–9.
55 Björkhem, I. and Danielsson, H., Anal. Biochem. 59, 508–516.
56 Sanghvi, A., Grassi, E., Bartman, C., Lester, R., Kienle, M.G. and Galli, G. (1981) J. Lipid Res. 22, 720–724.
57 Shefer, S., Cheng, F.W., Hauser, S., Batta, A.K. and Salen, G. (1981) J. Lipid Res. 22, 532–536.
58 Balasubramaniam, S., Mitropoulos, K.A. and Myant, N.M. (1973) Eur. J. Biochem. 34, 77–83.
59 Myant, N.B. and Mitropoulos, K.A. (1977) J. Lipid Res. 18, 135–153.
60 Katayama, K. and Yamasaki, K. (1968) Yonago Acta Med. 12, 103–109.
61 Balasubramaniam, S., Mitropoulos, K.A. and Myant, N.B. (1975) Biochim. Biophys. Acta 398, 172–177.
62 Shefer, S., Hauser, S. and Mosbach, E.H. (1968) J. Lipid Res. 9, 328–333.
63 Boyd, G.S., Brown, M.J.G., Hattersley, N.G. and Suckling, K.E. (1974) Biochim. Biophys. Acta 337, 132–135.
64 Aringer, L. and Eneroth, P. (1973) J. Lipid Res. 14, 563–572.

65 Aringer, L. (1978) J. Lipid Res. 19, 933–944.
66 Mitropoulos, K.A. and Venkatesan, S. (1977) Biochim. Biophys. Acta 489, 126–142.
67 Staple, E. and Gurin, S. (1954) Biochim. Biophys. Acta 15, 372–376.
68 Cronholm, T., Burlingame, A.L. and Sjövall, J. (1974) Eur. J. Biochem. 49, 497–510.
69 Björkhem, I. and Lewenhaupt, A. (1979) J. Biol. Chem. 254, 5252–5256.
70 Long, T.T., Jakoi, L., Stevens, R. and Qvarfordt, S. (1978) J. Lipid Res. 19, 872–878.
71 Mitropoulos, K.A., Balasubramaniam, S., Venkatesan, S. and Reeves, B.E.A. (1978) Biochim. Biophys. Acta 530, 99–111.
72 Mitropoulos, K.A., Venkatesan, S., Balasubramaniam, S. and Peters, T.J. (1978) Eur. J. Biochem. 82, 419–429.
73 Schwartz, C.C., Halloran, L.G., Vlahcevic, Z.R., Gregorey, D.H. and Swell, L. (1978) Science 200, 62–64.
74 Halloran, L.G., Schwartz, C.C., Vlahcevic, Z.R., Nisman, R.M. and Swell, L. (1978) Surgery 84, 1–7.
75 Wada, F., Hirata, K., Nakao, K. and Sakamoto, Y. (1969) J. Biochem. (Tokyo) 66, 699–703.
76 Boyd, G.S., Grimwade, A.M. and Lawson, M.E. (1973) Eur. J. Biochem. 37, 334–340.
77 Björkhem, I. and Danielsson, H. (1973) Biochem. Biophys. Res. Commun. 51, 766–773.
78 Holtzman, J.L., Gander, J.E. and Ericsson, R.R. (1983) J. Biol. Chem. 258, 5400–5404.
79 Björkhem, I. (1977) J. Pharm. Ther. (1977) 1, 327–348.
80 Björkhem, I. (1971) Eur. J. Biochem. 18, 299–304.
81 Björkhem, I., Danielsson, H. and Wikvall, K. (1974) Biochem. Biophys. Res. Commun. 3, 934–941.
82 Hansson, R. and Wikvall, K. (1979) Eur. J. Biochem. 93, 419–426.
83 Einarsson, K. and Johansson, G. (1968) Eur. J. Biochem. 6, 293–298.
84 Boström, H., Hansson, R., Jönsson, K:H. and Wikvall, K. (1981) Eur. J. Biochem. 120, 29–32.
35 Hansson, R. and Wikvall, K. (1980) J. Biol. Chem. 255, 1643–1649.
86 Boström, H. and Wikvall, K. (1982) J. Biol. Chem. 257, 11755–11759.
87 Einarsson, K. and Johansson, G. (1968) FEBS Lett. 1, 219–222.
88 Danielsson, H. and Wikvall, K. (1981) Biochem. Biophys. Res. Commun. 103, 46–51.
89 Kalles, I. and Wikvall, K. (1981) Biochem. Biophys. Res. Commun. 100, 1361–1369.
90 Sanghvi, A., Grassi, E., Warty, V., Diven, W., Wight, C. and Lester, R. (1981) Biochem. Biophys. Res. Commun. 103, 886–892.
91 Goodwin, C.D., Cooper, B.W. and Margolis, S. (1982) J. Biol. Chem. 257, 4469–4472.
92 Kwok, C.T., Burnett, W. and Hardie, I.R. (1981) J. Lipid Res. 22, 580–589.
93 Spence, J.T. and Gaylor, J.L. (1977) J. Biol. Chem. 252, 5852–5858.
94 Craig, J.F., Boyd, G.S., McLeod, R.J. and Suckling, K.E. (1979) Biochem. Soc. Trans. 7, 967–969.
95 Danielsson, H., Kalles, I. and Wikvall, K. (1980) Biochem. Biophys. Res. Commun. 97, 1459–1466.
96 Björkhem, I. (1969) Eur. J. Biochem. 8, 337–344.
97 Wikvall, K. (1981) J. Biol. Chem. 256, 3376–3380.
98 Björkhem, I., Einarsson, K. and Gustafsson, J.Å. (1972) Steroids 471–476.
99 Suzuki, M., Mitropoulos, K.A. and Myant, N.B. (1968) Biochem. Biophys. Res. Commun. 30, 516–521.
100 Bernhardsson, C., Björkhem, I., Danielsson, H. and Wikvall, K. (1973) Biochem. Biophys. Res. Commun. 54, 1030–1038.
101 Hansson, R. and Wikvall, K. (1982) Eur. J. Biochem. 125, 423–429.
102 Björkhem, I. (1975) Eur. J. Biochem. 51, 137–143.
103 Danielsson, H., Kalles, I., Lidström, B., Lundell, K. and Wikvall, K. (1983) Biochem. Biophys. Res. Commun. 113, 212–219.
104 Ali, S.S. and Elliott, W.H. (1976) J. Lipid Res. 17, 386–392.
105 Mui, M.M. and Elliott, W.H. (1971) J. Biol. Chem. 246, 302–304.
106 Blaskiewicz, R.J., O'Neil Jr., G.J. and Elliott, W.H. (1974) Proc. Soc. Exp. Biol. Med. 146, 92–95.
107 Shaw, R. and Elliott, W.H. (1979) J. Biol. Chem. 254, 7177–7182.
108 Mitropoulos, K.A., Suzuki, M., Myant, N.B. and Danielsson, H. (1968) FEBS Lett. 1, 13–15.
109 Björkhem, I., Danielsson, H. and Gustafsson, J. (1973) FEBS Lett. 31, 20–22.
110 Danielsson, H. (1973) Steroids 22, 667–676.

111 Ahlberg, J., Angelin, B., Björkhem, I., Einarsson, K., Gustafsson, J.-Å. and Rafter, J. (1980) J. Lab. Clin. Med. 95, 188–194.
112 Berséus, O. (1967) Eur. J. Biochem. 2, 493–502.
113 Berséus, O. (1967) Thesis, Opusc. Med. Suppl. VI.
114 Berséus, O. and Björkhem, I. (1967) Eur. J. Biochem. 2, 503–507.
115 Björkhem, I. and Holmberg, I. (1973) Eur. J. Biochem. 33, 364–367.
116 Björkhem, I. (1969) Eur. J. Biochem. 7, 413–417.
117 Berséus, O. (1965) Acta Chem. Scand. 19, 325–328.
118 Mitropoulos, K.A. and Myant, N.B. (1965) Biochem. J. 97, 26c–28e.
119 Popják, G., Edmond, J., Anet. F.A.L. and Easton Jr., N.R. (1977) J. Am. Chem. Soc. 99, 931–935.
120 Batta, A.K., Salen, G., Shefer, S., Dayal, B. and Tint, G.S. (1983) J. Lipid Res. 24, 94–96.
121 Hanson, R.F., Szczepanik, P. and Williams, G.C. (1980) J. Biol. Chem. 255, 1483–1485.
122 Haslewood, G.A.D. (1978) in: The Biological Importance of Bile Salts, Frontiers of Biology, Vol. 47, p. 61, North-Holland, Amsterdam.
123 Atsuta, Y. and Okuda, K. (1981) J. Biol. Chem. 256, 9144–9146.
124 Shefer, S., Cheng, F.W., Batta, A.K., Dayal, B., Tint, S., Salen, G. and Mosbach, E.H. (1978) J. Biol. Chem. 253, 6386–6392.
125 Gustafsson, J. and Sjöstedt, S. (1978) J. Biol. Chem. 253, 199–201.
126 Björkhem, I. and Gustafsson, J. (1973) Eur. J. Biochem. 36, 201–212.
127 Gustafsson, J. (1978) J. Lipid Res. 19, 237–243.
128 Björkhem, I., Danielsson, H. and Wikvall, K. (1976) J. Biol. Chem. 251, 3495–3499.
129 Hansson, R., Holmberg, I. and Wikvall, K. (1981) J. Biol. Chem. 256, 4345–4349.
130 Björkhem, I. and Gustafsson, J. (1974) J. Biol. Chem. 249, 2528–2535.
131 Taniguchi, S., Hoshita, N. and Okuda, K. (1973) Eur. J. Biochem. 40, 607–617.
132 Gustafsson, J. (1976) J. Lipid Res. 17, 366–372.
133 Pedersen, J.I., Björkhem, I. and Gustafsson, J. (1979) J. Biol. Chem. 254, 6464–6469.
134 Okuda, K., Weber, P. and Ullrich, V. (1977) Biochem. Biophys. Res. Commun. 74, 1071–1076.
135 Pedersen, J.I., Oftebro, H. and Vänngård, T. (1977) Biochem. Biophys. Res. Commun. 76, 666–673.
136 Sato, R., Atsuta, Y., Imai, Y., Taniguchi, S. and Okuda, K. (1977) Proc. Natl. Acad. Sci. (U.S.A.) 74, 5477–5481.
137 Pedersen, J.I., Holmberg, I. and Björkhem, I. (1979) FEBS Lett. 98, 394–398.
138 Björkhem, I., Holmberg, I., Oftebro, H. and Pedersen, J.I. (1980) J. Biol. Chem. 255, 5244–5249.
139 Atsuta, Y. and Okuda, K. (1982) J. Lipid Res. 23, 345–351.
140 Okuda, K. and Danielsson, H. (1965) Acta Chem. Scand. 19, 2160–2165.
141 Masui, T., Herman, R. and Staple, E. (1966) Biochim. Biophys. Acta 117, 266–268.
142 Okuda, K. and Takigawa, N. (1969) Biochim. Biophys. Acta 176, 873–879.
143 Okuda, K. and Takigawa, N. (1968) Biochem. Biophys. Res. Commun. 33, 788–793.
144 Okuda, K. and Takigawa, N. (1970) Biochim. Biophys. Acta 222, 141–148.
145 Björkhem, I., Jörnvall, H. and Åkesson, Å. (1974) Biochem. Biophys. Res. Commun. 57, 870–875.
146 Okuda, A. and Okuda, K. (1983) J. Biol. Chem. 258, 2899–2905.
147 Fukuba, R. (1974) Biochim. Biophys. Acta 341, 48–55.
148 Okuda, K., Higuchi, E. and Fukuba, R. (1973) Biochim. Biophys. Acta 293, 15–25.
149 Gustafsson, J. (1975) J. Biol. Chem. 250, 8243–8247.
150 Pedersen, J.I. and Gustafsson, J. (1980) FEBS Lett. 121, 345–348.
151 Kase, F., Björkhem, I. and Pedersen, J.I. (1983) J. Lipid Res. 24, 1560–1567.
152 Cass, O.W., Williams, G.C. and Hanson, F. (1980) J. Lipid Res. 21, 186–191.
153 Siperstein, M.D. and Murray, A.W. (1955) Science 138, 377–378.
154 Bremer, J. (1956) Acta Chem. Scand. 10, 56–71.
155 Elliott, W.H. (1955) Biochim. Biophys. Acta 17, 440–441.
156 Scherstén, T. (1967) Biochim. Biophys. Acta 141, 144–154.
157 Polokoff, M.A. and Bell, R.M. (1977) J. Biol. Chem. 252, 1167–1171.
158 Killenberg, P.G. (1978) J. Lipid Res. 19, 24–31.
159 Danielsson, H., Kallner, A. and Sjövall, J. (1963) J. Biol. Chem. 238, 3846–3852.

160 Kallner, A. (1967) Acta Chem. Scand. 21, 87–92.
161 Kallner, A. (1967) Acta Chem. Scand. 21, 315–321.
162 Kallner, A. (1967) Ark. Kemi 26, 567–576.
163 Karavolas, H.J., Elliott, W.H., Hsia, S.L., Doisy Jr., E.A., Matschiner, J.T., Thayer, S.A. and Doisy, E.A. (1965) J. Biol. Chem. 240, 1568–1577.
164 Hofmann, A.F. and Mosbach, E.H. (1964) J. Biol. Chem. 239, 2813–2821.
165 Björkhem, I. and Gustafsson, J. (1971) Eur. J. Biochem. 18, 207–213.
166 Noll, B.W., Ziller, S.A., Doisy, E.A. and Elliott, W.H. (1973) J. Lipid Res. 14, 229–234.
167 Mui, M.M. and Elliott, W.H. (1970) Fed. Proc. 29, 909.
168 Björkhem, I. and Einarsson, K. (1970) Eur. J. Biochem. 13, 174–179.
169 Björkhem, I. (1969) Eur. J. Biochem. 8, 345–351.
170 Hoshita, T., Shefer, S. and Mosbach, E.H. (1968) J. Lipid Res. 9, 237–243.
171 Andersson, K.E., Kok, E. and Javitt, N.B. (1972) J. Clin. Invest. 51, 112–117.
172 Mitropoulos, K.A. and Myant, N.B. (1967) Biochem. J. 103, 472–479.
173 Mitropoulos, K.A., Avery, M.D., Myant, N.B. and Gibbons, G.F. (1972) Biochem. J. 130, 363–371.
174 Makino, I., Sjövall, J., Norman, A. and Strandvik, B. (1971) FEBS Lett. 15, 161–164.
175 Back, P. (1973) Clin. Chim. Acta 44, 199–207.
176 Ayaki, Y. and Yamasaki, K. (1970) J. Biochem. 68, 341–346.
177 Yamasaki, K., Ayaki, Y. and Yamasaki, H. (1971) J. Biochem. 70, 715–718.
178 Ayaki, Y. and Yamasaki, K. (1972) J. Biochem. 71, 85–89.
179 Ikawa, S., Ayaki, Y., Ogura, M. and Yamasaki, K. (1972) J. Biochem. 71, 579–587.
180 Schwartz, C.C., Cohen, B.I., Vlahcevic, Z.R., Gregory, D.H., Halloran, L.G., Kuramoto, T., Mosbach, E.H. and Swell, L. (1976) J. Biol. Chem. 251, 6308–6314.
181 Vlahcevic, Z.R., Schwartz, C.C., Gustafsson, J., Haloran, L.G., Danielsson, H. and Swell, L. (1980) J. Biol. Chem. 255, 2925–2933.
182 Swell, L., Gustafsson, J., Schwartz, C.C., Halloran, L.G., Danielsson, H. and Vlahcevic, Z.R. (1980) J. Lipid Res. 21, 455–466.
183 Björkhem, I., Oftebro, H., Skrede, S. and Pedersen, J.I. (1981) J. Lipid Res. 22, 191–200.
184 Shefer, S., Cheng, F.W., Dayal, B., Hauser, S., Tint, G.S., Salen, G. and Mosbach, E.H. (1976) J. Clin. Invest. 57, 897-903.
185 Salen, G., Shefer, S., Cheng, F.W., Dayal, B., Batta, A.K. and Tint, G.S. (1979) J. Clin. Invest. 63, 38–44.
186 Hanson, R.F., Staples, A.B. and Williams, G.C. (1979) J. Lipid Res. 20, 489–493.
187 Salen, G. (1971) Ann. Intern.. Med. 75, 843–851.
188 Salen, G. and Grundy, S. (1973) J. Clin. Invest. 52, 2822–2835.
189 Setoguchi, T., Salen, G., Tint, G.S. and Mosbach, E.H. (1974) J. Clin. Invest. 53, 1393–1401.
190 Salen, G., Shefer, S., Mosbach, E.H., Hauser, S., Cohen, B.I. and Nicolau, G. (1979) J. Lipid Res. 20, 22–30.
191 Shore, V., Salen, G., Cheng, F.W., Forte, T., Shefer, S., Tint, G.S. and Lindgren, F.T. (1981) J. Clin. Invest. 68, 1295–1304.
192 Tint, G.S. and Salen, G. (1982) J. Lipid Res. 23, 597–603.
193 Oftebro, H., Björkhem, I., Skrede, S., Schreiner, A. and Pedersen, J.I. (1980) J. Clin. Invest. 65, 1418–1430.
194 Javitt, N.B., Kok, E., Cohen, B. and Burstein, S. (1982) J. Lipid Res. 23, 627–630.
195 Björkhem, I., Fausa, O., Hopen, G., Oftebro, H., Pedersen, J.I. and Skrede, S. (1983) J. Clin. Invest. 71, 142–148.
196 Shefer, S., Hauser, S. and Mosbach, E.H. (1966) J. Biol. Chem. 241, 946–952.
197 Shefer, S., Hauser, S. and Mosbach, E.H. (1966) J. Lipid Res. 7, 763–771.
198 Björkhem, I. and Karlmar, K.-E. (1974) Biochim. Biophys. Acta 337, 129–131.
199 Björkhem, I. and Skrede, S. (1982) J. Biol. Chem. 257, 8363–8367.
200 Goldfischer, S., Moore, C.L., Johnson, A.B., Spiro, A.J., Valsamis, M.P., Wisniewski, H.K., Ritch, R.H., Norton, W.T., Rapin, L. and Gartner, L.M. (1973) Science 182, 62–64.

201 Brown, F.R., McAdams, A.J., Cummins, J.W., Konkoi, R., Singh, I., Moser, A.B. and Moser, H.W. (1982) Johns Hopkins Med. J. 151, 344–361.
202 Parmentier, G.G., Janssen, G.A., Eggermont, E.A. and Eyssen, H.J. (1979) Eur. J. Biochem. 102, 173–183.
203 Mathis, R.K., Watkins, J.B., Szczepanik, P. and Lott, I.T. (1980) Gastroenterology 79, 1311–1317.
204 Hanson, R.F., Szczepanik, P., Williams, G.C., Grabowski, G. and Sharp, H.L. (1979) Science 203, 1107–1108.
205 Hanson, R.F., Isenberg, J.N., Williams, G.C., Hachey, D., Szczepanik, P., Klein, P.D. and Sharp, H.L. (1975) J. Clin. Invest. 56, 577–587.
206 Thompson, J.C. and Vars, H.M. (1953) Proc. Soc. Exp. Biol. Med. 83, 246–248.
207 Eriksson, S. (1957) Proc. Soc. Exp. Biol. Med. 94, 578–582.
208 Bergström, S. and Danielsson, H. (1958) Acta Physiol. Scand. 43, 1–7.
209 Shefer, S., Hauser, S., Berkesy, I. and Mosbach, E.H. (1970) J. Lipid Res. 11, 404–411.
210 Mosbach, E.H., Rotshild, M.A., Bekersy, I., Oratz, M. and Mongelli, J. (1971) J. Clin. Invest. 50, 1720–1730.
211 Shefer, S., Hauser, S., Bekersy, I. and Mosbach, E.H. (1969) J. Lipid Res. 10, 646–655.
212 Shefer, S., Hauser, S., Lapar, V. and Mosbach, E.H. (1973) J. Lipid Res. 14, 573–580.
213 Danzinger, R.G., Hofmann, A.F., Thistle, J.L. and Shoenfield, J.L. (1973) J. Clin. Invest. 52, 2809–2821.
214 Einarsson, K., Hellström, K. and Kallner, M. (1973) Metabolism 22, 1477–1483.
215 Boyd, G.S. and Lawson, M.E. (1976) FEBS Lett. 64, 435–439.
216 Dowling, R.H., Mack, E. and Small, D.M. (1970) J. Clin. Invest. 49, 232–242.
217 Dowling, R.H. (1972) Gastroenterology 62, 122–140.
218 Small, D.M., Dowling, R.H. and Redinger, R.N. (1972) Arch. Intern. Med. 130, 552–573.
219 Angelin, B., Björkhem, I., Einarsson, K. and Ewerth, S. (1982) Gastroenterology 83, 1097–1101.
220 Davis, R.A., Hyde, P.M., Kuan, J.-C.W., Malone McNeal, M. and Schexnayder, J.A. (1983) J. Biol. Chem. 258, 3661–3667.
221 Myant, N.B. and Eder, H.A. (1961) J. Lipid Res. 2, 363–368.
222 Mitropoulos, K.A., Balasubramaniam, S. and Myant, N.B. (1973) Biochim. Biophys. Acta 326, 428–438.
223 Balasubramaniam, S., Press, C.M., Mitropoulos, K.A., Magide, A.A. and Myant, N.B. (1976) Biochim. Biophys. Acta 441, 308–315.
224 Ewerth, S., Björkhem, I., Einarsson, K. and Öst, L. (1982) J. Lipid Res. 23, 1183–1186.
225 Björkhem, I., Blomstrand, R., Lewenhaupt, A. and Svensson, L. (1978) Biochem. Biophys. Res. Commun. 85, 532–540.
226 Gielen, J.J., VanCantford, J., Robaye, B. and Renson (1969) C.R. Acad. Sci. Paris 269, 731–732.
227 Danielsson, H. (1972) Steroids 20, 63–72.
228 Mitropoulos, K.A., Balasubramaniam, S., Gibbons, G.F. and Reeves, B.E.A. (1972) FEBS Lett. 27, 203–206.
229 Back, P., Hamprecht, B. and Lynen, F. (1969) Arch. Biochem. Biophys. 133, 11–21.
230 Kandutsch, A.A. and Saucier, S.E. (1969) J. Biol. Chem. 244, 2299–2305.
231 Balasubramaniam, S., Mitropoulos, K.A. and Myant, N.B. (1972) in: Bile acids in Human Diseases II, Bile Acid Meeting, Freiburg in Br., 1972 (Back, P. and Gerock, W., Eds.) pp. 97–102, Schattauer Verlag, Stuttgart.
232 Mayer, D. (1972) in: Bile Acids in Human Diseasès II, Bile Acid Meeting, Freiburg in Br., 1972 (Back, P. and Gerock, W., Eds.) pp. 103–109, Schattauer Verlag, Stuttgart.
233 Van Cantford, J. (1974) J. Interdiscip. Cycle Res. 5, 89–94.
234 Balasubramaniam, S., Mitropoulos, K.A. and Myant, N.B. (1975) in: Advances in Bile Acid Research, III, Bile Acid Meeting, Freiburg in Br., 1974 (Matern, S., Hackenschmidt, J., Back, P. and Gerock, W., Eds.) pp. 61–67, Schattauer Verlag, Stuttgart.
235 Mayer, D. (1975) in: Advances in Bile Acid Research III, Bile Acid Meeting, Freiburg in Br., 1974 (Matern, S., Hackenschmidt, J., Back, P. and Gerock, W., Eds.) pp. 53–59, Schattauer Verlag, Stuttgart.

236 Van Cantford, J. (1973) Biochemie 55, 1171–1173.
237 Takeuchi, N., Ito, M. and Yamamura, Y. (1974) Atherosclerosis 20, 481–494.
238 Van Cantford, J. (1972) C.R. Acad. Sci. Paris 275, 1015–1017.
239 Raicht, R.F., Cohen, B.I., Shefer, S. and Mosbach, E.H. (1975) Biochim. Biophys. Acta 388, 374–384.
240 Boyd, G.S., Brown, M.J., Hattersley, N.G., Lawson, M.E. and Suckling, K.E. (1974) in: Advances in Bile Acid Research III, Bile Acid Meeting, Freiburg in Br., 1974 (Matern, S., Hackenschmidt, J., Back, P. and Gerock, W., Eds.) pp. 45–51, Schattauer Verlag, Stuttgart.
241 Mosbach, E.H. (1972) in: Bile Acids in Human Diseases II, Bile Acids Meeting, Freiburg in Br.,1972 (Back, P. and Gerock, W., Eds.) pp. 89–96, Schattauer Verlg, Stuttgart.
242 Björkhem, I. and Kallner, A. (1976) J. Lipid Res. 17, 360–365.
243 Björkhem, I., Kallner, A. and Löf, A. (1978) IRCS Med. Sci. 6, 230.
244 Guchait, R. and Ganguli, N.C. (1960) Abstr. Symp. Biochem. Aspects of Cholesterol Metabolism and Arteriosclerosis, p. 8.
245 Bucher, N.L.R., Overath, P. and Lynen, F. (1960) Biochim. Biophys. Acta 40, 491–501.
246 Brown, M.S. and Goldstein, J.L. (1980) J. Lipid Res. 21, 505–517.
247 Weis, H.J. and Dietschy, J.M. (1969) J. Clin. Invest. 48, 2398–2408.
248 Hamprecht, B., Roscher, R., Waltinger, G. and Nussler, C. (1971) Eur. J. Biochem. 18, 15–19.
249 Scallen, T.J. and Sanghvi, A. (1983) Proc. Natl. Acad. Sci. (U.S.A.) 80, 2477–2480.
250 Strand, O. (1962) Proc. Soc. Exp. Biol. Med. 109, 668.
251 Strand, O. (1963) J. Lipid Res. 4, 305–311.
252 Johansson, G. (1970) Eur. J. Biochem. 17, 292–295.
253 Ahlberg, J., Angelin, B., Björkhem, I., Einarsson, K. and Leijd, B. (1979) J. Lipid Res. 20, 107–115.
254 Björkhem, I., Eriksson, M. and Einarsson, K. (1983) J. Lipid Res. 24, 1451–1456.
255 Mitropoulos, K.A., Myant, N.B., Gibbons, G.F., Balasubramaniam, S. and Reeves, B.E.A. (1974) J. Biol. Chem. 249, 6052–6056.
256 Schwartz, C.C., Vlahcevic, Z.R., Halloran, L.G., Nisman, R. and Swell, L. (1977) Proc. Soc. Exp. Biol. Med. 156, 261–264.
257 Einarsson, K., Ahlberg, J., Angelin, B. and Holmström, B. (1978) in: The Liver, Quantitative Aspects of Structure and Function (Preisig, R. and Bircher, J., Eds.) pp. 233–238, Editio Cantor, Aulendorf.
258 Liscum, L., Luskey, K.L., Chin, D.J., Ho, Y.K., Goldstein, J.L. and Brown, M.S. (1983) J. Biol. Chem. 258, 8450–8455.
259 Hui, D.Y., Innerarity, T.L. and Mahley, R.W. (1981) J. Biol. Chem. 256, 5646–5655.
260 Angelin, B., Raviola, C.A., Innerarity, T.L. and Mahley, R.W. (1983) J. Clin. Invest. 71, 816–833.

H. Danielsson and J. Sjövall (Eds.), *Sterols and Bile Acids*

CHAPTER 10

Bile alcohols and primitive bile acids

TAKAHIKO HOSHITA

Institute of Pharmaceutical Sciences, Hiroshima University School of Medicine, Hiroshima (Japan)

(I) Introduction

The bile acids in bile of mammals are taurine and glycine conjugates of derivatives of cholanoic acid. The bile of evolutionarily more primitive vertebrates contain other types of bile salts, i.e., sulfuric acid esters of bile alcohols and taurine-conjugated or unconjugated bile acids with more than 24 carbon atoms (higher bile acids). Although both types of compounds have the bile acid type of nuclear structure, they are chemically closer to cholesterol than the common bile acids. Until recently, bile alcohols and higher bile acids were supposed to occur only in the primitive vertebrates. However, it is now realized that they are present in mammals, including healthy and diseased humans. In addition C_{24} bile acids having a 3β-hydroxyl group and a double bond at position 5 have been found in humans. In this chapter, these cholenoic acid derivatives as well as higher bile acids are defined as primitive bile acids. The occurrence in nature of bile alcohols and primitive bile acids is especially interesting since these compounds appear to represent not only evolutionary precursors but also biosynthetic intermediates in the formation of the common C_{24} bile acids.

This chapter reviews the natural distribution, the chemical structure, and the metabolism of bile alcohols and primitive bile acids.

(II) Occurrence and structure of bile alcohols in lower vertebrates

Bile alcohols found in lower vertebrates are polyhydric derivatives of cholestane (C_{27}), 27-norcholestane (C_{26}), 26,27-dinorcholestane (C_{25}) or cholane (C_{24}). The trivial names of the bile alcohols include as a prefix part of the Latin name of the genus of the animal from which they were first isolated. When both isomers differing in the configuration at C-5 are known, the prefix 5α or 5β is then used with the

TABLE 1

Bile alcohols of lower vertebrates

Trivial name of bile alcohol	Systematic name	Natural source
Arapaimol-B	5β-Cholestane-2β,3α,7α,12α,26,27-hexol	*Arapaima gigas*
Scymnol	5β-Cholestane-3α,7α,12α,24,26,27-hexol	Sharks and rays
5α-Dermophol	5α-Cholestane-3α,7α,12α,25,26,27-hexol	Some amphibians
5β-Dermophol	5β-Cholestane-3α,7α,12α,25,26,27-hexol	Some amphibians
Arapaimol-A	5β-Cholestane-2β,3α,7α,12α,26-pentol	*Arapaima gigas*; some frogs
5α-Chimaerol	5α-Cholestane-3α,7α,12α,24,26-pentol	White sucker and related fishes; lungfish
5β-Chimaerol	5β-Cholestane-3α,7α,12α,24,26-pentol	*Chimaera monstrosa*; some sharks and rays
5α-Bufol	5α-Cholestane-3α,7α,12α,25,26-pentol	Newt; some frogs; lungfishes; coelacanth
5β-Bufol	5β-Cholestane-3α,7α,12α,25,26-pentol	Toads of genus Bufo; some frogs
5α-Cyprinol	5α-Cholestane-3α,7α,12α,26,27-pentol	Carp and related fishes; lungfish; coelacanth; some frogs
Latimerol	5α-Cholestane-3β,7α,12α,26,27-pentol	Coelacanth
5β-Cyprinol	5β-Cholestane-3α,7α,12α,26,27-pentol	Several bony fishes; some frogs
26-Deoxy-5α-chimaerol	5α-Cholestane-3α,7α,12α,24-tetrol	Some fishes
27-Deoxy-5α-cyprinol	5α-Cholestane-3α,7α,12α,26-tetrol	Some fishes; some frogs and toads
27-Deoxy-5β-cyprinol	5β-Cholestane-3α,7α,12α,26-tetrol	Some frogs and toads
Myxinol	5α-Cholestane-3β,7α,16α,26-tetrol	Hagfish
3-Epimyxinol	5α-Cholestane-3α,7α,16α,26-tetrol	Hagfish
16-Deoxymyxinol	5α-Cholestane-3β,7α,26-triol	Hagfish
3-Epi-16-deoxymyxinol	5α-Cholestane-3α,7α,26-triol	Hagfish
5α-Ranol	(24*R*)-27-Nor-5α-cholestane-3α,7α,12α,24,26-pentol	Some frogs
5β-Ranol	(24*R*)-27-Nor-5β-cholestane-3α,7α,12α,24,26-pentol	Some frogs
26-Deoxy-5α-ranol	(24*S*)-27-Nor-5α-cholestane-3α,7α,12α,24-tetrol	Some frogs
24-Epi-26-deoxy-5α-ranol	(24*R*)-27-Nor-5α-cholestane-3α,7α,12α,24-tetrol	Some frogs
26-Deoxy-5β-ranol	(24*S*)-27-Nor-5β-cholestane-3α,7α,12α,24-tetrol	Some frogs
24-Epi-26-deoxy-5β-ranol	(24*R*)-27-Nor-5β-cholestane-3α,7α,12α,24-tetrol	Some frogs
24-Dehydro-26-deoxy-5α-ranol	3α,7α,12α-Trihydroxy-27-nor-5α-cholestan-24-one	Bullfrog
24-Dehydro-26-deoxy-5β-ranol	3α,7α,12α-Trihydroxy-27-nor-5β-cholestan-24-one	Bullfrog
25-Nor-26-deoxy-5α-ranol	26,27-Dinor-5α-cholestane-3α,7α,12α,24-tetrol	Some frogs
25-Nor-26-deoxy-5β-ranol	26,27-Dinor-5β-cholestane-3α,7α,12α,24-tetrol	Some frogs
5α-Petromyzonol	5α-Cholane-3α,7α,12α,24-tetrol	Lamprey; lungfish
5β-Petromyzonol	5β-Cholane-3α,7α,12α,24-tetrol	Lungfish

original name. Table 1 lists all the known bile alcohols found in the bile of lower vertebrates.

Bile alcohols are present in the bile of lower vertebrates as the sodium salts of the monosulfuric acid ester of a hydroxyl group in the side chain, except in the case of hagfishes, where they exist as disulfates. Since the isolation of each individual bile alcohol sulfate is difficult, the chemical structure of bile alcohols has been elucidated after hydrolysis of the sulfates. Saponification was used in earlier studies, but the alkaline treatment of the sulfate esters may lead to a number of artifacts [1,2]. Therefore, solvolysis has been employed in recent studies as a better method to obtain native bile alcohols [3]. Chromatographic procedures are used almost exclusively for isolation and identification of bile alcohols. Systematic studies of separation and identification of bile alcohols by thin-layer, column and paper chromatography have been reported by Kazuno and Hoshita [4]. Bile alcohols differing in number and position of hydroxyl groups, in A/B ring junction, and in length of the side chain are separable by these methods. Gas-liquid chromatography permits a very satisfactory separation of bile alcohols on a microscale. Since the retention times are structure dependent, these values are often used to arrive at tentative structural conclusions for unidentified bile alcohols. Combined gas-liquid chromatography–mass spectrometry is the most powerful method for the identification of bile alcohols. This technique is capable of discovering and identifying small amounts of bile alcohols without their isolation. Further characterization of separated bile alcohols may be achieved by infrared spectroscopy, nuclear magnetic resonance spectroscopy, and mass spectrometry.

The existence of bile alcohols in nature was first demonstrated in 1898 by O. Hammarsten who isolated a bile alcohol named "scymnol" from the alkaline hydrolyzate of the bile of a shark, *Scymnus borealis* [5]. The structure of "scymnol" was finally established in 1961 as 24,26-epoxy-5β-cholestane-3α,7α,12α,27-tetrol (II) [1] (Fig. 1). It was concluded that "scymnol" was an artifact formed from the naturally occurring scymnol sulfate (I) during alkaline hydrolysis. The 4-membered oxide ring in the molecule of the artifact (II) is formed by the elimination of sulfate ion between the $-OSO_3^-$ group at C-26 and the hydroxyl group at C-24. Thus, Hammarsten's scymnol was renamed anhydroscymnol. The native scymnol was obtained from the solvolyzed bile and its structure was confirmed as 5β-cholestane-3α,7α,12α,24,26,27-hexol (III) by comparison with a synthetic sample [3]. The configuration of the hydroxyl group at C-24 remains to be established. Scymnol sulfate has been found in all sharks and rays examined but not in any other vertebrate, and is now recognized as the characteristic component of the bile of elasmobranchii, one of the oldest vertebrate groups.

Kihira et al. have found that the principal bile salt of the caecilian, *Dermophis mexicanus,* is a sulfate ester of 5β-dermophol, 5β-cholestane-3α,7α,12α,25,26,27-hexol [6]. 5β-Dermophol was also found as a minor constituent of the bile of the toad, *Bufo vulgaris formosus* [6].

5α-Dermophol was detected as a minor bile alcohol in solvolyzed bile of the newt, *Diemyctylus pyrrhogaster,* the congo eel, *Amphiuma means,* and the giant sala-

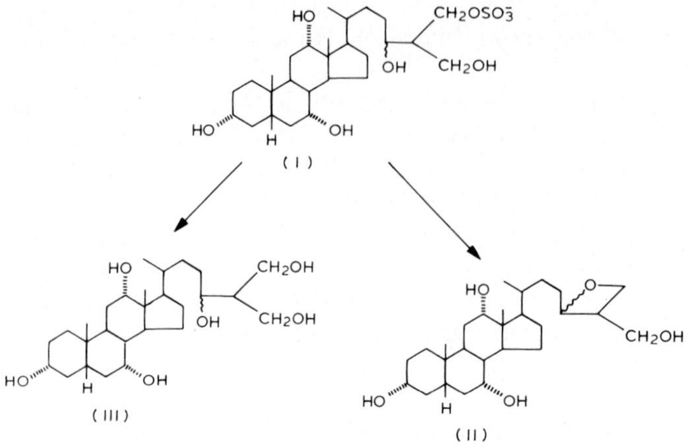

Fig. 1. Scymnol sulfate(I), anhydroscymnol(II) and scymnol(III).

mander, *Megalobactrachus japonicus* [6]. The structure of 5α-dermophol has been verified as 5α-cholestane-3α,7α,12α,25,26,27-hexol by partial synthesis [7].

A principal bile salt of *Arapaima gigas*, the very large South American fresh-water teleost of the family Osteoglossidae, is a sulfate ester of arapaimol-A [8]. The bile also contains a sulfate ester of a second bile alcohol, arapaimol-B [8]. Spectral analysis indicated that arapaimol-A and -B are 5β-cholestane-2β,3α,7α,12α,26-pentol and 5β-cholestane-2β,3α,7α,12α,26,27-hexol, respectively [8]. Arapaimol-A also occurs in the bile of some species of frogs [9].

5β-Chimaerol sulfate is the chief bile salt of *Chimaera monstrosa* [10], and also occurs as a minor companion of scymnol sulfate in the bile of elasmobranchii [11,12]. 5β-Chimaerol was characterized as 5β-cholestane-3α,7α,12α,24,26-pentol by comparison with synthetic samples prepared from cholic acid [3] and from anhydroscymnol [1].

A principal bile salt of the white sucker, *Catostomus commersoni*, is 5α-chimaerol sulfate [13]. Two other Catostomus species and the lungfish, *Neoceratodus forsteri*, also have 5α-chimaerol sulfate [14]. Spectral analysis of 5α-chimaerol supported the structure 5α-cholestane-3α,7α,12α,24,26-pentol.

5β-Bufol sulfate is the principal component in the bile of toads of the genus Bufo [9,15]. The structure of this bile alcohol was deduced as 5β-cholestane-3α,7α,12α,25,26-pentol by its conversion with lead tetraacetate oxidation to formaldehyde and 3α,7α,12α-trihydroxy-27-nor-5β-cholestan-25-one [15] and also by comparison with synthetic material [16]. The sulfate ester in 5β-bufol sulfate was shown to be at C-26 by ^{13}C nuclear magnetic resonance spectroscopy [17]. 5β-Bufol sulfate also occurs in some species of frogs as a major or minor biliary component [9,18,19].

5α-Bufol sulfate is the major component in bile of the newt, *Diemyctylus pyrrhogaster* [20], the frog, *Rana erythrea* [19], and the South American lungfish, *Lepidosiren paradoxa* [14]. It also occurs in lesser amounts in bile of the Australian

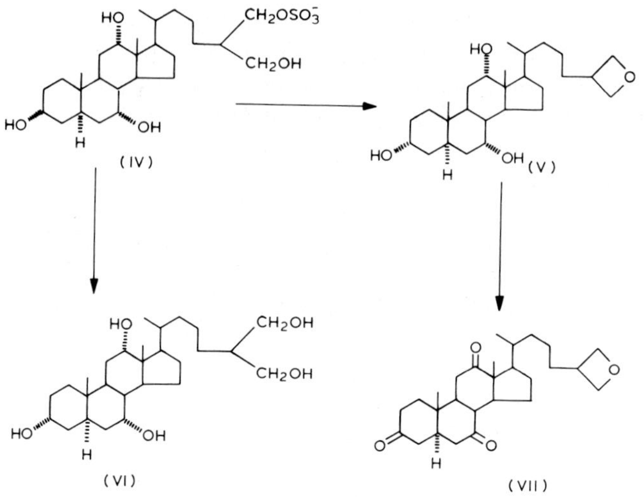

Fig. 2. 5α-Cyprinol sulfate(IV), anhydro-5α-cyprinol(V), 5α-cyprinol(VI) and dehydroanhydro-5α-cyprinol(VII).

lungfish, *Neoceratodus forsteri* [14], the coelacanth, *Latimeria chalumnae* [14], and some species of frogs [9]. The characterization and partial synthesis of 5α-bufol was accomplished by Hoshita et al. [20].

5α-Cyprinol sulfate (IV) (Fig. 2) is the principal bile salt of the carp, *Cyprinus carpio,* and related fishes [21,22]. It also occurs in bile of the lungfish [14], the coelacanth [23], the giant salamander [24], and some species of frogs [9,18,19]. Characterization of 5α-cyprinol was first reported by Hoshita et al. [21]. Alkaline hydrolysis of carp bile gave chiefly anhydro-5α-cyprinol, 26,27-epoxy-5α-cholestane-3α,7α,12α-triol (V) [2]. The structure of the artifact, anhydro-5α-cyprinol, suggested that the native bile alcohol, 5α-cyprinol, is 5α-cholestane-3α,7α,12α,26,27-pentol (VI). Solvolysis of carp bile gave chiefly 5α-cyprinol, whose spectral data were completely consistent with the structure VI [21]. The same structure for 5α-cyprinol was independently proposed by Anderson et al. [25].

5β-Cyprinol sulfate was first found in bile of the eel, *Conger myriaster*, the principal bile salts of which are taurocholate and taurochenodeoxycholate [26]. 5β-Cyprinol sulfate was later found in the bile of some species of frogs as their principal bile salt [9,18,19,27], and was also detected in bile of some fishes as their minor bile salt [28,29]. The structure of 5β-cyprinol was determined as 5β-cholestane-3α,7α,12α,26,27-pentol by direct comparison with the synthetic sample prepared by Hoshita et al. before its isolation from natural sources [30]. Partial synthesis of 5β-cyprinol was also reported by Haslewood and Tammar [29].

A principal bile salt of the ancient bony fish, the coelacanth, *Latimeria chalumnae*, is a sulfate ester of a bile alcohol named latimerol [23]. Alkaline hydrolysis of the coelacanth bile salts gave chiefly anhydrolatimerol along with some latimerol. Chromic oxide oxidation of anhydrolatimerol gave a product identical with dehydroanhydro-5α-cyprinol, 26,27-epoxy-5α-cholestane-3,7,12-trione (VII), prepared from anhydro-5α-cyprinol (V) by treatment with the same oxidant. Comparison of the infrared spectrum of latimerol with that of synthetic 3β,7α,12α-trihydroxy-5α-cholan-24-oic acid, showed that the former alcohol had the same nucleus as the latter acid. These results indicated that latimerol is the 3β epimer of 5α-cyprinol, 5α-cholestane-3β,7α,12α,26,27-pentol [23].

27-Deoxy-5α-cyprinol, 5α-cholestane-3α,7α,12α,26-tetrol, has been identified as a minor companion of 5α-cyprinol in the carp bile [31]. This tetrahydroxy-5α-bile alcohol was prepared from anhydro-5α-cyprinol (VII) by lithium aluminum hydride reduction [2]. 27-Deoxy-5α-cyprinol also occurs in bile of fishes [32], toads [9,33], and frogs [9].

27-Deoxy-5β-cyprinol, 5β-cholestane-3α,7α,12α,26-tetrol, is present in some species of frogs [9,19] and toads [9,33]. Two stereoisomers at C-25 of this bile alcohol have been prepared from (25*R*)- and (25*S*)-3α,7α,12α-trihydroxy-5β-cholestan-26-oic acids, respectively [13].

26-Deoxy-5α-chimaerol, 5α-cholestane-3α,7α,12α,24-tetrol, was detected as a minor constituent in solvolyzed bile of some fishes by gas-liquid chromatography–mass spectrometry [14,32].

A principal bile salt of the hagfishes, *Myxine glutinosa* and *Eptatretus stoutii*, is the disulfuric acid ester of myxinol, 5α-cholestane-3β,7α,16α,26-tetrol [34,35]. A second bile alcohol of the most primitive marine cyclostomes is 16-deoxymyxinol, 5α-cholestane-3β,7α,26-triol, which also occurs in the bile as the disulfate [36]. The positions of the sulfate moieties in myxinol disulfate were established to be C-3 and C-26 by oxidation and subsequent solvolysis [34]. Une et al. studied another species of the hagfish, *Heptatretus burgeri*, and found two new alcohols along with myxinol and 16-deoxymyxinol [37]. These were identified as 3-epimyxinol, 5α-cholestane-3α,7α,16α,26-tetrol, and 3-epi-16-deoxymyxinol, 5α-cholestane-3α,7α,26-triol. The occurrence of the 3α epimers along with myxinol and 16-deoxymyxinol in the same species suggests that the 3β-hydroxy bile alcohols arise from cholesterol by a route which involves 3-oxo intermediates rather than by a route which maintains the 3β-hydroxyl group of cholesterol.

5α-Ranol sulfate is the sole or principal bile salt of the frog, *Rana temporaria* [38]. The structure of 5α-ranol was shown to be 27-nor-5α-cholestane-3α,7α,12α,24,26-pentol [38]. The position of the sulfate moiety was established to be C-24 by oxidation with subsequent solvolysis [38]. 5α-Ranol sulfate also occurs in bile of various species of frogs as a major component [18,19].

5β-Ranol sulfate is a major bile salt of the bullfrog, *Rana catesbeiana* [39]. 5β-Ranol was identified as (24*R*)-27-nor-5β-cholestane-3α,7α,12α,24,26-pentol by comparison with synthetic material [39,40]. 5β-Ranol sulfate also occurs in bile of various species of frogs [9,18,19].

In a thorough analysis of solvolyzed material from bullfrog bile, Noma et al. isolated 4 new C_{26} bile alcohols along with 5α-ranol, 5β-ranol, and 5α-cyprinol [41]. Comparison with synthetic samples showed that these were 4 diastereoisomers at C-5 and C-24 of 26-deoxyranol, 27-norcholestane-3α,7α,12α,24-tetrol [41]. The deoxyranols also occur in various species of frogs as minor companions of 5α- or 5β-ranol [9,19].

Noma et al. found 2 keto bile alcohols in unconjugated form in bullfrog bile [42]. Their structures were determined as 24-dehydro-26-deoxy-5α-ranol and its 5β isomer by comparison with synthetic 3α,7α,12α-trihydroxy-27-nor-5α- and 5β-cholestan-24-ones, prepared from allocholic acid and cholic acid, respectively [41].

25-Nor-26-deoxy-5α- and 5β-ranols, 26,27-dinor-5α- and 5β-cholestane-3α,7α,12α,24-tetrols, were detected by gas-liquid chromatography–mass spectrometry as minor constituents in the bile of a few species of frogs [9].

The sole or principal bile salt of the lamprey, *Petromyzon marinus*, is the sulfate ester of a C_{24} bile alcohol [43]. The parent bile alcohol, 5α-petromyzonol, was characterized as 5α-cholane-3α,7α,12α,24-tetrol by comparison with a synthetic sample prepared from allocholic acid [43]. The position of the sulfate moiety in 5α-petromyzonol sulfate was deduced to be C-24 because the oxidation of the sulfate followed by solvolysis gave a trioxocholanol [43]. A small amount of 5α-petromyzonol sulfate has been found in bile of the Australian lungfish, *Neoceratodus forsteri*, whose major bile salts are sulfate esters of 5α-chimaerol and 27-deoxy-5α-cyprinol [14]. The African lungfish, *Protopterus aethiopicus*, also has minor amounts of this 5α-C_{24} bile salt and its 5β isomer, 5β-petromyzonol sulfate, along with the major bile salt, 5α-cyprinol sulfate [14].

(III) Occurrence and structure of primitive bile acids in lower vertebrates

Most primitive bile acids found in lower vertebrates possess the carbon skeleton of cholesterol. Differences within these C_{27} bile acids are associated with number, position, and configuration of hydroxyl groups and with side-chain unsaturation. In addition, some C_{28} bile acids have been found in bile of a few species of amphibians. Cholenoic acid derivatives have not been found in lower vertebrates. A list of primitive bile acids in lower vertebrates is given in Table 2.

The higher bile acids occur as taurine conjugates or in unconjugated form in the native bile of lower vertebrates. There is no evidence for the presence in these animals of glycine-conjugated higher bile acids. This seems reasonable since, even in the case of the common bile acids, glycine conjugates occur only in mammalian species. The natural occurrence of unconjugated bile acids in the bile of some lower vertebrates suggests that enzyme systems catalyzing conjugation are absent or present in low concentration in such species.

Unconjugated bile acids in bile may be obtained by extraction with ether or ethyl acetate of diluted and acidified bile. Taurine-conjugated higher bile acids, like conjugates of C_{24} bile acids, may be hydrolyzed by heating with alkali, but cannot be hydrolyzed by the bacterial enzymes which split conjugates of C_{24} bile acids (see Chapter 12). Batta et al. have reported that hydrolysis of conjugated higher bile acids can be achieved by incubation with rat fecal suspensions [44]. The separation and identification of higher bile acids may be achieved by the same methods used for bile alcohols. In addition, high-performance liquid chromatography is a powerful

TABLE 2
Primitive bile acids of lower vertebrates

Systematic name of primitive bile acid (trivial name)	Natural source
3α,7α,12α,24-Tetrahydroxy-24-methyl-5β-cholestan-26-oic acid	Toad
3α,7α,12α-Trihydroxy-24-methyl-5β-cholestan-26-oic acid	Bullfrog
3α,7α,12α-Trihydroxy-5α-cholest-22-ene-24-carboxylic acid	Toad
3α,7α,12α-Trihydroxy-5β-cholest-22-ene-24-carboxylic acid	Toad
2β,3α,7α,12α-Tetrahydroxy-5β-cholestan-26-oic acid (arapaimic acid)	*Arapaima gigas*
3α,7α,12α,22-Tetrahydroxy-5β-cholestan-26-oic acid	Turtles and tortoises
3α,7α,12α,24-Tetrahydroxy-5α-cholestan-26-oic acid	Bullfrog
(24R,25S)-3α,7α,12α,24-Tetrahydroxy-5β-cholestan-26-oic acid (varanic acid)	Some frogs; lizards
3α,7α,12α,26-Tetrahydroxy-5α-cholestan-27-oic acid	Bullfrog
3α,7α,12α,26-Tetrahydroxy-5β-cholestan-27-oic acid	Some frogs
3α,7α,12α-Trihydroxy-5α-cholestan-26-oic acid	Iguana; alligator; some frogs
(25R)-3α,7α,12α-Trihydroxy-5β-cholestan-26-oic acid	Some amphibians; reptiles; kite
(25S)-3α,7α,12α-Trihydroxy-5β-cholestan-26-oic acid	Some frogs; reptiles
3β,7α,12α-Trihydroxy-5β-cholestan-26-oic acid	Alligator feces
3α,7α,12α-Trihydroxy-5α-cholest-23-en-26-oic acid	Toad
(25R)-3α,7α,12α-Trihydroxy-5β-cholest-23-en-26-oic acid	Toad; lizard
3α,7α,12α-Trihydroxy-5β-cholest-24-en-26-oic acid	Lizard
3α,7α,24-Trihydroxy-5β-cholestan-26-oic acid	Lizard
3α,12α,22-Trihydroxy-5β-cholestan-26-oic acid	Turtle
3α,7α-Dihydroxy-5β-cholestan-26-oic acid	Alligator; kite
3α,7α-Dihydroxy-5β-cholest-23-en-26-oic acid	Lizard
3α,7α-Dihydroxy-5β-cholest-24-en-26-oic acid	Lizard
3α,7β-Dihydroxy-5β-cholestan-26-oic acid	Alligator feces
3β,7β-Dihydroxy-5β-cholestan-26-oic acid	Alligator feces
3α,12α-Dihydroxy-5β-cholestan-26-oic acid	Alligator feces
3β,12α-Dihydroxy-5β-cholestan-26-oic acid	Alligator feces
3α-Hydroxy-5β-cholestan-26-oic acid	Alligator feces
3β-Hydroxy-5β-cholestan-26-oic acid	Alligator feces
3α,12α-Dihydroxy-7-oxo-5β-cholestan-26-oic acid	Alligator
7α,12α-Dihydroxy-3-oxo-5α-cholestan-26-oic acid	Alligator
7α,12α-Dihydroxy-3-oxo-5β-cholestan-26-oic acid	Alligator

tool for the separation of diastereoisomers differing only in the configuration of the functional group in the side chain [45].

3α,7α,12α-Trihydroxy- and 3α,7α,12α,24-tetrahydroxy-24-methyl-5β-cholestan-26-oic acids have been found in bile of the bullfrog [42] and the toad [46], respectively. These C_{28} bile acids were partially synthesized before their isolation from natural sources [47].

In 1934, Shimizu and Oda isolated a major bile acid from the toad, *Bufo vulgaris formosus*, which they named "trihydroxybufosterocholenic acid" [48]. The structure of this bile acid was elucidated in 1967 by Hoshita et al. as 3α,7α,12α-trihydroxy-

5β-cholest-22-ene-24-carboxylic acid [49]. The Δ^{22} double bond was shown to be *trans* by infrared spectroscopy [50]. The stereochemistry at C-24 is still unknown.

Another unsaturated C_{28} bile acid was recently detected as a minor component in toad bile [46]. Its structure was established as 3α,7α,12α-trihydroxy-5α-cholest-22-ene-24-carboxylic acid by mass spectrometry and gas-liquid chromatography.

The bile of *Arapaima gigas*, whose major bile salts are sulfate esters of arapaimol-A and -B, contains small amounts of a higher bile acid, arapaimic acid [8]. Spectral analysis indicates that arapaimic acid is the bile acid corresponding to arapaimol-B, 2β,3α,7α,12α-tetrahydroxy-5β-cholestan-26-oic acid.

The major bile acid in all turtles and tortoises examined is 3α,7α,12α,22-tetrahydroxy-5β-cholestan-26-oic acid [51,52]. This higher bile acid may be considered a characteristic bile acid of Testudinidae.

Haslewood and Wootton isolated varanic acid, 3α,7α,12α,24-tetrahydroxy-5β-cholestan-26-oic acid, from bile of the monitor lizard, *Varanus niloticus* [53]. Varanic acid was later found in bile of the frog, *Bombina orientalis*, where it occurs in the unconjugated form [18]. Une et al. synthesized 4 diastereoisomers at C-24 and C-25 of 3α,7α,12α,24-tetrahydroxy-5β-cholestan-26-oic acid. Comparisons with these synthetic bile acids of known absolute configuration showed that the varanic acid in frog bile is (24*R*,25*S*)-3α,7α,12α,24-tetrahydroxy-5β-cholestan-26-oic acid [54].

Noma et al. studied minor bile acids of the bullfrog and found 4 different tetrahydroxycholestanoic acids [42]. These were identified as varanic acid, its 5α isomer, and 3α,7α,12α,26-tetrahydroxy-5α- and 5β-cholestan-27-oic acids by comparison with synthetic samples [42]. 3α,7α,12α,26-Tetrahydroxy-5β-cholestan-27-oic acid also occurs in bile of the frog, *Rana plancyi* [19].

In 1939, Kurauti and Kazuno isolated a major higher bile acid from the bile of the bullfrog, *Rana catesbeiana* [55]. This bile acid was later isolated from bile of *Alligator mississippiensis* [56]. Its structure was deduced as a 3α,7α,12α-trihydroxy-5β-cholestan-26-oic acid by its degradation to cholic acid [57] and by its conversion to the stem acid, 5β-cholestan-26-oic acid [58].

Another higher bile acid was isolated from the bullfrog bile as a minor component [59]. This compound was also characterized as a 3α,7α,12α-trihydroxy-5β-cholestan-26-oic acid since the partially synthesized trihydroxy-5β-cholestanoic acid was identical with the minor bile acid but not with the major bile acid [60].

The relation of these higher bile acids was solved by Bridgwater who synthesized the two C-25 stereoisomers of trihydroxy-5β-cholestanoic acid [61]. From comparison with the synthetic standards, it was concluded that the major bile acid of the bullfrog has the 25*R* and the minor bile acid the 25*S* configuration [61]. This conclusion was recently confirmed by X-ray crystallography [62]. Mendelsohn and Mendelsohn also isolated both (25*R*)- and (25*S*)-trihydroxy-5β-cholestanoic acids from the bile of *Crocodylus niloticus* [63]. The occurrence of both isomers in the same species at once arouses the suspicion that one is an artifact formed from the other. This is particularly possible in the case of the Crocodylidae, in which the bile acids occur as taurine conjugates. The drastic procedures involved in the hydrolysis of the taurine conjugates might cause racemization at C-25, giving rise to both diastereoisomers. However, the natural occurrence of both (25*R*)- and (25*S*)-trihydroxy-5β-cholestanoic acids in bullfrog bile was recently shown by Une et al. [45]. Since the bile acids of the bullfrog occur in unconjugated form, they could be isolated without use of drastic procedures. High-performance liquid chromatography revealed that bullfrog bile contains both 25*R* and 25*S* isomers in the ratio of about 20 : 1. Taurine-conjugated or unconjugated 3α,7α,12α-trihydroxy-5β-cholestan-26-oic acid also occurs in bile of various species of amphibians [9,18,19], crocodilians [64], and the kite, *Milvus lineatus lineatus* [65].

Okuda et al. isolated a higher bile acid from the bile of *Iguana iguana* [66]. The structure was shown to be 3α,7α,12α-trihydroxy-5α-cholestan-26-oic acid by lithium aluminum hydride reduction to 27-deoxy-5α-cyprinol [66]. The 5α-C_{27} bile acid was also partially synthesized from 27-deoxy-5α-cyprinol [67]. 3α,7α,12α-Trihydroxy-5α-cholestan-26-oic acid also occurs in bile of some species of frogs [18,19] and the alligator [68].

The 12-deoxy derivative of varanic acid, 3α,7α,24-trihydroxy-5β-cholestan-26-oic acid was detected in the bile of *Varanus monitor*, as a minor companion of varanic acid, the major bile acid of this lizard [69].

The presence of small amounts of 3α,12α,22-trihydroxy-5β-cholestan-26-oic acid as taurine conjugate in *Chelonia mydas* was reported by Haslewood et al. [52]. This bile acid is the 7-deoxy derivative of 3α,7α,12α,22-tetrahydroxy-5β-cholestan-26-oic acid, the major bile acid of this turtle, and is most likely formed by bacterial 7α-dehydroxylation (Chapter 12).

A trihydroxycholestenoic acid was isolated as a major bile acid from bile of the toad, *Bufo vulgaris formosus* [70] and was characterized as (25*R*)-3α,7α,12α-trihydroxy-5β-cholest-23-en-26-oic acid by oxidation to 23-norcholic acid and hydrogenation to (25*R*)-3α,7α,12α-trihydroxy-5β-cholestan-26-oic acid [71]. The 5α isomer, 3α,7α,12α-trihydroxy-5α-cholest-23-en-26-oic acid, was recently detected as a minor bile acid in toad bile [46]. The bile of *Varanus monitor* contains as minor constituents 3α,7α,12α-trihydroxy-5β-cholest-23- and 24-enoic acids [69]. The Δ^{24} acid has been synthesized prior to its detection in nature [72].

3α,7α-Dihydroxy-5β-cholestan-26-oic acid was isolated from alligator bile as a minor companion of 3α,7α,12α-trihydroxy-5β-cholestan-26-oic acid [73]. The bile of the kite contains considerable amounts of the dihydroxy- and trihydroxy-5β-cholestanoic acids [65]. Two dihydroxy-C_{27} bile acids with unsaturation in the side chain were recently found as minor bile acids of *Varanus monitor* [69]. Based on chromatographic behavior and mass spectral fragmentation, these bile acids were assigned the structures 3α,7α-dihydroxy-5β-cholest-23- and 24-en-26-oic acids [69]. The Δ^{24} acid has been partially synthesized [74].

Three higher bile acids possessing a keto group were detected in the bile of *Alligator mississippiensis*, and characterized as 7α,12α-dihydroxy-3-oxo-5β-cholestan-26-oic acid, 3α,12α-dihydroxy-7-oxo-5β-cholestan-26-oic acid, and 7α,12α-dihydroxy-3-oxo-5α-cholestan-26-oic acid [68]. Nothing is known about the formation of these bile acids.

Tint et al. studied bile acids excreted in the feces of *Alligator mississippiensis* [75].

Although small amounts of the biliary bile acids, 3α,7α,12α-trihydroxy- and 3α,7α-dihydroxy-5β-cholestan-26-oic acids, were detected, the major fecal bile acids were their 7-deoxy derivatives, 3α,12α-dihydroxy- and 3α-hydroxy-5β-cholestan-26-oic acids. Small amounts of 3β,7α,12α-trihydroxy-5β-cholestan-26-oic acid, 3α,7β-, 3β,7β- and 3β,12α-dihydroxy-5β-cholestan-26-oic acids, and 3β-hydroxy-5β-cholestan-26-oic acid were found as well [75]. Since intestinal bacterial in mammals are known to 7α-dehydroxylate C_{24} bile acids and to interconvert α- and β-hydroxyl groups (Chapter 12), these C_{27} bile acids may be products of the intestinal flora in the alligator.

(IV) Occurrence and structure of bile alcohols in mammals

In 1974, Setoguchi et al. found that patients with cerebrotendinous xanthomatosis had an impaired synthesis of bile acids and excreted large amounts of C_{27} bile alcohols in bile and feces [76]. Since then, a number of investigations have revealed the occurrence of bile alcohols in mammals. It is now recognized that, when new analytical methods are applied, traces of bile alcohols can be detected even in biological fluids from healthy humans. Table 3 lists all the known bile alcohols identified in mammals.

Since bile alcohols in mammals may be present in unconjugated form or as glucuronides or sulfate esters, studies of these compounds require techniques for group separation of the different forms. Ion-exchange chromatography has been used for this purpose [77–79]. Bile alcohol glucuronides may be deconjugated by

TABLE 3

Mammalian bile alcohols

Systematic name of bile alcohols	Natural source
(23*S*)-5β-Cholestane-3α,7α,12α,23,25-pentol	Bile and feces from CTX patients
(24*R*)-5β-Cholestane-3α,7α,12α,24,25-pentol	Bile and feces from CTX patients
5β-Cholestane-3α,7α,12α,25,26-pentol	Rabbit bile; human urine
(23*R*)-5β-Cholestane-3α,7α,12α,23-tetrol	Bile and feces from CTX patients
(24*S*)-5α-Cholestane-3α,7α,12α,24-tetrol	Rabbit bile
(24*R*)-5β-Cholestane-3α,7α,12α,24-tetrol	Bile and feces from CTX patients
(24*S*)-5β-Cholestane-3α,7α,12α,24-tetrol	Bile and feces from CTX patients; rabbit bile
5β-Cholestane-3α,7α,12α,25-tetrol	Bile and feces from CTX patients; rabbit bile
5α-Cholestane-3β,7α-diol	Bile from CTX patients
27-Nor-5β-cholestane-3α,7α,12α,24,25-pentol	Human urine
24-Nor-5β-cholestane-3α,7α,12α,25-tetrol	Bile from a patient with cholestasis; rabbit bile
26,27-Dinor-5β-cholestane-3α,7α,12α,24,25-pentol	Bile from a patient with cholestasis
3α,7α,12α-Trihydroxy-26,27-dinor-5β-cholestan-24-one	Bile from a patient with cholestasis

commercially available β-glucuronidase [80], and bile alcohol sulfates may be hydrolyzed by a number of methods [81–83].

Cerebrotendinous xanthomatosis (CTX) is a rare familial sterol storage disease (cf. Chapter 9). The excessive accumulation of cholesterol and cholestanol in tissues of patients with CTX [84], focuses the interest on abnormalities in sterol and bile acid metabolism. Salen and Grundy found that the total bile acid production is significantly decreased in CTX [85]. Paradoxically the activity of cholesterol 7α-hydroxylase is significantly higher than normal [86]. This discrepancy was explained, at least in part, by the finding that appreciable quantities of bile alcohols are excreted in bile and feces of CTX patients [76]. Up to now the following bile alcohols have been isolated and identified by comparison with synthetic samples: 5β-cholestane-3α,7α,12α,25-tetrol [76]; (23*R*)-5β-cholestane-3α,7α,12α,23-tetrol [87]; (24*R*)- and (24*S*)-5β-cholestane-3α,7α,12α,24-tetrols [87]; (23*S*)-5β-cholestane-3α,7α,12α,23, 25-pentol [88,89]; (24*R*)-5β-cholestane-3α,7α,12α,24,25-pentol [76,88]; 5α-cholestane-3β,7α-diol [90]. No bile alcohol possessing a hydroxyl group at the end of the side chain has been found. In all patients examined, the 25-tetrol is the major bile alcohol. The absolute configurations at C-23 of the 23-tetrol and at C-24 of the 24,25-pentol were determined by X-ray crystallography [91] and circular dichroism [92], respectively. The bile alcohols are excreted in unconjugated form in feces, whereas the biliary bile alcohols occur as glucuronoconjugates [80]. The position of the glucuronide moiety is presumably C-3 [80].

In 1980, Kibe et al. found considerable amounts of bile alcohol sulfates in the bile of a patient with cholestasis [81]. Solvolysis of the bile salts gave 3 different bile alcohols which were identified as 24-nor-5β-cholestane-3α,7α,12α,25-tetrol, 26,27-dinor-5β-cholestane-3α,7α,12α,24,25-pentol, and 3α,7α,12α-trihydroxy-26,27-dinor-5β-cholestan-24-one, by comparison with synthetic standards [81]. Nothing is known about the biosynthesis of these C_{25} and C_{26} bile alcohols. Since the accumulation of bile alcohols has not been found in other cases with cholestasis, it seems unlikely that cholestasis is the primary cause of the formation of bile alcohols with unusual side chains.

Trace amounts of bile alcohols resembling those excreted in CTX and in the patient with cholestasis were found in the bile of normal rabbit [93]. The following compounds were identified: 5β-cholestane-3α,7α,12α,25,26-pentol; 5β-cholestane-3α,7α,12α,25-tetrol; (24*S*)-5α- and 5β-cholestane-3α,7α,12α,24-tetrols; 24-nor-5β-cholestane-3α,7α,12α,25-tetrol [93]. This result and our unpublished observations on the presence of bile alcohols in the bile of healthy humans suggest that bile alcohols can be produced even in healthy mammals although in much smaller quantities.

The presence of bile alcohols in human urine was first demonstrated in 1981 by Karlaganis et al. [78]. Studying metabolic profiles of bile acids in urine, they found a number of bile alcohols in the steroid glucuronide fraction. The major compound was identified as 27-nor-5β-cholestane-3α,7α,12α,24,25-pentol [78]. Excretion of this C_{26} bile alcohol as the major bile alcohol in urine from healthy and diseased humans was confirmed by Karlaganis et al. [79] and by Ludwig-Köhn et al. [94]. The latter authors also identified 5β-cholestane-3α,7α,12α,25,26-pentol in human urine [94].

(V) Occurrence and structure of primitive bile acids in mammals

Primitive bile acids in mammals may be classified by carbon numbers as higher bile acids and as cholenoic acid derivatives. A list of primitive bile acids from mammalian sources is given in Table 4.

Higher bile acids and cholenoic acid derivatives in bile of mammals may be conjugated with taurine or glycine. Cholenoic acid derivatives in human urine, meconium, and amniotic fluid may also be present as sulfuric acid esters of the 3β-hydroxyl group. Sulfated and nonsulfated bile acids can be separated by column chromatography using Sephadex LH-20 [95] or the lipophilic anion exchanger, DEAP Sephadex LH-20 [82].

TABLE 4

Mammalian primitive bile acids

Systematic name of primitive bile acid	Natural source
3α,7α,12α-Trihydroxy-27*a*,27*b*-dihomo-5β-cholestane-26,27*b*-dioic acid	Serum of patients with intrahepatic bile duct anomalies
3α,7α,12α,24-Tetrahydroxy-5β-cholestan-26-oic acid	Bile of patients with intrahepatic bile duct anomalies; urine from Zellweger's syndrome
3α,7α,12α,25-Tetrahydroxy-5β-cholestan-26-oic acid	Gastric contents from neonates with high intestinal obstruction
3α,7α,12α,26-Tetrahydroxy-5β-cholestan-27-oic acid	Gastric contents from neonates with high intestinal obstruction
3α,7α,12α-Trihydroxy-5β-cholestan-26-oic acid	Human bile; baboon bile; bile, serum, urine, and feces from patients with intrahepatic bile duct anomalies; bile, serum, and urine from patients with Zellweger's syndrome
3α,7α-Dihydroxy-5β-cholestan-26-oic acid	Human bile; bile, serum, urine, and feces from patients with intrahepatic bile duct anomalies; bile, serum, and urine from patients with Zellweger's syndrome
3α-Hydroxy-5β-cholestan-26-oic acid	Serum of patients with intrahepatic bile duct anomalies
3β-Hydroxycholest-5-en-26-oic acid	Bile and serum of patients with intrahepatic bile duct anomalies
3β-Hydroxychol-5-en-24-oic acid	Human bile, meconium, amniotic fluid, and urine; bile and feces from newborn and fetal guinea pigs
3β,7α-Dihydroxychol-4-en-24-oic acid	Human bile
3β,7α-Dihydroxychol-5-en-24-oic acid	Human bile
3β,12α-Dihydroxychol-5-en-24-oic acid	Human urine and meconium
7α,12α-Dihydroxy-3-oxochol-4-en-24-oic acid	Gastric contents from neonates with high intestinal obstruction

In 1963, Carey and Haslewood isolated trace amounts of (25R)-3α,7α,12α-trihydroxy-5β-cholestan-26-oic acid from human fistula bile [96]. The stereochemistry at C-25 of this bile acid was recently confirmed by direct comparison with reference compounds of known absolute configuration [97]. This trihydroxy-5β-cholestanoic acid also occurs in baboon bile [98]. Hanson and Williams found the corresponding dihydroxy C_{27} bile acid, 3α,7α-dihydroxy-5β-cholestan-26-oic acid, in human bile [99]. The occurrence of these higher bile acids, quantitatively of minor importance, is of interest because they are biosynthetic precursors of two primary bile acids of mammalian species, cholic acid and chenodeoxycholic acid, respectively (Chapter 9).

Eyssen et al. found large quantities of 3α,7α,12α-trihydroxy-5β-cholestan-26-oic acid in the duodenal fluid from two unrelated infants with intrahepatic bile duct anomalies [100]. Hanson et al. have confirmed the presence of this bile acid in elevated amounts in bile, serum, urine, and feces from 2 siblings with the same syndrome [101]. Considerable amounts of 3α,7α-dihydroxy-5β-cholestan-26-oic acid were found by Parmentier et al. in bile, serum, urine, and feces from 3 other children with the same syndrome [102]. Varanic acid was also detected in the bile [102]. In addition, the serum of these patients contained significant amounts of an unusual C_{29} bile acid and small amounts of 3α-hydroxy-5β-cholestan-26-oic acid and 3β-hydroxycholest-5-en-26-oic acid [102,103]. The structure of the C_{29} bile acid was shown to be 3α,7α,12α-trihydroxy-27a,27b-dihomo-5β-cholestane-26,27b-dioic acid (3α,7α,12α-trihydroxy-27-carboxymethyl-5β-cholestan-26-oic acid) [104].

Hanson et al. [105] found increased amounts of 3α,7α,12α-trihydroxy-5β-cholestan-26-oic acid, 3α,7α-dihydroxy-5β-cholestan-26-oic acid, and varanic acid in the urine of 3 infants with Zellweger's syndrome [106]. The same observation was reported by Mathis et al. in 2 other patients with this syndrome [107]. Furthermore, Monnens et al. found an increased amount particularly of the trihydroxy C_{27} bile acid and also of the dihydroxy C_{27} bile acid in bile and serum from 2 infants with this syndrome [108]. The increased concentrations of higher bile acids may be explained by mitochondrial abnormalities in the liver of patients with Zellweger's syndrome [109]. More recent studies indicate that the occurrence of C_{27} bile acids is related to the absence of peroxisomes in this disease (cf. Chapter 9).

Clayton et al. found small amounts of 2 tetrahydroxy C_{27} bile acids along with a number of C_{24} bile acids in gastric contents from neonates with high intestinal obstruction [110]. One of the higher bile acids was identified as 3α,7α,12α,25-tetrahydroxy-5β-cholestan-26-oic acid; another was tentatively identified as 3α,7α,12α,26-tetrahydroxy-5β-cholestan-27-oic acid by its reduction with lithium aluminum hydride to 5β-cyprinol (5β-cholestane-3α,7α,12α,26,27-pentol) [110].

In 1971, Makino et al. found that considerable amounts of 3β-hydroxychol-5-en-24-oic acid were excreted in urine of children with extrahepatic biliary atresia [111]. Since then, the unsaturated C_{24} bile acid has been identified in human meconium [112,113], amniotic fluid [114,115], gallbladder bile from premature and term infants [116], urine from children and adults, both healthy and with liver disease [82,117], and bile and feces from newborn and fetal guinea pigs [118]. The natural occurrence of 3β-hydroxychol-5-en-24-oic acid suggests that the side chain of cholesterol is degraded before modification of the steroid ring system (Chapter 9).

3β,7α-Dihydroxychol-5-en-24-oic acid and its isomer, 3β,7α-dihydroxychol-4-en-24-oic acid, were found in the fistula bile from some patients with cholelithiasis [119]. These bile acids, at least the former, seem to be intermediates in an alternative pathway of chenodeoxycholic acid biogenesis in mammals [119, Chapter 9].

3β,12α-Dihydroxychol-5-en-24-oic acid has been found as a minor bile acid in human meconium [113] and urine [82], and 7α,12α-dihydroxy-3-oxochol-4-en-24-oic acid in gastric contents from neonates with high intestinal obstruction [110].

(VI) Metabolism of bile alcohols and primitive bile acids in mammals

The natural distribution and the chemical structure of bile alcohols and primitive bile acids indicate that these compounds found in lower vertebrates are evolutionary precursors of the common bile acids found in mammalian species. Haslewood proposed that the mechanism of conversion of cholesterol to the common bile acids in mammals is a recapitulation of the evolution of bile salts and thus would entail the intermediary formation of bile alcohols and primitive bile acids similar to or the same as those found in lower species [120]. Thus, studies have been carried out to test whether the naturally occurring bile alcohols and primitive bile acids are intermediates in the biosynthetic pathway between cholesterol and the C_{24} bile acids in mammals. There is no doubt that such studies contributed to the elucidation of the sequence of reactions in the biosynthesis of the mammalian C_{24} bile acids.

At the present time, it is believed that in the major pathway for the formation of cholic acid in mammals, elaboration of the cholesterol nucleus precedes the degradation of the side chain, forming 5β-cholestane-3α,7α,12α-triol (VIII) as an intermediate (Chapter 9) (Fig. 3). The oxidative cleavage of the side chain of VIII to yield cholic acid (XIV) entails an ω-oxidation followed by a β-oxidation. 3α,7α,12α-Trihydroxy-5β-cholestan-26-oic acid (X) was the first naturally occurring primitive bile acid shown to be a biosynthetic intermediate in this sequence. In 1955, Komatsubara administered this bile acid (X), isolated from frog bile, to bile fistula guinea pigs, whose bile does not contain cholic acid, and found cholic acid in the hydrolyzed fistula bile [121]. This conversion was confirmed using radioactive trihydroxy-5β-cholestanoic acid in bile fistula rats [122] and rat liver homogenates [123]. The formation of the trihydroxy-5β-cholestanoic acid from cholesterol in man was demonstrated by Staple and Rabinowitz, who isolated labeled trihydroxy-5β-cholestanoic acid from the fistula bile of patients receiving [26-^{14}C]cholesterol [124]. Carey isolated labeled trihydroxy-5β-cholestanoic acid from the bile of a patient given [4-^{14}C]cholesterol and showed that when the labeled bile acid was administered again to a second bile fistula patient, it was converted efficiently to cholic acid [125].

Masui and Staple [126] and Gustafsson [127] isolated labeled varanic acid (3α,7α,12α,24-tetrahydroxy-5β-cholestan-26-oic acid) (XII) after incubation of [^{3}H]3α,7α,12α-trihydroxy-5β-cholestan-26-oic acid with rat liver preparations. This acid is converted to cholic acid in rat and human in vivo [126,128] as well as in rat

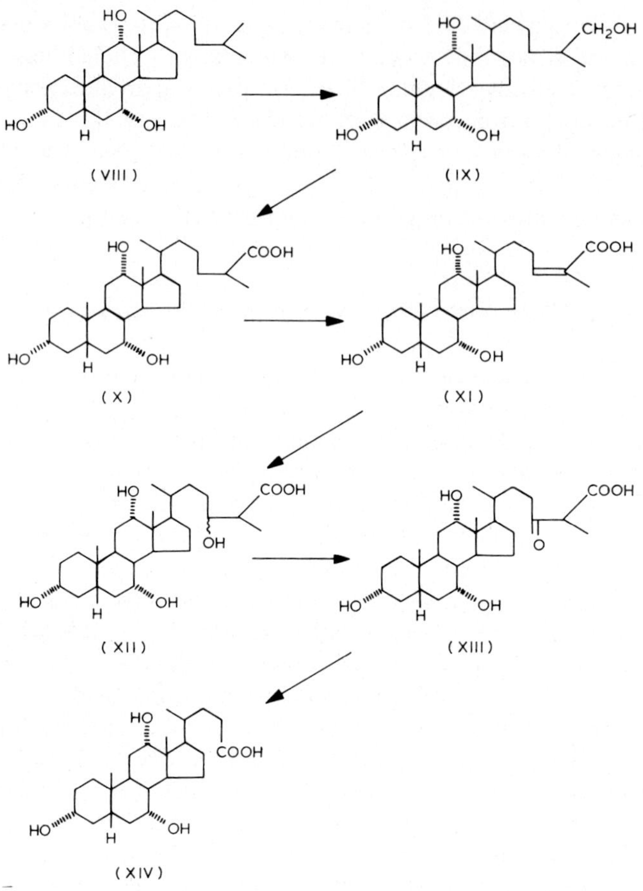

Fig. 3. Biosynthesis of cholic acid(XIV) from 5β-cholestane-3α,7α,12α-triol(VIII).

liver preparations [126,129]. Varanic acid has asymmetric carbons at positions 24 and 25 and thus there are 4 possible diastereoisomers. 3α,7α,12α-Trihydroxy-5β-cholest-24-en-26-oic acid (XI), which is also a probable intermediate in the pathway to cholic acid, has a trisubstituted double bond between C-24 and C-25, giving 2 possible geometrical isomers. Recently, Une et al. have analyzed the labeled products formed in incubations of [7β-^{3}H]3α,7α,12α-trihydroxy-5β-cholestan-26-oic acid (X) with rat liver homogenates [130]. (24E)-3α,7α,12α-Trihydroxy-5β-cholest-24-en-26-oic acid (XI) and (24R,25S)-varanic acid (XII) were identified as the products formed from either (25R)- or (25S)-trihydroxy-5β-cholestanoic acid (X). Neither the 24Z isomer of the α,β-unsaturated acid (XI) nor the other 3 isomers of the β-hydroxy acid (XII) were detected. It is interesting that the stereochemistry of varanic acid biosynthesized by the mammalian liver is identical with that of varanic acid occurring in the lower species.

The major pathway for the formation of chenodeoxycholic acid is thought to be the same as that for cholic acid, with the exception that no 12α-hydroxylation occurs. Thus, 3α,7α-dihydroxy-5β-cholestan-26-oic acid is a probable intermediate, and Hanson has shown that this acid can be made from cholesterol and is efficiently converted to chenodeoxycholic acid but only to a very limited extent to cholic acid [131].

As shown in Fig. 3, the initial reaction in the conversion of 5β-cholestane-3α,7α,12α-triol (VIII) to cholic acid is 26-hydroxylation, forming 27-deoxy-5β-cyprinol (5β-cholestane-3α,7α,12α,26-tetrol) (IX). The in vitro formation from the triol (VIII) and the in vitro conversion of trihydroxy-5β-cholestanoic acid (X) of 27-deoxy-5β-cyprinol (IX) were demonstrated before the detection of this tetrol in nature [132].

5β-Chimaerol, 5β-bufol, 5β-cyprinol, and scymnol are the 24-, 25-, and 27-hydroxylated, and 24,27-dihydroxylated derivatives of 27-deoxy-5β-cyprinol (IX), respectively. It is possible that these naturally occurring bile alcohols could be intermediates in alternative pathways for the formation of cholic acid (XIV) from 27-deoxy-5β-cyprinol (IX). To test this possibility, these cholestanepolyols were labeled with tritium and given to guinea pigs or rats with a biliary fistula [133–136]. Of the tested bile alcohols, 5β-chimaerol and 5β-cyprinol were converted efficiently to cholic acid [135,136]. However, these results do not provide conclusive evidence for alternative pathways of cholic acid formation since the conversion of these bile alcohols to cholic acid may merely reflect a lack of specificity of the enzyme systems involved in the conversion of 27-deoxy-5β-cyprinol (IX) to cholic acid (XIV) via trihydroxy-5β-cholestanoic acid (XII).

Danielsson and Kazuno have shown that 5β-ranol is an efficient precursor of cholic acid in bile fistula rats while 26-deoxy-5β-ranol is not [134]. The mechanism of the side-chain degradation of 5β-ranol is not known but probably an oxidation of the 26-hydroxyl group to a carboxyl group followed by a β-oxidation.

In steroid hormone biosynthesis, cholesterol is degraded to pregnenolone and isocaproic aldehyde via the intermediary formation of 20-hydroxy- and 20,22-dihydroxycholesterols. If the side chain of 5β-cholestane-3α,7α,12α-triol (VIII) were cleaved by an analogous mechanism, the pathway would be initiated by 25-hydroxylation. This proposal is supported by the finding that rat and human liver microsomes can convert 5β-cholestanetriol (VIII) into 5β-cholestane-3α,7α,12α,25-tetrol [137,138]. Moreover, Setoguchi et al. have isolated considerable amounts of the 25-tetrol from bile and feces of patients with CTX [76]. Salen et al. have shown that the 25-tetrol is converted into cholic acid in normal human subjects and CTX patients [139]. However, Yamada has found that in bile fistula rats and guinea pigs 5β-cholestane-3α,7α,12α,25-tetrol is an inefficient precursor of cholic acid compared with 5β-cholestane-3α,7α,12α-triol [140]. Hanson et al. have shown that 27-deoxy-5β-cyprinol (IX) is converted into cholic acid 6 times as efficiently as 5β-cholestane-3α,7α,12α,25-tetrol [141]. These results indicate that the pathway initiated by 25-hydroxylation is unlikely to be important in the formation of cholic acid in normal mammals.

The accumulation of bile alcohols in CTX may be explained by the finding that mitochondria isolated from the liver of CTX patient were completely devoid of 26-hydroxylating activity [142]. The consequences of this defect are discussed in detail in Chapter 9.

In 1967, Mitropoulos and Myant showed that rat liver mitochondria catalyze the conversion of cholesterol into 3β-hydroxychol-5-en-24-oic acid via the intermediates cholest-5-ene-3β,26-diol and 3β-hydroxycholest-5-en-26-oic acid [143]. In favor of the existence of this pathway in man, particularly in the fetus and newborn infants, high concentrations of 3β-hydroxychol-5-en-24-oic acid have been found in biological fluids from the fetus and newborn [111–118]. The conversion of 3β-hydroxychol-5-en-24-oic acid to chenodeoxycholic acid (but not to cholic acid) was demonstrated in rat liver mitochondria and in rats and hamsters with a biliary fistula [144,145].

Yamasaki and his co-workers have proposed an alternative pathway to chenodeoxycholic acid via the side chain degradation of cholest-5-ene-3β,7α-diol to form 3β,7α-dihydroxychol-5-en-24-oic acid [119]. The formation of chenodeoxycholic acid from 3β,7α-dihydroxychol-5-en-24-oic acid was demonstrated in rats [146] and hamsters [147].

(VII) Metabolism of bile alcohols and primitive bile acids in lower vertebrates

Studies on the biosynthesis of bile alcohols and primitive bile acids in lower vertebrates will provide additional information on the formation of the common bile acids in mammals and will help to clarify the molecular evolution of bile salts. However, such studies have been carried out only in a few species of lower vertebrates.

The major bile salt of the carp, *Cyprinus carpio*, is 5α-cyprinol sulfate [21]. When [4-^{14}C]cholesterol was injected intraperitoneally into the carp, radioactive 5α-cyprinol was isolated from gallbladder bile [148]. It has been shown that the initial step in the major pathway for the formation of 5α-cyprinol (VI) from cholesterol (XV) is the 7α-hydroxylation of cholesterol to form cholest-5-ene-3β,7α-diol (XVI) [149] (Fig. 4). It has also been shown that the Δ^5 double bond is isomerized to the Δ^4 position before being reduced [150]. These in vivo studies suggest that until the intermediary formation of a Δ^4 compound, presumably 7α,12α-dihydroxycholest-4-en-3-one (XVII), the sequence of reactions in the biosynthesis of 5α-cyprinol (VI) in the carp is the same as that in the conversion of cholesterol (XV) to cholic acid (XIV) in mammals. 7α,12α-Dihydroxycholest-4-en-3-one (XVII) was found to be converted into 5α-cholestane-3α,7α,12α-triol (XVIII) by the microsomal fraction of carp liver fortified with NADPH [151]. The conversion of the triol (XVIII) to 5α-cyprinol (VI) via 27-deoxy-5α-cyprinol (XIX) was also established. The 26-hydroxylation of the triol (XVIII) was catalyzed by the microsomal fraction fortified with NADPH, and the 27-hydroxylation of 27-deoxy-5α-cyprinol (XIX) was catalyzed by the mitochondrial fraction fortified with NADPH [151].

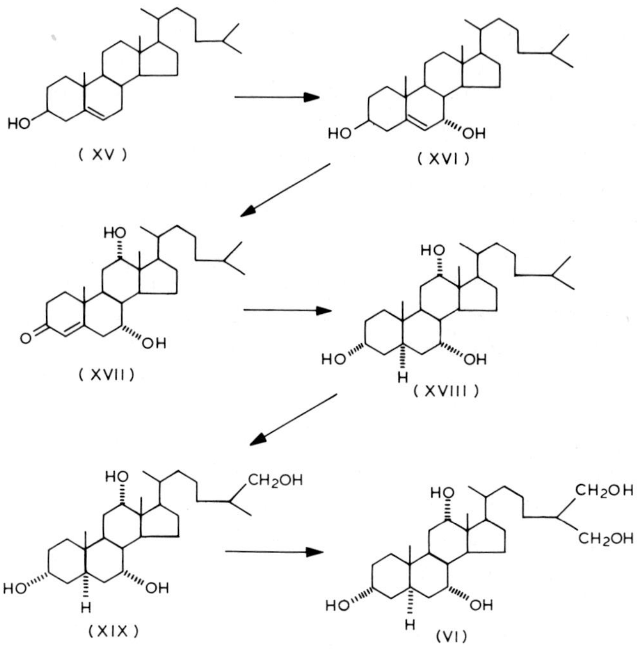

Fig. 4. Biosynthesis of 5α-cyprinol(VI) from cholesterol(XV).

The major bile salts of the giant salamander, *Megalobactrachus japonicus*, are 5α-cyprinol sulfate and tauroallocholate [24]. Amimoto has shown that in this amphibian 27-deoxy-5α-cyprinol (XIX) is efficiently converted into both 5α-cyprinol (VI) and allocholate, while 5α-cyprinol (VI) is an inefficient precursor of allocholate [152,153]. These results suggest that 27-deoxy-5α-cyprinol probably represents a branching point of the biosynthetic pathways leading to either 5α-cyprinol (VI) or to allocholic acid.

The major bile salt of the toad, *Bufo vulgaris formosus*, is 5β-bufol sulfate [15]. It has been shown that in vivo 5β-bufol and 27-deoxy-5β-cyprinol (IX) are formed from cholesterol [33,154] and also from 5β-cholestane-3α,7α,12α-triol (VIII) [155]. In vitro, the cholestanetriol (VIII) was converted into 27-deoxy-5β-cyprinol (IX) [156]. From these results, the following sequence of reactions for the formation of 5β-bufol was proposed: cholesterol (XV) → 5β-cholestane-3α,7α,12α-triol (VIII) → 27-deoxy-5β-cyprinol (IX) → 5β-bufol. Kuramoto et al. injected [2-^{14}C]mevalonate into toads and after 2 weeks isolated radioactive 5β-bufol from gallbladder bile [157]. The isolated labeled 5β-bufol was oxidized with lead tetraacetate to 3α,7α,12α-trihydroxy-27-nor-5β-cholestan-25-one with the liberation of formaldehyde. The C_{26} ketone had the same specific radioactivity as the 5β-bufol, but the formaldehyde was not labeled. The C_{26} ketone was further oxidized to 25-homocholic acid with loss of the terminal methyl group and loss of radioactivity corresponding to 0.8 atom of ^{14}C. These results indicate that the terminal hydroxyl-bearing carbon atom (C-26) of

5β-bufol is derived from C-3′ of mevalonate and the terminal methyl carbon atom (C-27) from C-2. This shows that in the biosynthesis of 5β-bufol the hydroxylation at the end methyl group of the cholesterol side chain is stereospecific as it is in the biosynthesis of the common bile acids in mammals [158].

In the in vivo studies with labeled cholesterol [33] as well as mevalonate [157], the label was incorporated into the minor bile acids of the toad, cholic acid (XIV) and 3α,7α,12α-trihydroxy-5β-cholestan-26-oic acid (X). In contrast, the major bile acids, 3α,7α,12α-trihydroxy-5β-cholest-22-ene-24-carboxylic acid and 3α,7α,12α-trihydroxy-5β-cholest-23-en-26-oic acid, did not become labeled and their biochemical origin is still obscure. The formation of labeled cholic acid and trihydroxy-5β-cholestanoic acid suggests that in the toad 27-deoxy-5β-cyprinol (VIII) is converted to cholic acid (XIV) via the C_{27} bile acid (X) by the same pathway as that in mammals.

The major bile salts of the bullfrog, *Rana catesbeiana*, are the sulfate esters of 5β-ranol and 26-deoxy-5β-ranol [39,41]. Bullfrog bile also contains unconjugated 3α,7α,12α-trihydroxy-5β-cholestan-26-oic acid (X) [45]. Masui has shown that cholesterol (XV) is the source of these bile alcohols and the higher bile acid [159,160]. Betsuki has shown that 5β-ranol and 26-deoxy-5β-ranol are formed from 5β-cholestane-3α,7α,12α-triol (VIII) as well as from varanic acid (XII), and has proposed the following pathway involving decarboxylation of the β-keto acid (XIII): 5β-cholestane-3α,7α,12α-triol (VIII) → 3α,7α,12α-trihydroxy-5β-cholestan-26-oic acid (X) → varanic acid (XII) → 3α,7α,12α-trihydroxy-24-oxo-5β-cholestan-26-oic acid (XIII) → 24-dehydro-26-deoxy-5β-ranol → 26-deoxy-5β-ranol → 5β-ranol [161,162]. This pathway is further supported by the finding that bullfrog bile contains the postulated intermediate 24-dehydro-26-deoxy-5β-ranol as a normal constituent [42].

The conversion of cholesterol to primitive bile acids in lower vertebrates was first demonstrated in 1959 by Briggs et al. in *Alligator mississippiensis* [163]. [26-^{14}C]Cholesterol was given to a bile fistula alligator, and two labeled products were isolated from bile. The major product was identified as 3α,7α,12α-trihydroxy-5β-cholestan-26-oic acid, the major bile acid of the reptile, and the minor one was identical with the second bile acid, later identified as 3α,7α-dihydroxy-5β-cholestan-26-oic acid.

Hoshita et al. have shown that liver microsomes from the green iguana, in which the major biliary bile salt is tauroallocholate, convert 7α,12α-dihydroxycholest-4-en-3-one (XVII) into 5α-cholestane-3α,7α,12α-triol (XVIII) rather than into 5β-cholestane-3α,7α,12α-triol (VIII) which is involved in cholic acid biosynthesis [164]. On the basis of this result and that obtained from studies with carp liver [151], it can be assumed that 5α-bile acids and alcohols are formed from cholesterol by a modification of the biosynthetic pathway to the corresponding 5β isomers in which the only difference is the stereospecific saturation of the Δ^4 double bond of the intermediate XVII.

In summary, the information so far available indicates that the sequence of reactions for the formation of bile alcohols and primitive bile acids in lower vertebrates is very similar to or the same as that for the formation of the intermediates between cholesterol and the common bile acids in mammalian species.

References

1 Cross, A.D. (1961) J. Chem. Soc. 2817–2821.
2 Hoshita, T. (1962) J. Biochem. (Tokyo) 52, 125–130.
3 Bridgwater, R.J., Briggs, T. and Haslewood, G.A.D. (1962) Biochem. J. 82, 285–290.
4 Kazuno, T. and Hoshita, T. (1964) Steroids 3, 55–65.
5 Hammarsten, O. (1898) Z. Physiol. Chem. 24, 322–350.
6 Kihira, K., Yasuhara, M., Kuramoto, T. and Hoshita, T. (1977) Tetrahedron Lett. 687–690.
7 Kihira, K., Une, M., Kuramoto, T. and Hoshita, T. (1979) Hiroshima J. Med. Sci. 28, 167–172.
8 Haslewood, G.A.D. and Tökés, L. (1972) Biochem. J. 126, 1161–1170.
9 Anderson, I.G., Haslewood, G.A.D., Oldham, R.S., Amos, B. and Tökés, L. (1974) Biochem. J. 141, 485–494.
10 Bridgwater, R.J., Haslewood, G.A.D. and Watt, J.R. (1963) Biochem. J. 87, 28–31.
11 Okuda, K., Enomoto, S., Morimoto, K. and Kazuno, T. (1962) J. Biochem. (Tokyo) 51, 441–442.
12 Kouchi, M. (1964) Hiroshima J. Med. Sci. 13, 341–350.
13 Anderson, I.G. and Haslewood, G.A.D. (1970) Biochem. J. 116, 581–587.
14 Amos, B., Anderson, I.G., Haslewood, G.A.D. and Tökés, L. (1977) Biochem. J. 161, 201–204.
15 Okuda, K., Hoshita, T. and Kazuno, T. (1962) J. Biochem. (Tokyo) 51, 48–55.
16 Hoshita, T. (1962) J. Biochem. (Tokyo) 52, 176–179.
17 Kuramoto, T., Kihira, K., Matsumoto, N. and Hoshita, T. (1981) Chem. Pharm. Bull. (Tokyo) 29, 1136–1139.
18 Kuramoto, T., Kikuchi, H., Sanemori, H. and Hoshita, T. (1973) Chem. Pharm. Bull. (Tokyo) 21, 952–959.
19 Une, M., Matsumoto, N., Kihira, K., Yasuhara, M., Kuramoto, T. and Hoshita, T. (1980) J. Lipid Res. 21, 269–276.
20 Hoshita, T., Hirofuji, S., Nakagawa, T. and Kazuno, T. (1967) J. Biochem. (Tokyo) 62, 62–66.
21 Hoshita, T., Nagayoshi, S. and Kazuno, T. (1963) J. Biochem. (Tokyo) 54, 369–374.
22 Hoshita, T., Nagayoshi, S., Kouchi, M. and Kazuno, T. (1964) J. Biochem. (Tokyo) 56, 177–181.
23 Anderson, I.G. and Haslewood, G.A.D. (1964) Biochem. J. 93, 34–39.
24 Amimoto, K. (1966) J. Biochem. (Tokyo) 59, 340–343.
25 Anderson, I.G., Briggs, T. and Haslewood, G.A.D. (1964) Biochem. J. 90, 303–308.
26 Hoshita, T., Yukawa, M. and Kazuno, T. (1964) Steroids 4, 569–574.
27 Kazuno, T., Betsuki, S., Tanaka, Y. and Hoshita, T. (1965) J. Biochem. (Tokyo) 58, 243–247.
28 Sasaki, T. (1966) J. Biochem. (Tokyo) 60, 56–62.
29 Haslewood, G.A.D. and Tammar, A.R. (1968) Biochem. J. 108, 263–268.
30 Hoshita, T., Kouchi, M. and Kazuno, T. (1963) J. Biochem. (Tokyo) 53, 291–294.
31 Hoshita, T., Sasaki, T. and Kazuno, T. (1965) Steroids 5, 241–247.
32 Anderson, I.G., Banister, K.E., Haslewood, G.A.D., Cho, D. and Tökés, L. (1980) Zool. J. Linn. Soc. 68, 41–51.
33 Hoshita, T., Sasaki, T., Tanaka, Y., Betsuki, S. and Kazuno, T. (1965) J. Biochem. (Tokyo) 57, 751–757.
34 Haslewood, G.A.D. (1966) Biochem. J. 100, 233–237.
35 Anderson, I.G., Haslewood, G.A.D., Cross, A.D. and Tökés, L. (1967) Biochem. J. 104, 1061–1063.
36 Anderson, I.G. and Haslewood, G.A.D. (1969) Biochem. J. 112, 763–765.
37 Une, M., Kihira, K., Kuramoto, T. and Hoshita, T. (1978) Tetrahedron Lett. 2527–2530.
38 Haslewood, G.A.D. (1964) Biochem. J. 90, 309–313.
39 Kazuno, T., Masui, T. and Okuda, K. (1965) J. Biochem. (Tokyo) 57, 75–80.
40 Kuramoto, T., Noma, Y. and Hoshita, T. (1983) Chem. Pharm. Bull. (Tokyo) 31, 1330–1334.

41 Noma, Y., Noma, Y., Kihira, K., Yasuhara, M., Kuramoto, T. and Hoshita, T. (1976) Chem. Pharm. Bull. (Tokyo) 24, 2686–2691.
42 Noma, Y., Une, M., Kihira, K., Yasuda, M., Kuramoto, T. and Hoshita, T. (1980) J. Lipid Res. 21, 339–346.
43 Haslewood, G.A.D. and Tökés, L. (1969) Biochem. J. 114, 179–184.
44 Batta, A.K., Salen, G., Cheng, F.W. and Shefer, S. (1979) J. Biol. Chem. 254, 11907–11909.
45 Une, M., Nagai, F. and Hoshita, T. (1983) J. Chromatogr. 257, 411–415.
46 Une, M., Kuramoto, T. and Hoshita, T. (1983) J. Lipid Res. 24, 1468–1474.
47 Hoshita, T. (1959) J. Biochem. (Tokyo) 46, 507–511.
48 Shimizu, T. and Oda, T. (1934) Z. Physiol. Chem. 227, 74–83.
49 Hoshita, T., Okuda, K. and Kazuno, T. (1967) J. Biochem. (Tokyo) 61, 756–759.
50 Hoshita, T. (1959) J. Biochem. (Tokyo) 46, 1551–1552.
51 Amimoto, K., Hoshita, T. and Kazuno, T. (1965) J. Biochem. (Tokyo) 57, 565–570.
52 Haslewood, G.A.D., Ikawa, S., Tökés, L. and Wong, D. (1978) Biochem. J. 171, 409–412.
53 Haslewood, G.A.D. and Wootton, V. (1950) Biochem. J. 47, 584–597.
54 Une, M., Nagai, F., Kihira, K., Kuramoto, T. and Hoshita, T. (1983) J. Lipid Res. 24, 924–929.
55 Kurauti, Y. and Kazuno, T. (1939) Z. Physiol. Chem. 262, 53–60.
56 Haslewood, G.A.D. (1952) Biochem. J. 52, 583–587.
57 Mabuti, H. (1941) J. Biochem. (Tokyo) 33, 117–130.
58 Bridgwater, R.J. and Haslewood, G.A.D. (1952) Biochem. J. 52, 588–590.
59 Mabuti, H. (1941) J. Biochem. (Tokyo) 33, 131–135.
60 Komatsubara, T. (1954) Proc. Jpn. Acad. 30, 618–621.
61 Bridgwater, R.J. (1956) Biochem. J. 64, 593–599.
62 Batta, A.K., Salen, G., Blount, J.F. and Shefer, S. (1979) J. Lipid Res. 20, 935–940.
63 Mendelsohn, D. and Mendelsohn, L. (1969) Biochem. J. 114, 1–3.
64 Shah, P.P., Staple, E. and Rabinowitz, J.L. (1968) Arch. Biochem. Biophys. 123, 427–428.
65 Kuramoto, T. and Hoshita, T. (1972) J. Biochem. (Tokyo) 72, 199–201.
66 Okuda, K., Horning, M.G. and Horning, E.C. (1972) J. Biochem. (Tokyo) 71, 885–890.
67 Kamat, S.Y. and Elliott, W.H. (1972) Steroids 20, 279–294.
68 Tint, G.S., Dayal, B., Batta, A.K., Shefer, S., Joanen, T., McNease, L. and Salen, G. (1980) J. Lipid Res. 21, 110–117.
69 Ali, S.S., Stephenson, E. and Elliott, W.H. (1982) J. Lipid Res. 23, 947–954.
70 Hayakawa, S. (1953) Proc. Jpn. Acad. 29, 279–284.
71 Hayakawa, S. (1953) Proc. Jpn. Acad. 29, 285–288.
72 Okuda, K. and Danielsson, H. (1965) Acta Chem. Scand. 19, 2160–2165.
73 Dean, P.D.G. and Aplin, R.T. (1966) Steroids 8, 565–579.
74 Hoshita, N. and Okuda, K. (1967) J. Biochem. (Tokyo) 62, 655–657.
75 Tint, G.S., Dayal, B., Batta, A.K., Shefer, S., Joanen, T., McNease, L. and Salen, G. (1981) Gastroenterology 81, 114–119.
76 Setoguchi, T., Salen, G., Tint, G.S. and Mosbach, E.H. (1974) J. Clin. Invest. 53, 1393–1401.
77 Setchell, K.D.R., Almé, B., Axelson, M. and Sjövall, J. (1976) J. Steroid Biochem. 7, 615–629.
78 Karlaganis, G., Almé, B., Karlaganis, V. and Sjövall, J. (1981) J. Steroid Biochem. 14, 341–345.
79 Karlaganis, G., Nemeth, A., Hammarskjörd, B., Strandvik, B. and Sjövall, J. (1982) Eur. J. Clin. Invest. 12, 399–405.
80 Hoshita, T., Yasuhara, M., Une, M., Kibe, A., Itoga, E., Kito, S. and Kuramoto, T. (1980) J. Lipid Res. 21, 1015–1021.
81 Kibe, A., Nakai, S., Kuramoto, T. and Hoshita, T. (1980) J. Lipid Res. 21, 594–599.
82 Almé, B., Bremmelgaard, A., Sjövall, J. and Thomassen, P. (1977) J. Lipid Res. 18, 339–362.
83 Parmentier, G. and Eyssen, H. (1975) Steroids 26, 721–729.
84 Salen, G. (1971) Ann. Intern. Med. 75, 843–851.
85 Salen, G. and Grundy, S.M. (1973) J. Clin. Invest. 52, 2822–2835.
86 Nicolau, G., Shefer, S., Salen, G. and Mosbach, E.H. (1974) J. Lipid Res. 15, 146–151.
87 Yasuhara, M., Kuramoto, T., Hoshita, T., Itoga, E. and Kito, S. (1978) Steroids 31, 333–345.

88 Shefer, S., Dayal, B., Tint, G.S., Salen, G. and Mosbach, E.H. (1975) J. Lipid Res. 16, 280–286.
89 Hoshita, T., Yasuhara, M., Kihira, K. and Kuramoto, T. (1976) Steroids 27, 657–664.
90 Björkhem, I., Buchmann, M.S. and Skrede, S. (1983) Biochim. Biophys. Acta 753, 220–226.
91 Kihira, K., Ohira, S., Kuramoto, M., Kuramoto, J., Nakayama, M. and Hoshita, T. (1982) Chem. Pharm. Bull. (Tokyo) 30, 3040–3041.
92 Dayal, B., Salen, G., Tint, G.S., Toome, V., Shefer, S. and Mosbach, E.H. (1978) J. Lipid Res. 19, 187–190.
93 Murata, M., Kuramoto, T. and Hoshita, T. (1978) Steroids 31, 319–332.
94 Ludwig-Köhn, H., Henning, H.V., Sziedat, A., Matthaei, D., Spiteller, G., Reiner, J. and Egger, E.J. (1983) Eur. J. Clin. Invest. 13, 91–98.
95 Makino, I., Hashimoto, K., Shinozuka, K., Yoshino, K. and Nakagawa, S. (1972) Gastroenterology 68, 545–553.
96 Carey Jr., J.B. and Haslewood, G.A.D. (1963) J. Biol. Chem. 238, PC855–PC856.
97 Batta, A.K., Salen, G., Shefer, S., Dayal, B. and Tint, G.S. (1983) J. Lipid Res. 24, 94–96.
98 Shah, P.P., Staple,. E., Shapiro, I.L. and Kritchevsky, D. (1969) Lipids 4, 82–83.
99 Hanson, R.F. and Williams, G. (1971) Biochem. J. 121, 863–864.
100 Eyssen, H., Parmentier, G., Compernolle, F., Boon, J. and Eggermont, E. (1972) Biochim. Biophys. Acta 273, 212–221.
101 Hanson, R.F., Isenberg, J.N., Williams, G.C., Hachey, D., Szczepanik, P., Klein, P.D. and Sharp, H.L. (1975) J. Clin. Invest. 56, 577–587.
102 Parmentier, G.G., Janssen, G.A., Eggermont, E.A. and Eyssen, H.J. (1979) Eur. J. Biochem. 102, 173–183.
103 Janssen, G. and Parmentier, G. (1981) Steroids 37, 81–89.
104 Janssen, G., Toppet, S. and Parmentier, G. (1982) J. Lipid Res. 23, 456–465.
105 Hanson, R.F., Szczepanik-van Leeuwen, P., Williams, G.C., Grabowski, G. and Sharp, H.L. (1979) Science 203, 1107–1108.
106 Bowen, P., Lee, C.S.N., Zellweger, H. and Lindenburg, R. (1964) Bull. Johns Hopk. Hosp. 114, 402–414.
107 Mathis, R.K., Watkins, J.B., Szczepanik-van Leeuwen, P. and Lott, I.T. (1980) Gastroenterology 79, 1311–1317.
108 Monnens, L., Bakkeren, J., Parmentier, G., Janssen, G., van Haelst, U., Trijbels, F. and Eyssen, H. (1980) Eur. J. Pediat. 133, 31–35.
109 Goldfisher, S., Moore, C.L., Johnson, A.B., Spiro, A.J., Valsamis, M.P., Wisniewaki, H.K., Ritch, R.H., Norton, W.T. and Gartner, L.H. (1973) Science 182, 62–64.
110 Clayton, P.T., Muller, D.P.R. and Lawson, A.M. (1982) Biochem. J. 206, 489–498.
111 Makino, I., Sjövall, J., Norman, A. and Strandvik, B. (1971) FEBS Lett. 15, 161–164.
112 Back, P. and Ross, K. (1973) Z. Physiol. Chem. 354, 83–89.
113 Back, P. and Walter, K. (1980) Gastroenterology 78, 671–676.
114 Délèze, G., Sidiropoulos, D. and Paumgartner, G. (1977) Pediatrics 59, 647–650.
115 Délèze, G., Paumgartner, G., Karlaganis, G., Giger, W., Reinhard, M. and Sidiropoulos, D. (1978) Eur. J. Clin. Invest. 8, 41–45.
116 Nittono, H. (1979) Acta Pediat. Jpn. 21, 25–33.
117 Back, P. (1973) Clin. Chim. Acta 44, 199–207.
118 Li, J.R., Marai, L., Dinh, D.M. and Subbiah, M.T.R. (1977) Steroids 30, 815–825.
119 Harano, K., Harano, T., Yamasaki, K. and Yoshioka, D. (1976) Proc. Jpn. Acad. 52, 453–456.
120 Haslewood, G.A.D. (1967) J. Lipid Res. 8, 535–550.
121 Komatsubara, T. (1955) Seikagaku (in Japanese) 27, 519–522.
122 Bridgwater, R.J. and Lindstedt, S. (1957) Acta Chem. Scand. 11, 409–413.
123 Bergström, S., Bridgwater, R.J. and Gloor, U. (1957) Acta Chem. Scand. 11, 836–838.
124 Staple, E. and Rabinowitz, J.L. (1962) Biochim. Biophys. Acta 59, 735–736.
125 Carey Jr., J.B. (1964) J. Clin. Invest. 43, 1443–1448.
126 Masui, T. and Staple, E. (1966) J. Biol. Chem. 241, 3889–3893.
127 Gustafsson, J. (1975) J. Biol. Chem. 250, 8243–8247.

128 Swell, L., Gustafsson, J., Danielsson, H., Schwartz, C.C. and Vlahcevic, Z.R. (1981) J. Biol. Chem. 256, 912–916.
129 Gustafsson, J. (1980) Lipids 15, 113–121.
130 Une, M., Morigami, I., Kihira, K. and Hoshita, T. (1984) J. Biochem. (Tokyo) 96, 1103–1107.
131 Hanson, R.F. (1971) J. Clin. Invest. 50, 2051–2055.
132 Danielsson, H. (1960) Acta Chem. Scand. 14, 348–352.
133 Danielsson, H., Kallner, A., Bridgwater, R.J., Briggs, T. and Haslewood, G.A.D. (1962) Acta Chem. Scand. 16, 1765–1769.
134 Danielsson, H. and Kazuno, T. (1964) Acta Chem. Scand. 18, 1157–1163.
135 Yukawa, M. (1965) Hiroshima J. Med. Sci. 14, 187–194.
136 Yamada, T. (1966) Hiroshima J. Med. Sci. 15, 179–191.
137 Cronholm, T. and Johansson, G. (1970) Eur. J. Biochem. 16, 373–381.
138 Björkhem, I., Gustafsson, J., Johansson, G. and Persson, B. (1975) J. Clin. Invest. 55, 478–486.
139 Salen, G., Shefer, S., Setoguchi, T. and Mosbach, E.H. (1975) J. Clin. Invest. 56, 226–231.
140 Yamada, T. (1966) Hiroshima J. Med. Sci. 15, 375–390.
141 Hanson, R.F., Staples, A.B. and Williams, G.C. (1979) J. Lipid Res. 20, 489–493.
142 Oftebro, H., Björkhem, I., Skrede, S., Schreiner, A. and Pedersen, J.I. (1980) J. Clin. Invest. 65, 1418–1430.
143 Mitropoulos, K.A. and Myant, N.B. (1967) Biochem. J. 103, 472–479.
144 Mitropoulos, K.A. and Myant, N.B. (1967) Biochim. Biophys. Acta 144, 430–439.
145 Kok, E., Burstein, S., Javitt, N.B., Gut, M. and Byon, C.Y. (1981) J. Biol. Chem. 256, 6155–6159.
146 Usui, T. and Yamasaki, K. (1964) Steroids 3, 147–161.
147 Kulkarni, B. and Javitt, N.B. (1982) Steroids 40, 581–589.
148 Hoshita, T. (1964) Steroids 3, 523–529.
149 Hoshita, T. (1967) J. Biochem. (Tokyo) 61, 440–449.
150 Hoshita, T. (1967) J. Biochem. (Tokyo) 61, 633–635.
151 Hoshita, T. (1969) J. Biochem. (Tokyo) 66, 313–319.
152 Amimoto, K. (1966) Hiroshima J. Med. Sci. 15, 213–224.
153 Amimoto, K. (1966) Hiroshima J. Med. Sci. 15, 225–237.
154 Kazuno, T. and Okuda, K. (1961) J. Biochem. (Tokyo) 50, 352–354.
155 Enomoto, S. (1962) J. Biochem. (Tokyo) 51, 393–397.
156 Enomoto, S. (1962) J. Biochem. (Tokyo) 52, 1–4.
157 Kuramoto, T., Itakura, S. and Hoshita, T. (1974) J. Biochem. (Tokyo) 75, 853–859.
158 Atsuta, Y. and Okuda, K. (1981) J. Biol. Chem. 256, 9144–9146.
159 Masui, T. (1961) J. Biochem. (Tokyo) 49, 211–216.
160 Masui, T. (1962) J. Biochem. (Tokyo) 51, 112–118.
161 Betsuki, S. (1966) J. Biochem. (Tokyo) 60, 411–416.
162 Betsuki, S. (1966) Hiroshima J. Med. Sci. 15, 25–33.
163 Briggs, T., Whitehouse, M.W. and Staple, E. (1959) Arch. Biochem. Biophys. 85, 275–277.
164 Hoshita, T., Shefer, S. and Mosbach, E.H. (1968) J. Lipid Res. 9, 237–243.

H. Danielsson and J. Sjövall (Eds.), *Sterols and Bile Acids*

CHAPTER 11

Metabolism of bile acids in liver and extrahepatic tissues *

WILLIAM H. ELLIOTT

Edward A. Doisy Department of Biochemistry, St. Louis University School of Medicine, St. Louis, MO 63104 (U.S.A.)

(I) Introduction

Bile acids synthesized in the liver are primarily derivatives of 5β-cholanic acid; however, bile acids of lower animals and some fishes may be predominantly of the 5α or allo series. A significant feature of these two types of bile acids lies in the planar structure of the 5α-acids as opposed to the 5β-acids where ring A is extended below the planes of rings B, C, and D (Fig. 1). As noted below small quantities of allo acids are now detected from mammalian sources.

(1) Enterohepatic circulation

Eutherian mammals usually synthesize cholic and chenodeoxycholic acids as primary bile acids, which are conjugated in the liver with glycine or taurine; in the remainder of the animal kingdom only taurine conjugates are found. These "bile salts" are secreted by the liver as constituents of bile which is carried via the biliary duct system to the gallbladder. Bile is concentrated in the gallbladder for ultimate discharge into the duodenum where the bile salts are intimately associated with

* This review is limited primarily to C_{24} bile acids, derivatives of 5β- or 5α-cholanic acids. The IUPAC system of nomenclature properly indicates by number of position of the carboxyl group, e.g., 5β-cholan-24-oic acid. The name "cholanic acid" proposed by Wieland is used here instead of the longer IUPAC designation as 24-oic acid. The term "allo" applied to the 5α-bile acids is also used. Since bile acids exist largely as anions in physiological fluids and tissues, they are designated with the suffix "ate", as in cholate, glycocholate, lithocholate-3-sulfate, and chenodeoxycholate-3-glucuronide. The meaning of the term "bile acid" has been addressed recently by Lester et al. [1]. The term "bile salts" will be limited here to those conjugates of bile acids derivatized through the carboxyl group primarily with glycine or taurine. Tables of bile acids or bile alcohols and their types of conjugates in animals (identified by class and species [2,3,4–6] are recommended.

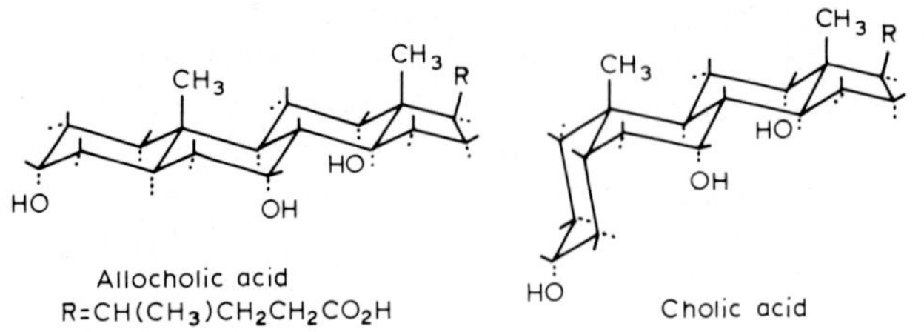

Fig. 1. Comparison of structures of 5α- and 5β-bile acids. Allocholic acid (3α,7α,12α-trihydroxy-5α-cholanic acid); cholic acid (3α,7α,12α-trihydroxy-5β-cholanic acid).

dietary lipids and its various digestive products. While most of the latter constituents are absorbed in the upper 100 cm of the small intestine, conjugated bile acids are absorbed passively from all sites of the gastrointestinal tract, pass through the duodenum–jejunum, and are largely absorbed in the ileum, by active transport mechanisms [7,8]. The lower section of the small intestine contains microorganisms, as does the large intestine which receives the constituents of the small bowel. Bacteria at these sites biotransform bile salts by 3 principal types of reactions: hydrolysis of the amide linkage of the conjugate to liberate free bile acid, removal of the C-7 hydroxyl group and oxidation–reduction of existing hydroxyl or generated keto groups (Chapter 12). After absorption, this mixture of modified bile acids is returned almost completely to the liver by the hepatic portal circulation in the process known as enterohepatic circulation (Fig. 2). This process of recycling is not restricted to bile salts or bile acids. A small fraction (0.2–0.6 g in man) of bile acids is not absorbed in the process and is lost to the body as fecal bile acid. Many of the products returned to the liver are chemically modified before they are recycled as bile salts. Products which survive this cycle several times as new entities compared to the primary bile acids are known as secondary bile acids. Prominent among these in human bile are deoxycholic and lithocholic acids. Each is a product of the action of those bacteria which promote loss of the 7α-hydroxyl group; deoxycholic is derived from cholic, and lithocholic from chenodeoxycholic acid. The term tertiary bile acids is applied to products of hepatic or intestinal metabolism of secondary bile acids which differ from the primary bile acid. Reviews on enterohepatic circulation are available [7,8]. It should be noted that the rat is one of a few species which does not have a gallbladder.

(2) Subcellular location

Results of studies over a period of about 20 years confirm that cytoplasm is the major subcellular location of bile acids in rat liver [9–11] and that cholic acid is the major bile acid. Kurtz et al. [10] reported 64% of hepatic bile acids in cytosol, 33% in microsomes, and 3% in mitochondria of male rats, and 69%, 26% and 6%, respectively in these fractions of female rat liver. Table 1 shows the relative proportions of 7 non-sulfated bile acids in these fractions of liver from male and female rats [10].

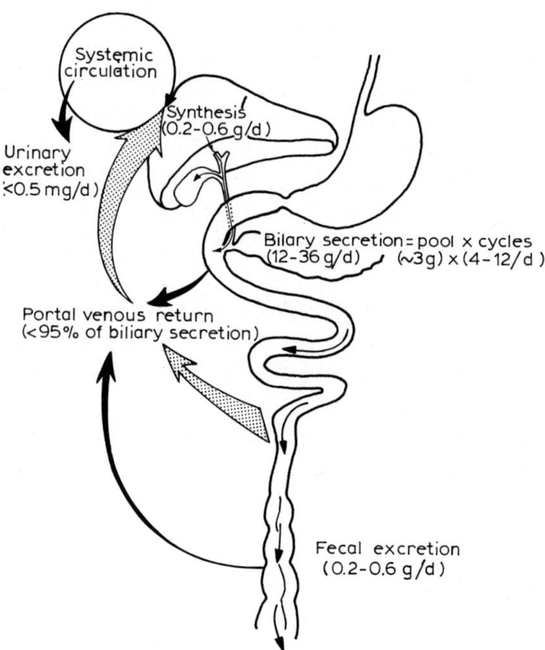

Fig. 2. The enterohepatic circulation in man. Reprinted with permission from ref. 7.

TABLE 1

Percentage of non-sulfated bile acids in rat liver subcellular fractions [a]

Fraction	LC	DC	CDC	HDC	β-MC	α-MC	C	Others
Mitochondria								
Male (8) ($\bar{x}$)	1.2	13.0	3.9	8.6	3.7	–	49.2	20.4
Female (6) ($\bar{x}$)	14.2	16.5	16.0	5.2	–	–	41.9	6.2
$p <$	0.025	N.S.	0.025	N.S.	0.0005	–	N.S.	–
Microsomes								
Male ($\bar{x}$)	4.2	10.5	10.6	14.7	11.1	3.0	30.8	15.1
Female ($\bar{x}$)	3.2	7.7	17.2	14.5	5.1	3.4	38.0	10.9
$p <$	N.S.	N.S.	0.025	N.S.	0.05	N.S.	N.S.	–
Cytosol								
Male ($\bar{x}$)	1.4	3.9	4.5	6.4	13.3	7.1	40.9	22.5
Female ($\bar{x}$)	4.2	7.0	9.0	5.3	4.1	6.8	48.2	15.4
$p <$	0.05	0.0125	0.0125	N.S.	0.0005	N.S.	0.025	–

[a] LC, lithocholate; DC, deoxycholate; CDC, chenodeoxycholate; HDC, hyodeoxycholate; β-MC, β-muricholate; α-MC, α-muricholate; C, cholate; Others, unidentified by difference to equal 100%; $\bar{x}$ = mean value; values considered significant if p was less than 0.05; N.S., not significant.

Sex differences were marked: in the male all fractions contained higher proportions of β-muricholate and lower percentages of chenodeoxycholate; in the female larger amounts of deoxycholate and cholate appeared in cytosol, and greater quantities of lithocholate were found in cytosol and mitochondria. An increase of hepatic β-muricholate from 10% in normal male rats to 72% of the bile acids after 8–10 days of bile duct ligation has been reported [12]. The concentration of hepatic bile acids in neonatal rats (0–1 to 60 days) increased after birth with a concomitant increase in chenodeoxycholate and β-muricholate and a decrease in cholate until the 60th day of life [13].

In normal human liver (7 samples) identified bile acids were cholate (54%), chenodeoxycholate (28%), and deoxycholate (18%) [12]. With a more sensitive system of analysis (glass capillary gas chromatography–mass spectrometry and selected ion monitoring) the values reported for 5 bile acids from 10 samples of normal human bile [14] were cholate (41%), chenodeoxycholate (39%), deoxycholate (15%), ursodeoxycholate (4%), and lithocholate (1%).

(3) Transport and hepatocytes

Bile acids and their conjugates are transported in the liver by carrier processes which are largely not understood. It has been demonstrated that the process is dependent on sodium ions and requires metabolic energy. Papers of Anwer et al. [15], Kitani and Kanai [16] and Erlinger [17] summarize current concepts.

Biochemical studies with isolated rat hepatocytes have largely been concerned with transport mechanisms [15], secretion of bile acids [17–19], or biosynthesis of bile acids [20]. The capacity of cultured hepatocytes to convert tauro- or glycochenodeoxycholate to α- and β-muricholates [19,21] and to produce bile salts (glycine or taurine conjugates) during the dark phase of the diurnal cycle [21] has been established. Demonstrations of other metabolic transformations by hepatocytes are included in the following sections.

(II) Conjugation

(1) Amino acids and proteins

Conjugation of bile acids with glycine has been observed in mammals, whereas non-mammals generally produce only taurine conjugates [2]. The ratio of glycine to taurine varies with the species [2] and is influenced by diet, vitamins, hormones [22] or other factors [23]. In organ culture, fragments of human fetal liver formed conjugates with cholic acid in preference to chenodeoxycholic acid. Taurine conjugates of primary bile acids predominate throughout gestation and remain the major bile salt synthesized until well into the first year of life. Supplementation of the culture medium with taurine resulted in enhanced taurocholate production with reduced synthesis of glycocholate; supplementation of the medium with hydrocortisone reversed the glycine–taurine ratio [24].

Ornithine and arginine have been detected in conjugation with bile acids. Ornithocholic acid has been identified in bile of oxen and humans [25], particularly in patients infected with *Klebsiella pneumoniae,* and in bile of guinea pigs treated with *K. pneumoniae* [26]. Argininocholate was characterized from bile of isolated perfused rat liver [27[]. Ciliatine (2-aminoethylphosphonic acid, the phosphoric analog of taurine), found free and combined in phospholipids of protozoa, marine, fresh water vertebrates and in mammalian tissue, has been identified in bovine gallbladder bile in conjugation with cholic acid, which was named ciliatocholic acid [28].

The rather insoluble lithocholic acid was reported bound to hepatic protein [29] probably via the ϵ-amino group of lysine [30,31]. Lithocholate was liberated from the protein via the action of cholylglycine hydrolase [32], and thus differs from the binding of bile acids associated with albumin. The biological importance of tissue-bound lithocholate has yet to be established.

(a) Preparation and analyses of CoA derivatives

Coenzyme A (CoA) derivatives of bile acids were prepared [33,34] by a modification of the mixed anhydride procedure for the synthesis of palmityl CoA. A yield of 70% was calculated from the quantity of cholylhydroxamate formed after treatment of the CoA derivative with hydroxylamine. By modification of this procedure and purification of the products by chromatography on Sephadex LH-20, aqueous solutions of CoA derivatives of cholic, chenodeoxycholic, deoxycholic, and lithocholic acids were pbtained, frozen at $-70°C$, and shown to be free from hydrolysis for several months [35].

Separation of bile acid-CoA derivatives from unreacted coenzyme A can be effected by high-performance liquid chromatography. With a radial compression C_{18} column containing 5-μm particles, coenzyme A was eluted with or immediately following the solvent front with a solvent system of 2-propanol/50 mM phosphate buffer (pH 7.0) (160/340) and a UV-detector set at 254 nm. Capacity factors for the above CoA derivatives are 1.50, 3.50, 4.18 and 9.50. CoA derivatives of comparable 5α-bile acids, purified and separated in a similar manner were eluted just prior to the comparable 5β-derivative [36]. CoA derivatives of 5β- and 5α-cholate and deoxycholate were separable with this solvent system.

(b) Bile acid: CoA synthetase (bile acid CoA ligase) and bile acid CoA: glycine/taurine-N-acyltransferase

A mechanism for hepatic formation of amino acid conjugates of bile acids developed from early investigations of Siperstein and Murray [37], Bremer [38], and Elliott [39] is summarized as follows:

$$\text{Bile acid} + \text{ATP} + \text{CoASH} \rightleftharpoons \text{bile acid-SCoA} + \text{AMP} + \text{PP}_i \quad (1)$$

$$\text{Bile acid-SCoA} + \text{amino acid} \rightleftharpoons \text{bile acid-NH-amino acid} + \text{CoASH} \quad (2)$$

Bremer and Gloor [40] concluded that enzymes for both reactions were present in hepatic microsomes, but recent studies with microsomes of rat [40–42] and human liver [43] have confirmed the presence of only one enzyme, CoA ligase. The assay system, essentially that for long-chain acyl-CoA ligase [42,43], includes 50 mM NaF, a phosphate buffer (pH 7.5), the enzyme preparation, and constituents of Eqn. 1. Product formation was linear up to 12 min with added protein (between 0.1 and 1.2 mg) from a crude microsomal fraction. Sterol carrier protein [44], cysteine or nicotinamide [38,40] were without effect. This rate-limiting enzyme in the two-step sequence catalyzing conjugation of bile acids exhibits a diurnal variation such that the time of maximum enzyme activity coincides with predicted maximum activity of cholesterol 7α-hydroxylase and the time of maximal biosynthesis of bile acids [45]. The enzyme has not been purified.

Amino acid-*N*-acyltransferase [37,40,41,44] has been purified 90-fold from the soluble fraction of rat liver [46], and 900-fold from the soluble fraction of bovine liver [47]; the preparations were capable in each case of utilizing taurine or glycine. The enzyme obtained from rat liver showed significant activity in the presence of 50 μM deoxycholyl-CoA or cholyl-CoA with glycine, taurine, β-alanine, and aminomethanesulfonate. No significant activity was noted with D- or L-alanine, L-glutamine, L-ornithine, L-arginine, or L-lysine [46]. Similarly, no significant activity was noted with the bovine liver enzyme preparation [48] with the first four of these amino acids, or with L-serine or β-alanine; the latter may represent a species difference. No significant activity was found with palmitoyl-CoA, succinyl-CoA, acetyl-CoA, benzoyl-CoA or phenylacetyl-CoA [46]. The relative activity of the enzyme with glycine and bile acid CoA derivatives was cholyl-CoA (100%), deoxycholyl-CoA (106%), lithocholyl-CoA (75%), and chenodeoxycholol-CoA (58%). A bisubstrate kinetic analysis of the bovine enzyme preparation showed a Tetra Uni ping-pong mechanism which was supported by the demonstration that the enzyme catalyzed the release of CoA from cholyl-CoA in the absence of glycine. The preparation was considered to have a purity of about 80%.

A study of the specificity of bile acid-CoA : glycine/taurine *N*-acyltransferase from bovine liver to form glycine conjugates with 16 different bile acid-CoA analogs showed that norcholyl-CoA failed to form a conjugate; homocholyl-CoA (the analog of cholic acid with an additional CH_2 in the side chain) exhibited a 30-fold decrease in activity compared to cholyl-CoA [34].

The formation of conjugates of taurine or glycine is induced by glucocorticoids, specifically dexamethasone [49]. In primary cultures of rat fetal liver dexamethasone increased and maintained taurine conjugation of cholate, chenodeoxycholate, and deoxycholate; short-term cultures of adult rat hepatocytes maintained conjugation of bile acids with glycine and taurine [49]. Enzymatic activity was stimulated by low doses of ethynylestradiol [50], and has been verified in fetal liver [51].

(c) Metabolism

Hydrolysis of glyco- or tauroconjugates provides the free amino acids [52]. Glycine is degraded in mitochondria to CO_2 and 5,10-methylene-H_4 folate, which reacts with another molecule of glycine to provide serine, a precursor of pyruvate. Thus, from 2 moles of glycine, 1 mole of CO_2 and 1 mole of pyruvate are formed. Studies in humans with [1-^{14}C]glycine conjugates of cholate, chenodeoxycholate and deoxycholate in which the bile acids were labeled with ^{3}H showed that $^{14}CO_2$ was expired. ^{3}H was largely retained in the bile acid. The daily fractional turnover of the glycine moiety was 3 times greater than that of the bile acid, and glycocholate could be dehydroxylated in the intestine to glycodeoxycholate without deconjugation [53,54]. Measurement of $^{14}CO_2$ production is the basis of a simple breath test for patients with increased bile acid deconjugation [55]. The metabolism of taurine is limited to a few known biochemical reactions, namely, conversion to inorganic sulfate by intestinal microorganisms but not by mammalian tissue.

(2) Sulfates

Palmer [56–58] first reported the presence in human bile of a sulfate ester of lithocholate in as much as 40–80% of the small amounts of available glyco- and taurolithocholate. Following intragastric or intraduodenal intubation of glyco-[24-^{14}C]lithocholic acid 3-sulfate to rats with bile fistulas, 70–89% of the radioactivity was recovered in bile [59]; allolithocholate 3-sulfate was also reported in rat bile [60]. The radioactive conjugate was absorbed intact without loss of the sulfate, and was not metabolized in the liver (e.g., to the muricholates or chenodeoxycholate) [58,59]. Similarly, chenodeoxycholate 3-sulfate was not metabolized after intravenous infusion into rats or hamsters with or without obstruction of the biliary tract [58,59,61]. Lithocholate 3-sulfate is efficiently removed from the body [62].

Sulfated allo bile acids occur more abundantly or exclusively in bile of female rats compared to male rats [63]. Allochenodeoxycholate monosulfate was the major sulfated allo acid from the female; none was detected in bile of the male. Other monosulfates identified include allocholate, and the 3β epimers of allochenodeoxycholate and allocholate. From female rat bile collected 48–60 h after cannulation allochenodeoxycholate constituted about 63% of the mono- and disulfate fractions; none was found in bile from male rats. Sulfates of allocholate and the 3β epimers of allochenodeoxycholate and allocholate were present in smaller amounts. Initial collections of bile (0–12 h) contained allodeoxycholate and its 3β epimer in the monosulfate fraction.

A cytosolic sulfotransferase has been identified in rat liver and kidney which utilizes 3′-phosphoadenosine-5′-phosphosulfate (PAPS) and shows a greater rate of sulfation for glycolithocholate than lithocholate. In an assay with the enzyme preparation, PAPS, and conjugated bile acids, 3 unidentified products were formed from taurocholate suggesting multiple sulfation of more polar conjugated bile acids [64]. The enzyme from liver, proximal intestine or adrenals of hamster produced only glycochenodeoxycholate 7-sulfate. Comparable results with the enzyme from kidney will be discussed in Section VI.3. Hepatic enzyme from the female hamster shows 4-fold greater activity than that of the male [65].

A partially purified preparation from cytosol of human liver utilized PAPS and showed activity toward estrone, dehydroepiandrosterone and phenol; the product formed from chenodeoxycholate was identified as the 7-sulfate, whereas that from deoxycholate was the 12-sulfate. No disulfates were detected [66]. The enzyme in rat fetal liver was induced by glucocorticoids to promote synthesis of deoxycholate 3-sulfate from deoxycholate [49]. Greater activity was observed in the female rat [67] which was stimulated by low doses of ethinylestradiol [50]. Rat hepatic sulfotransferase showed a diurnal variation for glycolithocholate, but not for lithocholate, suggesting multiple hepatic sulfotransferases for bile acids [45]. Perinatal hamsters exhibited hepatic sulfotransferase activity for the free bile acid (lithocholate) or the glycine or taurine conjugate [68].

(3) Glucuronides

Glucuronides of bile acids were first reported [69] in urine of jaundiced patients. Material in the "sulfate fraction" of bile acids removed from urine was more polar in thin-layer chromatography (TLC), and was hydrolyzed with a β-glucuronidase preparation. Glucuronides identified (in mg/24 h) were cholic (3.0), chenodeoxycholic (1.48), deoxycholic (0.57) and 3β-hydroxy-5-cholenic acid (0.64). Chenodeoxycholic acid 3-glucuronide was identified by mass spectrometry [70] and chemical synthesis [71]. The hepatic origin of these conjugates was demonstrated by incubation of labeled bile acids and UDP-glucuronic acid with hepatic microsomal protein derived from rats given phenobarbital. Labeled product from lithocholate, chenodeoxycholate and cholate was more polar by TLC than the parent bile acid. The activity of the glucuronyltransferase decreased with the number of hydroxyl groups in the bile acid; lithocholate and chenodeoxycholate were 9.1 and 4.4 times more active than cholate. Induction of enzyme activity was enhanced by pretreatment with phenobarbital, or in vitro with bile salts or Triton X-100, and was reduced with methylcholanthrene [72]. A microsomal UDP-glucuronosyltransferase (UDP-glucuronate: β-D-glucuronosyltransferase, EC 2.4.1.17) obtained from human liver was active toward bile acids, bilirubin and estradiol. Enzymatic activity decreased with an increasing number of hydroxyl groups in the bile acid [73]. The enzyme, purified 50-fold from rat liver microsomes, catalyzed the conjugation of chenodeoxycholate and of testosterone with UDP-glucuronic acid, but did not glucuronidate estrone, bilirubin, 4-nitrophenol or morphine [74]. Other evidence supports the existence of additional hepatic UDP-glucuronyltransferases for other substrates. Bile acid glucuronides identified from urine will be considered in Section VI.3.

(III) Hydroxylation of the steroid nucleus

Evidence for a specific nuclear hydroxylation of a bile acid is frequently associated with similar information pertinent to another position of the bile acid. Thus, the topics in this section are titled separately, but evidence may also be cited under headings for other nuclear positions; e.g. β-muricholic acid, a $3\alpha,6\beta,7\beta$-trihydroxy acid, will be included in sections dealing with hydroxylation at 3α, 6β and 7β positions.

(1) 3α-Hydroxylation

Bile acids formed in the liver from cholesterol have a 3α-hydroxyl group [75]. Several investigations have been carried out to ascertain whether the liver can 3α-hydroxylate a C_{24} bile acid devoid of that group. Initial experiments designed to study intestinal absorption of 5β-cholanic acid showed that male rats given the radioactive acid intraperitoneally excreted unidentified more polar metabolites [76]. The experiment was repeated with rats and guinea pigs with biliary fistula. Radioactive metabolites identified from rat bile were: 7α-hydroxy-5β-cholanic acid (I) (5%); 7-oxo-5β-cholanic acid (II) (6%), chenodeoxycholic acid (6%), β- and α-muricholic acids (III) (13 and 2.5%, respectively) [77,78]. From guinea pig bile the labeled metabolites were: compounds I (21%), II (8%), III (15%), and 7-oxolithocholic acid (2%) [79,80]. The ability of the rat and guinea pig to 3α-hydroxylate was inferred by the presence of labeled chenodeoxycholate in the bile of each species, and the identification of metabolites of this acid, α- and β-muricholates in rat bile, and 7-oxolithocholate in guinea pig bile [81]. The presence of labeled 7α-hydroxy- and 7-oxo-5β-cholanate and chenodeoxycholate, and the absence of lithocholate in the bile of each species suggested that initial hydroxylation of 5β-cholanate occurred at C-7. No 12α-hydroxylated metabolites were identified from either species, in accord with the concept that hepatic 12α-hydroxylation does not occur once the cholesterol-like side chain has been modified [82].

In a similar study of the metabolism of [24-^{14}C]12α-hydroxy-5β-cholanic acid given intraperitoneally to male rats with bile fistulas [83], the identified biliary metabolites were 7α,12α-dihydroxy-5β-cholanic acid (26%), deoxycholic acid (18%), cholic acid (15%), 6β,12α-hydroxy-5β-cholanic acid (0.8%), and 12% of unchanged 12α-hydroxy-5β-cholanic acid. Thus, 5β-cholanic acid and 12α-hydroxy-5β-cholanic acids are hydroxylated in vivo preferentially in the order 7α, 3α, and 6β. The preference for 7α-hydroxylation may be related to the concentration and properties of the active enzyme. Although no in vitro studies have been carried out, these studies infer the ability of hepatic tissue to provide characteristic 3α-hydroxy bile acids from derivatives devoid of a C-3 oxygen. How often this activity is required is questionable, because of the abundance of 3-hydroxylated sterol derivatives provided to and by the liver.

(2) 6β- and 6α-hydroxylation

The conversion of lithocholate to 3α,6β-dihydroxy-5β-cholanate by the rat [84–86], mouse [87] and chicken [88] confirmed the presence of an active hepatic 6β-hydroxylase. Earlier studies reported the metabolism of chenodeoxycholate [89,90] in the rat and mouse [81,91,92] to α-murocholic acid (3α,6β,7α-trihydroxy-5β-cholanic acid) and to β-muricholic acid [89,90,93,94] (3α,6β,7β-trihydroxy-5β-cholanic acid).

Other precursors of the muricholates via 6β-hydroxylation include 5β-cholanic acid [78], lithocholic acid [84–86], 7-oxolithocholic acid [95,96], and ursodeoxycholic acid (3α,7β-dihydroxy-5β-cholanic acid) [97]. The rat metabolized 12α-hydroxy-5β-cholanic acid to 6β,12α-dihydroxy-5β-cholanic acid [83] and a small amount of 6β,7α,12α-trihydroxy-5β-cholanic acid [98]. 3α,6β,12α-Trihydroxy-5β-cholanic acid was isolated from urine of surgically jaundiced rats after administration of deoxycholate [99]. A series of bile acids from rat bile of unconfirmed structures but containing the 6β,7β-diol will be reviewed in Section III.3.

The male rat is more efficient than the female in conversion of chenodeoxycholate to α-muricholate [100], and of taurochenodeoxycholate to tauro-α-muricholate [101]. Taurochenodeoxycholate is preferred to chenodeoxycholate as substrate for microsomal enzyme preparations. The 6β-hydroxylase system requires NADPH and O_2 for activity and is a cytochrome-P-450-dependent system [91,102]. Enzymatic activity is inhibited by carbon monoxide [103], and is stimulated about 20% by a high carbohydrate diet [104], 3–4-fold following treatment with phenobarbital [86,105,106], and 2–3-fold after biliary obstruction [107]. A higher activity of 6β-hydroxylase with respect to lithocholate has been observed in germ-free compared to conventional rats; the metabolite was 3α,6β-dihydroxy-5β-cholanate [108]. This enzyme preparation also produced 6β-hydroxy-4-pregnene-3,20-dione from progesterone. A reconstituted system containing partially purified cytochrome P-450 and NADPH–cytochrome P-450 reductase catalyzed 6β-hydroxylation of lithocholate and of taurochenodeoxycholate [105]. An active 6β-hydroxylase has been considered to be rather exclusive to the rat and mouse, but β-muricholate has been recently reported as a constituent of bile of a child with intrahepatic cholestasis [109]. β-Muricholate and other 6β-hydroxylated bile acids found in extrahepatic sources will be treated in Section VI.3.

Microsomal preparations from hog or human liver [110–112] fortified with an NADPH-generating system 6α-hydroxylate lithocholate or taurolithocholate to hyodeoxycholate or taurohyodeoxycholate, respectively. The major bile acids of the pig are hyocholic acid (the 3α,6α,7.α-triol) [113,114], chenodeoxycholic acid and hyodeoxycholic acid. Early studies [115] demonstrated that chenodeoxycholate is 6α-hydroxylated to hyocholate, and that hyodeoxycholate disappeared from pig bile after interruption of enterohepatic circulation; thus, hyodeoxycholate is derived from hyocholate by 7α-dehydroxylation via intestinal microflora [115,116]. After administration of radioactive hyodeoxycholate to the pig with a bile fistula, the only identifiable radioactive produce was the conjugate acid. In 1971 Haslewood [117] reported the identification of hyodeoxycholate from bile of germ-free pigs, constituting about 4% of the total biliary bile acids. To explain this apparent contradiction with earlier work, Haslewood [3] suggested that the germ-free pigs may have become adapted to a special vegetarian diet.

An uncertainty also exists with human hepatic 6α-hydroxylase. Hyodeoxycholate has not been isolated from human bile. Despite the above-reported conversion of taurolithocholate to taurohyodeoxycholate [112], investigators have been unable to demonstrate hydroxylation of conjugated or free mono- or dihydroxy bile acids with human liver homogenates. With radioactive taurolithocholate and human hepatic microsomes fortified with NADPH, less than 1% of the radioactivity was found in fractions more polar than the substrate [118], whereas with lithocholate less than 0.5% change occurred; these results are comparable to thoseof Carey and Williams [119] and Normal and Palmer [120]. Metabolites of hyodeoxycholate were not detected in bile of women with asymptomatic non-calcified gallstones receiving hyodeoxycholate (0.75–1 g/day) for 4 months [121]. Thus, hyodeoxycholate is not metabolized in the pig or human. 3β,6α-Dihydroxy-5β-cholanic acid was reported as a constituent of pig bile and gallstones [122], but it may also be a product of the action of intestinal bacteria recycled via enterohepatic circulation. Urinary 6α-hydroxy bile acids including hyocholate, hyodeoxycholate, 3α,6α/β,12α-trihydroxy- and 3α,6α,7α,12α-tetrahydroxy-5β-cholanate [123–125] will be reviewed in Section VI.3.

In the bile fistula rat administered radioactive hyodeoxycholate was recovered largely unchanged [106]. However, from urine of surgically jaundiced rats a small amount of a more polar labeled metabolite was isolated and identified as ω-muricholate (the 3α,6α,7β-triol) [127]. The presence of other metabolites (α- and β-muricholates, 3α,6β-dihydroxy-5β-cholanate and 6-oxo-allolithocholate) suggested that the 6-oxo derivative was a common intermediate in the epimerization of the 6α-hydroxyl of hyodeoxycholate to the 6β-hydroxyl of α-, β- and ω-muricholates and of 3α,6β-dihydroxy-5β-cholanate [127]. The importance of the role of the 6-oxo derivative was confirmed by Einarsson [128] and Thomas et al. [129] in similar experiments with 3α,6β-dihydroxy-5β-cholanate. Thus, the rat differs from the pig in ability to synthesize the 6β-hydroxylated bile acids (α- and β-muricholates and 3α,6β-dihydroxy-5β-cholanate) rather than the 6α-hydroxylated acids. ω-Muricholate has been shown to be also a metabolite of β-muricholate in the rat due to intestinal microorganisms [130] (cf. Chapter 12). The 6α-hydroxylase of rat liver hydroxylates allochenodeoxycholate to provide small amounts of allohyocholate (the 3α,6α,7α-triol of the 5α series) [131].

(3) 7α- and 7β-hydroxylation

7α-Hydroxylation of lithocholate occurs in the rat [84,85], guinea pig [84], hamster [132], dog [87], and the pig [110]. Similarly allolithocholate is hydroxylated to allochenodeoxycholate by the rat [133]; 5β-cholanic acid [97] and 12α-hydroxy-5β-cholanic acid [83] were also 7α-hydroxylated. 3α,6β-Dihydroxy-5β-cholanate is metabolized by the rat with a bile fistula mainly to β-muricholate (35%) and not more than 0.2% of α-muricholate [129]. Deoxycholate is 7α-hydroxylated to cholate by the rat [90,134], chicken [135] and as the taurine conjugate by cod fish [136]. There is no evidence of 7α-hydroxylation of bile acids by human liver [118,139]. Bile acid 7α-hydroxylase activity has not been detected in the dog, guinea pig, and a number of other species which retain substantial quantities of deoxycholate in bile [2,3].

Because of the importance of this enzyme in the rat, extensive studies have been carried out in this species. Like the activity of 6β-hydroxylase on taurochenodeoxycholate, taurodeoxycholate is 7α-hydroxylated much more efficiently than deoxycholic acid. Enzymatic activity is inhibited by carbon monoxide, is stimulated about 3-fold by prior treatment of the animal with phenobarbital, but is not stimulated by biliary drainage, starvation or prior treatment with cholestyramine [103]. A reconstituted system of partially purified cytochrome P-450 and NADPH–cytochrome P-450 reductase efficiently catalyzed 7α-hydroxylation of taurodeoxycholate [103,138]. From rats treated with phenobarbital, the microsomal enzyme was purified about 7 times based on P-450, or 12-fold based on specific activity; the partially purified enzyme exhibited a single band on sodium dodecyl sulfate–polyacrylamide gel electrophoresis, and a molecular weight of about 54000. Assay of this purified material with NADPH–cytochrome P-450 reductase, dilauroylglyceryl-3-phosphocholine and NADPH showed that the preparation was free from 12α-, 25- and 26-hydroxylase activities [139].

7β-Hydroxylated acids found naturally include ursodeoxycholate (the 3α,7β-diol), 3α,7β,12α-trihydroxy-5β-cholanate, and β-muricholate. Although ursodeoxycholate is well known as a constituent of bear bile, no experiments have been reported to ascertain the mechanism of biosynthesis in this species. Small amounts of conjugates of ursodeoxycholate and 3α,7β,12α-trihydroxy-5β-cholanate have been identified as constituents of human gallbladder or duodenal bile [140]. Current evidence indicates that these materials are products of bacterial synthesis (cf. Chapter 12). 3α,7β,12α-Trihydroxy-5β-cholanate is not metabolized by rat liver, but is modified in the cecum to deoxycholic acid [141]. The mechanism of conversion of α-muricholate to β-muricholate in the rat has not been elucidated. A ketol (6β-hydroxy-7-one) has been postulated as an intermediate [93,94], but this axial ketol is labile to rearrangement to the 6-oxo-7β-hydroxy configuration, neither of which has been isolated [94]. From metabolic studies of 5β-cholanic acid [77], the ratio of quantities of the metabolites chenodeoxycholate, β-muricholate and α-muricholate (10 : 24 : 5) was markedly different from the ratio of these acids derived from radioactive chenodeoxycholate (11 : 3 : 4), suggesting that the pathway to β-muricholate from 5β-cholanate was different from that through chenodeoxycholate.

Strong evidence for hepatic 7β-hydroxylase was obtained from studies with isolated rat hepatocytes, in which a 10–15-fold increase in production of tauro-β-muricholate over conjugated chenodeoxycholate was obtained [142], in agreement with the observations of Kemper et al. [143]. Since the liver cells are in suspension and have lost their "secretory mechanism", chenodeoxycholate served as a continuing substrate for production of the 3α,6β,7β-triol. Six new bile acids related to β-muricholate containing unsaturation in the steroid nucleus or in the side chain have been isolated from bile of Sprague–Dawley rats given daily injections of ethynylestradiol [144]. Two of these may be similar to unsaturated 6β,7β-diols found with β-muricholate in male rat bile only in the first 12 h after cannulation [145].

Ikawa [146] suggested that the presence in rat bile of an equal mixture of sulfate and taurine conjugates of 3β,7β-dihydroxy-5-cholenate indicates that 7β-hydroxy bile acids make little contact with hepatic microsomal enzymes and are therefore excreted into bile much faster without significant change to the bile acid or to the main components of the bile. Recall that the 7β-hydroxyl projects upward on the non-polar side of the bile acid.

(4) 12α-Hydroxylation

With few exceptions 12α-hydroxylation is carried out on C_{27}-sterol substrates by a hepatic microsomal enzyme (cf. Chapter 9). Those exceptions include 12α-hydroxylation of chenodeoxycholic acid in the python [147], eel [148], chicken [149] and trout [150]. Perfusion of isolated rat liver with chenodeoxycholic acid was reported to provide about 30% of the biliary acids as cholic acid [151]. Taurochenodeoxycholate was hydroxylated to taurocholate by liver homogenates of cod fish [1[36].

In the 5α series allochenodeoxycholate is 12α-hydroxylated to allocholate in the bile fistula rat [131] or with a hepatic microsomal preparation from rat, rabbit or human liver fortified with NADPH [152,153]. Kallner [133] noted that small amounts of more polar derivatives were present in rat bile, with largely unchanged allochenodeoxycholate. Allohyocholate was identified as a minor metabolite [154]. With rabbit liver microsomal preparations, allochenodeoxycholate is a competitive inhibitor for 12α-hydroxylation of 7α-hydroxy-cholest-4-en-3-one and 5α-cholestane-3α,7α-diol, precursor of cholic and allocholic acids, respectively [155]. Allocholic acid has also been characterized as a metabolite of 3β,7α-dihydroxy-5-cholenic acid after intraperitoneal injection into carp [156].

(5) 16α-Hydroxylation

The boa constrictor and python (species Boidae) are unique in that the major bile acid is pythocholic acid (3α,12α,16α-trihydroxy-5β-cholanic acid) along with varying

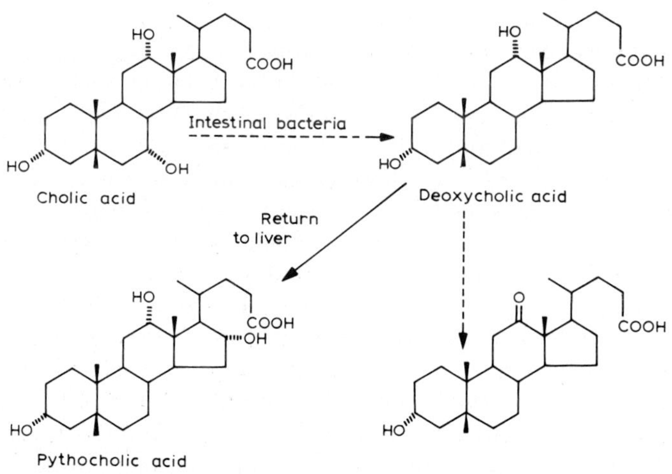

Fig. 3. Biosynthesis of pythocholic acid.

amounts of cholic acid [157]. The pathway of metabolism developed from studies with radioactive cholesterol, deoxycholate, and cholate is shown in Fig. 3.

Two unusual processes occur in the liver of these snakes: 12α-hydroxylation of chenodeoxycholate to form cholate and 16α-hydroxylation of deoxycholate to produce pythocholate. Labeled cholesterol afforded labeled cholic and chenodeoxycholic acids, but not labeled pythocholic acid. Labeled pythocholic acid was obtained following administration of labeled deoxycholate. There was evidence for the presence of a radiometabolite corresponding to 3α,12α-dihydroxy-16-oxocholanic acid in feces after oral administration of labeled cholesterol, cholic or deoxycholic acid, but the material was absent from bile [147].

(IV) Hydroxylation in the side chain

22S. Haemulcholic acid ([22*S*]-3α,7α,22-trihydroxy-5β-cholanic acid) isolated from bile of *Parapristipoma trilineatum* (Haemulidae, marine teleost), and recently *Mormyrus cabbalus* [158] has been synthesized and characterized as a 22*S*-hydroxy bile acid, one of a few with an extranuclear hydroxyl group [159]. Chenodeoxycholate, cholate and haemulcholate are present as taurine conjugates in bile of the fish. The origin of this acid is unknown, but it has been suggested that the acid may represent a product of β-oxidation of chenodeoxycholate.

23. Three naturally occurring bile acids hydroxylated at position 23 are 3α,7α,23-trihydroxy-5β-cholanic acid from bile of seals, sea-lions, and walruses (order Pinnipedia), 3α,12α,23-trihydroxy-5β-cholanic acid (bitocholic acid) from bile of snakes such as the Gaboon viper (*Bitus gabonica*) and Puff adder (*B. arietans*), and 3α,7α,12α,23-tetrahydroxy-5β-cholanic acid from bile of sea-lions, walruses, seals, the above viper and adder and certain Colubridae [2]. Specimens of seal bile obtained by Hammarsten in 1899 re-examined about 60 years later provided chenodeoxycholate, cholate, "α-phocaecholic acid" (3α,7α,12α,23-tetrahydroxy-5β-cholanic acid) and "β-phocaecholic acid" (3α,7α,23-trihydroxy-5β-cholanic acid) [160]. Recent investigations of samples of biliary acids from Antarctic seals have established that these two derivatives have the 23α configuration [161]. Haslewood has utilized the term phocaecholic acid for the 3α,7α,23α-triol, and has discontinued [162] use of the prefixes "α-" and "β-". If phocaecholic acid is shown to be a primary bile acid in Pinnipedia, Haslewood [2,3] has suggested that chenodeoxycholate is the probable precursor, whereas deoxycholic should be the precursor of bitocholate, analogous to the formation of pythocholic acid from deoxycholate.

The origin of the 3α,7α,12α,23ξ-tetrahydroxy-5β-cholanic has been studied [163] with subcellular fractions of adder (*Vipera berua*) liver with the following conclusions: the active microsomal enzyme requires NADPH and O_2; deoxycholate is not converted to cholate, but to 3α,7β,12α-trihydroxy-5β-cholanate. Bitocholic acid could result from two pathways: (a) cholate is converted to 3α,7α,12α,23ξ-tetrahydroxy-5β-cholanate by hepatic 23-hydroxylase; the tetrahydroxy acid is 7α-dehydroxylated by intestinal microorganisms to produce bitocholate (the 3α,12α,23ξ-trihydroxy acid) and returned to the liver by enterohepatic circulation; (b) cholate is 7α-dehydroxylated by intestinal microorganisms to deoxycholate which is returned to the liver for 23-hydroxylation. Pathway (a) was favored since less than 5 times as much bitocholate was produced from [24-^{14}C]deoxycholate as from [24-^{14}C]cholate.

Products identified from incubation of [24-^{14}C]deoxycholate with a microsomal fraction of adder liver included 12α-hydroxy-3-oxo-5β-cholanate, 3α,7β,12α-trihydroxy-5β-cholanate and bitocholate, but no bitocholate was detected from similar incubations with [24-^{14}C]cholate [163].

3α,7α,12α,23-Tetrahydroxy-5β-cholanic acid has also been identified by mass spectrometry as a significant constituent of the taurine fraction from urine of cholestatic subjects [164]. Further comment will be found in Section VI.3.

(V) Oxidoreduction

Ketonic bile acids are returned to the liver via enterohepatic circulation, but only 9% of the bile acids of fasting human serum are monooxo acids [165]; little or none of these derivatives is found in bile. Reduction of these ketonic bile acids is carried out in the liver apparently by cytosolic hydroxysteroid dehydrogenases. The major products are the α-hydroxy derivatives (e.g., 3α-, 7α-, and 12α-hydroxyl groups) regardless of the configuration at position 5. From in vitro studies with synthetic 3-oxo-5β-cholanates and rat liver homogenates Usui and Yamasaki [166] found that variable amounts of 3α- and 3β-hydroxy products were formed. Kallner [167] concluded that the ratio of such products was related to the ratio of concentrations of substrate to enzyme used. Thus, as the ratio [substrate]/[enzyme] was increased, an increase in the proportion of 3β epimer was found. Berséus [168] purified a 3α-hydroxysteroid dehydrogenase from the $100\,000 \times g$ supernatant fraction of rat liver up to 70-fold and showed that the preparation fortified with NADPH catalyzed reduction of 3-oxo-5β- or 5α-cholanates, 7α-hydroxy-3-oxo-, 7α,12α-dihydroxy-3-oxo-5β-cholanates and appropriate C_{27}-, C_{21}- or C_{19}-steroids to the 3α derivatives; 5α derivatives showed a slower rate of reaction. Ikeda et al. [169] reported that a similar preparation had a molecular weight of 32 500 dalton, was active on C_{19}-, C_{21}-, and C_{23}–C_{26}-sterols, and was inhibited by reagents containing Hg^{2+}.

The stereochemistry of the reduction was elucidated by use of [4A-^{3}H]NADPH, [4B-^{3}H]NADPH or the comparable forms of NADH; only the tritium from the [4A-^{3}H]NADPH or [4A-^{3}H]NADH was incorporated into the product, probably in the 3β position [170]. Whether more than one 3-hydroxysteroid dehydrogenase active on 3-oxo-bile acids exists in cytosol of liver cells remains to be determined.

Microsomal fractions contain 3α- and 3β-hydroxysteroid dehydrogenases which do not appear to be derived from cytosol [171]. Thus, microsomal 3α-hydroxysteroid dehydrogenase preferentially utilized [4B-^{3}H]NADH instead of [4A-^{3}H]NADPH preferred by the cytosolic enzyme. Microsomal 3β-hydroxysteroid dehydrogenase was inactive toward ethanol, and thus is not an active component of alcohol dehydrogenase [172]. These dehydrogenases were active with C_{19}, C_{21}, C_{24} and C_{27}

3-oxosteroids, and showed a higher ratio of $3\alpha/3\beta$ products from C_{19}- and C_{21}-steroids with microsomal preparations from female rats than from male rats regardless of the configuration at C-5. Only 3-oxo-5β-cholanate was studied in these experiments, where the rate of product formation and ratio of epimers ($3\alpha/3\beta$) was greater with NADH + microsomes from females, whereas the rate was greater with NADPH + microsomes from males [171].

A study of the reduction of [24-^{14}C]3-oxo-5β-cholanic acid in bile fistula rats given [1-$^{2}H_2$]ethanol showed that all metabolites had a 3α-hydroxy group and all radioactive products (lithocholate, 3α,6β-dihydroxy-5β-cholanate, chenodeoxycholate and β-muricholate) contained about 13 atom% excess deuterium in the 3β position. Thus, the 3β-hydroxy-5β-steroid dehydrogenase isoenzyme of alcohol dehydrogenase [172] has no function in the reductive metabolism of bile acids. Cholic acid was not radioactive but contained deuterium at the 3β, 5β and other positions, probably because of the transfer of deuterium from ethanol via NADH to NADPH, which it utilized in the biosynthesis of cholesterol and bile acids and in oxido reduction of the 3-hydroxyl group of the latter [173].

Although cholesterol is the major source of 5β-bile acids, an unsaturated acid, 3β-hydroxy-5-cholenic acid [174] has been found in meconium, mainly as the sulfate [175], in bile of a boy with a deficiency of 3β-hydroxysteroid dehydrogenase [176], and in urine of healthy persons and individuals with liver disease [164]. The details of metabolism of 3β-hydroxy-5-cholenic acid to lithocholate have not been entirely elucidated, but the mechanism for conversion of the 3β-hydroxy-Δ^5 to the 3-oxo-Δ^4 derivative has been formulated in the C_{27} series (cf. Chapter 9). Briefly, the 3β-ol is dehydrogenated by a microsomal enzyme fortified with NAD to provide the 3-oxo-Δ^4 system [177,178]. Whether a $\Delta^5 \rightarrow \Delta^4$ isomerase is essential is not known, since there is no direct evidence for the formation of the intermediary 3-oxo-Δ^5 system; the rate-limiting step is the dehydrogenation of the 3β-ol which may prevent accumulation of the 3-oxo-Δ^5 system [177]. The reduction of the double bond at 4–5 to the 5β- or 5α-bile acid is catalyzed by the respective Δ^4-3-oxosteroid 5β- or 5α-reductase obtained from liver cytosol [170], and has been purified about 10-fold [178]. The formation of the 3-oxo-5β derivative requires the enzyme and NADPH; the proton from the A side (4A-NADPH) appeared in the product as the 5β-H, whereas the proton at C-4 is derived from the aqueous medium. Formation of the 5α derivative requires (4B-NADPH) in a similar mechanism (Fig. 4) [179]. Reduction of the 3-oxo product is then catalyzed by 3α-hydroxysteroid dehydrogenase as discussed above.

3β,7α-Dihydroxy-5-cholenic acid, postulated as an intermediate in the mitochondrial synthesis of chenodeoxycholate from 7α-hydroxycholesterol [180,181], and a closely allied product, 3α,7α-dihydroxy-4-cholenic acid, have each been isolated from bile of hens and humans. Incubation of 3β,7α-dihydroxy-5-cholenic acid with rat or carp hepatic microsomal preparations fortified with NADPH provided 3-oxo-7α-hydroxy-4-cholenic acid. Administration of the Δ^5 acid to rats with cannulated bile ducts provided biliary metabolites identified as chenodeoxycholate, α- and β-muricholates. Similar incubation of 3-oxo-7α-hydroxy-4-cholenic

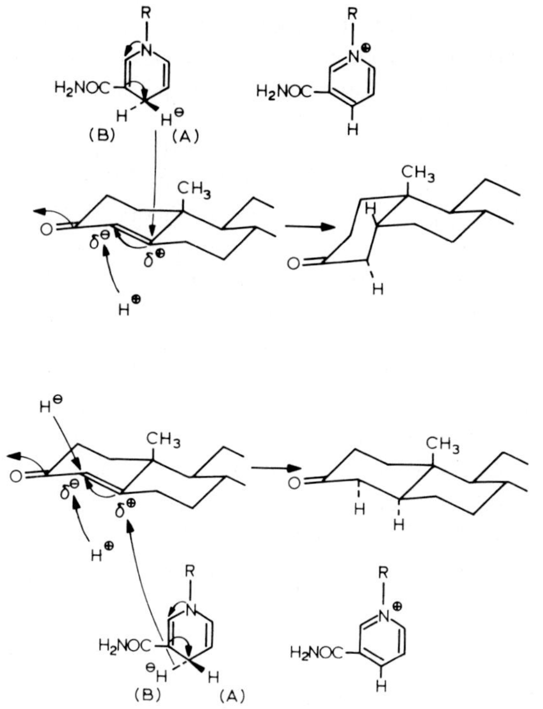

Fig. 4. Mechanism and stereochemistry of enzymatic reduction of a 3-oxo-Δ^4-steroid to a 3-oxo-5β-steroid (upper) and a 3-oxo-5α-steroid (lower section). Reprinted with permission from ref. 179.

acid with the 105 000 $\times g$ supernatant fraction from liver provided acidic metabolites as chenodeoxycholate (7.8%), trihydroxy (6%) and monohydroxy (16%) acids [182]. The activities of the microsomal enzyme, 3β-hydroxy-Δ^5-steroid dehydrogenase, and the two cytosolic enzymes, Δ^4-3-oxosteroid 5β-reductase and 3α-hydroxysteroid dehydrogenase are consonant with the above observations. Reduction by microsomal enzymes of 3-oxo-4-cholenic acid provided all 4 isomers of 3ξ-hydroxy-5ξ-cholanic acid by the male rat, whereas only allolithocholate (excreted as the sulfate) was formed by the female rat [183]. With an active 5α-reductase in female rat liver, allochenodeoxycholate may be derived from 3-oxo-7α-hydroxy-4-cholenic acid or its precursors in the female rat as reported by Eriksson et al. [145]. The metabolism of 3β,7α-dihydroxy-5-cholenic acid to allocholate by carp was noted in Section III.4.

3β-Hydroxy derivatives of bile acids (iso-bile acids) are generally products of the action of intestinal microorganisms [184] (see Chapter 12). Bile from female rats contained the 3β epimers of allocholate and allochenodeoxycholate in the sulfate fraction collected 48–60 h after cannulation, presumably free of material carried in enterohepatic circulation; more was found in comparable samples of male rat bile. From bile collected in the first 12 h after cannulation the sulfate fraction of male and female rats contained the above two derivatives and the sulfate of the 3β

epimers of allodeoxycholate [145]. A study of the metabolism of 3β isomers of [24-^{14}C]chenodeoxycholate and [3α-^{3}H]ursodeoxycholate was carried out in rats with cannulated bile ducts. After intraduodenal infusion of the free acids or their taurine conjugates, 97% of the radioactive materials in either case was present in portal blood as the administered iso derivative, whereas in bile 97% ofthe radioactivity was present in the naturally occurring 3α derivatives. The tritium from [3α-^{3}H]isoursodeoxycholate was found completely in the 3β position in biliary ursodeoxycholate [185].

Prior to and during a lengthy assessment of the effects of oral administration of relatively large amounts of ursodeoxycholate on humans with gallstones, extensive studies were initiated on the chronic toxicity and metabolism of this bile acid in humans [196]. Analyses of human bile during the period of ingestion of the bile acid showed that about 50% of bile acids was ursodeoxycholate. Apparently, through the course of enterohepatic circulation, dehydrogenation of dihydroxy bile acids provides 7-oxolithocholate, which is a precursor of biliary chenodeoxycholate and ursodeoxycholate by a ratio of at least 10 : 1; some evidence suggests that biliary chenodeoxycholate derived from administered 7-oxolithocholate is itself a source of biliary ursodeoxycholate. An extensive review on this topic is available [186].

(VI) Extrahepatic studies

Metabolic changes in the structure of bile acids may occur in other tissues. This section considers those areas where modified bile acids have been identified or where bile acids have been found for the first time. In many cases definitive information is lacking as to the exact site where these modifications in structure have occurred.

(1) Brain

Lithocholic acid has been detected in trace amounts in brain of guinea pigs with experimental allergic encephalomyelitis and in multiple sclerosis brain tissue. Incubation of radioactive lithocholate for long periods with homogenates of rat brain promoted dehydrogenation to 3-oxo-5β-cholanate or provided 3α,6β-dihydroxy-5β-cholanate in 1–6% yield [187]. The reduction of 3-oxo-5β-cholanate to lithocholate was effected with the supernatant from brain of rat [188] or guinea pig; lithocholate was rapidly removed from brain and excreted in feces [187,189]. Since there was suggestive evidence of the presence in guinea pig brain of 3β-hydroxy-5-cholenic acid, consideration of an alternative mitochondrial pathway of degradation of cholesterol to lithocholate via 3β-hydroxy-5-cholenic acid [174, Chapter 9] may be warranted. Further studies are needed to clarify these observations.

(2) Cecum

Modifications of bile acids in the cecum may be attributed to intestinal bacterial metabolism, although there have been no studies to ascertain whether mucosal cells of the cecum may contain the necessary enzymes. The conversion of deoxycholate to allodeoxycholate in rat cecum was studied [190] with labeled 12α-hydroxy-3-oxo-5β-cholanate (I), 12α-hydroxy-3-oxo-5α-cholanate (II), 12α-hydroxy-3-oxo-4-cholenic acid (III) and allodeoxycholate (IV). After intraperitoneal administration of each of the above materials, the distribution of dihydroxy acids in rat bile was: I, 98% deoxycholate; II, 98% allodeoxycholate; and III, 55% deoxycholate and 45% allodeoxycholate. After intracecal administration the distribution in bile was: I, 88% deoxycholate; II, 41% deoxycholate and 59% allodeoxycholate; IV, 66% allodeoxycholate and 34% deoxycholate. The relative amounts of these two acids were similar in bile and feces after intracecal administration. A probable mechanism can be written as follows:

Deoxycholate ⇌ 12α-hydroxy-3-oxo-5β-cholanate ⇌ 12α-hydroxy-3-oxo-4-cholenic acid

Allodeoxycholate ⇌ 12α-hydroxy-3-oxo-5α-cholanate ⇌ 12α-hydroxy-3-oxo-4-cholenic acid

Similarly, after intracecal administration of allocholic acid to rats, bile contained allocholate, cholate, allodeoxycholate and deoxycholate; from allochenodeoxycholate, chenodeoxycholate and allochenodeoxycholate were the products, and from allolithocholate mainly allochenodeoxycholate and chenodeoxycholate were obtained [133].

(3) Urine

Reports of bile acid sulfates in human urine [56,57] have prompted studies of urinary bile acids under various conditions [164,191,192], and have stimulated investigators to develop new analytical systems to ascertain their chemical composition. Although most of the 37 bile acids in Table 2A have assigned structures with hydroxyl groups at positions 1, 2, 3, 6, 7, 12 and 23, a rather large number of minor urinary bile acids not included in the table await structural elucidation. Data in Table 2A were compiled from studies of urinary samples from healthy patients [164], patients with hepatobiliary diseases [109,123–125,164,191–197], late pregnancy and recurrent cholestasis of pregnancy [125,198], and healthy newborn children [199].

1ξ-Hydroxylation. Hydroxylation at C-1 of major human biliary acids has been demonstrated. 1β,3α,12α-Trihydroxy-5β-cholanate is a product [200] of metabolism of deoxycholate by Penicillium sp. ATCC 12556, and a urinary metabolite in patients given [24-^{14}C]deoxycholate [123]. Similar experiments with [24-^{14}C]cholate afforded the tetrol, now characterized as 1β,3α,7α,12α-tetrahydroxy-5β-cholanate [123,201]. This tetrol has also been tentatively identified in gastric contents of neonates with duodenal atresia [202]. A urinary 1-hydroxylated derivative of chenodeoxycholate has been obtained from patients with hepatitis [194]. Very likely 1β-hydroxylation occurs in the liver [203].

TABLE 2

Bile acids identified from (A) human urine, or (B) human meconium

A Bile acid [a]	Fraction [b]	References	GL [b]	B Meconium
23-nor-5β-3α,7α,12α-ol	U, G, T	164,193–195,198		209
Tetrol [c]	U, G, T	164,198		209 [d]
5β-3α,6α,7α,12α-ol	U, G, T	123,164,193,194,197 [d]–199 [d]		
5α-3α,7α,12α-ol	G, T, MoS	164,194,195,198		209
5β-1β,3α,7α,12α-ol	G, T	123,164,193,194,197 [d]–199 [d]		209 [d]
5β-3α,7α,12α,23-ol	G, T	164,193,194,198		
5β-3α,7α,12α-ol	U, G, T, MoS	109,124,164,192–194,196–199		175, 209
5α-3α,7β,12α-ol	U, G, T	124,164,195		
5β-3α,6β,12α-ol [d]	U, G	164,193,194,198	193	
5α-3α,12α-ol	G, MoS	164,193,194		
5β-3α,6α,12α-ol [d]	U, G, T, MoS	125,198	125,193	
5β-3β,7α-ol	MoS	124,164,194,198		
5β-1β,3α,12α-ol	U, G, T, MoS	123,164,193–195,198,200		
5α-3α,7α-ol	MoS	164,194,195,198		
5β-3β,12α-ol	MoS	164,194,198		
5β-3α,6α,7α-ol	U, G, T, MoS	109,123,124,164,193–195,197–199	125,193	209
5β-3β,7β,12α-ol	U, G	164,194,198		
5β-3α,7β,12α-ol	U, G, T	124,164,194,195,198		175 [d]

2β-Hydroxylation. The 2β-hydroxylated derivative of cholic acid, 2β,3α,7α,12α-tetrahydroxy-5β-cholanate, was characterized as a minor component of gastric contents of neonates with duodenal atresia [202]. Identification was facilitated by the availability of the authentic compound, arapaimic acid, which was isolated from bile of *Arapaima gigas* (Chapter 10) and was synthesized [204]. This tetrol is also a minor urinary metabolite of cholate in patients with intrahepatic cholestasis [123]. A polar bile acid formulated as a 2,3,6,7-tetrol obtained from urine of healthy newborn infants [199] apparently differs from an unidentified urinary tetrol from patients with cholestasis [164].

6-Hydroxylation. Urinary acids hydroxylated at position 6, especially 6α, include hyodeoxycholate, hyocholate, 3α,6α/β,12α-trihydroxy- and 3α,6α,7α,12α-tetrahydroxy-5β-cholanates. Hyocholate, the major bile acid in urine, serum and duodenal fluid of a child with intrahepatic cholestasis [109], is a major urinary metabolite of chenodeoxycholate in patients with intrahepatic cholestasis, while 3α,6α,12α-trihydroxy-5β-cholanate is only a minor metabolite of deoxycholate [123]. The 3α,6α,7α,12α-tetrahydroxy acid, obtained from urine of patients with liver diseases [194] and from gastric contents of neonates with duodenal atresia [203] is another metabolite of cholic acid [123]; several unidentified tetrols have yet to be char-

TABLE 2 (continued)

A Bile acid [a]	Fraction [b]	References	GL [b]	B Meconium
5β-3α,12α-ol	U, G, T, MoS	164,192–194,196,198	125,193	175,209
5β-3α,12β-ol	U, G, T, MoS	164,193,194,198		
5β-3α,7α-ol	U, G, T, MoS	109,124,164,192–194,196–199	125,193	175,209
5β-3α,6β-ol	G, Mos	164,193,194,198		
5α-3α-ol	MoS	164,191,193,194,198		
Δ-diol [c]	MoS	164,193,198		209 [d]
5β-3α,6α-ol	T, MoS	124,164,193,194,198	125,193	209
Δ^5-3β,12α-ol	G, MoS	164,193,194,198		209
5α-3β,12α-ol	T, MoS	164,193,194,198		
5β-3α-ol	MoS	124,164,191,192,194,196,198	125	175,209
5β-3α,7β-ol	MoS	124,164,192–194,198		175
Δ^5-3β-ol	MoS	164,191–194,198,199		175,209
5β-3β-ol-12-one	G, MoS	164,194		
5β-3α-ol-12-one	G, MoS	164,193–196,198		
5β-3α,6β,7β-ol	–	109		
2,3,6,7-tetrol [c]	–	199		
5β-3α,7α-ol-12-one	–	196		
5β-3α,12α-ol-7-one	–	196		
5β-3α-ol-7,12-dione	–	196		

[a] Configuration at C-5 and of hydroxyl groups are indicated by Greek letters; Δ indicates double bond; superscript denotes position of double bond.
[b] U, unconjugated; G, glycine conjugated; T, taurine conjugated; MoS, monosulfate; GL, glucuronide.
[c] Positions of substituents not known.
[d] Stereochemistry of hydroxyl groups is tentative.

acterized, but it is likely that these 6α-hydroxylated bile acids are also products of hepatic metabolism [123].

In patients treated with phenobarbital, tetrahydroxy bile acids become major urinary bile acids; the ratio of the 1β,3α,7α,12α-tetrol to the 3α,6.α,7α,12α-tetrol was about 4:1. Stimulation of 6α-hydroxylase was evident from the presence of hyocholate in urine and plasma after 1.5–4.5 weeks on phenobarbital. Thus, phenobarbital stimulates 1β- and 6α-hydroxylation [197].

23-Hydroxylation. Common to the reports of 3 papers [164,194,198] was identification of the urinary acid 3α,7α,12α,23-tetrahydroxy-5β-cholanate, present as the taurine and glycine conjugates. Whether this is a precursor of norcholate (23-nor-3α,7α,12α-trihydroxy-5β-cholanate) remains to be determined.

Sulfates. All urinary monohydroxy and most dihydroxy bile acids were monosulfated. Position 3 was sulfated in the major bile acids which were also conjugated with glycine or taurine [164]. Allo bile acids derived from 5β-acids (Section V.2) or from cholestanol [154,205] were present in urine as sulfates [164]. The unsaturated acids, 3β-hydroxy-5-cholenic [191,192], 3β,12α-dihydroxy-5-cholenic and the unidentified "Δ-diol" were each present in the sulfate fraction; the origin of 3β,12α-dihydroxy-5-cholenic acid is unknown.

After administration of radioactive bile acids to patients with cholestasis, most of the urinary bile acids were sulfated [206]. However, the relatively large percentage of disulfates has not been noted by other investigators. Perfusion of an isolated rat kidney with various bile acids showed a decreasing production of monosulfates in relation to an increased number of hydroxyl groups [207]. Perfusion of chenodeoxycholate afforded the 7-sulfate (71%) and a trace of the 3-sulfate (2%); no disulfate was found [208]. With the successful synthesis of various isomeric sulfates of the common bile acids, definitive identification of the sulfates found in human urine can be anticipated.

Glucuronides. Progress in identification of urinary glucuronides of bile acids has not kept pace with studies of other bile acids. The new method of fast atom bombardment mass spectrometry will undoubtedly be an important aid in the structure determination of both glucuronides and other conjugates. The glucuronide moiety is attached at C-6 in hyodeoxycholate, whereas in cholate and chenodeoxycholate it is coupled at C-3. Of 22 urinary bile acid glucuronides representing 12–36% of the urinary bile acids, seven were identified [125] (Table 2A); 76% of urinary hyodeoxycholate was present as glucuronide in a case of malabsorption [191].

(4) Meconium

Bile acids in meconium also reflect "atypical" synthesis. Back and Walter [209] reported on the presence of 14 bile acids obtained from meconium of 6 healthy infants (Table 2B). On the average 21% of chenodeoxycholate and of hyocholate and 8% of cholate were sulfated. Deoxycholate was the major bile acid of the sulfate fraction; lithocholate, 3β-hydroxy-5-cholenate [175] and 3β,12α-dihydroxy-5-cholenate were found only in the sulfate fraction, but quantities of lithocholate (range 0.3–1.4%) and 3β,12α-dihydroxy--5-cholenate were small. The amount of 1β,3α,7α,12α-tetrahydroxy acid (79% as the taurine conjugate and 21% unconjugated) ranged from 3.6 to 11.1% of the total bile acids [209]. The fetal bile acids of a number of animals, normal, adrenalectomized, thyroidectomized, or diabetic, are reviewed by Subbiah and Hassan]210].

Acknowledgement

The author is pleased to acknowledge support from the National Institutes of Health, Public Health Service, U.S.A., through Grant HL-07878.

This review constitutes Paper LXXV in the series on Bile Acids from Saint Louis University.

References

1 Lester, R., St. Pyrek, J., Little, J.M. and Adcock, E.W. (1983) Am. J. Physiol. 244, G107–G110.
2 Haslewood, G.A.D. (1967) Bile Salts, pp. 82–107, Methuen, London.
3 Haslewood, G.A.D. (1978) The Biological Importance of Bile Salts, pp. 161–182, North-Holland, Amsterdam.
4 Tammar, A.R. (1974) in: Chemical Zoology (Florkin, M. and Scheer, B.T., Eds.) Vol. VIII, Bile Salts in Fishes, pp. 595–612, Academic Press, New York.
5 Tammar, A.R. (1974) in: Chemical Zoology (Florkin, M. and Scheer, B.T., Eds.) Vol. IX, Bile Salts of Amphibia, pp. 67–76, Academic Press, New York.
6 Tammar, A.R. (1974) in: Chemical Zoology (Florkin, M. and Scheer, B.T., Eds.) Vol. IX, Bile Salts in Reptilia, pp. 337–351, Academic Press, New York.
7 Carey, M.C. (1982) in: The Liver, Biology and Pathobiology (Arias, I., Popper, H., Schachter, D. and Shafritz, D.A., Eds.) pp. 429–465, Raven Press, New York.
8 Hofmann, A.F. (1977) Clin. Gastroenterol. 6, 3–24.
9 Okishio, T. and Nair, P.P. (1966) Biochemistry 5, 3662–3668.
10 Kurtz, W., Leuschner, U., Hellstern, A. and Janka, P. (1982) Hepato-gastroenterology 29, 227–231.
11 Strange, R.C., Chapman, B.T., Johnston, J.D., Nimmo, I.A. and Percy-Robb, I.W. (1979) Biochim. Biophys. Acta 573, 535–545.
12 Greim, H., Trülzsch, D., Czygan, P., Hutterer, F., Schaffner, F., Popper, H., Cooper, D.Y. and Rosenthal, O. (1973) Ann. N.Y. Acad. Sci. 212, 139–147.
13 Yousef, I.M. and Tuchweber, B. (1982) Biol. Neonate 42, 105–112.
14 Yanagisawa, I., Itoh, M., Ishibashi, M., Miyazaki, H. and Nakayama, F. (1980) Anal. Biochem. 104, 75–86.
15 Anwer, M.S., Kroker, R. and Hegner, D. (1976) Biochem. Biophys. Res. Commun. 73, 63–71.
16 Kitani, K. and Kanai, S. (1981) Life Sci. 29, 269–275.
17 Erlinger, S. (1981) Hepatology 1, 352–359.
18 Boyer, J.L. (1980) Physiol. Rev. 60, 303–326.
19 Davis, R.A., Hyde, P.M., Krean, J.-C.W., Malone-McNeal, M. and Archambault-Schexnayder, J. (1982) J. Biol. Chem. 258, 3661–3667.
20 Botham, K.M., Beckett, G.J., Percy-Robb, I.W. and Boyd, G.S. (1980) Eur. J. Biochem. 103, 299–305.
21 Botham, K.M., Lawson, M.E., Beckett, G.J., Percy-Robb, I.W. and Boyd, G.S. (1981) Biochim. Biophys. Acta 666, 238–245.
22 Danielsson, H. and Einarsson, K. (1969) in: The Biological Basis of Medicine (Bittar, E.E. and Bittar, N., Eds.) Vol V, p. 279, Academic Press, New York.
23 Garbutt, J.J., Lack, L. and Tyor, M.P. (1971) Am. J. Clin. Nutr. 24, 218–228.
24 Haber, L.R., Vaupshas, V., Vitullo, B.B., Seemayer, T.A. and de Belle, R.C. (1978) Gastroenterology 74, 1214–1223.
25 Gordon, B.A., Kuksis, A. and Beveridge, J.M.R. (1963) Can. J. Biochem. 41, 77–89.
26 Peric-Golia, L. and Jones, R.S. (1963) Science 142, 245–246.
27 Yousef, I.M. and Fisher, M.M. (1975) Can. J. Physiol. Pharmacol. 53, 880–887.
28 Tamari, M., Ogawa, M. and Kametaka, M. (1976) J. Biochem. 80, 371–377.
29 Nair, P.P., Mendeloff, A.I., Vocci, M., Bankoski, I., Gorelik, M., Herman, G. and Plapinger, R. (1977) Lipids 12, 922–929.
30 Nair, P.P., Solomon, R., Bankoski, J. and Plapinger, R. (1978) Lipids 13, 966–970.
31 Turjman, N., Mendeloff, A.I., Jacob, C., Guidry, C. and Nair, P.P. (1981) J. Steroid Biochem. 14, 1237–1240.
32 Nair, P.P., Gordon, M. and Reback, J. (1967) J. Biol. Chem. 242, 7–11.
33 Shah, P.P. and Staple, E. (1968) Steroids 12, 571–576.
34 Czuba, B. and Vessey, D.A. (1982) J. Biol. Chem. 257, 8761–8765.
35 Killenberg, P.G. and Dukes, D.F. (1976) J. Lipid Res. 17, 451–455.

36 Elliott, W.H., Abbott, D.A., Schlarman, D.E. and Tal, D.M. (1983) Fed. Proc. 42, 1835.
37 Siperstein, M.D. and Murray, A.W. (1955) Science 138, 377–378.
38 Bremer, J. (1956) Acta Chem. Scand. 10, 56–71.
39 Elliott, W.H. (1955) Biochim. Biophys. Acta 17, 440–441.
40 Bremer, J. and Gloor, V. (1955) Acta Chem. Scand. 9, 689–698.
41 Killenberg, P.G. (1978) J. Lipid Res. 19, 24–31.
42 Polokoff, M.A. and Bell, R.M. (1977) J. Biol. Chem. 252, 1167–1171.
43 Schersтén, T. (1967) Biochim. Biophys. Acta 141, 144–154.
44 Vessey, D.A., Crissey, M.H. and Zakin, D. (1977) Biochem. J. 163, 181–183.
45 Kirkpatrick, R.B., Robinson, S.F. and Killenberg, D.G. (1980) Biochim. Biophys. Acta 620, 627–630.
46 Killenberg, P.G. and Jordan, J.T. (1978) J. Biol. Chem. 253, 1005–1010.
47 Vessey, D.A. (1979) J. Biol. Chem. 254, 2059–2063.
48 Czuba, B. and Vessey, D.A. (1980) J. Biol. Chem. 255, 5296–5299.
49 Lambiotte, M. and Thierry, N. (1980) J. Biol. Chem. 255, 11324–11331.
50 Kirkpatrick, R.B. and Killenberg, P.G. (1980) J. Lipid Res. 21, 895–901.
51 Jordan, J.T. and Killenberg, P.G. (1980) Am. J. Physiol. 238, G429–G433.
52 Norman, A. (1970) Scand. J. Gastroenterol. 5, 231–236.
53 Hepner, G.H., Hofmann, A.F. and Thomas, P.J. (1972) J. Clin. Invest. 51, 1889–1897.
54 Hepner, G.H., Hofmann, A.F. and Thomas, P.J. (1972) J. Clin. Invest. 51, 1898–1905.
55 Fromm, H. and Hofmann, A.J. (1971) Lancet 2, 621–625.
56 Palmer, R.H. (1967) Proc. Natl. Acad. Sci. (U.S.A.) 58, 1047–1050.
57 Palmer, R.H. and Bolt, M.G. (1971) J. Lipid Res. 12, 671–679.
58 Palmer, R.H. (1971) J. Lipid Res. 12, 680–687.
59 Eng, C. and Javitt, N.J. (1981) Gastroenterology 80, 1331.
60 Cronholm, T., Makino, I. and Sjövall, J. (1971) Eur. J. Biochem. 26, 251–258.
61 Eyssen, H.J., Parmentier, G.G. and Mertens, J.A. (1976) Eur. J. Biochem. 66, 507–514.
62 Cowen, A.E., Korman, M.G., Hofmann, A.F., Cass, O.W. and Coffin, S.B. (1975) Gastroenterology 69, 67–76.
63 Eriksson, H., Taylor, W. and Sjövall, J. (1978) J. Lipid Res. 19, 177–186.
64 Chen, L.J., Bolt, R.J. and Admirand, W.H. (1977) Biochim. Biophys. Acta 480, 219–227.
65 Barnes, S., Burhol, P.G., Zander, R., Haggstrom, G., Settine, R.L. and Hirschowitz, B.I. (1979) J. Lipid Res. 20, 952–959.
66 Lööf, L. and Hjertén, S. (1980) Biochim. Biophys. Acta 617, 192–204.
67 Hammerman, K.J., Chen, L.J., Fernandez-Corugedo, A. and Earnest, D.L. (1978) Gastroenterology 75, 1021–1025.
68 Jordan, J.T. and Killenberg, P.G. (1980) Biochim. Biophys. Acta 620, 627–630.
69 Back, P., Spacynski, K. and Gerok, W. (1974) Hoppe-Seyler's Z. Physiol. Chem. 355, 749–752.
70 Back, P. (1976) Hoppe-Seyler's Z. Physiol. Chem. 357, 213–217.
71 Back, P. and Bowen, D.V. (1976) Hoppe-Seyler's Z. Physiol. Chem. 357, 219–234.
72 Fröhling, W., Stiehl, A., Czygan, P. and Kommerell, B. (1976) Biochim. Biophys. Acta 444, 525–530.
73 Matern, H., Matern, S., Schelzig, C. and Gerok, W. (1980) FEBS Lett. 118, 251–254.
74 Matern, H., Matern, S. and Gerok, W. (1982) J. Biol. Chem. 257, 7422–7429.
75 Fieser, L.F. and Fieser, M. (1959) Steroids, pp. 421–443, Reinhold, New York.
76 Sjövall, J. and Åkesson, I. (1955) Acta Physiol. Scand. 34, 279–286.
77 Ray, P.D., Doisy Jr., E.A., Matschiner, J.T., Hsia, S.L., Elliott, W.H., Thayer, S.A. and Doisy, E.A. (1961) J. Biol. Chem. 236, 3158–3162.
78 Ray, P.D. (1962) Ph. D. Dissertation, Saint Louis University.
79 Wells, L.W., Ray, P.D. and Thayer, S.A. (1961) Fed. Proc. 20, 283.
80 Wells, L.W. (1964) Ph. D. Dissertation, Saint Louis University.
81 Danielsson, H. and Kazuno, T. (1959) Acta Chem. Scand. 13, 1141–1148.
82 Bergström, S., Danielsson, H. and Samuelsson, B. (1960) in: Lipid Metabolism (Bloch, K., Ed.) p. 291, Wiley, New York.

83 Sonders, R.C., Hsia, S.L., Doisy Jr., E.A., Matschiner, J.T. and Elliott, W.H. (1969) Biochemistry 8, 405–413.
84 Okuda, K. and Kazuno, T. (1961) J. Biochem. 50, 20–23.
85 Thomas, P.J., Hsia, S.L., Matschiner, J.T., Doisy Jr., E.A., Elliott, W.H., Thayer, S.A. and Doisy, E.A. (1964) J. Biol. Chem. 239, 102–105.
86 Einarsson, K. and Johansson, G. (1969) FEBS Lett. 4, 177–180.
87 Kurata, Y. (1967) Hiroshima, J. Med. Sci. 16, 281–285.
88 Johansson, G. (1966) Acta Chem. Scand. 8, 611–616.
89 Bergström, S. and Sjövall, J. (1954) Acta Chem. Scand. 8, 611–616.
90 Mahowald, T.A., Matschiner, J.T., Hsia, S.L., Richter, R., Doisy Jr., E.A., Elliott, W.H. and Doisy, E.A. (1957) J. Biol. Chem. 225, 781–793.
91 Hsia, S.L. (1971) in: The Bile Acids (Kritchevsky, P. and Nair, P.P., Eds.) Vol. 1, pp. 95–120, Plenum, New York.
92 Ziboh, V.A., Matschiner, J.T., Doisy Jr., E.A., Hsia, S.L., Elliott, W.H., Thayer, S.A. and Doisy, E.A. (1961) J. Biol. Chem. 236, 387–390.
93 Samuelsson, B. (1959) Acta Chem. Scand. 13, 976–983.
94 Cherayil, G.D., Hsia, S.L., Matschiner, J.T., Doisy Jr., E.A., Elliott, W.H., Thayer, S.A. and Doisy, E.A. (1963) J. Biol. Chem. 238, 1973–1978.
95 Mahowald, T.A., Yin, M.A., Matschiner, J.T., Hsia, S.L., Doisy Jr., E.A., Elliott, W.H. and Doisy, E.A. (1958) J. Biol. Chem. 230, 581–588.
96 Samuelsson, B. (1959) Acta Chem. Scand. 13, 236–240.
97 Samuelsson, B. (1959) Acta Chem. Scand. 13, 970–975.
98 Sonders, R.C. (1965) Ph. D. Dissertation, Saint Louis University.
99 Ratliff, R.L., Matschiner, J.T., Doisy Jr., E.A., Hsia, S.L., Thayer, S.A., Elliott, W.H. and Doisy, E.A. (1959) J. Biol. Chem. 234, 3133–3136.
100 Yousef, I.M., Magnusson, R., Price, V.M. and Fisher, M.M. (1973) Can. J. Physiol. Pharmacol. 51, 418–423.
101 Einarsson, K., Gustafsson, J.-Å. and Goldman, A.S. (1972) Eur. J. Biochem. 31, 345–353.
102 Voigt, W., Thomas, P.J. and Hsia, S.L. (1968) J. Biol. Chem. 243, 3494–3499.
103 Björkhem, I. and Danielsson, H. (1974) Mol. Cell. Biochem. 4, 79–95.
104 Carella, M., Björkhem, I., Einarsson, K. and Hellström, K. (1976) Br. J. Nutr. 36, 273–279.
105 Björkhem, I., Danielsson, H. and Wikvall, K. (1974) J. Biol. Chem. 249, 6439–6445.
106 Voigt, W., Hsia, S.L., Cooper, D.Y. and Rosenthal, O. (1978) FEBS Lett. 2, 124–126.
107 Danielsson, H. (1973) Steroids 22, 567–579.
108 Einarsson, K., Gustafsson, J.-Å. and Gustafsson, B. (1973) J. Biol. Chem. 248, 3623–3630.
109 Huang, C.T.L., Szczepanik-Van Leeuwen, P., Strickland, A., Calvin, R. and Nichols, B.L. (1979) Fed. Proc. 38, 1118.
110 Kurata, Y. (1963) J. Biochem. 53, 295–298.
111 Kurata, Y. (1964) J. Biochem. 54, 415–419.
112 Trülzsch, D., Roboz, J., Greim, H., Czygan, P., Rudick, J., Hutterer, F., Schaffner, F. and Popper, H. (1974) Biochem. Med. 9, 158–166.
113 Haslewood, G.A.D. (1954) Biochem. J. 56, 581–587.
114 Ziegler, P. (1956) Can. J. Chem. 34, 1528–1531.
115 Bergström, S., Danielsson, H. and Göransson, A. (1959) Acta Chem. Scand. 13, 776–783.
116 Samuelsson, B. (1960) Ark. Kemi 15, 425–432.
117 Haslewood, G.A.D. (1971) Biochem. J. 123, 15–18.
118 Björkhem, I., Einarsson, K. and Hellers, G. (1973) Eur. J. Clin. Invest. 3, 459–465.
119 Carey Jr., J.B. and Williams, G. (1962) J. Clin. Invest. 42, 450–455.
120 Norman, A. and Palmer, R.H. (1964) Lab. Clin. Med. 63, 986–1000.
121 Thistle, J.L. and Schoenfield, L.J. (1971) Gastroenterology 61, 488–496.
122 Kimura, T. (1937) Z. Physiol. Chem 248–284.
123 Bremmelgaard, A. and Sjövall, J. (1980) J. Lipid Res. 21, 1072–1081.
124 Summerfield, J.A., Billing, B.H. and Shackleton, C.H.L. (1976) Biochem. J. 154, 507–516.

125 Almé, B. and Sjövall, J. (1980) J. Steroid Biochem. 13, 907–916.
126 Matschiner, J.T., Mahowald, T.A., Hsia, S.L., Doisy Jr., E.A., Elliott, W.H. and Doisy, E.A. (1957) J. Biol. Chem. 225, 803–810.
127 Matschiner, J.T., Ratliff, R.L., Mahowald, T.A., Doisy Jr., E.A., Eilliott, W.H., Hsia, S.L. and Doisy, E.A. (1958) J. Biol. Chem. 230, 589–596.
128 Einarsson, K. (1966) J. Biol. Chem. 241, 534–549.
129 Thomas, P.J., Hsia, S.L., Matschiner, J.T., Thayer, S.A., Elliott, W.H., Doisy Jr., E.A. and Doisy, E.A. (1965) J. Biol. Chem. 240, 1059–1063.
130 Sacquet, E.C., Raibard, P.M., Mejean, C., Rittot, J.M., Leprince, C. and Leglise, P.C. (1979) Appl. Environ. Microbiol. 37, 1127–1131.
131 Mui, M.M. and Elliott, W.H. (1971) J. Biol. Chem. 246, 302–304.
132 Emmerman, S. and Javitt, N.B. (1967) J. Biol. Chem. 242, 661–664.
133 Kallner, A. (1967) Ark. Kemi 26, 567–576.
134 Bergström, S., Rottenberg, M. and Sjövall, J. (1953) Hoppe-Seyler's Z. Physiol. Chem. 295, 278–285.
135 Hirofuji, S. (1965) Hiroshima J. Med. Sci. 14, 93–100.
136 Kallner, A. (1968) Acta Chem. Scand. 22, 2361–2370.
137 Knodell, R.G., Kinsey, M.D., Boedeker, E.C. and Collin, D.P. (1976) Gastroenterology 71, 196–201.
138 Hansson, R. and Wikvall, K. (1980) J. Biol. Chem. 255, 1643–1649.
139 Murakami, K. and Okuda, K. (1981) J. Biol. Chem. 256, 8658–8662.
140 Sjövall, J. (1959) Acta Chem. Scand. 13, 711–716.
141 Samuelsson, B. (1960) Acta Chem. Scand. 14, 21–27.
142 Botham, K.M. and Boyd, G.S. (1983) Eur. J. Biochem. 134, 191–196.
143 Kemper, H.J.M., Vos-Van Holstein, M.P.N. and de Lange, J. (1982) J. Lipid Res. 23, 823–830.
144 Kern Jr., F., Eriksson, H., Curstedt, T. and Sjövall, J. (1977) J. Lipid Res. 18, 623–634.
145 Eriksson, H., Taylor, W. and Sjövall, J. (1978) J. Lipid Res. 19, 177–186.
146 Ikawa, S. (1977) J. Biochem. 82, 1093–1102.
147 Bergström, S., Danielsson, H. and Kazuno, T. (1960) J. Biol. Chem. 235, 983–988.
148 Masui, T., Ueyama, F., Yashima, H. and Kazuno, T. (1967) J. Biochem. 62, 650–654.
149 Ahlberg, J.W., Ziboh, V.A., Sonders, R.C. and Hsia, S.L. (1961) Fed. Proc. 20, 283.
150 Denton, J.E., Yousef, M.K., Yousef, I.M. and Kuksis, A. (1974) Lipids 9, 945–951.
151 Yousef, I.M. and Fisher, M.M. (1975) Lipids 10, 571–573.
152 Blaskiewicz, R.J., O'Neil Jr., G.J. and Elliott, W.H. (1974) Proc. Soc. Exp. Biol. Med. 146, 92–95.
153 Mui, M.M. and Elliott, W.H. (1975) Biochemistry 14, 2712–2717.
154 Elliott, W.H. (1976) in: The Hepatobiliary System (Taylor, W., Ed.) pp. 469–481, Plenum, New York.
155 Joyce, M.J. and Elliott, W.H. (1982) Fed. Proc. 41, 883.
156 Yamaga, N. (1971) J. Biochem. 70, 125–131.
157 Haslewood, G.A.D. and Wootton, V. (1951) Biochem. J. 49, 67–71.
158 Anderson, I.G., Banister, K.E., Haslewood, G.A.D., Cho, D. and Tökés, L. (1980) Zool. J. Lennein Soc. 68, 41–51.
159 Kihira, K., Morioka, Y. and Hoshita, T. (1981) J. Lipid Res. 22, 1181–1187.
160 Bergström, S., Krabisch, L. and Lindeberg, O.G. (1959) Acta Soc. Med. Upsaliensis 64, 160–164.
161 Kutner, A., Jaworska, R., Kutner, W. and Grzeszkiewicz, A. (1981) in: Advances in Steroid Analysis (Görög, S., Ed.) pp. 333–337, Akadémiai Kiadó, Budapest.
162 Haslewood, G.A.D. (1964) Biol. Rev. 39, 537–574.
163 Ikawa, S. and Tammer, A.R. (1976) Biochem. J. 153, 343–350.
164 Almé, B., Bremmelgaard, A., Sjövall, J. and Thomassen, P. (1977) J. Lipid Res. 18, 339–362.
165 Björkhem, I., Angelin, B., Einarsson, K. and Ewerth, S. (1982) J. Lipid Res. 23, 1020–1025.
166 Usui, T. and Yamasaki, K. (1964) Steroids 3, 147–161.
167 Kallner, A. (1967) Ark. Kemi 26, 553–565.
168 Berséus, O. (1967) Eur. J. Biochem. 2, 493–502.
169 Ikeda, M., Hayakowa, S., Ezaki, M. and Ohmori, S. (1981) Hoppe-Seyler's Z. Physiol. Chem. 362, 511–520.

170 Björkhem, I. and Danielsson, H. (1970) Eur. J. Biochem. 12, 80–84.
171 Björkhem, I., Danielsson, H. and Wikvall, K. (1973) Eur. J. Biochem. 36, 8–15.
172 Waller, G., Theorell, H. and Sjövall, J. (1965) Arch. Biochem. Biophys. 111, 671–684.
173 Cronholm, T., Makino, I. and Sjövall, J. (1972) Eur. J. Biochem. 24, 507–519.
174 Mitropoulos, K.A. and Myant, N.B. (1967) Biochem. J. 103, 472–479.
175 Back, P. and Ross, K. (1973) Hoppe-Seyler's Z. Physiol. Chem. 354, 83–89.
176 Laatikainen, T., Perheentupa, J., Vihko, R., Makino, I. and Sjövall, J. (1972) J. Steroid Biochem. 3, 715–719.
177 Berséus, O. and Einarsson, K. (1967) Acta Chem. Scand. 21, 1105–1108.
178 Björkhem, I. (1969) Eur. J. Biochem. 8, 337–344.
179 Björkhem, I. (1969) Doctoral Thesis, Opuscula Medica, Stockholm.
180 Yamasaki, K. (1978) Kawasaki Med. J. 4, 227–264.
181 Kulkarni, B. and Javitt, N.B. (1982) Steroids 40, 581–589.
182 Ikawa, S., Ayaki, Y., Ogura, M. and Yamasaki, K. (1972) J. Biochem. 71, 579–587.
183 Ogura, M. and Yamasaki, K. (1967) Steroids 9, 607–622.
184 Macdonald, I.A., Bokkenheuser, V.D., Winter, J.D., McLerson, A.M. and Mosbach, E.H. (1983) J. Lipid Res. 24, 675–700.
185 Shefer, S., Salen, G., Hauser, S., Dayal, B. and Batta, A.K. (1982) J. Biol. Chem. 257, 1401–1406.
186 Bachrach, W.H. and Hofmann, A.F. (1982) Digest. Dis. Sci. 27, 737–856.
187 Ramsey, R.B. and Nicholas, H.J. (1982) Adv. Lipid Res. 10, 143–232.
188 Martin, C.W. and Nicholas, H.J. (1973) Steroids 21, 633–646.
189 Naqvi, S.H.M. and Nicholas, H.J. (1973) Lipids 8, 651–653.
190 Kallner, A. (1967) Acta Chem. Scand. 21, 315–321.
191 Makino, I., Sjövall, J., Norman, A. and Strandvik, B. (1971) FEBS Lett. 15, 161–164.
192 Back, P. (1973) Clin. Chim. Acta 44, 199–207.
193 Almé, B., Norden, Å. and Sjövall, J. (1978) Clin. Chim. Acta 86, 251–259.
194 Bremmelgaard, A. and Sjövall, J. (1979) Eur. J. Clin. Invest. 9, 341–348.
195 Amuro, Y., Hayashi, E., Endo, T., Higashino, K. and Kishimoto, S. (1983) Clin. Chim. Acta 127, 61–67.
196 Amuro, Y., Endo, T., Higashino, K., Uchida, K. and Yamamura, Y. (1981) Clin. Chim. Acta 114, 137–147.
197 Back, P. (1982) Klin. Wochenschr. 60, 541–549.
198 Thomassen, P.A. (1979) Eur. J. Clin. Invest. 9, 425–432.
199 Strandvik, B. and Wikström, S.-Å. (1982) Eur. J. Clin. Invest. 12, 301–305.
200 Carlström, K., Kirk, D.N. and Sjövall, J. (1981) J. Lipid Res. 22, 1225–1234.
201 Tohma, M., Takeshita, H., Mahara, R. and Makino, I. (1983) Koenshu-Iyo Masu Kenkyukai 10, 77–84.
202 Clayton, P.T., Muller, D.P.R. and Lawson, A.N. (1982) Biochem. J. 206, 489–498.
203 Schneider, J.J. and Bhacca, N.S. (1966) J. Biol. Chem. 241, 5313–5324.
204 Haslewood, G.A.D. and Tökés, L. (1972) Biochem. J. 126, 1161–1170.
205 Karavolas, H.J., Elliott, W.H., Hsia, S.L., Doisy Jr., E.A., Matschiner, J.T., Thayer, S.A. and Doisy, E.A. (1965) J. Biol. Chem. 240, 1568–1572.
206 Stiehl, A. (1974) Eur. J. Clin. Invest. 4, 59–63.
207 Czygan, P., Ast, E., Fröhling, W., Stiehl, A. and Kommerall, B. (1977) in: Bile Acid Metabolism in Health and Disease (Paumgartner, G. and Stiehl, A., Eds.) pp. 83–87, MIT Press, Lancaster.
208 Summerfield, J.A., Gollan, J. and Billing, B.H. (1976) Biochem. J. 156, 339–345.
209 Back, P. and Walter, K. (1980) Gastroenterology 78, 671–676.
210 Subbiah, M.T.R. and Hassan, A.S. (1982) Adv. Lipid Res. 19, 137–161.

H. Danielsson and J. Sjövall (Eds.), *Sterols and Bile Acids*

CHAPTER 12

Metabolism of bile acids in intestinal microflora

PHILLIP B. HYLEMON

Department of Microbiology and Immunology, Medical College of Virginia, Virginia Commonwealth University, Richmond, VA 23298 (U.S.A.)

(I) Introduction

The intestinal microflora of man and animals can biotransform bile acids into a number of different metabolites. Normal human feces may contain more than 20 different bile acids which have been formed from the primary bile acids, cholic acid and chenodeoxycholic acid [1–5]. Known microbial biotransformations of these bile acids include the hydrolysis of bile acid conjugates yielding free bile acids, oxidation of hydroxyl groups at C-3, C-6, C-7 and C-12 and reduction of oxo groups to give epimeric hydroxy bile acids. In addition, certain members of the intestinal microflora 7α- and 7β-dehydroxylate primary bile acids yielding deoxycholic acid and lithocholic acid (Fig. 1). Moreover, 3-sulfated bile acids are converted into a variety of different metabolites by the intestinal microflora [6,7].

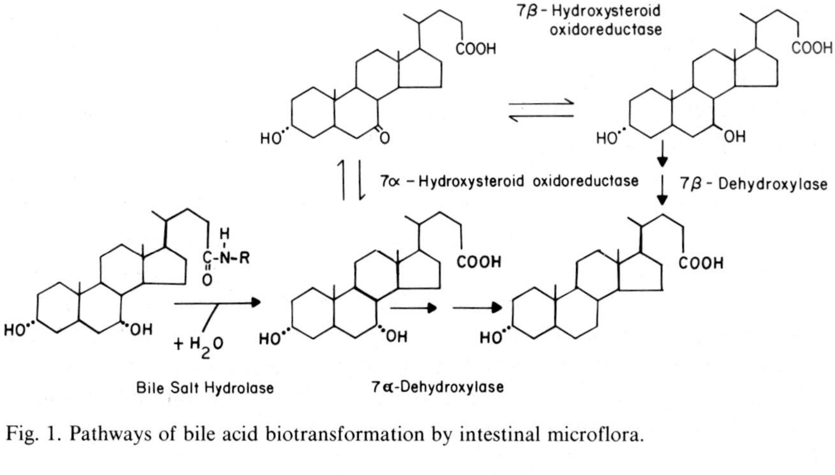

Fig. 1. Pathways of bile acid biotransformation by intestinal microflora.

The hydrolysis of bile acid conjugates is probably the initial reaction catalyzed by intestinal bacteria. Therefore, primarily free bile acids are isolated from the feces of man and animals [1–5]. The bulk of the free bile acids in feces of man is deoxycholic acid and lithocholic acid which are generated by the 7α-dehydroxylation of cholic acid and chenodeoxycholic acid, respectively. A portion of fecal acids is absorbed from the intestinal tract, returned to the liver where they are conjugated and again secreted via biliary bile. Therefore, the final composition of biliary bile acids is the result of a complex interaction between liver enzymes and enzymes in intestinal bacteria.

(II) Composition of intestinal microflora

The adult human body is composed of approximately 10^{13} eukaryotic animal cells [8]. However, there are 10^{14} or 10 times as many prokaryotic cells on the body surfaces and in the gastrointestinal tract of man [9]. These organisms are capable of carrying out hundreds of enzymatic reactions that the host animal cell cannot catalyze. Indeed, the combined activities of both mammalian and bacterial enzymes are often required to form various metabolic end products of certain endogenous and exogenous compounds [10]. In contrast to the liver, the intestinal microflora tends to hydrolyze conjugated metabolites and reduce the polarity of these compounds. The extent of degradation is usually limited by the constraints inherent to the anaerobic environment of the large bowel, where reductive sequences are strongly favored.

Our concept of the composition of the indigenous intestinal microflora of man has changed markedly in recent years. It has been discovered that greater than 99% of all intestinal bacteria are obligate anaerobes. Perhaps the most extensive investigation of the human fecal flora are those of Moore and Holdeman [11] and Holdeman et al. [12]. These investigators isolated the predominant microflora of 20 adult Japanese–Hawaiians and characterized some 1147 strains of bacteria which represented 113 different species. The average direct microscopic count in these specimens was 5×10^{11} organisms/g wet weight feces and it was possible to culture 80–90% of these bacteria. Greater than two-thirds of the isolates were the following species: Bacteroides species, *Eubacterium aerofaciens, E. eligens, E. biforme, E. rectale, Fusobacterium prausnitzii, Bifidobacterium adolescentis, B. longum, Peptostreptococcus productus* and *Gemmiger formicilis*. The species of *Bacteroides* isolated in the highest viable numbers included: *vulgatus, thetaiotaomicron* and *distasonis*. The remaining one third of the bacterial isolates described by Moore and Holdeman [11] included more than 100 different kinds of bacteria, many of which could not be classified below the genus level. The results of this study also showed considerable variation in the fecal flora from one individual to another. It was estimated statistically that there may be more than 400 different species of bacteria in the human gastrointestinal tract at any given time [12]. Furthermore, the study by Moore and Holdeman [11] was carried out using non-selective media and probably approximates the true state of the human fecal flora.

(III) Deconjugation

The ability to hydrolyze the peptide bond in conjugated bile acids (Fig. 1) is widely distributed among intestinal bacteria. Conjugated bile acid hydrolase (CBH) (EC 3.5) activity has been detected in members of the genera Bacteroides, Bifidobacterium, Fusobacterium, Clostridium, Lactobacillus, Peptostreptococcus and Streptococcus [13–17]. However, there is considerable variation in occurrence of this enzymatic activity among species and strains.

Although certain properties of this enzyme have been described in whole cells of intestinal bacteria, deconjugation activity has been purified only from *Clostridium perfringens* [18] and *Bacteroides fragilis* [19]. There were considerable differences in the characteristics of this enzyme isolated from these bacteria (Table 1). One major difference was their kinetic properties. The CBH from *C. perfringens* showed typical Michaelis–Menten kinetics for all substrates assayed. However, the CBH from *B. fragilis* showed biphasic kinetics in substrate versus velocity plots, except for glycocholic acid, and inhibition of activity at high (2–4 mM) substrate concentrations for most substrates. The estimated K_m values for the enzyme isolated from *B. fragilis* were at least 10-fold lower than those determined for the *C. perfringens* CBH, using similar assay techniques. The enzyme from either *C. perfringens* or *B. fragilis* hydrolyzed both dihydroxy and trihydroxy glycine- and taurine-conjugated bile acids. Little activity was found with taurolithocholic acid using the purified enzyme. However, crude extracts of *C. perfringens* slowly hydrolyzed this compound.

CBH has been reported to be synthesized constitutively in most intestinal bacteria. However, Hylemon and Stellwag [20] detected a 300-fold increase in total units of activity in *B. fragilis* after the cells entered the stationary phase of growth. CBH activity was detected in the periplasmic space, membrane fraction and soluble extracts. Hence, the synthesis of this enzyme in *B. fragilis* appears to be under genetic regulation.

TABLE 1

Characteristics of conjugated bile acid hydrolase from intestinal bacteria [a]

Organism [b]	M_r	pH optimum	Apparent K_m (mM)				Kinetic properties
			GC	TC	GCDC	TCDC	
Bacteroides fragilis	250000	4.2–4.5	0.35	0.45	0.26	0.29	Non-Michaelis–Menten
Clostridium perfringens	ND	5.6	3.6	3.7	1.4	3.0	Michaelis–Menten

[a] ND, not determined; GC, glycocholic acid; TC, taurocholic acid; GCDC, glycochenodeoxycholic acid; TCDC, taurochenodeoxycholic acid.

[b] *B. fragilis* [19] and *C. perfringens* [18].

(IV) Desulfation

Lithocholic acid is formed in the large bowel by the microbial 7α-dehydroxylation of chenodeoxycholic acid (Section VI) and returned to the liver where the C-24 carboxyl group is conjugated with either glycine or taurine. The 3α-hydroxyl group is conjugated to sulfate prior to biliary excretion. Conjugated lithocholate 3-sulfate is poorly absorbed from the gastrointestinal tract. The unabsorbed lithocholate sulfate is metabolized by the intestinal microflora into a variety of products. Desulfation appears to occur either by elimination or hydrolysis. Following the original work of Palmer [6], Kelsey et al. [7,21] showed that mixed human fecal cultures converted lithocholic acid 3-sulfate to lithocholic acid, its 3β epimer (isolithocholic acid), the 3β-yl palmitate, 3-cholenoic acid and 5β-cholanoic acid. The formation of the 3-cholenoic acid and the 3-palmitate of isolithocholic acid represents novel microbial biotransformations, but the mechanism(s) of formation and enzymology are not understood. Borriello and Owen [22] demonstrated that many species of intestinal clostridia converted lithocholic acid sulfate to isolithocholic acid, 3-cholenoic acid and 5β-cholanoic acid. Kinetic studies showed that isolithocholic acid was converted into 3-cholenoic acid and 5β-cholanoic acid. These observations suggest that intestinal clostridial species may have 3β-dehydroxylating activity.

Huijghebaert et al. [23] isolated a bile salt sulfatase-producing strain designated, Clostridium S_1 from rat feces. This bacterium hydrolyzed the 3-sulfates of lithocholic acid, chenodeoxycholic acid, deoxycholic acid and cholic acid but not the 7- or 12-monosulfates. Sulfatase activity required the 3-sulfate group to be in the equatorial position. A free C-24 or C-26 carboxyl group was also required for sulfatase activity in whole cells of this bacterium. The 3-sulfate of cholesterol, C_{19}- and C_{21}-steroids were not hydrolyzed by Clostridium S_1 [24]. Nevertheless, C_{19}- and C_{21}-steroid sulfates are hydrolyzed in the gut by microbial activity suggesting that the intestinal microflora may contain bacteria with steroid sulfatases possessing different substrate specificities. However, it should be noted that enzyme substrate specificity studies carried out in whole cells may reflect both cell wall permeability and enzyme specificity.

(V) Epimerization of hydroxyl groups

Bile acid hydroxysteroid dehydrogenases (oxidoreductases) (HSDH) are pyridine nucleotide-linked enzymes found in certain species of intestinal bacteria. The major transformation of bile acids resulting from HSDH activities is the epimerization of various hydroxyl groups through oxo intermediates which may represent a significant fraction of human fecal bile acids. The epimerization of bile acids can be carried out by a single organism containing both α- and β-HSDHs (intraspecies epimerization) or by a collaboration of two organisms (interspecies epimerization) one species containing the α-HSDH and a second containing the β-HSDH (Fig. 1).

HSDH activities are found rather widely distributed among intestinal bacteria including members of the genera: Bacteroides, Eubacterium, Clostridium, Bifidobacterium and Escherichia [25–29]. In the human intestinal microflora, 7α-HSDH appears to be much more widely distributed than 3α-HSDH or 12α-HSDH [17]. Individual species may contain from 1 to 3 different stereospecific HSDHs. However, there is considerable variation between strains regarding the presence and extent of HSDH activity.

(1) 3α- and 3β-hydroxysteroid dehydrogenase

The epimerization of the 3α-hydroxyl group by the intestinal microflora has been suggested by the presence of 3β epimers in feces of man and laboratory animals. The epimerization of the 3α-hydroxyl group of bile acids has been demonstrated only in members of the genera Clostridium and Eubacterium [13,30–33]. Neither the 3α- nor the 3β-HSDH has been purified from anaerobic bacteria, although 3α-HSDH has been studied in crude cell extracts of *C. perfringens* and certain strains of *Eubacterium lentum*. The enzyme characterized from *E. lentum* [32] was NADP linked and heat labile. Both enzymes showed alkaline pH optima and exhibited broad substrate specificity toward 3α-hydroxy bile acids and neutral steroids. Moreover, 3α-HSDH oxidized the 3α-hydroxyl group of both 5α- and 5β-steroids. A relative molecular weight was estimated by gel filtration to be 205 000 for the enzyme in *E. lentum*.

3β-HSDH has not been measured in cell extracts of either *C. perfringens* or *E. lentum*. However, whole cells of these bacteria produced 3α- and 3β-hydroxy bile acids from 3-oxo bile acid substrates. Aeration of whole cell suspensions or growing cultures favored the formation of 3-oxo bile acids; whereas, anaerobic conditions increased the rate of formation of 3β-hydroxy bile acids [34].

(2) 6α- and 6β-hydroxysteroid dehydrogenase

β-Muricholic acid (3α,6β,7β-trihydroxy-5β-cholanoic acid) is present in the feces of germ-free rats, mice and pigs [17]. However, ω-muricholic acid (3α,6α,7β-trihydroxy-5β-cholanoic acid) is present in feces of conventional animals. These observations suggested that the intestinal microflora can epimerize the 6β-hydroxyl group of β-muricholic acid.

Sacquet et al. [35] isolated a Clostridium sp. (R6 X 76) from the feces of rats that was capable of forming ω-muricholic acid from β-muricholic acid. Eyssen et al. [36] isolated a gram-positive bacterium (strain R 1) from rats that oxidized the 6β-hydroxyl group of β-muricholic acid, yielding the 6-oxo derivative. This bacterium was identified as a strain of *Eubacterium lentum*. Two different species of the genus Fusobacterium were also isolated that reduced the 6-oxo group to 6α-hydroxyl bile acids. When grown as a mixed culture, these bacteria could epimerize the 6β-hydroxyl group of β-muricholic acid. Thus, the epimerization of the 6β-hydroxyl group of bile acids can occur either by intra- or interspecies mechanisms. However, neither the 6α- nor the 6β-hydroxysteroid dehydrogenase has been purified or characterized in cell extracts prepared from intestinal bacteria.

TABLE 2

Characteristics of 7α- and 7β-hydroxysteroid dehydrogenase (HSDH) from intestinal bacteria [a]

HSDH	Organism [b]	Pyridine nucleotide	M_r	pH optimum	Apparent K_m (mM)			
					CDC	GCDC	UDC	GUDC
7α	*Escherichia coli*	NAD	105 000	9.8	0.060	0.10	–	–
	Bacteriodes	NAD	320 000	8.5–9	0.048	0.083	–	–
	thetaiotaomicron	NADP	127 000	9.0	ND	ND	–	–
7β	*Peptostreptococcus productus*	NADP	52 000	9.8–10	–	–	0.022	0.238
	Eubacterium aerofaciens	NADP	45 000	10 –10.5	–	–	0.108	0.909
	Clostridium absonum	NADP	200 000	9.5	–	–	0.0095	–

[a] ND, not determined; CDC, chenodeoxycholic acid; GCDC, glycochenodeoxycholic acid; UDC, ursodeoxycholic acid; GUDC, glycoursodeoxycholic acid.

[b] *E. coli* [37], *B. thetaiotaomicron* [39], *P. productus* and *E. aerofaciens* [43], *C. absonum* [40–42].

(3) 7α-Hydroxysteroid dehydrogenase

The epimerization of the 7α-hydroxyl group can occur either by intra- or interspecies mechanisms [16]. However, it is difficult to quantitatively assess the degree of 7-hydroxy epimerization in vivo because this transformation competes with the irreversible 7-dehydroxylation of bile acids (Section VI). 7α-HSDH activity has been reported in several genera of intestinal bacteria; however, the most complete characterization of this enzyme has been carried out with the enzyme isolated from *Escherichia coli* [37] and Bacteroides sp. [29,38,39] (Table 2). Both enzymes used both free and conjugated bile acids as substrates, showed alkaline pH optima and lower K_m values for dihydroxy than for trihydroxy bile acids. However, cell extracts prepared from Bacteriodes sp. contained both NAD- and NADP-dependent 7α-HSDH activities; whereas, extracts from *E. coli* contained only an NAD-dependent enzyme activity. Additional studies showed that the two 7α-HSDH activities detected in Bacteriodes sp. differed in molecular weight, differential heat inactivation and Mn^{2+} requirement, suggesting the presence of two distinct enzymes [29].

The NAD-dependent 7α-HSDH was found to be associated with both cytoplasmic and cell membrane fractions during the preparation of spheroplasts of *B. fragilis* [20]. Moreover, the activity of this enzyme in *B. fragilis* increased 3–5-fold as the cultures entered stationary growth phase. However, the mechanism of regulation of enzyme synthesis is not yet known.

(4) 7β-Hydroxysteroid dehydrogenase

The 7β epimers of cholic and chenodeoxycholic acid are frequently detected in feces and bile of man. However, the epimerization of the 7β-hydroxy bile acids by intestinal bacteria has been directly demonstrated only recently. 7β-Hydroxysteroid dehydrogenase activity has been detected in cell extracts prepared from *Clostridium absonum* [40–42], *Eubacterium aerofaciens* [43,44], *Peptostreptococcus productus* [44] and certain lecithinase–lipase-negative human intestinal clostridia [45]. *C. absonum* is normally isolated from soil. Both *C. absonum* and *E. aerofaciens* will oxidize ursodeoxycholic (3α,7β-dihydroxy-5β-cholanoic) acid and 3α,7α,12α-trihydroxy-5β-cholanoic acid to 7-oxo bile acids when the E_h (redox potential) of the culture medium is relatively high (> −100 mV). *C. absonum* has both 7α-HSDH (NAD- and NADP-linked) and 7β-HSDH (NADP-linked) activities in cell extracts and epimerizes chenodeoxycholic acid to ursodeoxycholic acid under anaerobic conditions. In *C. absonum* the 7α- and 7β-HSDHs are inducible by certain bile acids including chenodeoxycholic acid and deoxycholic acid, but not ursodeoxycholic acid. The induction of these enzymes by deoxycholic acid was unexpected because this bile acid is not metabolized by *C. absonum* [42]. The lecithinase–lipase-negative intestinal clostridia will also catalyze the epimerization of the 7α-hydroxyl group of bile acids but the regulation of these activities has not been studied.

The physiological role for the conversion of chenodeoxycholic acid to ursodeoxycholic acid by *C. absonum* or other intestinal bacteria is unknown. However, ursodeoxycholic acid is more polar than chenodeoxycholic acid (Chapter 13) and should be less toxic to bacterial cell membranes than the latter. Indeed, *C. absonum* will readily grow in media containing 1 mM ursodeoxycholic acid but not 1 mM chenodeoxycholic acid [42]. Therefore, the epimerization of the axial 7α-hydroxyl group may represent a detoxication process for *C. absonum* and would provide a physiological explanation for these enzymes.

P. productus and *E. aerofaciens* contain only a constitutive 7β-HSDH and these organisms participate in interspecies 7β-hydroxy epimerization when co-cultured with bacteria producing 7α-HSDH. The characteristics of the enzyme isolated from different anaerobic bacteria are compared in Table 2. The enzyme isolated from *P. productus* has a much higher specific activity than the extracts prepared from *E. aerofaciens* and *C. absonum*.

(5) 12α-Hydroxysteroid dehydrogenase

12-Oxo bile acids can be detected when cholic acid is incubated with mixed fecal flora [46]. Moreover, the occurrence of 12-oxo and 12β-hydroxy bile acids in human feces [1–5], suggests the presence of 12α- and 12β-HSDH activities in bacteria. However, intestinal bacteria having 12β-HSDH have not been isolated. 12α-HSDH has been conclusively demonstrated only in the genera Eubacterium and Clostridium [13,47–49]. 12α-HSDH has been characterized from *E. lentum* [48], *Clostridium leptum* [49] and Clostridium sp. ATCC 29733 [47] (Table 3). The enzyme from *E. lentum* is unstable in the absence of reducing agents, has a pH optimum of 8–10.5 and a molecular weight of 125 000 as determined by gel filtration chromatography. The enzyme has lower K_m values for cholic and deoxycholic acid than for their glycine conjugates.

TABLE 3

Characteristics of 12α-hydroxysteroid dehydrogenase from intestinal anaerobic bacteria [a]

Organism [b]	M_r	pH optimum	Pyridine nucleotide	Apparent K_m (mM)			
				C	DC	GC	GDC
E. lentum	125 000	8–10.5	NAD	0.059	0.028	0.25	0.16
C. leptum	225 000	8.5–9	NADP	7.0	1.6	2.7	0.57
Clostridium sp.	100 000	7.8	NADP	0.67	0.40	2.5	0.30

[a] C, cholic acid; DC, deoxycholic acid, GC, glycocholic acid; GDC, glycodeoxycholic acid.
[b] *E. lentum* [47], *C. leptum* [52], Clostridium sp. [46].

Harris and Hylemon [49] purified (63-fold) a 12α-HSDH from *C. leptum*. The pH optimum was 8.5–9.0 with deoxycholic acid as the substrate. The enzyme from *C. leptum* has lower K_m values for conjugated than free 12α-hydroxy bile acids. Moreover, the K_m values were much higher (10–100-fold) than those of the enzyme from *E. lentum*. The 12α-HSDH had a molecular weight of approximately 225 000 as estimated by gel filtration chromatography. Cell extracts of Clostridium sp. ATCC 29733 also contained 12α-HSDH activity. This enzyme had a pH optimum of 7.8 and a molecular weight of approximately 100 000 as estimated by gel filtration chromatography. 12α-HSDH from all 3 intestinal bacteria were synthesized constitutively during growth.

(VI) 7α- and 7β-dehydroxylase

Quantitatively, the most important bile acid microbial transformation of cholic and chenodeoxycholic acid is the 7α-dehydroxylation yielding the secondary bile acids deoxycholic acid and lithocholic acid, respectively. The 7α-dehydroxylation alters markedly the physical properties and physiological effects of the bile acid molecule. There is a decrease in the solubility of secondary bile acids in aqueous solutions and an alteration of the critical micellar concentration (Chapter 13).

Intestinal bacteria capable of 7α-dehydroxylating bile acids have been isolated by several laboratories [16,50]. Most intestinal bacteria that carry out 7-dehydroxylation have been identified as members of the genera Clostridium [50–52] or Eubacterium [51,53]. Stellwag and Hylemon [52] and Ferrari et al. [54] demonstrated that the fecal population of 7α-dehydroxylating intestinal bacterial in man and rats is in the range of 10^3–10^5 viable organisms/g wet weight feces.

The reaction mechanism for 7α-dehydroxylation of bile acids was first investigated by Samuelsson [55] using doubly labeled cholic acid fed to conventional rats. The reaction was reported to occur by a diaxial *trans* elimination of water (6β-H, 7α-OH) yielding a postulated Δ^6-steroid intermediate followed by *trans* hydrogenation at the 6α and 7β positions generating the secondary bile acids (Fig. 2). Studies

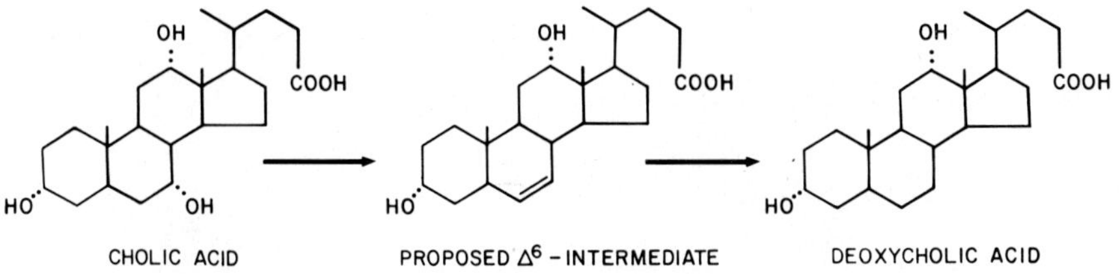

Fig. 2. Reaction mechanism for 7α-dehydroxylation of cholic acid.

by Ferrari et al. [56] and White et al. [57–59] supported this mechanism by demonstrating the reduction of the chemically synthesized 3α,12α-dihydroxy-5β-chol-6-enoic acid intermediate to deoxycholic acid by cell extracts of *C. bifermentans* and Eubacterium sp. V.P.I. 12708, respectively. Hydration of the Δ^6 intermediate to either 7α- or 7β-hydroxy bile acids was not detected. Surprisingly, both whole cells and cell extracts of Eubacterium sp. V.P.I. 12708 were able to directly 7β-dehydroxylate ursodeoxycholic acid [59]. It is not known if this activity involves *cis* or *trans* elimination of water.

White et al. [60] reported that 7-dehydroxylase activity was inducible in Eubacterium sp. 12708. There was a 90-fold increase in the specific activity of 7α-dehydroxylase following the addition of cholic acid to growing cultures. The inductive mechanism is highly specific, requiring a free C-24 carboxyl group and an unhindered 7α-hydroxyl (but not 7β-hydroxyl) group on the B ring of the steroid nucleus. Interestingly, there was no detectable uptake of [24-^{14}C]cholic acid into whole cells of this bacterium. The addition of cholic acid resulted in the differential synthesis of at least 5 new polypeptides with molecular weights of 77000, 56000, 56000, 27000 and 23500 as determined by two-dimensional sodium dodecyl sulfate–polyacrylamide gel electrophoresis (Fig. 3). The relative molecular weight of the catalytically active enzyme was 114000, estimated by gel filtration. Moreover, 7α- and 7β-dehydroxylase and Δ^6-reductase activities all co-eluted suggesting that all 3 activities may reside in the same complex (Table 4).

An NADH–flavin oxidoreductase was also induced by cholic acid in this bacterium [61]. The physiological function of this enzyme in 7-dehydroxylation is presently unknown. Moreover, it is not known which of the induced polypeptides constitute 7-dehydroxylase; however, the polypeptides of 56000 and 27000 molecular weight co-purify with enzymatic activity upon anaerobic high-performance gel filtration.

Both 7α/β-dehydroxylase and Δ^6-steroid reductase activities are stimulated by adding NAD to anaerobically dialyzed cell extracts of Eubacterium sp. V.P.I. 12708. NADH inhibited all 3 activities at high concentrations (0.5 mM) but stimulated 7α-dehydroxylase activity at lower concentrations ($<$ 0.10 mM). Double reciprocal plots of NADH inhibition of 7α-dehydroxylase activity suggested negative cooperativity. The effect of low concentrations of NADH on the kinetics of 7β-dehydroxylase and Δ^6-steroid reductase activity is presently unknown. The activity of 7α-dehy-

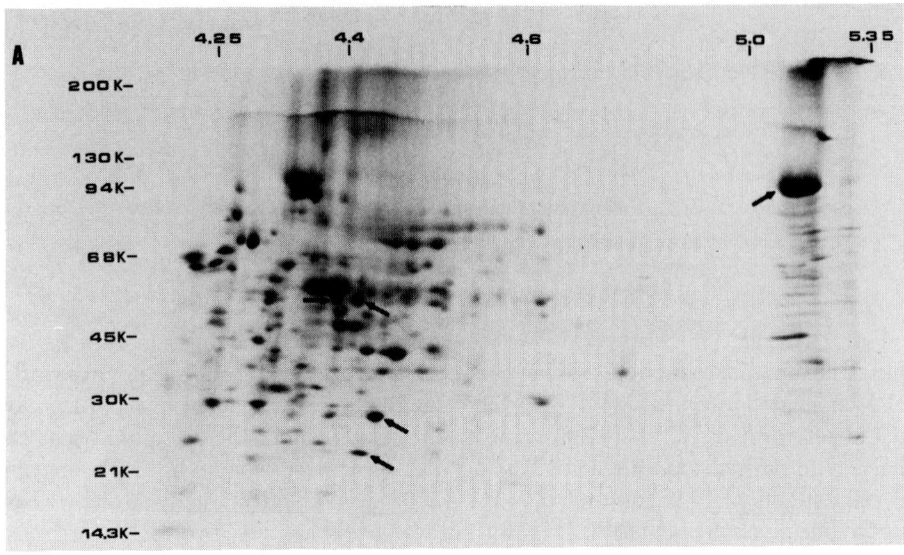

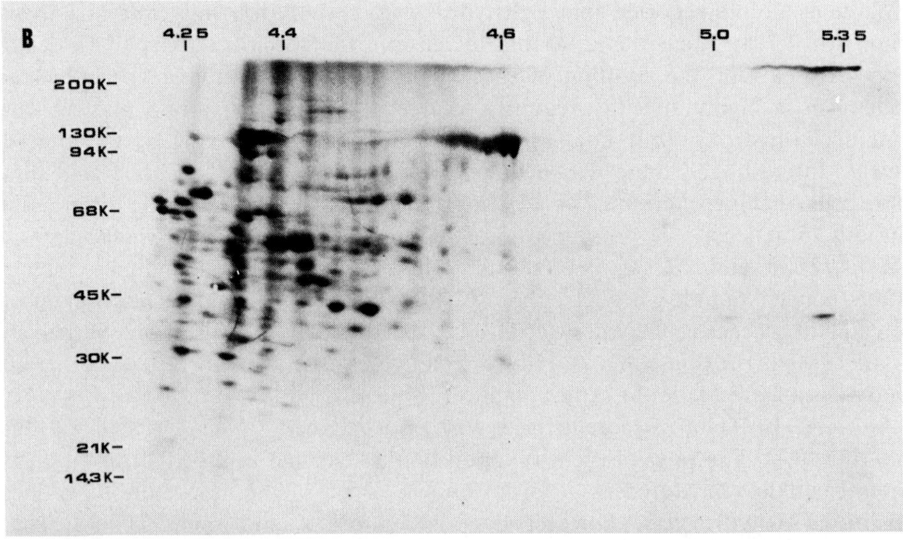

Fig. 3. Two-dimensional sodium dodecyl sulfate–polyacrylamide gel electrophoresis of [^{35}S]methionine polypeptides from cholic acid-induced (A) and control (B) cultures of Eubacterium V.P.I. 12708. Arrows indicate the synthesis of new polypeptides.

droxylase was regulated by the NAD/NADH ratio, with maximum activity at an NAD mole fraction of 0.70–0.85 [58].

Clostridium leptum V.P.I. 10900, *C. sordellii, C. bifermentans* [62] and several additional clostridial species 7α-dehydroxylate primary bile acids. Whole cells of *C.*

TABLE 4

Characteristics of 7-dehydroxylase in cell extracts of Eubacterium sp. V.P.I. 12708 [a]

Activity measured [b]	Cofactor requirement(s)	Bile acid K_m (μM)	Spec. act. (nmoles/h/ mg protein)	Inhibition by NADH (0.5 mM) (%)	M_r	Inducer of enzyme activity
7α-Dehydroxylase (CDC)	NAD	49	780	57	114000	C, CDC
7β-Dehydroxylase (UDC)	NAD	15	300	36	114000	C, CDC
Δ^6-Reductase	NAD + $FMNH_2$	ND	743	78	114000	C, CDC

[a] ND, not determined; C, cholic acid; CDC, chenodeoxycholic acid; UDC, ursodeoxycholic acid; Δ^6, 3α-hydroxy-5β-chol-6-enoic acid.
[b] 7α [57], 7β [59], Δ^6 [58].

leptum carried out 7α- but not 7β-dehydroxylation of free bile acids. Conjugated bile acids were not substrates for 7α-dehydroxylase in either *C. leptum* or Eubacterium sp. V.P.I. 12708. All detectable 7α-dehydroxylation activity was lost when whole cells of *C. leptum* were broken under strictly anaerobic conditions [52]. Therefore, it appears that the 7α-dehydroxylase in *C. leptum* V.P.I. 10900 may have quite different properties from those of the enzyme in Eubacterium sp. V.P.I. 12708. Bile acid substrate specificity studies showed that 7-dehydroxylase from Eubacterium sp. V.P.I. 12708 was highly specific requiring a free C-24 carboxyl group and an unhindered 7α- or 7β-hydroxyl group. The Δ^6-steroid reductase activity reduced either 3α-hydroxy-5β-chol-6-enoic acid or 3α,12α-dihydroxy-5β-chol-6-enoic acid.

The biotransformations described in this chapter are not required for growth of the bacteria and their physiological importance is currently unknown. However, the 7α-hydroxy epimerization of chenodeoxycholic acid by *C. absonum* may represent a detoxication mechanism [42] and the 7-dehydroxylating reaction might serve as an ancillary electron acceptor for bacteria having this enzyme. The absence of critical data necessary to address these questions stems, in part, from the paucity of work on genetic exchange systems in anaerobic bacteria containing these enzymes. The biochemical characterization of mutant strains deficient in a given bile acid biotransformation may reveal some physiological basis for these enzymes. Research along these lines should help explain how the regulation of synthesis and activity of these enzymes occur in the organism's natural ecosystem.

Acknowledgement

The author is pleased to acknowledge support from the National Institutes of Health, Public Health Service, U.S.A. through Grant CA-17747.

References

1 Eneroth, P., Gordon, B., Ryhage, R. and Sjövall, J. (1966) J. Lipid Res. 7, 511–523.
2 Eneroth, P., Gordon, B. and Sjövall, J. (1966) J. Lipid Res. 7, 524–530.
3 Ali, S.S., Kuksis, A. and Beveridge, J.M.R. (1966) Can. J. Biochem. 44, 967–969.
4 Subbiah, M.T.R., Tyler, N.E., Buscablia, M.D. and Maria, L. (1976) J. Lipid Res. 17, 78–84.
5 Setchell, K., Lawson, A., Tanida, N. and Sjövall, J. (1983) J. Lipid Res. 24, 1085–1100.
6 Palmer, R. (1972) in: Bile Acids in Human Diseases (Back, P. and Gerok, W., Eds.) pp. 65–69, Schattauer Verlag, Stuttgart.
7 Kelsey, M.I., Molina, J.E., Huang, S.K.S. and Shaikh, B. (1980) J. Lipid Res. 21, 751–759.
8 Dobzhansky, T. (1971) Genetics of the Evolutionary Process, Vol. I, Columbia University, New York.
9 Lucky, T.D. (1972) Am. J. Clin. Nutr. 25, 1292–1295.
10 Goldman, P. (1978) Annu. Rev. Pharmacol. Toxicol. 18, 523–539.
11 Moore, W.E.C. and Holdeman, L.V. (1974) Appl. Microbiol. 27, 961–979.
12 Holdeman, L.V., Good, I.J. and Moore, W.E.C. (1976) Appl. Environ. Microbiol. 31, 359–375.
13 Midvedt, T. and Norman, A. (1967) Acta Pathol. Microbiol. Scand. 71, 629–638.
14 Masada, N. (1981) Microbiol. Immunol. 25, 1–11.
15 Kobaski, K., Nishizawa, I., Yamada, T. and Hase, J. (1978) J. Biochem. (Tokyo) 84, 495–497.
16 Hylemon, P.B. and Glass, T.L. (1983) in: Human Intestinal Microflora in Health and Disease (Hentges, D.J., Ed.) pp. 189–213, Academic Press, New York.
17 Macdonald, I.A., Bokkenheuser, V.D., Winter, J., McLeron, A.M. and Mosbach, E.H. (1983) J. Lipid Res. 24, 675–700.
18 Nair, P.P., Gordon, M. and Reback, J. (1976) J. Biol. Chem. 242, 7–11.
19 Stellwag, E.J. and Hylemon, P.B. (1976) Biochim. Biophys. Acta 452, 165–176.
20 Hylemon, P.B. and Stellwag, E.J. (1976) Biochem. Biophys. Res. Commun. 69, 1088–1094.
21 Kelsey, M.I., Hwang, K.K., Huang, S.K. and Shaikh, B. (1981) J. Steroid Biochem. 14, 205–211.
22 Borriello, S.P. and Owen, R.W. (1982) Lipids 17, 477–482.
23 Huijghebaert, S.M., Mertans, I.A. and Eyssen, H.J. (1982) Appl. Environ. Microbiol. 43, 185–192.
24 Huijghebaert, S.M. and Eyssen, H.J. (1982) Appl. Environ. Microbiol. 44, 1030–1034.
25 Aries, V. and Hill, M.J. (1970) Biochim. Biophys. Acta 202, 535–543.
26 Macdonald, I.A., Jellett, J.F., Mahony, D.E. and Holdemon, L.V. (1979) Appl. Environ. Microbiol. 37, 992–1000.
27 Edenharder, R. and Deser, H.J. (1981) Zentralbl. Bakteriol. Parasitenk. Infektionskr. Hyg. Abt. I: Orig. Reihe B174, 91–104.
28 Hirano, S. and Masuda, N. (1981) Appl. Environ. Microbiol. 42, 912–915.
29 Hylemon, P.B. and Sherrod, J.A. (1975) J. Bacteriol. 122, 418–424.
30 Dickinson, A.B., Gustafsson, B.E. and Norman, A. (1971) Acta Pathol. Microbiol. Scand., Sect. B 79B, 691–698.
31 Hirano, S., Masada, N. and Akimori, N. (1981) Acta Med. Univ. Kagoshima 23, 55–64.
32 Macdonald, I.A., Mahony, D.E., Jellett, J.F. and Meier, C.E. (1977) Biochim. Biophys. Acta 489, 466–476.
33 Macdonald, I.A., Meier, E.C., Mahony, D.E. and Costain, G.A. (1976) Biochim. Biophys. Acta 450, 142–153.
34 Macdonald, I.A., Hutchinson, D.M., Forrest, T.P., Bokkenheuser, V.D., Winter, J. and Holdeman, L.V. (1983) J. Steroid Biochem. 18, 97–104.
35 Sacquet, E.C., Raibard, P.M., Mejean, C., Riottot, M.J., Leprince, C. and Leglise, P.C. (1979) Appl. Environ. Microbiol. 37, 1127–1131.
36 Eyssen, H., DePauw, G., Stragier, J. and Verhulst, A. (1983) Appl. Environ. Microbiol. 45, 141–147.
37 Macdonald, I.A., Williams, C.N. and Mahony, D.E. (1973) Biochim. Biophys. Acta 309, 243–253.
38 Macdonald, I.A., Williams, C.N., Mahony, D.E. and Christe, W.M. (1975) Biochim. Biophys. Acta 384, 12–24.
39 Sherrod, J.A. and P.B. Hylemon (1977) Biochim. Biophys. Acta 486, 351–358.

40 Macdonald, I.A. and Roach, P.B. (1981) Biochim. Biophys. Acta 665, 262–269.
41 Macdonald, I.A., Hutchinson, D.M. and Forrest, T.P. (1981) J. Lipid Res. 22, 458–466.
42 Macdonald, I.A., White, B.A. and Hylemon, P.B. (1983) J. Lipid Res. 24, 1119–1126.
43 Hirano, S. and Masuda, N. (1982) Acta Med. Univ. Kagoshima 24, 43–47.
44 Hirano, S. and Masuda, N. (1982) Appl. Environ. Microbiol. 43, 1057–1063.
45 Edenharder, R. and Knaflic, T. (1981) J. Lipid Res. 22, 652–658.
46 Hirano, S., Masuda, N., Oda, H. and Immura, T. (1981) Microbiol. Immunol. 25, 271–282.
47 Macdonald, I.A., Jellet, J.F. and Mahony, D.E. (1979) J. Lipid Res. 20, 234–239.
48 Macdonald, I.A., Jellet, J.F., Mahony, D.E. and Holdeman, L.V. (1979) Appl. Environ. Microbiol. 37, 992–1000.
49 Harris, J.N. and Hylemon, P.B. (1978) Biochim. Biophys. Acta 528, 148–157.
50 Hayakawa, S. (1973) Adv. Lipid Res. 11, 143–192.
51 Hirano, S., Nakama, R., Tamaki, M., Masuda, N. and Oda, H. (1981) Appl. Environ. Microbiol. 41, 737–745.
52 Stellwag, E.J. and Hylemon, P.B. (1979) J. Lipid Res. 20, 325–333.
53 Gustafsson, B.E., Midtvedt, T. and Norman, A. (1966) J. Exp. Med. 123, 413–432.
54 Ferrari, A., Pacini, N., Canzi, E. and Brano, F. (1980) Curr. Microbiol. 4, 257–260.
55 Samuelsson, B. (1960) J. Biol. Chem. 235, 361–366.
56 Ferrari, A., Scolastinco, C. and Beretta, L. (1977) FEBS Lett. 75, 166–168.
57 White, B.A., Cacciapuoti, A.F., Fricke, R.J., Whitehead, T.R., Mosbach, E.H. and Hylemon, P.B. (1981) J. Lipid Res. 22, 891–898.
58 White, B.A., Paone, D.A.M., Cacciapuoti, A.F., Fricke, R.J., Mosbach, E.H. and Hylemon, P.B. (1983) J. Lipid Res. 24, 20–27.
59 White, B.A., Fricke, R.J. and Hylemon, P.B. (1982) J. Lipid Res. 23, 145–153.
60 White, B.A., Lipsky, R.H., Fricke, R.J. and Hylemon, P.B. (1980) Steroids 35, 103–109.
61 Lipsky, R.H. and Hylemon, P.B. (1980) Biochim. Biophys. Acta 612, 328–336.
62 Hayakawa, S. and Hattori, T. (1970) FEBS Lett. 6, 131–133.

H. Danielsson and J. Sjövall (Eds.), *Sterols and Bile Acids*

CHAPTER 13

Physical–chemical properties of bile acids and their salts

MARTIN C. CAREY *

Department of Medicine, Harvard Medical School, Division of Gastroenterology, Brigham and Women's Hospital, Boston, MA 02115 (U.S.A.)

(I) Introduction

In a review bearing this title, it has become axiomatic to stipulate that most of the physiologic, pathophysiologic and metabolic properties of bile acids and their salts can be attributed to their multifaceted physical–chemical characteristics. A fundamental understanding of the surface-active and detergent-like properties of this family of amphiphilic steroids is therefore crucial for comprehending their functions and malfunctions in biological systems [1]. The physical–chemical properties of bile acids and their salts have been extensively reviewed a number of times past [2–6], most notably in a comprehensive treatise from 1971 by Donald M. Small [5]. This chapter will cover only those aspects of the physical chemistry of bile acids and their salts that have progressed substantially during the intervening years. For a critical overview of recent experimental approaches employed in the study of detergent-like molecules with particular reference to bile acids and their salts, a short exposition by this writer should be consulted [6].

(II) Molecular structures

(1) Chemistry

The common bile acids and salts possess a characteristic molecular structure shown schematically for sodium cholate in Fig. 1 [7]. In contrast to the all *trans* arrangement of the alicyclic ring systems in allo bile salts, a crucial feature of the

* Correspondence to: Department of Medicine, Brigham and Women's Hospital, 75 Francis Street, Boston, MA 02115, U.S.A. Telephone: (617) 732-5822.

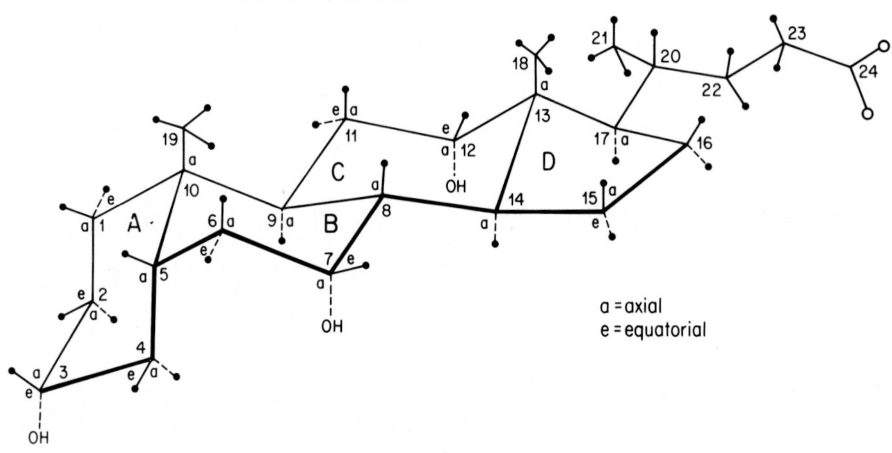

Fig. 1. Schematic diagram of the molecular structure of sodium cholate. The oxygens of the ionized carboxyl group of the side chain are depicted by open circles. The sodium ion is not displayed. (Redrawn from refs. 7 and 9 with permission.)

alicyclic saturated ring systems of the common bile salts is the *cis* fusion of the A/B rings [8]. Barnes and Geckle [9], employing 400 MHz ^{1}H-nuclear magnetic resonance (NMR) spectroscopy, successfully resolved and assigned all the proton resonances of sodium cholate in dilute aqueous (^2H_2O) solution. The availability of high-field-strength superconducting magnets resolved the resonances between 1.0 and 2.3 δ which had hitherto remained enveloped within a broad peak [10,11]. The assignments of the individual methylene protons were made by consideration of the expected couplings based on the molecular structure [7, and Section III.2] and ^{1}H-nuclear Overhauser enhancement experiments; verification of the assignments of the methine protons was carried out by of single frequency ^{1}H-decoupled ^{13}C-NMR. The orientation of each proton with respect to the plane of the molecule (Fig. 1) is given by the dashed (α, below the plane) or solid (β, in or above the plane) lines. Orientation with respect to each ring is denoted in terms of e (equatorial, in the plane) and a (axial, out of the plane). The 1α, 3α, 6α, 11α and 15α orientations are equatorial while other α orientations are axial; 2β, 4β, 7β, and 12β are equatorial, while other β orientations are axial. No axial–equatorial assignments can be made for the protons on C-16; they have been proven equivocal by all physical methods, including X-ray [7] and NMR analysis [9].

The orientation of the mobile side chain at C-17 has not been unambiguously resolved for alkali salts of bile acids in aqueous solutions. However, evidence adduced from the differences in calculated molecular areas of surface-adsorbed bile salts versus spread monomolecular layers of insoluble bile acids at their collapse pressures [12] suggest that the side chain, when ionized, lies α-axial with respect to the plane of the molecule, but when undissociated lies parallel to the surface. Effects of systematic variations in pH between 1 and 13 on the surface areas of spread and adsorbed glycocholate molecules suggest that the difference between the two surface

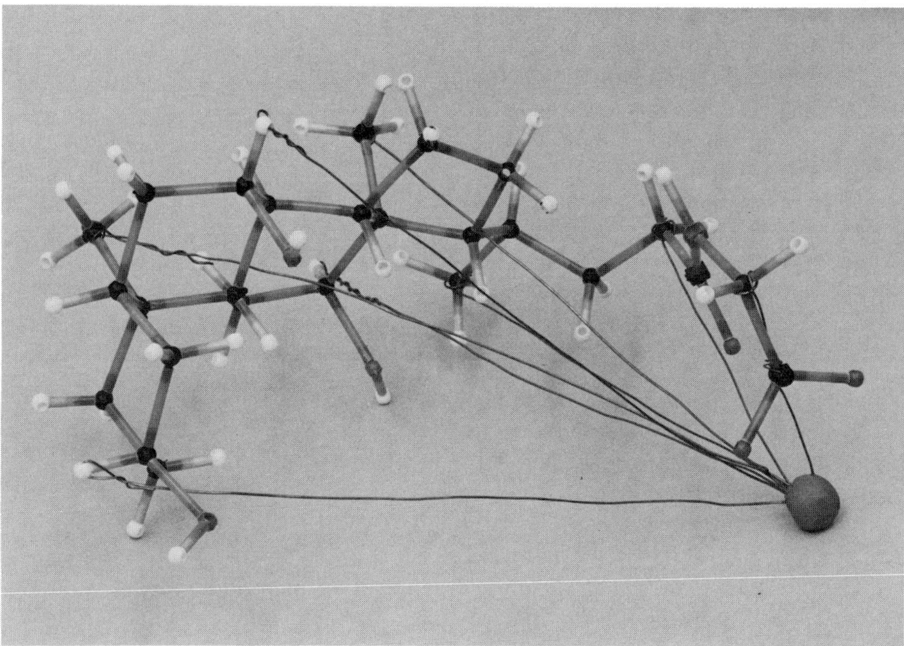

Fig. 2. Solution structure of dysprosium glycocholate, 1:1 complex — the dysprosium ion is the large sphere at the bisector of the carboxyl group; the hydrophilic side of the molecule faces the observer. (Modified from ref. 14, courtesy of Dr. Stephen Barnes.)

areas is 26 Å^2, in agreement with equatorial and α-axial configurations of the glycine group in the undissociated and dissociated states, respectively [13].

Recently, the side chain structure of glycocholate monomers was resolved by NMR employing the paramagnetic lanthanide, dysprosium [14]. Dysprosium chloride interacted with 0.5 mM sodium glycocholate in ^2H_2O to form a 1:1 salt complex (binding constant, K_D, 3 ± 0.1 mM). Lanthanide probe NMR indicated the structural features depicted in Fig. 2: (a) the dysprosium atom is situated on the bisector of the O–C = O group; (b) the distances between all 3 hydroxyl functions and the dysprosium ion (10–14 Å) are incompatible with lanthanide–steroid hydroxyl coordination; (c) the aliphatic side chain lies in the plane of the B, C and D rings whereas the carboxylate and amide carbonyl groups are in the plane of the A ring; (d) the side chain apparently shows a high degree of order, possibly because the dysprosium ion and the amide carbonyl group are coordinated through intercalated water (^2H_2O) molecules. These results confirm the general consensus based on the surface monolayer studies [12,13] that in aqueous solutions all polar groups of the bile salt nucleus and ionized side chain lie on the same face of the molecule forming the α or hydrophilic surface. Since the lanthanides are isomorphous with calcium [15], similar results might be expected with ^{43}Ca-NMR of calcium bile salts.

Based on sodium ion activities [16] and conductance studies [17,18] it appears that, below their respective critical micellar concentration (CMC) values, all sodium bile salts behave as fully dissociated 1 : 1 electrolytes. In contrast, using calcium-specific electrodes, Moore et al. [19] found high-affinity binding of Ca to sodium taurocholate monomers below the CMC. With sodium cholate in 25–100 mM solutions, multicomponent self-diffusion and ^{23}Na-NMR studies [20] suggest that counterion binding to micellar solutions is low (~ 18%) compared with typical detergents (~ 50–60%) [21] and that the hydration numbers are higher, ~ 20–30 water molecules per cholate ion. Once extensive self-aggregation takes place in the 100–400 mM range, these values increase to about 45% and 40, respectively. In the high-field NMR studies [9], titration of a 4 mM sodium cholate solution to pH 6.0 where the system is supersaturated with cholic acid [5] (equilibrium precipitation pH 6.5), the only spectral change noted was a small (0.01 δ) upfield shift in the resonances from C-23–CH_2, i.e. from protons next to the C-24 COO^- group. This is most probably related to the undissociated form of cholate, since it was eliminated once cholic acid precipitated with a subsequent rise in pH to 6.4. At pH 7, peak broadening was observed above a sodium cholate concentration of 5 mM, indicative of the initiation of self-association. Although ^{1}H-NMR peak broadening has also been attributed to increased microviscosity or other inter- and intramolecular phenomena rather than to significant self-aggregation in sodium cholate solutions [22], the correct interpretation of these data is probably self-aggregation. The 400 MHz ^{1}H-NMR spectrum of 23-norcholate [9] was almost identical to that of cholate with the exception that the proton resonances were shifted down-field slightly; this was most marked for the protons on the carbon atom adjacent to the carboxyl group.

(2) Hydrophilic–hydrophobic balance

All of the common bile salts possess a 3α-hydroxyl function and one or two other hydroxyl functions at positions 6α/β, 7α/β, 12α; many other permutations, such as hydroxylations at unusual positions can occur in nature [8,23] (cf. Chapter 11). In addition, hydroxyl groups may be sulfated or glucuronidated and the side chain may be unconjugated or amide-linked to taurine and glycine or other amino acids [1,23,24]. Moreover, di-, tri- and tetra-conjugates have been synthesized and chemically and physico-chemically characterized [25]. Finally, each hydroxyl function can be dehydrogenated to give oxo bile acids and salts [1]. Such modifications can greatly alter the polarity of both the steroid nucleus and that of the side chain. The relative overall potency of the hydrophilic functional groups versus the contiguous surface cavity area of hydrocarbon exposed to water and the topological relationships of each is conventionally known as the hydrophilic–hydrophobic balance (HHB) [26]. Because of increasing awareness that the HHB properties of bile salts are important predictors of physical–chemical [6,12,27–29] and ultimately pathophysiological functions [6], the use of reversed-phase HPLC (high-performance liquid chromatography) has been employed to quantify this property of the entire molecule in the monomeric state [26,30]. However, with respect to certain membrane-binding functions, the HHB of the steroid nucleus may be more relevant than that of the overall molecule [31,32]; this partial HHB property is not easily quantified directly.

Taurine-conjugated bile salts are more hydrophilic than the corresponding glycine conjugates, as evident from the mobilities in HPLC [6,26] and conventional partition chromatography [8,23]. The free bile salts are the least hydrophilic. Polarity increases with number of hydroxyl groups. For monohydroxy bile salts the polarity (HPLC mobility) falls in the order 3-OH ~ 6-OH > 7-OH > 12-OH [30]. Equatorial hydroxyl functions are more polar than axial and the 5α-H (allo) are more polar than the 5β-H (normal) bile salts. Oxo substituents have intermediate polarities which lie between α- and β-hydroxyl groups at the corresponding positions. However, in terms of predicting and rationalizing HPLC elution patterns, both the contiguous non-polar surface and the environment of polar constituents on the steroid nucleus must also be considered. For example, both 3α,7β,12α-trihydroxy-5β-cholanoate and ursodeoxycholate are highly polar due to the greater water solvation of the unhindered equatorial 7β-hydroxyl function. In addition, this orientation facilitates binding of extensive layers of water, which also reduces the effective contiguous hydrocarbon area on the β face of the molecule. The equatorial 6α-hydroxyl group is somewhat less polar than the 7β-hydroxyl group whereas a 6β-hydroxyl function is more polar due to less steric constraint. Similar connotations apply to allo bile salts which have an axial 3α-hydroxyl function and are more polar because of the *trans* A/B ring juncture. In both allo and normal bile salts, 7α- and 12α-hydroxyl functions are less polar than axial or equatorial 3-hydroxyl functions due to steric constraint, engendering less water binding. Many of these trends, inferred by HPLC analysis, have been corroborated by CMC data [33]. Further, it also appears that when the 3, 7, 12 polar functions are all epimerized simultaneously, polarity falls again since now the conventional hydrophilic side of the molecule has become the least polar face [33]. For a further discussion of exceptions to these principles in relation to HPLC retention values, the reader should consult Elliot and Shaw's excellent review [30]. Sulfation and/or glucuronidation renders the bile salts strikingly more polar; in recent studies ([25], J.M. Donovan, I.M. Yousef and M.C. Carey, unpublished data) on fully sulfated unconjugated and glycine- or taurine-conjugated bile salts, the polarity of the molecules by thin-layer chromatography was in the rank order cholate > ursodeoxycholate > chenodeoxycholate ~ deoxycholate > lithocholate, suggesting that pansulfation obliterates the high HPLC polarity induced by an unsulfated 7β-hydroxyl group.

(3) Miscellaneous physical constants

A compilation of critical physical constants for the common bile acids and their salts is given in Table 1. The vast majority of literature values for melting points (m.p.) fall between the limits given in this table [34,35]. However, certain bile acids are notorious in forming crystalline polymorphs [36–38], and most dihydroxy bile acids form stable crystalline solvates with a wide variety of solvent molecules

TABLE 1

Physical constants of bile acids and their alkali salts

Common name (acid)	m.p. [a] (acid, °C)	Density by			V_{ap} (cm^3/g) [e]	ϕ_v^0 app. molal vol. (cm^3/mole) [f]		Mol. vol [g] (Å^3/molecule of anion)
		Crystal data [b]	Flotation [c]	Densimetry [d]		Na^+/K^+ salt	Anion	
Lithocholic	184(−2)→186(+3)	1.121	1.125	–	(0.789)	314.3	320.9	533
Deoxycholic	176(−6)→178	1.16 1.37 (Rb)	1.16 1.36 (Rb)	0.997	0.762	316.0 315.8	322.6 322.4	536
Chenodeoxycholic	172(−7, +1)	1.162	–	0.997	0.772	320.1	326.7	542
Ursodeoxycholic	203(−7, +2)	1.185	1.174	0.997	0.780	323.5	330.1	548
Cholic	198(+4)	1.153 1.191 (Na^+) 1.245 (Na^+, H_2O)	1.156 1.167 (Na^+) 1.22 (Na^+, H_2O)	0.997 1.105 (^2H_2O)	0.730	314.4 327.6 (K^+)	321.0 324.0	536
Dehydrocholic	237	–	–	–	0.761	323.0 320.0 (K^+)	316.4 316.4	525

[a] Values as in Merck Index, 10th Edn. [34] with literature ranges excluding solvates and low m.p. polymorphs (see ref. 35).
[b] From refs. 5, 7, 43–47 and 51.
[c] From refs. 5, 7, 43–47 and 51.
[d] From Vadnere et al. [50], infinite dilution, 0.2 M Tris, 25°C.
[e] Calculated from molecular weight of sodium salt and data in column to right (infinite dilution).
[f] From refs. 50 and 52 extrapolated to infinite dilution. Data for lithocholate based on 1.6 cm^3/mole difference between cholate and deoxycholate [52]. Anionic data based on additivity. ϕ_v^0 (K^+) = 3.6 cm^3/mole; ϕ_v^0 (Na^+) = −6.6 cm^3/mole.
[g] Calculated from apparent molal volume of anion at infinite dilution (f) and Avogadro's number (6.023×10^{23} molecules/mole).

[37,39–41]. In these cases m.p. values alone are not an adequate criterion for identification or purity of a specific bile acid, since when solvate molecules are present in a fixed stoichiometry, a sharp but lower m.p. value is usually obtained. Finally, certain bile acids, most notably deoxycholic acid [5,42], form stable mixed crystalline complexes, so-called "choleic acids" with a variety of macromolecular guest molecules in a fixed bile acid : guest stoichiometry (see Section III.3).

Since density is crucially influenced by molecular packing, the physical state of a bile acid or salt appreciably influences its density. Of the two columns of density values for the crystalline state in Table 1 [5,43–47], the density by direct methods (generally flotation) and complete or partial crystal data (with water and/or ethanol) are in excellent agreement, as are those for two rarer bile acids not tabulated here: 3α,7α,12α-trihydroxy-5β-cholestan-26-oic acid, 1.135 g/cm^3 [48] and hyodeoxycholic acid, 1.17 g/cm^3 [49], but those for monomers in solution at infinite dilution by precision densimetry (Table 1) are much lower [50]. Solid bile acids are generally more dense than water and their crystalline alkaline metal salts (Rb, Na) are more dense than the corresponding acids [7,51]. The solution values for sodium salts reported earlier by pycnometry [5] refer to estimates for 1–19 g/dl (i.e. concentrated micellar solutions) and are appreciably larger than those for the monomeric state since density of bile salts is now known to increase dramatically upon self-aggregation [50]. Density is lowest with lithocholic acid (LC) and increases stepwise within the dihydroxy series in the rank order deoxycholic acid (DC) < chenodeoxycholic acid (CDC) < ursodeoxycholic acid (UDC) indicating proportionally greater exposure of the second hydroxyl function to hydration (see Section II.2). The value for cholic acid (C) falls again, suggesting a tightly bound semi-crystalline H-bonding structure between 3α-, 7α- and 12α-hydroxyl functions. For this reason the sodium salt of cholic acid is less dense than the rubidium salt of deoxycholic acid.

The values for apparent molar volumes (ϕ_v^0) at infinite dilution (Table 1) have been extrapolated from highly precise measurements well below the CMC [50,52]. Using the reported values for ϕ_v^0 of the K^+ and Na^+ counterions [52], a determination of ϕ_v^0 for the anions alone can be made. The difference of 1.6 cm^3/mole between C and DC ions is in agreement with literature data [52] for the substitution of a hydrogen atom by a hydroxyl group. However, CDC and UDC are quite anomalous as noted earlier, suggesting the powerful hydrating effect of α- and especially β-hydroxyl groups at C-7 [30]. The decrease in volume of 4–8 cm^3/mole between the ϕ_v^0 for cholic and dehydrocholic acid is also expected for the volume decrement upon substitution of CHOH groups with C = O functions [52]. Since the molecular volume calculations (Å^3/mole) given by Small [5] for the sodium salts at finite (micellar) concentration differ appreciably from those shown in Table 1 for the anions (at infinite dilution), it is a likely inference that unhydrated monomers of bile salt anions are more voluminous (in water) than when incorporated into micelles. This conclusion is verified by other data summarized later.

(III) Crystalline structures

This hitherto neglected area is now receiving major attention and the crystalline structures of many common and uncommon bile acids [43,44,48,49], their alkaline and alkaline metal salts [7,51,53] have been defined. "Choleic acids" have been the subject of much activity in this field. A summary of the earlier work on "choleic acids" can be found in Sobotka [42] and Small [5].

(1) Bile acids and their derivatives

The crystal and molecular structures of 3 solvate-free natural bile acids [43,44,49] and the *p*-bromoanilide derivative of DC [54] have been elucidated. Crystallographic data are given in summary form in Table 2 and a single projection of the molecular packing in each unit cell is given in Fig. 3. Of the bile acid crystals, all are orthorhombic except for CDC [43], which is monoclinic. There are 4 molecules in each unit cell, with the packing arrangement and intermolecular H-bonding pattern in the case of CDC being distinctly different from the others. The details of the highly complex H-bond network for CDC are listed in Table 2 and involve 8 distinct H-bonding patterns. In the asymmetric unit cell, there are two separate orientations denoted by molecules I and II (Fig. 3, Table 2). While the geometry of each steroid nucleus is that expected for a cholane derivative, there are subtle differences in intramolecular bond lengths and angles and other details of the molecular geometry for both molecules such as the orientation of the carboxyl group in the asymmetric unit. Both molecules have complete intermolecular hydrogen bonding, forming helices of type II molecules linked indirectly as rotamers through chains of type I molecules. In the orthorhombic crystals of LC [44], the packing and H-bond network is simpler, involving all O atoms (Table 2) with each layer of molecules being identical and only related by rotation, inversion and translation. In hyodeoxycholic acid (HDC) [49], the H-bonding pattern involves O(3) and O(6) as well as O(24–1). However, there are no H bonds with the carboxyl O(24–2) group (Table 2). Only the molecular association in the crystal structure of DC *p*-bromoanilide [54] (Table 2, Fig. 3) reveals a cage-like dimeric structure with a polar interior cavity and a non-polar exterior surface. In this respect, the molecular packing resembles "choleic acids" rather than true bile acid crystals.

(2) Bile salt hydrates

Crystal and molecular structures of 3 bile salt hydrates have been solved [7,51,53]. The crystallographic data (Table 2) show that all are monoclinic with 2 molecules in each unit cell. Whereas the anions are held together mainly by ion–ion and ion–dipole interactions between the counterions and the carboxylate and hydroxyl groups to which water molecules contribute, the crystal packing patterns are remarkably similar (Figs. 4 and 5). The crystal packing upon looking down the b

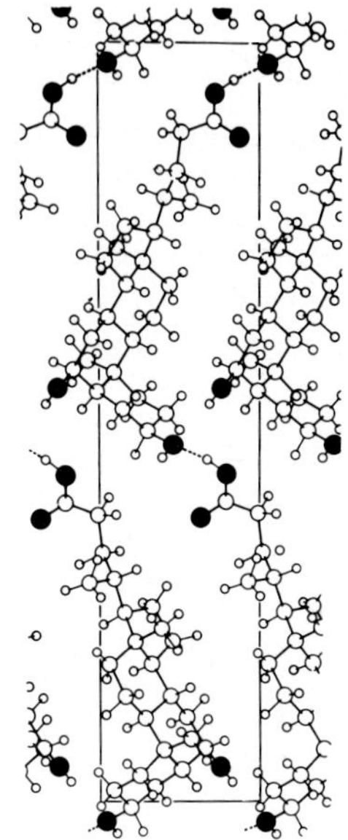

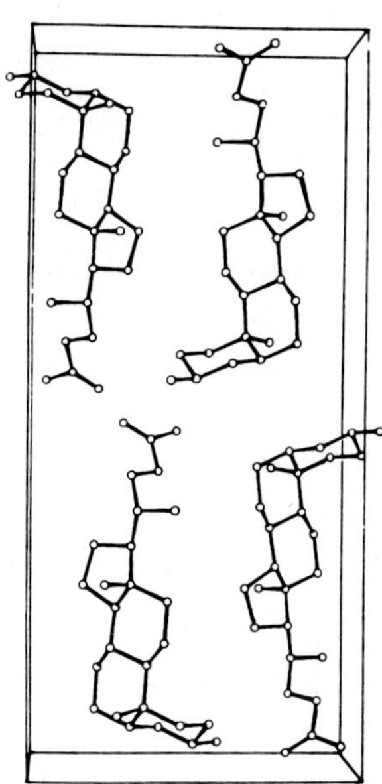

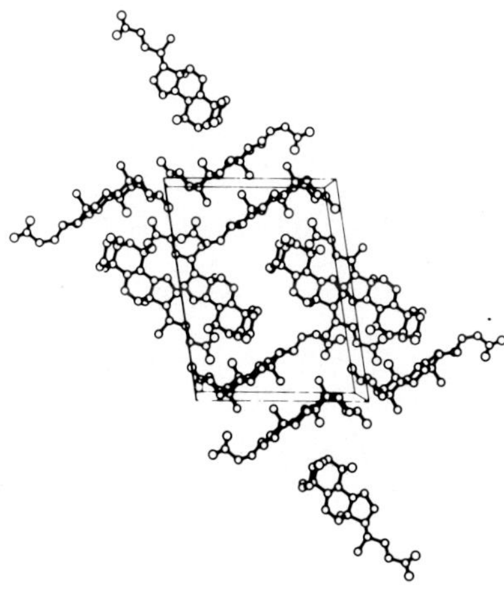

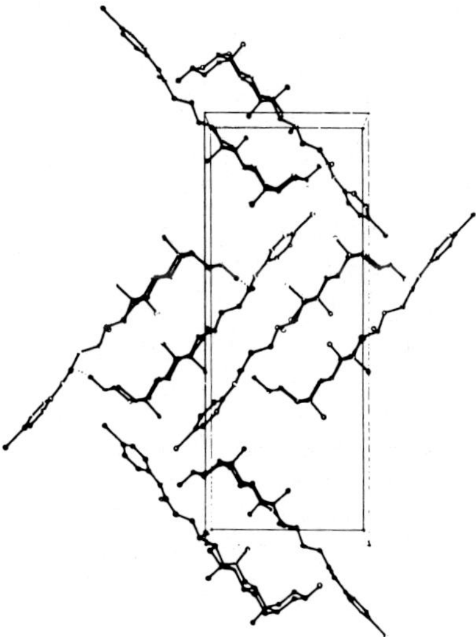

Fig. 3. Crystal packing and structural configurations of bile acids (α-axis projection). (From refs. 43, 44, 49 and 54 with permission.)

TABLE 2

Crystallographic data for bile acids and salts

Bile acids	Habit	Space group	Unit cell					
			Dimensions (Å)			Angles (°)		
			a	*b*	*c*	α	β	γ
Hyodeoxycholic [49]	Orthorhombic	$P2_12_12_1$	11.574	29.921	6.443	90	90	90
Lithocholic [44]	Orthorhombic	$P2_12_12_1$	6.807	12.178	26.779	90	90	90
Chenodeoxycholic [43]	Monoclinic	$P2_1(C_2^2$, No. 4)	18.785	8.120	14.889	90	99.1	90
Deoxycholic *p*-bromoanilide [54]	Orthorhombic	$P2_12_12_1$	11.942	30.62	7.585	90	90	90
Sodium cholate monohydrate [7]	Monoclinic	$P2_1$	12.197	8.214	12.559	90	108.07	90
Rubidium deoxycholate monohydrate [51]	Monoclinic	$P2_1$	13.118	7.817	11.788	90	97.74	90
Calcium cholate chloride heptahydrate [53]	Monoclinic	$P2_1$	11.918	8.636	15.302	90	97.93	90

Molecules	H bonding		Other observations
	C number	Length (Å)	
Z			
4	O(3)–O(6) O(3)–O(24-1)	2.794 2.683	1/2H-bonding potential utilized; no C = O–H bonds; C(20) in R configuration
4	O(3)–O(24-1) O(3)–O(24-2)	2.712 2.597	All O atoms involved in H bonding; C(20) in R configuration
4	*Mol. I – I* O(3)–O(24-1) O(3)–O(24-2) *Mol. II – II* O(3′)–O(24-1′) *Mol. I – II* O(7′)– O(3′) O(7′)– O(24-2′)	*I – I* 2.74 2.90 *II – II* 2.86 2.74 2.71	Highly complex H-bond network; all O atoms involved Also I–II in reversed linkages
	Mol. I – II O(7′)–O(24-2)	 2.87	
4	O(3)–O(24)	2.96	No H bonding involving O(12); all *trans* side chain
2	Na^+–5-O atoms 3 OHs of different anions C = O of 4th to O of H_2O	2.344 – 2.509	All O atoms involved in H bonding. H bonding to form zig-zag spirals parallel to b-axis. Further H bonding across ends of molecules to give sandwich sheet structure with non-polar exteriors. Na and H_2O inside hydrophilic bilayers. Van der Waals' contact of hydrophobic bilayers. Counterion steroid–OH bonding
2	Rb^+–6-O atoms 3 to 2 O–C = O 3 to OH 3,7 and 3′ H_2O coordinated to O(3)(7′)	2.86 – 3.18 2.75–2.79	Similar to Na cholate
2	Ca in bidentate coordination with 2 COO^-, hydrated with $5H_2O$	2.363– 2.59	Similar to Na cholate with the exception of no counterion–steroid OH bonding

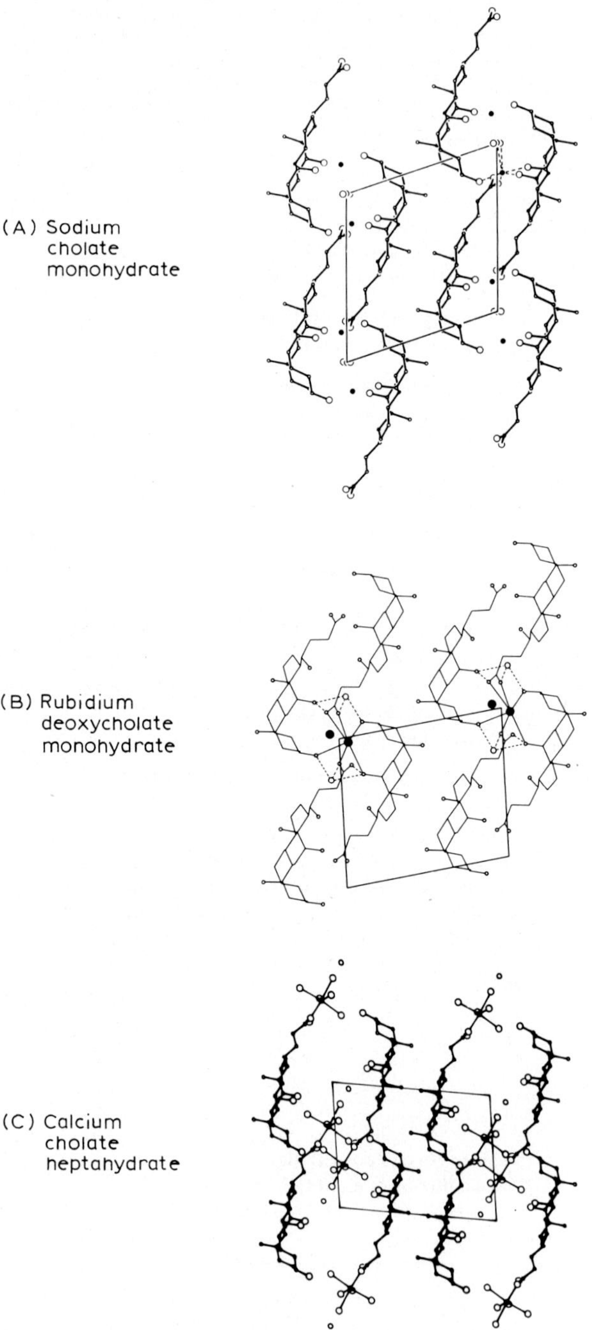

Fig. 4. Crystal packing and structural configurations of bile salts to show bilayer arrangement. The solid circles represent the position and coordination of the cations. Reprinted in modified form from refs. 7, 51 and 53 with permission.)

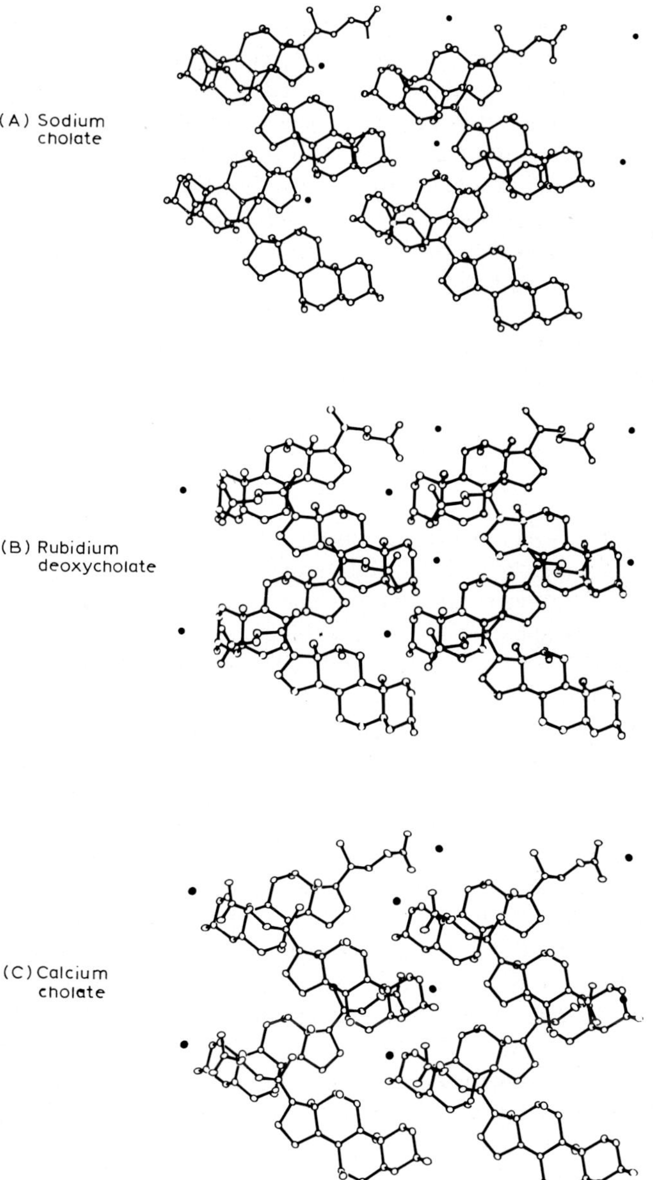

Fig. 5. Crystal packing of bile salts showing overlapping of side chains with A/B rings. (Reprinted in modified form from ref. 53 with permission.)

axis is characterized by an assembly of bilayers with the hydrophilic faces of the molecules in apposition forming a "sandwich" of counterions and water molecules while, on the hydrophobic faces, neighboring molecules interact in bilayers with apparently close van der Waals' contacts between the inverted convex hydrocarbon surfaces. The hydrophobic interactions in all 3 crystal structures involve contacts between the hydrophobic portions of the carboxylate side chains and the A and B rings (Fig. 5). This unexpected finding results in a staggered "zig-zag" pattern in all bile salt hydrates that is likely to find relevance in the packing of bile salt molecules to form simple micelles in aqueous solution [53]. This arrangement, together with the fact that in all cases the carboxylate side chain displays two different conformations, is consistent with the finding that calcium, sodium and rubidium ions interact with the polar faces of the bilayers in grossly similar but with different details in the bonding configurations (Table 2). It is noteworthy that in all 3 structures the cations are coordinated to the carboxylate groups: whereas calcium interacts only with the oxygen atoms of the carboxylate group and directly with five of the water molecules of the hydrate, the Rb and Na ions also interact directly with one and two hydroxyl functions, respectively [7,51,53].

(3) "Choleic acids"

Deoxycholic acid and a few other bile acids display the unusual property of forming inclusion or canal complexes with a wide variety of organic compounds [5,42]. These stoichiometric crystalline complexes, or "choleic acids", have received much attention from crystallographers who, in the older work, have generally focused on guest molecules such as aliphatic and aromatic hydrocarbons, fatty acids, alcohols, esters, ethers, phenols, azo dyes, alkaloids, methyl orange, β-carotene and cholesterol [42,55–57]. These structures are characterized by channels covered inside with the non-polar groups of DC and the interaction between host and guest molecules are of a hydrophobic type. As a corollary, the DC molecules form hydrogen-bonded bilayers stacked in different arrays so as to leave hydrophobic channels between them. More recent work has focused on crystalline inclusion complexes formed between DC and bulky rather than elongated molecules such as (+)-camphor [58], norbornadiene [59], cyclohexenone [60], aromatic compact polarizable molecules, such as *p*-diiodobenzene and phenanthrene [61] and highly polar molecules such as ethanol/water [47], acetic acid [62], and even water itself [46]. These studies have demonstrated a rich variety of structures which highlight the versatility of DCA molecules to pack in crystals with the guest molecules in stoichiometric proportions. In all cases with hydrocarbons, hydrophobic channels are formed by the steroid bilayers interacting via their hydrophobic groups: however, remarkable versatility exists in that the steroid molecules are shifted parallel to each other in either or both of two directions, thus forming channels of differing sizes, shapes and orientations to accommodate the guest molecules with optimal van der Waals' guest–host interactions [58–61]. Variation in geometric and/or electronic structure of guest molecules yields different complexes. In the case of small polar molecules, DC molecules form hydrogen-bonded layers which contain channels filled by continuous or interrupted chains of single or mixed polar molecules [46,47]. The polar molecules are generally linked by H bonds with each other and with the hydrophilic functional groups of the DC molecules lining the channel walls. The channel walls are thus hydrophilic [46,47,62], unlike the hydrophobic channel walls found in the classical orthorhombic inclusion complexes of DC and hydrophobic molecules [55–61]. An "addition" compound of cholic acid and ethanol [45] does display these features partially and is crystallographically similar to DC *p*-bromoaniline (Fig. 3d). "Choleic acids", once mistakenly thought to be the molecular "principle" involved in fat absorption from the gut [63], are not entirely lacking in pathophysiological relevance. The rare human enteroliths (intestinal stones) consist chiefly of "choleic acid" complexes of DC and fatty acids in a molecular ratio of 8 : 1 [64]. In the few cases of cholic acid enteroliths examined chemically, no included fatty acids have been detected [65]. It is not known whether hydrophobic and hydrophilic guest molecules can be complexed bifunctionally with DC to form "mixed" "choleic acids".

(IV) Surface physical chemistry

(1) Bile acids

Surface studies of insoluble monolayers of all the common unconjugated bile acids, including the unsubstituted cholanoic acid, have been carried out by a number of workers and thoroughly reviewed [5]. Being insoluble non-swelling amphiphiles with limited aqueous solubility, their surface pressure–area (π-A) isotherms can be measured satisfactorily with a Langmuir–Pockels surface balance on an aqueous subphase containing 3–6 M NaCl to salt out polar functions and at sufficient acidic pH (1–3) to prevent ionization [5,6].

Bile acids appear in general to form gaseous and liquid monolayers, but not condensed or solid monomolecular films. π-A isotherms, typical of those shown for CDC and UDC (Fig. 6) [12] are found with most bile acids (representative monolayer data summarized in Table 3a). Upon compression of a bile acid surface film, the physical state changes from that of a two-dimensional gas ($A > 8000$ $Å^2$/molecule) to a two-dimensional liquid ($A = 90$–150 $Å^2$/molecule). Between a certain range of areas ($\sim$ 300-8000 $Å^2$) the isotherm is flat. Between about 200–300 $Å^2$ and about 80–100 $Å^2$, π begins to rise sharply upon compression ("lift off", Table 3a) and at about 75–120 $Å^2$ depending upon the bile acid species, there is a change in slope of the isotherm (Fig. 6) caused by a rearrangement or a secondary phase transformation in the two-dimensional liquid [5,12]. As molecular areas are reduced to less than 80–90 $Å^2$, the isotherms become flat again and this is due to collapse of the film which usually becomes three-dimensional with piling of one molecule on top of the other. As shown by Ekwall and Ekholm [66], the first two layers of molecules probably interact via their hydrophobic surfaces, while the third interacts with the second via their hydrophilic surfaces. It is possible, therefore, that the structure of the surface multilayer is similar to that in the crystalline conformation of the acids (Fig. 3). Analysis of π-A isotherms by the surface phase rule derived by Crisp [67,68] is detailed elsewhere [5,6] and its utility emphasized. While this

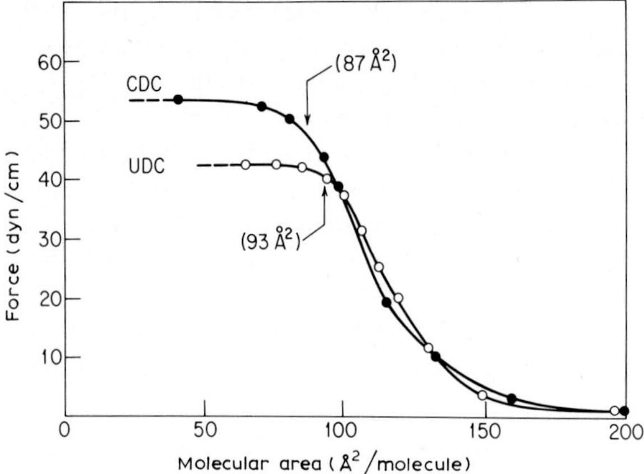

Fig. 6. Force–area isotherms for compression of monomolecular layers of the undissociated acid form of CDC and UDC at an air–0.6 M NaCl (pH 2) aqueous interface (25°C). The arrowed points represent the areas per molecule at the collapse pressures (~ 50 dyn/cm for CDC and ~ 40 dyn/cm for UDC). (From refs. 6 and 12 with permission.)

general outline applies to most common bile acids at air–water interfaces, molecules of cholanoic acid and lithocholic acid at pH 10.0 on 3 M NaCl subphases are oriented vertically (areas/molecule at collapse = 42–43 Å^2) (Table 3a) [5]. The isotherms of both are reminiscent of that of cholesterol [69] save for the fact that the isotherms remain liquid upon compression [5]. It is obvious that the unsubstituted steroid nucleus cannot be anchored to the interface; with lithocholic acid at pH 10, strong ionization anchors the molecule to the interface and 3 M NaCl dehydrates the single polar function on the A ring forcing the alicyclic rings out of the interface and as a result the molecule becomes vertically oriented [5]. The collapse pressures (Table 3a) generally increase as the hydrophilicity of the steroid nucleus increases. Collapse pressures of cholic acid are curiously much lower than expected. These results may be spurious, since on a subphase of 3 M NaCl, cholic acid is still too soluble to form stable monomolecular films [5]. The π-A isotherm given by Ekwall and Ekholm [66] confirms this suggestion since it does not become flat between molecular areas of 110 and 20 Å^2 suggesting progressive bulk solubility of this bile acid.

(2) Bile salts

Surface tensions of the soluble alkali salt of di- and tri-hydroxy bile salts have been widely employed [5,11,12,33,70–74] to measure CMCs of bile salts (see Section VI.1). Employing Gibbs' adsorption isotherm equation and the steep slope of the experimental surface tension versus bile salt concentration curve, the surface excess, i.e. concentration of bile salt molecules/cm^2 of interface, can be calculated accurately in high bulk ionic strength [12,70]. Using this value and Avogadro's number, the area per molecule at the interface can be calculated [6]. These values (Table 3b),

TABLE 3a

Surface physical chemistry of bile acids (17–23°C)

Spread films

Bile acid	Substrate		Areas (Å^2/molecule)		Pressure (mN/m)		Film state	Other
	pH	[NaCl] (M)	Lift-off	Collapse	Multilayer	Collapse		
Cholanoic acid	2	3	50	42	N.O.	20	Liquid	Isotherm similar to cholesterol
Lithocholic acid	1.5	0	125	80	23	13	Liquid	Multilayer film, solid
	"Acidic"	3	110	85	25	15	Liquid	Multilayer film, solid
	3.0	3	130	85	N.O.	15.5	Liquid	Multilayer film, solid
	10.0	3	130	43	N.O.	29	Liquid	2nd-order phase transition = 75Å^2
Deoxycholic acid	2	3	200	110	15	30	Liquid	Multilayer film, solid
	3	3	170	93	N.O.	23	Liquid	2nd-order phase transition = 120 Å^2
	3	2	150	80	N.O.	22	Liquid	2nd-order phase transition = 95 Å^2
Chenodeoxycholic acid	"Acidic"	3	150	86	N.O.	30	Liquid	N.R.
	2	5	180	87	N.O.	50	Liquid	N.R.
Ursodeoxycholic acid	2	5	180	93	N.O.	42	Liquid	N.R.
Cholic acid	"Acidic"	3	160	110 [a]	N.O.	14 [a]	Liquid	N.R.
	2	3	300	120 [a]	N.O.	14 [a]	Liquid	N.R.

N.O., not observed; N.R., not recorded.

[a] Probably spurious.

when compared with the area(s) of the acids at the collapse pressure, are generally smaller (see ref. 13 and Section II.1). The greatest lowering of the air–water interfacial tension is produced by the most hydrophobic bile salt [74]. Surface tension studies of taurine- and glycine-conjugated bile acids indicate that they induce an appreciably greater lowering of surface tension then the free species [12]. As is expected, bile salts align also at oil–water interfaces and reduce interfacial tension to about 5 mN/m [75–77], compared with ~ 40–50 mN/m at water–air interfaces [11,12,33,70–74]. The molecular areas at these interfaces are generally much larger (200–300 Å^2/molecule) than those observed for air–water interfaces in Table 3b.

A very interesting and novel approach, that of ellipsometry, has been applied recently to evaluate the interfacial thickness of bile salt films [74]. Ellipsometry is an optical non-destructive method used to examine properties of surface films such as refractive index, extinction coefficient, and thickness of the film [78]. The average area occupied by a DC anion at the air–water interface is 84 Å^2 measured by ellipsometry [74] which is identical to that calculated by the Gibbs adsorption isotherm [6,12] (Table 3b). Further, the average DC film thickness measured by ellipsometry was 6.3 Å in agreement with the vertical dimension of the DC ion from molecular models or estimated by dividing the molecular volume of the DC anion (Table 1) by the interfacial area (84 Å^2), which gives 6.38 Å for the vertical dimension. This remarkable agreement between both methods suggests that the molecular shapes of bile salts are more reminiscent of cylinders than saucers.

(3) Mixed monolayers

A large body of new information accumulated in the late 1960s and early 1970s on the molecular interactions in mixed films of bile acids and other insoluble lipids spread at both CCl_4– and air–water (pH 2–3, 3–5 M NaCl) interfaces [79–84]. Small [5] refers to the earlier surface balance work on bile acid–fatty acid and bile acid–lecithin mixtures, and extensively discussed his own studies of the interactions of cholic (C), deoxycholic (DC), and lithocholic (LC) acids with egg yolk lecithin with an analysis employing classical additivity diagrams. He concluded that C is only partially miscible in monolayers with egg lecithin and lies flat on the air–water surface. An analogous study carried out by Llopes et al. [83] employing dipalmitoyl glycero-3-phosphocholine showed a strong condensing effect of C and a negative deviation from additivity; partial areas of C were 133–150 Å^2/molecule. The results favored a lecithin-induced transition of C molecules lying flat to a vertical stacked dimer arrangement which would be consistent with the partial molecular areas. This interpretation appears more reasonable than Small's [5] view and corresponds to the crystalline packing of bile acids (Fig. 3) and the strong condensing effects upon mixed bile acid–lecithin monolayers. Small's [5] and Miñones Trillo et al.'s [82] studies on DC-, LC- and cholanoic acid–egg yolk lecithin monolayers are also consistent with this mode of packing, i.e. vertically oriented dimers of the hydroxylated bile acids and monomers of the parent compound (cholanoic acid) inter-

TABLE 3b

Surface physical chemistry of bile salts (23–25°C)

Adsorbed films

Bile salts	pH	[NaCl]	Calculated areas (Å^2/molecule) at surface saturation	Lowest surface tension (mN/m)	Ref.
Deoxycholate	10	0.15–0.5	84	44	74
Chenodeoxycholate	10	0.3–1.0	88	46	12
Ursodeoxycholate	10	0.3–1.0	85	48	12
Cholate	9	0.15	88	49	5, 33

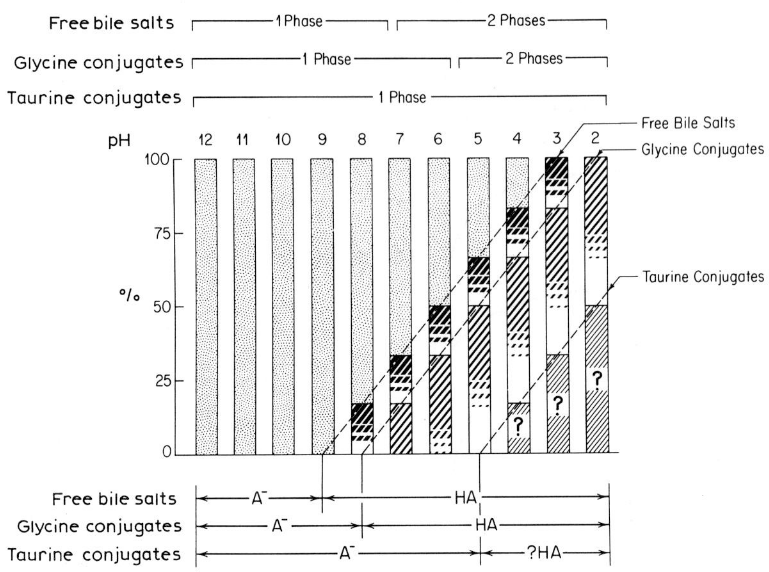

Fig. 10. Physical state and percent ionization of the common free, G-conjugated, and T-conjugated bile salts as functions of pH. (From ref. 6 with permission.)

GUDC (~ pK, 3.5). Similar pK_a values (5.02–5.08) have been obtained for C, DC, CDC, UDC, HDC and LC by extrapolation of pK_a values in various mole fractions of methanol in water at 25°C to zero methanol concentration [88]. This suggests that hydroxyl substitution does not affect the intrinsic acid strength of any of the bile acids, probably because of the distance separating the hydroxyl groups from the electrochemical center. Moreover, when monomeric solutions of pansulfated bile salts are titrated in water, the thermodynamic pK_a values of the carboxylate groups of the free acids and the glycine conjugates are within the 4.8–5.0 range, typical of both soluble short-chain monocarboxylic acids and bile salts at infinite dilution ([25], and J.M. Donovan, I.M. Yousef and M.C. Carey, unpublished data).

However, the pK_a value of each dihydroxy epimer increases sharply once the bile salt concentration exceeds its CMC (Fig. 8) [5,6,35]. In general, the aqueous pK_a values of all unconjugated bile salts in micelles are higher due to electrostatic effects and fall in the range of pH 5–6.5 depending upon bile salt concentration [5]. The pK_a values of the glycine conjugates fall in the range of pH 4–5 [5]. Because the acidity of even 10 M HCl is not adequate to titrate sulfonic acids to completion, the pK_a values of taurine (T)-conjugated bile salts are not yet known. They are likely to fall in the range pH -1.5 to $+1.5$ which are estimates for the free amino acid, taurine [89].

Fig. 10 summarizes these concepts [6]. From the graph, the percentage of free, glycine- and taurine-conjugated bile salts, which exist in ionized (A^-) and unionized (HA) form and the physical state of the systems, can be estimated at physiological pH values. Protonation of free bile salts begins at pH 9.0, glycine conjugates at pH

8.0 and taurine conjugates possibly at about pH 3–4. On account of the general high solubility of bile acids in bile salt micelles, precipitation of the HA form (indicated by the two-phase bracket) does not commence until pH 7.25 ± 0.85 (mean ± range) in the case of free bile salts, and pH 5.85 ± 1.5 in the case of the glycine conjugates.

(2) Bile acids — solubility behavior

Aqueous bile acid solubilities can be estimated from potentiometric titration curves. For example, in Fig. 9, below the apparent CMC values the horizontal slopes give an estimate of the HA solubilities in water. These values are close to those derived directly (37°C, pH 2.4) employing radiolabeled compounds (CDC, 256 μM; UDC, 53 μM) [35]. Only recently has this subject been reinvestigated in a systematic fashion employing sensitive and accurate analytic methods. Roda and associates [90] studied 10 highly purified unconjugated bile acids, and allowed them to equilibrate in bidistilled and decarbonated water at pH 3.0 for 60 days at temperatures which ranged between 10 and 50°C (±0.1°C). The results displayed in Fig. 11 show, as was expected, that trihydroxy bile acids are more soluble than the dihydroxy species which are in turn more soluble than the monohydroxy species. The lowest solubility observed was for LC at 10°C (5×10^{-8} M) and the highest (1.6×10^{-3} M) was for 3α,7β,12α-trihydroxy-5β-cholanoic acid, relatively independent of temperature. Within each series of isomers, subtle differences in both aqueous solubility and its dependence on temperature were noted.

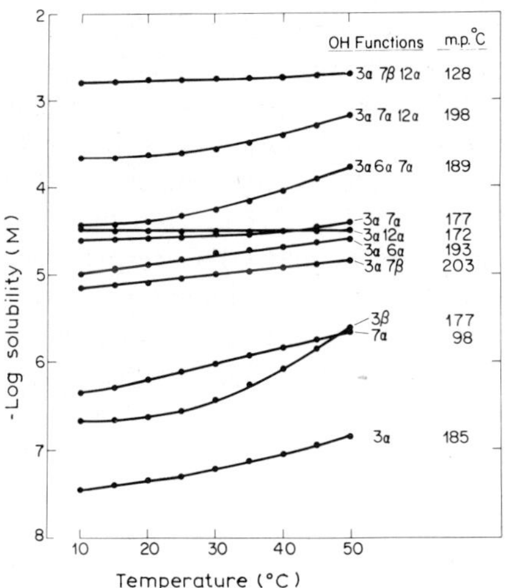

Fig. 11. Effects of temperature on water solubility (in negative logarithmic units, moles/l) of undissociated free bile acids at pH 3. (Modified from ref. 90.) Numbers and Greek letters denote position and orientation, respectively, of hydroxyl groups in each 5β-cholanoic acid. Mean m.p.s [34–41, and private communications from A. Roda and A.F. Hofmann] are indicated on each curve.

The thermodynamic functions associated with water solubility of the bile acids were uniformly associated with a positive enthalpy term ($+\Delta H^0_{25}$) and a negative entropy term ($-\Delta S^0_{25}$), suggesting that the solubilization process was endothermic and occurred with an increased structuring of the solvent molecules to envelop the bulky amphiphilic molecules [90]. In Dervichian's [91] words, "the difference in the behavior of the two parts of the amphiphilic molecules as regards water and with themselves in the crystal structure depend on whether, for each of the parts, the sum of the free energies for the passage of a molecule from the interior of a crystal into the molecules of the solvent is positive or negative". The different parts of this total energy are: (a) the work of removing each part of the amphiphilic molecule against the cohensive forces which bind that part to the corresponding part of neighboring molecules (i.e., H bonding, van der Waals' interactions); (b) the work required to separate the molecules of the solvent, against the cohesive forces in the interior of the solvent (H bonding in H_2O), so as to make room for one or the other part of the amphiphilic molecule; and (c) the energy of the affinity (or of wetting) of each part of the amphiphilic molecule for the solvent molecules. Hence, for molecules of similar size and structure, solubility will be related to: (a) the crystal energy which, if high, will tend to decrease solubility; (b) the intrinsic hydrophilicity of individual hydroxyl groups; and (c) the total contiguous hydrocarbon surface area exposed to water. The data in Fig. 11, taken together with the known m.p. values as an index of crystal energy and the hydrophilic/hydrophobic balance of the molecules [26,30,33], assist us in understanding the subtle difference in aqueous solubility between iso- and epi-meric bile acids. Within the trihydroxy class, the solubility of 3α,12α-hydroxy bile acids falls with the rank order of the third hydroxyl function 7β-OH > 7α-OH > 6α-OH. 3α,7β,12α-Trihydroxy-5β-cholanoic acid, the most soluble, has the lowest m.p. (128°C) and a very hydrophilic 7β function. Even though the m.p. of hyocholic acid (HC) is 9°C less than that of C, the crowding of its highly polar 6α-OH with the 7α-OH limits its hydrophilicity [30]. Within the dihydroxy class, the similarities of DC and CDC solubilities are anomalous and are not consistent with other studies [35]; CDC is probably more soluble than DC as would be expected in view of its 5°C lower m.p. and more polar 7α-OH (> 12α-OH in DC) function. Despite the more polar 6α- and 7β-OH functions of HDC and UDC, respectively, they are the least soluble of the 4 dihydroxy bile acids. This apparently occurs because of their high crystal energies which increase with decreasing order of the solubilities, i.e. 193°C (HDC) and 203°C (UDC). In the case of the monohydroxy species, solubilities increase with decreasing crystal energies (m.p.) and with increasing hydrophilicity of the 3α- > 3β-OH function. A formal thermodynamic analysis of these solubility values is given elsewhere [90].

(3) Temperature–solubility relations

As with conventional detergents, bile salt–aqueous mixtures exhibit a typical temperature (CMT) which transforms the system into a clear micellar phase [3,5,6]. For most of the common bile salts (an account of the phase relations of common bile

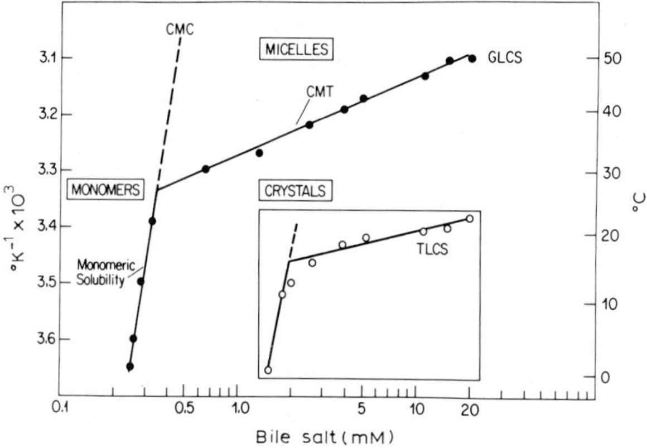

Fig. 12. Partial phase diagrams for the dilute region of aqueous solutions of the disodium salts of sulfated monohydroxy bile salts; glycolithocholate sulfate (GLCS at pH 10.0) and taurolithocholate sulfate (TLCS at pH 7.0, inset). The solid solubility curves and the interrupted CMC curves demarcate areas where crystals (and monomers), micelles (and monomers), and monomers alone are found. The critical micellar temperature (CMT) represents an equilibrium between micelles and hydrated crystals connected via the monomer concentration at the CMC. The Krafft point is a triple point and only represents the CMT at the CMC. (After ref. 6 with permission.)

salt–water systems can be found in ref. 4), water freezes before the detergent "freezes", hence the CMT lies below 0°C [4]. For most of the monohydroxy bile salts including their sulfates [86,87] and certain dihydroxy bile salts such as 7α,12α-dihydroxy-5β-cholanoate (M.C. Carey, unpublished observation), hyodeoxycholate [2], and the zwitterionic *N*-alkylsulfobetaine amide of deoxycholic acid [92], this temperature may lie above body temperature (see Fig. 12). The Krafft point is not synonymous with the CMT, but should be restricted to the CMT at the CMC [3,6]. Hence, in a two-component system, the Krafft point is a "triple point" where the CMC, CMT and monomeric solubilities intersect.

The CMT phenomenon may be explained on the basis of the coupling between the monomer–hydrated solid equilibrium and the monomer–micelle equilibrium [93,94]. This implies that as a suspension of bile salt crystals in water is heated, the monomeric solubility increases along the monomeric solubility curve in Fig. 12. Once the CMC is reached (dashed curve), the system attempts to continue to increase its monomeric solubility, but cannot do so owing to the flow of monomeric bile salts into micelles. Hence, the bile salt solubility curve demonstrates a sharp break point at the Krafft temperature because all monomers leaving the crystals are at concentrations above the CMC. The traditional crystal melting explanation proposed by Krafft and Wiglow [95,96] is obviously incorrect, since the alicyclic skeleton of bile salts is as rigid in the crystalline state as in solution; the crystals apparently "melt" at the CMT, because once the temperature-dependent monomeric solubility (CMC) is reached, the crystalline monomers are rapidly solubilized as micelles. In contrast to classic detergents, the CMT of bile salts shows a marked positive slope with increases in bile salt concentration [86,87]. It can be shown theoretically and experimentally that the smaller the micelle at the CMC, the greater the positive slope [97]; this is evidence for non-cooperative self-association with certain bile salt species (see Section VI.7).

(VI) Micelle formation in aqueous solvents

(1) Critical micellar concentrations

Bile salts carry extensive hydrophobic (hydrocarbon) portions in each molecule that attempt to reduce their contact with water (4). This is reflected in rapid, dynamic association–dissociation equilibrium to form "self-aggregates" or micelles as the total concentration of bile salt solute is increased (the CMC) [2–6]. Experimentally, micelles are undetectable in dilute solutions of the monomers, and are detected in increasing numbers and often size above the CMC [98]. Because bile salt micelles are often small (i.e., dimers) [5], and since self-aggregation continues to proceed in many cases with increasing concentration above the CMC [17,18,20,52,98], the detection of the lowest concentration at which the first aggregates form depends particularly upon the sensitivity of the experimental probes employed [98] and the physical–chemical conditions [3–5].

(a) Methods for determining bile salt CMC values

Over 50 methods have been employed in the literature to determine CMC values of bile salt solutions (reviewed in [6]). These can be divided into two broad categories: (a) methods requiring no physical or chemical additive in the bulk solution; and (b) methods involving the use of an additive in the bulk solution. The former methods, also called non-invasive, include surface tension and the measurements of a variety of colligative bulk properties (conductivity, turbidimetry, osmometry, self-diffusion, refractive index, modal volumes, electrometric force) or electromagnetic bulk properties (NMR, sound velocity and adsorption, etc.), all as functions of bile salt concentration. The second set of methods, also called invasive, depends upon a change in some physical or chemical property of an additive which occurs with the formation of micelles. These include the spectral change of a water-soluble dye, micellar solubilization of a water-insoluble dye, interfacial tension at liquid–liquid interfaces, and partition coefficients between aqueous and immiscible non-polar phases. Whereas a detailed discussion of the merits and demerits of both approaches can be found elsewhere [6], non-invasive methods which are correctly utilized provide the most reliable CMC values.

(b) Influence of variation in physical–chemical conditions

It should be obvious that to determine the CMC of a given bile salt, the material must be homogeneous and the amphiphile must be wholly in the salt form [2–6]. Most commercially available bile salts are impure; the contaminants are of many different kinds [6]. Many commonly available bile salts contain an excess of NaCl or even Ca^{2+} ions which not only influence the CMC, but in particular outrule accurate conductivity experiments [17,18]. Most important of all, the pH of the system must be sufficiently high so as to ensure complete ionization. Taurine conjugates are completely ionized at pH values > 2–4 [5,6] but glycine conjugates, and especially unconjugated bile salts, are not fully ionized unless the pH of the system is > 8 and > 9, respectively (see Fig. 10) [6]. Hence, all reported measurements of glycine-conjugated and unconjugated bile salts carried out at pH values below 8 and 9 respectively, represent the CMCs of the anions solubilizing a variable percentage of protonated bile acids [5,6,35]. Under these conditions, the reported CMCs are generally much lower than those of the pure bile salts. As in the case of all ionic amphiphiles, the CMC is generally increased with an elevation in temperature above ambient levels and is depressed with the addition of neutral electrolytes and with micellar solubilization of an otherwise insoluble lipid [3–6]. Thus, mixed micellar CMC values are generally much lower than those of the pure bile salts (16,99–102). The term "IMC" (intermicellar concentration) may be employed to denote the concentration of bile salt monomers found in such systems [102].

(c) Inventory of published data

NaC and NaTDC are the two bile salts that have been most extensively studied. A total of 86 examinations of NaC [5,9,17,22,33,50,52,71,72,76,98,103–138] and 48 examinations of NaTDC [5,16–18,33,70,76,100,101,103,104,111,115,117,139–145] have been carried out, giving an average CMC of 9.5 mM for NaC and 2.4 mM for NaTDC. Taking all values for NaC where the pH was > 8.0, the most important physical–chemical condition for an unconjugated bile salt [6], we obtain CMCs of 10.8, 6.9, and 3.3 mM, in water, 0.15 M Na^+ and 0.5 M Na^+ respectively, at 20–25°C. Control of the pH can be disregarded with NaTDC on account of its sulfonate side chain [6]; thus, we obtain CMCs of 3.8, 2.0 and 1.2 mM, in water, 0.15 M Na^+ and 0.5 M Na^+ respectively, at 20–25°C. It is obvious that the CMC values of both hydrophilic and hydrophobic bile salts are exquisitively sensitive to ionic strength. True cooperative aggregation probably does not occur with bile micelles in water and possibly not in physiological ionic strength; i.e., it is not a critical phenomenon. Thus, the concept of a CMC is fraught with definitional and interpretational problems for bile salts and as a result many values, depending upon the experimental technique and in many cases, arbitrary choices of values are quoted in the literature.

(2) Micellar size and polydispersity

The average size of bile salt micelles and the distribution of micellar sizes around the mean value are important physical–chemical characteristics of a bile salt solution [5,6]. Because bile salt micellar growth is sensitive to total detergent concentration within the micellar phase, with temperature and ionic strength, the physical–chemical conditions must be rigorously controlled and specified [5,6]. Further, most conventional methods of estimating micellar size require an extrapolation to the CMC and therefore are valid only at this concentration, provided it is accurately known [6]. The CMC literature cited shows how hazardous such an extrapolation may be. Furthermore, size estimates are influenced by the technique employed and some widely divergent values have been published [146]. In principle, all conventional thermodynamic methods (e.g. classical light scattering, analytical ultracentrifugation) give the anhydrous micelle molecular weight from which the mean aggregation number ($\bar{n}$) is derived utilizing the monomer weight [6]; the more recent technique of quasi-elastic light scattering (QLS) measures the mean hydrodynamic radius ($\bar{R}_h$) of micelles from which $\bar{n}$ can be derived from a knowledge of micellar shape [6,146].

(a) Unconjugated bile salts

The $\bar{n}$ values for the unconjugated bile salts NaC, NaUDC, NaCDC and NaDC have been evaluated by analytical ultracentrifugation (sedimentation/equilibrium) [147,148], surface tension/ellipsometry [74], classical light scattering [12,73,105,126,128,138,149], octanol–water partitioning [119], viscometry [22], molecular sieve chromatography [150], and QLS [12,112] in 0.1–0.15 M NaCl at 20–25°C. Excluding the results of studies where there was evidence of impurities in the compounds [73], incorrect pH, i.e., < 8–9 [105,148], and ignoring the invasive partitioning method [119], the literature results are in close agreement for finite 1–5% (w/v) concentrations. $\bar{n}$ values are 3 ± 1 (NaC), 6 ± 1 (NaUDC), 8 ± 3 (NaCDC) and 15 ± 3 (NaDC); the sizes of the micelles increase with decreasing hydrophilicity [6]. Where evaluated [147], the $\bar{n}$ values are ~ 1 unit smaller at 37°C. Whereas the concentration dependence of aggregation of unconjugated bile salts within the micellar phase has not been extensively studied by colligative methods, there appears to be a modest stepwise increase in $\bar{n}$ at higher bile salt concentrations, at least in water and physiological ionic strength [17,20,50,52,66,98]. Increases in ionic strength induce marked increases in micellar size, particularly in the case of the more hydrophobic bile salts (CDC, DC), and a greater sensitivity of $\bar{n}$ to higher detergent concentrations [77,81,126,128,138,147]. With the latter two hydrophobic bile salts, partial protonation leads to polymerization with enormous increases in aggregation numbers [105,147] and gel formation [151–153]. Studies carried out at pH values < 9.0 give abnormal rheological behavior and values for $\bar{n}$ [105,147,154] which cannot be considered true micelle formation in the classic sense. The relationship between pH (7.2–9.2) and concentration on the properties of DC solutions have been extensively discussed elsewhere [4,147,155–159].

(b) Glycine-conjugated bile salts

Under similar physical–chemical conditions, the aggregation of NaGC, NaGUDC, NaGCDC, and NaGDC seems to follow an identical pattern [147] with the exception that micellar $\bar{n}$ values are generally somewhat larger than the unconjugated species and the micelles grow in a more pronounced fashion with increases in ionic strength [147]. Typical $\bar{n}$ values for finite concentrations at 20–25°C in 0.15 M

NaCl at appropriate pH values (> 8) are 6 ± 2 (NaGC), 13 (NaGUDC), 17 ± 4 (NaGCDC) and 22 ± 4 (NaGDC) [5,11,12,70,73,126,138,145,147,149]. The latter two species are also exquisitely sensitive to pH; as the pH_{ppt} is approached, "micelles" of gigantic proportions are obtained [147].

(c) Taurine-conjugated bile salts

These species have been the most carefully studied owing to the availability of relatively pure materials and their insensitivity to pH [5,6]. Studies utilizing equilibrium ultracentrifugation [142,147,160], classical and quasi-elastic light scattering [12,70,71,138,145,146,149,161,162], ionic self-diffusion [163–165], and gel filtration [166] in 0.15 M NaCl at 20–25°C, give $\bar{n}$ values of 5 ± 3 (NaTC), 15 ± 2 (NaTUDC), 18 ± 2 (NaTCDC) and 22 ± 3 (NaTDC). NaTDC is capable of attaining the largest size of all bile salt micelles as functions of increases in bile salt concentration, decreases in temperature and added ionic strength [146,161]. It is clear that for comparable conditions, micellar size and growth potential increase from free to glycine-conjugated to taurine-conjugated homologs: within the dihydroxy species, hydrophilicity is correlated inversely with micellar size, but the trihydroxy species, although less hydrophilic than UDC species [26], form the smallest micelles under all physical-chemical conditions [147].

(d) Polydispersity

Polydispersity of simple bile salt micelles can only be assessed by modern QLS techniques employing the 2nd cumulant analysis of the time decay of the autocorrelation function [146,161]. These studies have shown, in the cases of the 4 taurine conjugates in 10 g/dl concentrations in both 0.15 M and 0.6 M NaCl, that the distribution in the polydispersity index (V) varies from ~ 20% for small $\bar{n}$ values to ~ 50% for large $\bar{n}$ values [6,146]. Others [112] have found much smaller V values (2–10%) for the unconjugated bile salts in 5% (w/v) solutions. Recently, the significance of QLS-derived polydispersities have been questioned on the basis of the rapid fluctuation in $\bar{n}$ of micellar assemblies; hence V may not actually represent a micellar size distribution [167–169]. This argument is specious, since a micellar size distribution and fast fluctuations in aggregation number are identical quantities on the QLS time scale (μsec–msec) [94].

(3) Micellar shape and hydration

At low concentrations just above the CMC and at low ionic strengths (< 0.2 M NaCl), nearly all simple bile salt micellar solutions contain spherical or nearly spherical micellar particles [5,6,12,146]. Intrinsic viscosity measurements [162,170–172] are in agreement with this and also indicate that the micelles are highly hydrated, cholates > DC [162,172]. The maximum size of these globular micelles falls in the range $\bar{R}_h$ = 10–16 Å with $\bar{n}$ = 10–12 [146]. In the case of NaTC, the water of hydration amounts to about 30 moles H_2O/mole of monomer in the micelle [162]. By employing the translational mobility of ^3H_2O, Lindman et al. [173]

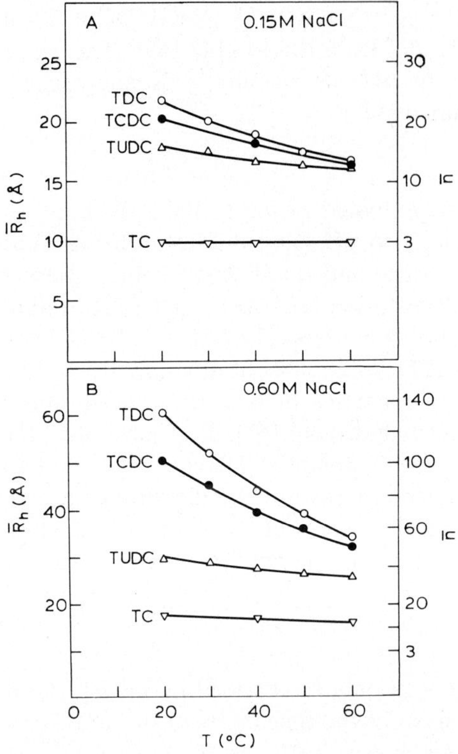

Fig. 13. Mean hydrodynamic radii ($\bar{R}_h$, in Å) and aggregation numbers ($\bar{n}$) for the taurine conjugates of 4 common bile salts in 0.15 M and 0.6 M NaCl as functions of temperature. (From ref. 6 with permission.)

found a hydration value of 35–40 for each NaC monomer over a wide range of concentrations above 10 mM. The more hydrophobic bile salts such as DC and CDC and their conjugates grow dramatically under conditions of high detergent concentration, high ionic strength and low temperatures (Fig. 13) [146,161]. For example, in 0.8 M NaCl, TDC micelles attain an $\bar{R}_h = 90$ [161]. These large sizes have been shown by light scattering techniques to be consistent with a rod-shaped geometry [146,161]. From this shape, the $\bar{n}$ values can be derived [6,146], and are shown to extend to > 100 (Fig. 13). Since only about 8–10 bile salt molecules are said to be accommodated in a primary micelle [147], this implies by necessity a polymerization between the hydrophilic surfaces of primary micelles to form secondary micelles [146,147]. Like the thermodynamic forces involved in primary micelle formation, the polymerization forces are also hydrophobic in nature and provide an explanation for the poor growth of NaC and NaUDC and their conjugates [146]. Intermicellar H bonding possibly stabilizes these large aggregates, which probably are very flexible elongated rods [146,147]. With all bile salts in low ionic strengths, this polymerization interaction does not occur readily, suggesting the importance of electrostatic shielding of the anionic charged side chains in facilitating the polymerization process [146]. Evidence is later discussed that secondary micelles form by a linear polymerization of primary micelles and probably not by successive addition of monomers to pre-existing primary micelles.

(4) Micellar structures

Since bile salt molecules have two distinct sides, a hydrophilic and a hydrophobic, they are planar amphiphiles and orient at interfaces with the hydrophobic surface facing upwards toward air and their hydrophilic surface anchored in the aqueous phase [5,6]. Since the initial proposal by Ekwall et al [103], more detailed by Small [147], it has been considered that the interaction of bile salt monomers to form primary micelles is due to agglomeration of hydrophobic surfaces in a back-to-back manner so as to maximize van der Waals' contacts between the alicyclic steroid rings on the convex (hydrophobic) side of the molecules [147]. The ionic side chains provide an opposing electrostatic force but these were considered to be staggered as much as possible to minimize electrostatic repulsion. Until recently, the side chains were considered to have no other function in the aggregation process. This schema has now come under close scrutiny and indeed challenged on both theoretical and experimental grounds ([53] and M.C. Carey, unpublished data).

(i) It is in fact difficult to pack up to 10 bile salt molecules into a globular aggregate so that they interact maximally via their steroid skeletons. Further, it is difficult in this mode of packing to avoid intramicellar cavities that could accommodate water molecules. Recent studies [174] utilizing the fluorescence of pyrene, solubilized in NaC, NaDC and NaTCDC micelles, suggest that bile salt packing is tight since the micellar environment is much more apolar in bile salt micelles than in classical detergent micelles.

(ii) The CMCs of bile salts are dependent on side chain length. In a series of $3\alpha,7\alpha,12\alpha$-trihydroxy bile salts (all with an identical steroid nucleus), the C_{27}, C_{24}, C_{23} and C_{22} derivatives display CMC values (in 0.15 M Na^+, 25°C) of 0.5 mM, 11 mM, 21 mM and 38 mM as evaluated by dye spectral shift and surface tension [33,175]. With respect to the common taurine, glycine and free species, the C_{24} series display CMCs of 6, 10 and 11 mM evaluated by the same methods [33]. Hogan et al. [53] have pointed out that in the crystal structures of bile salts [7,51,53] (see Section IV.2) the C residues are staggered within the bilayer to apparently maximize hydrophobic interactions between side chains and A/B rings. Hence, this interaction, if it is maintained in micelles, should be enhanced as the lengths of the hydrophobic side chains are increased. This is just what is found if the CMCs are taken as evidence of such interactions. If correct, this suggests that the hydrophobic part of the side chain may be intimately involved in hydrophobic interactions in bile salt self-aggregation. Indeed, it is possible that the bile salt homolog with no side chain (etianate) may not form micelles at all. The other interpretation is that the more elongated the side chains are, the further the ionic functions will be kept away from the steroid skeleton and this in turn will facilitate greater van der Waals' contact between the bulky steroid rings.

(iii) In the presence of equimolar ionic strengths and bile salt concentrations, primary micelles of free bile salts polymerize into secondary micelles less readily than glycine conjugates, and these are less polymerizable than the taurine conjugates [5,147]. If hydrophobic interactions of the hydrophobic sides of the steroid skeletons were the only factors involved, the trend should be the inverse function of the observed rank ordering, since free carboxylate groups are weaker than those of glycine which, in turn, are much weaker than sulfonate groups in taurine conjugates [6]. Again, this suggests that hydrophobic side chain–steroid interactions may be involved in not only primary micelle formation but also in the polymerization of primary micelles to form secondary micelles.

(5) Micellar charge and counterion binding

The fractional binding of counterions to ionic micelles is commonly denoted by the parameter β. It follows that the corresponding micellar charge is 1-β [176]. Work on classic micellar systems such as dodecyl sulfate and octanoate show that this subject is highly complicated and as yet not fully understood [176–179]. In the presence of different counterions (such as the alkali ions Li^+, Na^+, K^+, Rb^+ and Cs^+), micellar size and shape, CMC values and CMT values of dodecyl sulfate are altered and do not follow the order of atomic number of the alkali ions in the periodic table nor their hydrated radius (P.J. Missel, G.B. Benedek and M.C. Carey, unpublished observations). Hydrated radius bears an inverse relationship to atomic radius, viz. (in Å) Li^+ (2.35), Na^+ (1.85), K^+ (1.32), Cs^+ (1.27) and Rb^+ (1.26). A few examples of relevance to bile salt micelles are that K^+ ions are bound to classic micelles more than Na^+ ions [180,181] and induce a greater depression in the CMT compared with Na^+ salts [182]. Micelles of K^+ salts are also larger than those of Na^+ salts at a given ionic strength, detergent concentration and temperature (P.J. Missel, G.B. Benedek and M.C. Carey, unpublished observations). Possibly because of strong coulombic interactions, divalent ions such as Ca^{2+} and Mg^{2+} are more associated with alkyl sulfate micelles than the corresponding Na^+ ions [176,183], but the effects are strongly concentration dependent [183]. Further, CMCs of divalent salts of straight-chain amphiphiles are ~ 20% smaller than those of the sodium salts. In addition, the CMTs are elevated, and micellar sizes are doubled [183–186].

Much less is known about micellar charge and counterion binding in the case of bile salts. Based on the result of ionic self-diffusion measurements [20,163,173], conductance studies [17,18,187], Na^+, K^+ and Ca^{2+} activity coefficients [16,19,144,188,189] and NMR studies with ^{23}Na, ^{85}Rb and ^{133}Cs [190], a number of generalities can be made. Below the "operational" CMC, all bile salts behave as fully dissociated 1:1 electrolytes, yet interionic effects between cations and bile salt anions decrease the equivalent conductance of very dilute solutions [17,18,187]. With the onset of micelle formation, counterions become bound to a small degree: β values at this concentration are about < 0.07–0.13 and are not greatly influenced by the species of monovalent alkali cations [163,190]. At concentrations above the CMC, β values remain relatively constant to 100 mM in the case of C and this increases to 0.45 at 400 mM C [20,173]. As with classic detergents, binding of K^+ is greater than Na^+ and binding of Ca^{2+} is greater still [19,188]. However, no studies have appeared on the degree of dissociation/association of pure calcium bile salts — all published studies have been carried out with Ca^{2+} added to Na salts [189] or in the presence of a swamping excess of Na^+ ions (~ 0.3 M) [19]. The extent of Ca^{2+} binding is apparently determined both by the number and position of the hydroxyl groups on the steroid nucleus as well as the nature of the ionic side chain [189]. Ca^{2+} binding is also greatly decreased in proportion to the concentration of univalent electrolytes [189]. Recent studies suggest that Ca^{2+} has a much greater affinity for TC monomers compared to TC monomers in micelles [19]: however, in a swamping excess of Na^+ ions, Ca^{2+} ions must compete for binding to micelles, but not monomers; this explanation was not considered. Since Ca^{2+} ions are only weakly hydrated in solution [191], their coordination to both bile salt monomers and micelles may be different than for Na^+ ions (as in the crystal structures, Fig. 4) and may well be influenced by many factors in the aqueous environment such as ionic strength, univalent electrolyte species, temperature and other additives. It appears from recent studies that hydroxyl groups at C-7 and their orientation as well as the anionic side chain and hydrophilicity of the molecules may all influence Ca^{2+} binding, giving observed Ca^{2+} affinities in the rank order of CDC = DC > C > UDC [189,192] and free salts > glycine conjugates > taurine conjugates. Conclusions drawn from ^{133}Cs and ^{23}Na NMR studies suggest that the alkali ions are, in general, hydrated when bound to bile salt micelles [190].

(6) Rates of exchange of micellar and intermicellar components

Chemical relaxation methods (π-jump, T-jump, stopped flow, shock-tube and ultrasonic absorption) and NMR have been used to define the nature and number of relaxation processes in micellar solutions [193,194]. These include: (1) the counterion association/dissociation to/from micelles (ionization); (2) detergent ion association/dissociation to/from micelles (exchange); (3) micelle formation/dissolution; and (4) change of micellar shape and/or size. Very few points of agreement have been reached in the literature concerning the origin and characteristics of the relaxation processes [194]. The fastest relaxation process (well below 1 μsec) has been attributed to the exchange of detergent ions between solvent and micelles and a slower relaxation process (100–10 μsec) has been assigned to micelle formation–dissolution equilibria [194]. The former relaxation process has been measured for NaDC at concentrations well above the CMC [52]. The association rate constant (10^9/M/sec) is similar to that for exchange of detergent ions in classic detergent systems [193].

(7) Critical and non-critical self-association

Critical self-association implies a strong cooperative interaction of a large number of detergent ions to form micelles of a fairly uniform size over a narrow concentration range, conventionally called the CMC [195]. Non-critical self-association implies that the detergent interactions are non-cooperative and occur usually in a progressive fashion over a wide concentration range, often beginning as dimers [195]. Bile salt aggregates provide examples of both phenomena depending upon the bile salt species and the physical–chemical conditions: unfortunately, the more investigations that have been made, the more confusing the self-association picture has become [6]. The following principles can be formulated from the vast literature on the subject. In water and in low ionic strengths, all bile salts, whether free or conjugated with glycine or taurine, appear to self-associate in a non-cooperative-continuous manner. This process was first inferred from solubilization studies on cholates with both small (e.g. xylene) [103,124,125] and large (e.g. naphthalene) hydrophobic solubilizates [98,104]; it has been confirmed in other unconjugated and conjugated bile salt systems by NMR [9,22], fluorescent probe spectrometry [108,109], surface tension [33,140], osmotic coefficient [115], dye spectral shift [33,142], partial molal and specific volumes [50,52], activity of bile salt ions and counterions [16,144,173], viscosity [170–172], light scattering [12,134,146,161], and by electric conductivity [17,18]. Probably the most elegant example of the step-wise association process comes from two lines of evidence: electrical conductance of TDC in water [18] and by ultrasonic absorption spectra of NaDC and NaC in low ionic strengths [52]. Fig. 14 displays the equivalent conductance of dilute NaTDC solution in water at 25°C [18]. With increases in NaTDC concentration, the conductance curve

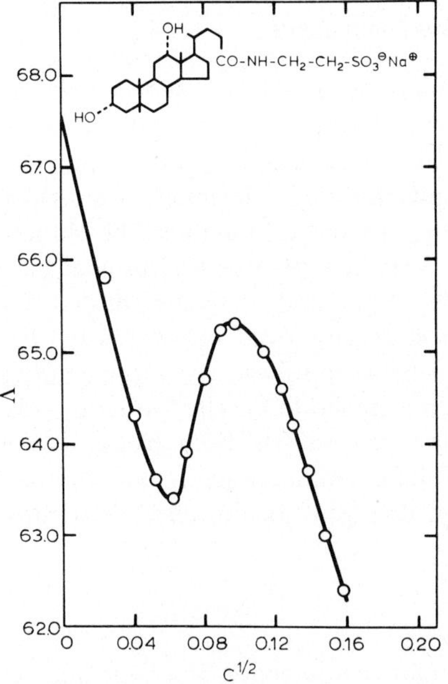

Fig. 14. Equivalent conductance (Λ) vs. square root ($C^{1/2}$) of NaTDC concentration in moles/l. The curve illustrates conductivity of NaTDC in the vicinity of the CMC. (From ref. 18 with permission.)

exhibits a steep decrease to a minimum at ~ 3.6 mM, then rises sharply again to a maximum at ~ 8.1 mM, only to fall again at higher concentrations. This behavior is much less marked with cholates, demonstrating no minimum in the conductance curve and no secondary peak [17]. Careful surface tension [140] and ionic activity [16] measurements of NaTDC in water show sharp breaks at 3.1 and 3.4 mM respectively and no significant change in activity thereafter (to 100 mM). In contrast, NaTC continues to change in anionic activity over the same concentration range [16,140]. The question then arises: why the marked change in NaTDC conductivity between 3.6 mM (i.e. the CMC by other methods) and 8.1 mM? It is most likely due to bile salt anion pairing without any significant counterion binding with the result that the effective radius of the spherical aggregate is considerably less than twice that of the single ions and results in an increase in conductance [18]. This is also consistent with hydrophobic interactions which, when aggregates form, must perforce be associated with dehydration of the opposing hydrophobic surfaces. Further, while the effective charge increases in proportion to the number of ions in the aggregates, the spherical radius increases only by a factor of 20% as a result of the

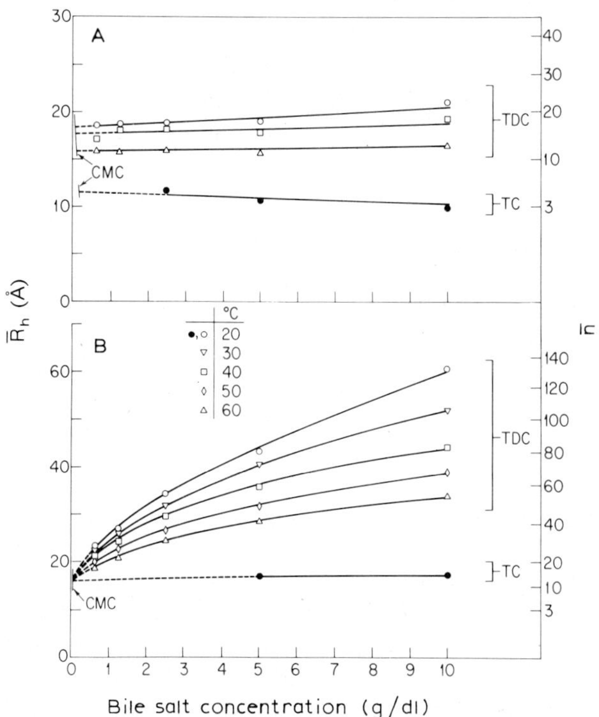

Fig. 15. Mean hydrodynamic radii ($\bar{R}_h$, in Å) and aggregation numbers ($\bar{n}$) of TC and TDC micelles as functions of bile salt concentration and temperature in (A) 0.15 M NaCl and (B) 0.6 M NaCl. In each panel the curves are extrapolated to the estimated CMC values. (From ref. 146 reprinted with permission.)

cubic dependence of radius on volume [18]. Counterion binding (β) to NaTCDC (and presumably NaTDC) increases progressively above the CMC [163]. The marked fall in conductance above 8.1 mM in Fig. 14 is probably due to a greater counterion effect and continued micellar aggregation ($\bar{n}$ being 22 at finite concentrations [147], see Section VI.2). Both effects overcome the rise in equivalent conductance which follows the initial aggregation. From the conductance of NaTC [17], ion pairing is initiated at ~ 10 mM but an increase in conductance does not occur, possibly because of immediate counterion binding which has been demonstrated ($\beta = 0.13$) at this concentration [163]. It is now evident from anion activity [16] and surface tension studies [140] that self-association of the TC anions continues to at least 100 mM (in water, 25°C). In high (~ 0.3–0.7 M) ionic strengths (NaCl), surface tension [12,140] and light scattering [146,161] studies suggest that micellization of the conjugated dihydroxy species is indeed cooperative over a narrow CMC range; with NaTC this does not appear to be the case [146]. The situation is confounded by the fact that in the higher ionic strength, conjugated dihydroxy bile salt micelles continue to grow continuously with increases in concentration, whereas NaTC micelles do not (Fig. 15) [146].

Chemical relaxation methods [52] show evidence of a distribution of relaxation frequencies rather than a single one as found with classic ion detergents [193]. Thus, in agreement with the above conclusions, NaC and NaDC apparently self-associate over a whole range of concentrations and not at some critical micellar concentration. Further, the relaxation frequencies are strongly concentration dependent, suggesting that the distribution of aggregate sizes is wide and shifts upwards as bile salt concentration is increased [52].

(VII) Reverse micelle formation in non-aqueous media

An understanding of the aggregation of bile salts, their acids and derivatives in non-aqueous media is crucial for providing insights into the interactions of bile salts and bile acids within hydrophobic domains such as biological membranes and mixed micelles.

(1) Bile acid esters

Earlier work [196–198] on bile acid methyl esters and hydroxylated cholane and cholestane derivatives by NMR, IR and UV spectroscopy, as well as osmometry revealed a singular pattern of self-association in CCl_4 and $CHCl_3$. (i) Trihydroxy substituents induced the greatest degree of self-association, cholanoates exhibiting the largest binding constants. (ii) Dihydroxy species were less well associated and monohydroxy species self-associated poorly. (iii) Steric hindrance with respect to the ease of OH–OH bonding was crucially important in that CDC derivatives associated more than DC compounds; further, β-oriented hydroxyls on the steroid skeleton were less effective in inducing self-association. (iv) Single hydroxyl groups in the side chain also hindered self-association. (v) Carbonyl groups in the side chain became involved in intermolecular H bonding only at very high solute concentrations. Hence, these spectrometric studies were apparently consistent with mainly intermolecular H bonding between α-oriented hydroxyl groups in the rings. The equilibria for methyl cholate involved dimers, tetramers and perhaps higher oligomers at the highest concentrations. By employing NMR spectrometry and vapor pressure osmometry, Fendler et al. [199,200] carried out a study on the reverse micellar aggregation and the equilibria of bile acid methyl and ethyl esters in several protic and aprotic organic solvents. They showed that methyl (Me) and ethyl esters of C and MeDC form small reversed micelles in CCl_4, CH_2Cl_2, CS_2 and $CHCl_3$. Overall, the self-association proceeded via a multiple stepwise equilibrium (monomer–dimer, monomer–dimer–trimer, monomer–dimer–tetramer, etc.) rather than via a monomer–*n*-mer equilibrium. In this regard, bile acid methyl esters behave like other reverse micellar systems [201] except that the aggregates of the steroid detergents are smaller [196–200]. As noted in earlier work [196–198], the behavior was markedly dependent on whether the solvent was capable of hydrogen bonding and upon the number of hydroxyl groups on the steroid nucleus [199,200]. The order of affinities for self-association decreased with decreasing hydrophilicity: MeC > MeDC $\gg$ MeLC — the latter being monomeric in the protic solvents ($CHCl_3$, CH_2Cl_2) and dimeric in the other two. Self-association in the aprotic solvents (CCl_4, CS_2) was consistently greater than in $CHCl_3$; in all cases hydrogen bonding of the 3α-hydroxyl group was the most prominent feature in stabilizing the aggregates.

As noted above, MeC trimerizes and MeLC does not self-associate in $CHCl_3$. Under these conditions, Foster et al. [202] used vapor pressure osmometry to show that solubilized cholesterol (which dimerizes in $CHCl_3$ [203]) heteroassociated with MeC but not with MeLC. The result was a 1 : 1 mixed dimer complex of cholesterol and MeC with a molar free energy of formation which was 33% that for the trimerization of MeC in the same solvent [202]. The bonding is presumably via the 3-hydroxyl functions in both steroids; this interaction may be of potential importance in the binding of cholesterol to bile acids and salts within membranes and mixed micelles.

(2) Bile acids and salts

Small [5] investigated, by IR spectroscopy, the hydrogen-bonding patterns of several bile acids in crystalline or amorphous melts and in Nujol mulls. He concluded that, in the crystalline state, cholanoic, LC and dehydrocholic acid form strong H-bonded carboxylic acid dimers; with LC, the 3α-hydroxyl group may be involved in polymeric self-association. Carboxylic acid dimers are less evident in di- and trihydroxy bile acid crystals but the 3α- and 7α-hydroxyl groups participate in various modes of H bonding. No hydrogen bonding of the 12α-hydroxyl group was detected by IR spectroscopy. In amorphous melts, H bonding of all hydroxyl groups occurs as well as COOH–COOH dimers. Many of these derived H-bonding patterns for the acids in the solid state have been revised and updated by rigorous crystallographic determinations (see Section III.1 and Table 2).

In aqueous–organic phase partitioning experiments, Vadnere and Lindenbaum [119] have shown that NaC, NaDC, NaCDC and NaUDC in concentrations reaching 0.1 M at pH 8 when all the salts are partially undissociated [6], distribute between the aqueous buffer and 1-octanol over the temperature range from 25°C to 55°C. As verified by vapor pressure osmometry, the bile salts (and/or acids) existed as monomers in 1-octanol, a water-immiscible, hydrogen-bonding solvent. In contrast, at pH 8.0 (25°C). NaDC distributed between aqueous and organic phases of isooctane/1-octanol (70 : 30 v/v) and isooctane/chloroform (80 : 20 v/v) forming reverse dimers in the former and most probably reverse tetramers and hexamers in the latter — all in equilibrium with monomers [204]. In this work it could not be verified whether the associated species in the organic phase was composed of bile salt anions or undissociated bile acid molecules, or both. Hydrogen-bonded pairs and higher aggregates are probably associated via the 3α- and 12α-hydroxyl groups, although if the free acids are the self-associating species, carboxylic acid linkages may also be involved [5]. Fontell [205] solved the phase relations of the 3-component systems, bile salt (NaC or NaDC), *n*-decanol and water at 20°C (pH 8–8.8). A conspicuous feature of these systems was that there was a continuous optically clear isotropic phase which extended from the water corner to the *n*-decanol corner. X-ray, light scattering, viscosity and conductivity studies [205] showed that the extensive 1 phase zone contained two different micellar structures. At high water contents, the micelles were of the "normal" type where water constituted the intermicellar solution and the micelles contained solubilized decanol. At high decanol contents, the micelles were of the reverse type, containing a water core, within which were located the counterions (Na^+) and the ionized groups of the bile salt molecules; in this region of the phase diagram, decanol was the main constituent of the intermicellar solution. Fabre et al. [206] pointed out the similarities in the phase equilibria of these systems to that of classic ternary microemulsion-forming systems. From measurements of the relative self-diffusion coefficients of sodium, cholate, decanol, water and chloride, Fabre et al. [206] concluded that both structures and properties of normal and reverse bile salt–decanol–water micelles differ markedly from those of typical oil–water–classic detergent systems; for example, no distinct transition was observed between the two types of aggregates; a progressive change apparently occurred at ~ 30–50 vol% decanol. Despite their importance, no detailed characterization of these normal or reversed bile salt micelles is available.

(3) Bile salts within the hydrophobic domains of liposomes and membranes

The classic X-ray diffraction work of Small et al. [5,207,208] pointed out the existence of inverted (reverse) bile salt micelles within mixed bile salt–phospholipid liquid crystalline bilayers. The aggregates were considered to consist of 2–4 molecules (of cholate) with their hydrophilic sides facing inwards bound by hydrogen bonds between the hydroxyl groups, leaving their hydrophobic sides facing outwards to interact with the acyl chains of the phospholipid. At saturation, about 1 molecule of cholate was present for every 2 molecules of lecithin. Appreciably more bile salts could be intercalated between the lecithin chains when conjugated bile salt mixtures isolated from ox bile were employed. When saturated, the hexagonal and cubic liquid crystalline phases of these systems contained 2 molecules of lecithin for every 3 molecules of bile salt. By X-ray diffraction, Small and Bourgès [207] found that the addition of NaC to a lamellar phase of egg lecithin caused an increase in the calculated thickness of the lipid bilayer, provided the percentage of water was above 25–30%; a decrease in the X-ray spacing occurred if the percentage of water was less. However, at a constant weight percentage of lecithin and NaC, the repeat distances of the lamellar phase swelled to a much greater extent with added water than pure lecithin alone. The former experiments indicated that NaC molecules fit into the lamellar structures with the long axis of the molecules normal to the plane of the bilayer; depending upon percent water, the lipid bilayer may become further disordered or more ordered, respectively, thus altering the X-ray spacings in either direction. The latter experiments are an example of the well known swelling behavior of zwitterionic phospholipid bilayers where an amphiphile with a net charge is introduced [209], i.e. much more water can be contained between the lamellae of mixed lipid bilayers when one component has a net charge compared with pure phospholipid bilayers. This results in a more extensive single-phase region before the appearance of a 2-phase system of swollen liquid crystals in excess water [209]. In the 4-component cholesterol–egg lecithin–sodium cholate–water systems [207,210], the lamellar phase is also able to hold up to about 25% by weight of cholesterol. At cholesterol saturation the content of NaC in the lamellar phase is reduced to ~ 2%, suggesting that cholesterol and cholate molecules compete for similar binding sites within the lamellar phase.

Several NMR spectroscopic probes have been employed to investigate the interactions of bile salts with model membranes. The results are in general agreement with the deductions above, and suggest additional details:

(i) Ulmius et al. [211] employed perdeuterated palmitoyloleoyl glycero-3-phosphocholine at 24°C, and showed that the deuterium order parameter (S) decreases with cholate incorporation into lamellar (and hexagonal) bilayers. At the lowest cholate : lecithin molar ratio (~ 0.1) there is no change in S of the lamellar phase between C-2 and C-8, but a monotonic decrease occurs between C-8 and C-18. With greater cholate incorporation (molar ratio ~ 0.8) there was a continuous monotonic reduction in the NMR order parameter from C-2 to C-18. This dramatic decrease in the order of the lamellar phase on addition of cholate is most likely due to the bulky nature of H-bonded cholate dimers intercalated normal to the surface of the bilayers. It was suggested [211] that the profound increase in lecithin chain mobility occurred because a substantial fraction of cholate molecules are placed flat on the bilayer surface. This interpretation appears unlikely. As inferred from Small's work [5,207,208], the hydrophobic domains of the lecithin bilayers would have been just saturated at the higher molar ratio (0.8); thus, it is not surprising that S values of all acyl carbons of lecithin are perturbed. For example, this phenomenon is also highlighted by the tendency of lipids surrounding irregular surfaces of proteins to be disordered [212]. It appears that both bile salts and proteins have common disordering properties in membranes; this effect is the reverse of that seen with incorporation of cholesterol into fluid phospholipid bilayers [209,213].

(ii) Employing the quadrupole splittings of selectively deuterated DC and CDC in lamellar multilayers of egg lecithin, Saitô et al. [214] reached the same conclusion. Also employing deuterium NMR, these authors found that the molecular motion of the terminal deuterium of the fatty acid chains of pure palmitic acid in erythrocyte ghosts was enhanced by the presence of 1 mM DC; since this lipid is crystalline at ambient temperatures, it is not surprising that bile salts increase the molecular motion of the ends of the chains.

(iii) Madden and Cullis [215] showed that unsaturated phosphotidylethanolamine, which adopts a reverse hexagonal (H_{II}) phase in water, can, by incorporating DC, adopt a stable lamellar structure. Again, this suggests intercalation of the steroid rings parallel with the acyl chains of phospholipid bilayers.

(iv) By observing the deuterium splitting of ^2H_2O-hydrated egg lecithin bilayers, Persson et al. [216] found that there is progressive decrease in the exchange of water with incorporation of NaC, consistent with tighter hydration. Similarly, ^{23}Na line widths decrease, suggesting a loosening of the interaction between sodium ions and the lamellar surface. The mixed bilayer affinities of univalent alkali ions fell in the sequence $K^+ > Na^+ > Rb^+ > Cs^+ \simeq Li^+$ [216].

(v) Additional information about the molecular structure of the hexagonal and cubic phases [211,217] obtained through measurements of phospholipid translational diffusion (by pulsed NMR) revealed that the lateral diffusion of lecithin in both phases was of the same order of magnitude as in the lamellar phase [211]. A reasonable conclusion from these studies is that the hydrocarbon region must also be continuous in the hexagonal and cubic phases as it is in the lamellar phase. This would appear to outrule Small's proposal [5,207,208,210] that the liquid crystalline structures are composed of discrete "mixed micellar" units.

(vi) By monitoring ^{1}H line widths by 500 MHz NMR, Stark and Roberts [218] concluded that the motion of TC in bile salt–egg lecithin vesicles becomes preferentially restricted while polar portions of lecithin remain mobile until large liposomes predominate. Again, these observations are consistent with all other deductions outlined above, but also suggest that TC molecules in vesicles at low bile salt to phospholipid ratios are probably buried deeply within the lecithin bilayers and apparently do not interact with the phosphocholine head groups. This conclusion is consistent with the deuterium order parameters obtained by Ulmius et al. [211] in systems containing C and deuterated lecithin at a molar ratio of 0.1.

The functional role of bile salts within model and native membranes has begun to be closely scrutinized in recent years [219–223]. This is not surprising in view of the wide use of bile salts to extract and reconstitute intrinsic membrane proteins [224] and their use in the formation of vesicles without sonication [225]. There is also scientific and clinical interest in the membrane-damaging properties of bile salts [226,227] and toxicity of bile acids used therapeutically [228].

Bangham and Lea [219] explored NaCl conductances of black lipid membranes of egg lecithin : cephalin (3 : 1) in the presence of varying concentrations of C and DC within the bilayers. Permeability was linearly related to the bile salt concentration beginning at ~ 0.07 mM in the case of NaDC and ~ 0.6 mM in the case of NaC. In these concentration ranges, the number of monomers forming the conducting unit was 1.03 (NaDC) and 1.37 (NaC); however, the data dispersion was very wide, suggesting that the conducting unit could be 1 or 2 bile salt monomers.

In a more rigorous study using black lipid membranes of oxidized cholesterol and egg lecithin–cholesterol (5 : 1 w/w), Abramson and Shamoo [220] showed that NaDC and NaC acted as selective divalent cation ionophores at concentrations greater than 0.4 mM and 1 mM, respectively. The relative permeability sequence for both anions was $Mn^{2+} > Ca^{2+} > Sr^{2+} <> Ba^{2+} > Mg^{2+}$ in oxidized cholesterol membranes and $Ca^{2+} <> Ba^{2+} > Mg^{2+} > Sr^{2+} > Mn^{2+}$ in lecithin–cholesterol membranes. From the exponent of the least square fits of conductivity vs. detergent concentration, the size of the conducting unit was deduced to be 3–4 monomers in the case of C and 6–7 monomers in the case of DC. Saturation was not observed at high $CaCl_2$ concentrations, suggesting that each reverse bile salt micelle did not act as a mobile carrier but as a channel. Further, the affinity of bile salts for divalent cations was much greater than sodium dodecyl sulfate in these systems. Both studies suggest that higher bile salt concentrations are required for permeability to cations compared with anions — the bile salt concentrations at which conductivity was initiated, i.e. 0.4 and 1 mM for DC and C in the presence of 5 mM $CaCl_2$ are possibly the reverse micellar "CMCs" within the hydrophobic domains of the membranes.

Hunt et al. [221,222] and Castellino and Violand [223] investigated by proton NMR and ^{31}P NMR the facilitated transport of Pr^{3+} and Eu^{3+}, respectively with different bile salts, in small unilamellar vesicles of several lecithins and lecithin–cholesterol mixtures. These lanthanides are isomorphous with Ca^{2+} and are probably good probe ions for Ca^{2+} transport [229]. They employed the time course of the downfield NMR shift of the intravesicular phosphocholine head group resonances following the addition of 5 mM and 0.4 mM extravesicular Pr^{3+} and Eu^{3+}, respectively. The permeability of the vesicles to the lanthanides increased by several orders of magnitude over the self-diffusion rates and were proportional to bile salt concentration [221–223]. Hunt's kinetic analysis [221,222] suggested a transbilayer movement of reverse micelles consisting of 4 monomers of NaC, NaGC, NaDC, NaCDC and NaTC. In these studies, transport virtually ceased at or below the phase transition temperature of dipalmitoylglycero-3-phosphocholine (~ 41°C) [222] and also ceased when fluidity of egg lecithin was decreased by incorporation of up to 40 mole% cholesterol [223]. These results argue for a carrier-type mechanism via diffusion or flip-flop of lanthanide–bile salt complexes [222] rather than a simple channel-type diffusion mechanism [223]. Thus, reverse bile salt micelles act as cation ionophores within artificial membranes but the exact mechanism (carrier or channel type) is in dispute. Further, bile salts in very low concentration within the hydrophobic domains of unilamellar vesicles induce rapid flip-flop of lecithin molecules from one side of the membrane to the other [230], and probably induce water, electrolyte and even macro-molecular flow through native membranes (see ref. 32).

(VIII) Mixed micelle formation

In an earlier review [3], mixed micelles formed by bile salts were classified into those with: (i) non-polar lipids (e.g., linear or cyclic hydrocarbons); (ii) insoluble amphiphiles (e.g., cholesterol, protonated fatty acids, etc.); (iii) insoluble swelling amphiphiles (e.g., phospholipids, monoglycerides, "acid soaps"); and (iv) soluble amphiphiles (e.g., mixtures of bile salts with themselves, with soaps and with detergents) and the literature up to that date (1970) was critically summarized. Much recent work has appeared in all of these areas, but the most significant is the dramatic advances that have taken place in our understanding of the structure, size, shape, equilibria, and thermodynamics of bile salt–lecithin [16,18,28,29,99–102,127, 144,218,223,231–238] and bile salt–lecithin–cholesterol [238,239] micelles which are of crucial importance to the solubility of cholesterol in bile [1]. This section briefly surveys recent results on the above subclasses. Information on solubilization, solubilization capacities or phase equilibria of binary, ternary or quaternary systems or structures of liquid crystalline phases can be found in several excellent reviews [5,85,207,208,210,211,213,216,217] and, where relevant, have been referred to earlier.

(1) Bile salt–hydrocarbon micelles

Montet et al. [240] monitored the chemical shift of C-18/C-19 angular methyl groups of NaDC, NaC and NaUDC in the presence of solubilized naphthalene. With the exception of NaUDC, the C-19 group was shifted markedly compared to the C-18 group. The results with NaUDC were consistent with changes in the molecular packing of bile salt micelles when the steroid amphiphile had an equatorial 7-hydroxy function; the bulky solubilized probe interacts as much with rings C/D as with rings A/B. Employing an analog, 2-methylnaphthalene, Leibfritz and Roberts [241] suggested on the basis of its ^{13}C NMR spectrum that there was considerable restriction in the molecular motion of the hydrocarbon in NaDC micelles, indicating that it resided in a micelle-"dissolved" state. In contrast, when NaDC micelles were saturated with *p*-xylene, its ^{13}C spectrum was not appreciably influenced, suggesting that it preferentially resided in a micelle-"adsorbed" state. Fung and Thomas [242] reached similar conclusions employing ^{2}H spin-lattice relaxation times of perdeuterobenzene and perdeuteronaphthalene in NaC and NaDC solutions. Benzene rotated rapidly about its C-6 axis but naphthalene did not rotate in its molecular plane. The reasons for micellar adsorption rather than hydrophobic solubilization of small polarizable aromatic molecules have been discussed in detail by Mukerjee [243,244]. By examining the basic hydrolysis rates of *p*-nitrophenyl esters in aqueous solution of NaDC and NaC at 25°C, Menger and McCreery [137] concluded that the more hydrophobic esters (octanoate, dodecanoate and longer esters) had very large binding constants (NaDC $\gg$ NaC) and their unreactivity to hydroxyl ions strongly suggested that they resided within the hydrocarbon interior of the micelles with folded chains protecting the reactive carbonyl groups. In contrast, the smaller, more hydrophilic *p*-nitrophenylacetate was reactive above the bile salt's CMC, suggesting that it was probably adsorbed near the micellar surface. These authors [137] also found that elevating the ionic strength of NaDC solutions (at pH 12.0) from 0.23 to 0.80 NaCl (which increases $\bar{n}$ from 5 to ~ 160) [147] increased the hydrolysis rate of *p*-nitrophenyl octanoate by only 19%. Such a small rate change accompanying a huge increase in $\bar{n}$ supports the idea that secondary micelles form by the aggregation of primary micellar units and not by a stepwise addition of monomers. Zana and Cuveli [174] reached similar conclusions by noting that the migration of solubilized pyrene by fluorescence lifetimes and excimer formation from one primary micelle to a neighboring one in secondary micelles (NaDC, NaTCDC) is very slow, suggesting that the bonding region must have a partly hydrophilic character, presumably from hydrogen bonds. Fung and Peden [245] concluded from ^2H NMR of [7,7-$^2H_2$]NaDC that secondary micelles are in equilibrium with primary micelles (tetramers) of NaDC. There are other confirmatory studies [108,246,247] suggesting the general schema that small planar molecules are free to rotate about an axis perpendicular to the plane in bile salt micelles whereas bulky planar or non-planar molecules are held in a rigid conformation. Most of the former are therefore in the micelle-adsorbed state; most of the latter are solubilized.

(2) Bile salt–insoluble amphiphile micelles

Bile salt–acyl alcohol micelles studied by Spink and Colgan [248] confirm that not all aggregates of NaDC or NaC solutions are capable of solubilizing action and that the surfactant aggregates build up gradually with increasing surfactant concentration. Small aliphatic alcohols and aromatic alcohols generally result in an initial decrease in bile salt micellar size before a sharp increase occurs [112]. The reduction in size monitored by QLS was considered to arise from a change in water structure which diminished the hydration layer around the micelles [112]. At high alcohol contents, the micelles become markedly swollen as the phase limit was approached. The smallest change was induced by alcohols of low volume, e.g. benzyl alcohol [112]. Again, micelle-adsorbed states are the rule with small alcohols, in contrast to solubilized states with large alcohols. Similarly, nitroxide-labeled long-chain fatty acids are held in a rigid solubilized state in bile salt micelles [108]. On the basis of a molecular and thermodynamic analysis of the very different cholesterol-solubilizing capacities of NaUDC vs. NaCDC micelles, it was concluded by Carey et al. [12] that cholesterol molecules did not interact with the micellar core of simple bile salt micelles but were bonded to the hydrophobic micellar exterior. This is consistent with other studies such as the low saturation ratios of bile salt micelles for this steroid alcohol [3–5,27], the fact that micellar size only increases 1–3 Å as cholesterol is solubilized up to the phase limit [239] and the proposed H-bonding interactions between OH groups of cholesterol and methyl cholate in $CHCl_3$ [202].

(3) Bile salt–swelling amphiphile micelles

It appears that evolutionary pressure designed the common bile salts to be remarkably efficient solubilizers of swelling amphiphiles, lipids which by themselves form a number of well-defined liquid crystalline phases in water [2–6]. The physical properties and equilibria of bile salt–natural lecithins [5,102,127,231–233], bile salt–sphingomyelin [249], bile salt–monoglyceride [5,250] and bile salt–"acid soap" micelles [5, and O. Hernell, J. Staggers, R. Stafford and M.C. Carey, unpublished data] have been characterized by a variety of physical–chemical methods. However, the most rigorous and systematic studies have been carried out on bile salt–egg lecithin systems [102,127,231–233]. Not surprisingly, the physical–chemical picture that emerges appears to be similar for all bile salt–swelling amphiphile systems examined.

Fig. 16 displays the $\overline{R}_{\mathrm{h}}$ values derived by QLS measurements of two bile salt–lecithin (BS–L) systems at 10 g/dl as fucntions of the L to BS ratio and 3 temperatures. As L/BS ratio is increased, micellar sizes vary markedly. In the

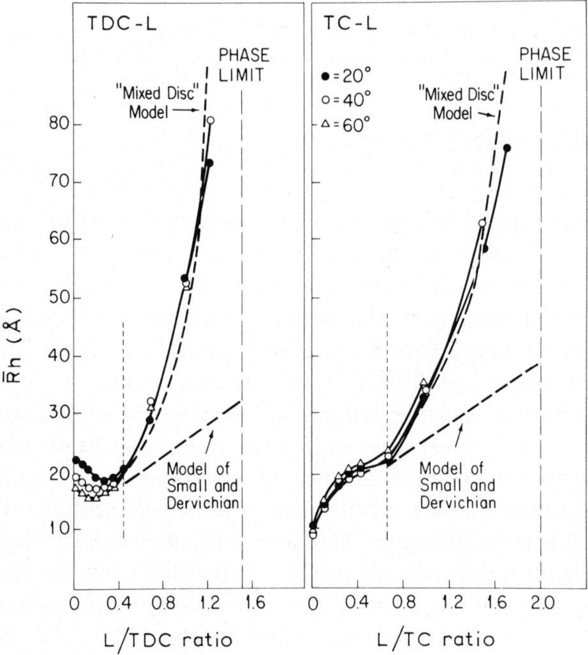

Fig. 16. Mean hydrodynamic radii ($\overline{R}_{\mathrm{h}}$, in Å) of TDC–L micelles (left) and TC–L micelles (right) as functions of L/BS ratio and 3 temperatures (other conditions, 10 g/dl total lipids, 0.15 M NaCl, pH 7.0). To the left of the short vertical dashed lines, the data are consistent with the coexistence of simple BS and mixed BS–L micelles in varying proportions. To the right of this line the data are consistent with a "mixed disk" molecular model for the micellar structure rather than the "plain disk" model proposed by Small and Dervichian. (From refs. 6 and 102 with permission.)

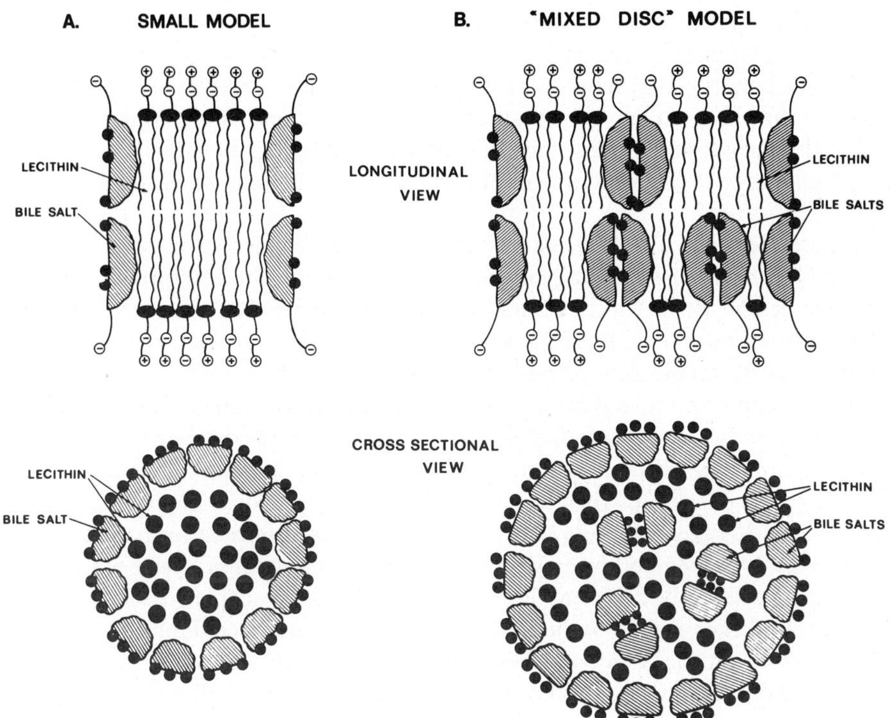

Fig. 17. Longitudinal and cross-sectional views of the proposed molecular models for the structure of bile salt–lecithin (BS–L) mixed micelles. All recent experimental data for BS–swelling amphiphile micelles are consistent with model B. In this model, reverse BS aggregates are present in high concentrations within the hydrophobic domains of L or other swelling amphiphile bilayers. BS also coat the perimeter of the disks as a bilayered "ribbon". (From ref. 102 with permission.)

TDC–L system there is an initial decrease in size and in the TC–L system an initial increase in size. Beyond the vertical dashed lines in the center of the plots the micellar sizes are seen to increase strongly to $\bar{R}_h > 80$ Å as the L/BS values reach the phase limit (broad dashed line). It is apparent that these micellar sizes are much larger than the sizes based on the micellar structures proposed by Small and Dervichian [5,6] (Fig. 17). This finding led us to propose a new molecular model (the "mixed disk" micelle) for these BS–L particles in which BS both coat the perimeter and are solubilized (probably as reverse dimers) within the disk-like fragments of L bilayers (Fig. 17). The marked divergence in micellar sizes as the phase limit is approached provides an explanation for the existence of the limit since at these lipid ratios the micelles become maximally swollen with L. As the L to BS ratio is increased beyond the phase limit, the excess L plus BS constitute a second lecithin-rich liquid crystalline phase [102,236,251].

The $\bar{R}_h$ values to the left of the narrow-dashed vertical lines (Fig. 16) show dissimilar behavior between the two systems. In addition, there is a pronounced temperature dependence, especially in the case of the TDC–L system. A mathematical analysis of these curves, taken together with the variance of the data (an index of micellar polydispersity) [102] shows that simple micelles and mixed BS–L micelles of fixed composition coexist in varying proportions over these BS–L ratios. Since physiological biliary lipid compositions fall within these lipid ratios, this hypothesis has crucial relevance to the structure and function of native human and animal biles [1].

The general features of these curves have been reproduced for other BS–L systems by QLS and classic light scattering [232], although the interpretation was considered to be consistent with the Small–Dervichian model. The estimated sizes of BS–sphingomyelin micelles [249], BS–"acid soap" micelles (O. Hernell et al., unpublished data) and BS–monoolein micelles [250] are more or less similar, indicating a coexistence of simple and mixed micelles at low swelling amphiphile to BS ratios and "mixed disk" micelles at high ratios. The hypothesis of a coexistence of pure BS micelles in equilibrium with mixed micelles at low swelling amphiphile to BS ratios has been disputed [233,252], whereas support for the mixed disk model has come from small-angle X-ray scattering [233], enthalpies of mixed micelle formation [231] and phase transition temperatures [234]. The coexistence region has been more difficult to probe directly by X-ray [233] and NMR spectroscopic methods [218], owing to the rapid exchange of monomers between simple and mixed micelles, giving an average picture on the X-ray and NMR time scales. However, strong inferential support is available in the equilibrium dialysis studies of Duane [99] and Borgström [100], the kinetic analysis of solid cholesterol crystal dissolution by BS–L systems by Higuchi et al. [253], and in the schlieren profiles of BS–sphingomyelin micelles by Yedgar and Gatt [249]. With regard to the shape of the mixed micelles, all methods (X-ray [233], QLS [102], NMR [235]) are in agreement that it is disk-like with a thickness equivalent approximately to a lecithin bilayer ($\sim$ 60 Å); as L to BS ratios are increased, the disks enlarge markedly [102,233].

The intermicellar BS concentration (IMC) is a key parameter in such systems since it is decreased in proportion to swelling amphiphile to BS ratios [99,100], is critically influenced by micelle size [102], and determines the swelling amphiphile–BS phase limit since it controls the lipid ratio in the micellar particles [102]. As a corollary, it is greatly influenced by BS species, being much higher with the more hydrophilic C and UDC than the less hydrophilic DC and CDC [99,100,254]. The actual values have been measured directly by surfactant ion electrodes [16,144], QLS-monitored dilution effects on preserving $\overline{R}_h$ [102], Sephadex G-10 exclusion [101], equilibrium dialysis [99,100], and others [6]. The trends are similar for all bile salts and show a pattern similar to that for TDC–L systems [100] displayed in Fig. 18.

The interior microenvironment of BS–L micelles has been probed by fluorescence spectroscopy using a variety of large probes with both common BS–egg and –synthetic L micelles as functions of temperature [223,232,238], NMR of [^{2}H]lecithins [235,237] differential scanning calorimetry [236], X-ray scattering [233], and electron spin resonance of spin-labels incorporated into lecithin and fatty acid chains [232].

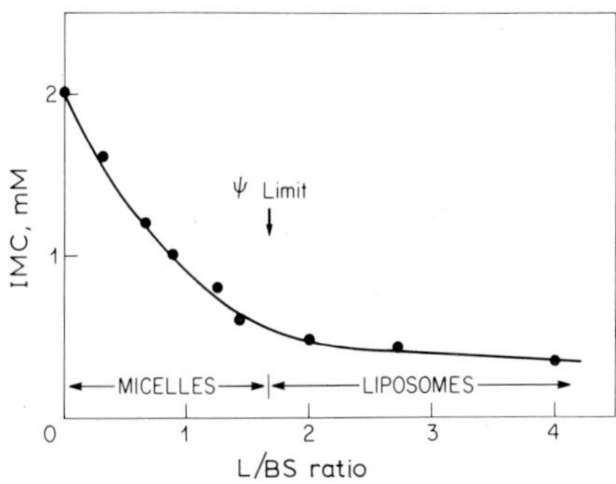

Fig. 18. Intermicellar (monomeric) bile salt concentrations (IMC) in TDC–L micelles and vesicle (liposome) systems as estimated by equilibrium dialysis. (Conditions: pH 7, 2 mM Tris–maleate, 1 mM $CaCl_2$, 150 mM NaCl, 0.2% NaN_3, 25°C, starting [TDC] = 12 mM.) ψ limit indicates "phase limit" of the TDC–L micellar phase, L/BS ratio represents the lipid ratio in the particles. (From ref. 6 with permission.)

In many instances the data for mixed micelles have been contrasted with those of BS–L vesicles. The general results and molecular implications are that the phase transitions of saturated lecithins in mixed micelles take place over a much larger temperature range than for the pure lecithin liposomes; the phase transition temperature (T_m) is depressed in proportion to bile salt content, and the enthalpy at T_m is reduced. This non-cooperative behavior and depression of T_m and ΔH are consistent with the "mixed disk" BS–L structure in which the incorporated BS fluidize the phospholipid matrix. In contrast, the melting behavior of L in BS-saturated vesicles (molar saturation ratio ~ 0.1) acts cooperatively. From fluorescence data [232,238], the packing density of lipid molecules is very similar in both mixed micelles and liposomes yet the diffusion of L molecules in micelles as evaluated by spin labeling is smaller than those in liposomes and the "microviscosity" evaluated by fluorescent probes is larger. Other NMR studies [223] with fluid-phase lecithins indicate considerable internuclear head group interactions of phospholipid within the micelles and indicate that segmented motions in this head group region are slow. These results suggest that mixed micelles involve tight molecular packing at the periphery, presumably because many BS molecules are deeply embedded within the bilayers. However, the segmented motion of the hydrocarbon chains toward the interior of the bilayer is fluidized in agreement with the work of Ulmius et al. [211] on C–L lamellar liquid crystals. Stark et al. [237] showed that this increase in fluidity is more marked at 4°C when palmitoyloleoylglycero-3-phosphocholine is in the gel state then at 51°C when it is in the liquid-crystalline state; these trends are similar to those found in other work [211].

(4) Bile salt–soluble amphiphile micelles

Since 1970, little work has been published on this subject. A kinetic dialysis study has been employed to determine the CMC and composition of mixed bile salt micelles of NaTC plus DC or TDC at pH 7.4 [255]. The results suggest that mixed micellar composition is largely predicted by the molar composition of the binary system; in all cases the CMC is decreased by the more hydrophobic species, i.e. that with the lower CMC, in agreement with previously reported values for TC plus TDC micelles [5]. Barry and Gray [256] studied the properties of mixed micelles in aqueous solutions of the alkyltrimethyl ammonium salt of C. This large cationic amphiphile forms a tight salt linkage with C when the stoichiometry is 1:1 but is partially dissociated and soluble. In an excess of C, the cationic detergent is "solubilized" to form mixed micelles. The mixed micelles are small ($\bar{n} = 19$–32) and spherical and only slightly charged. CMCs evaluated by non-equilibrium surface tension and conductivity studies [256] were similar, averaging 0.04–0.21 mM. Interfacial areas in 0.1 M NaBr (84–103 $Å^2$) calculated from the surface excess and Avogadro's number are in the range expected for BS molecules either lying flat or forming H-bonded surface dimers. This ambiguity has not been resolved. These authors [257] also showed that alkyltrimethyl ammonium salts of DC and CDC separated into two liquid phases (coacervation) in 1:1 molar ratios which were solubilized by an excess of either detergent or by an elevation of temperature, demonstrating an upper consolute point. Similar observations were made on the alkyltrimethyl ammonium salts of DC by Kellaway and Marriott [258,259] with the exception that short-chain alkyltrimethyl ammonium bromides did not form complexes but behaved in similar fashion to the addition of inorganic salts, i.e. a counterion effect with pronounced CMC lowering and micellar growth. These mixtures cannot be considered true examples of BS–soluble amphiphile micelles. Physical measurements carried out by Gatt et al. [143] showed that mixtures of NaTDC and G_{m1} ganglioside (a soluble amphiphile) in 3:1 and 2:1 molar ratios at 20°C formed mixed micelles with higher CMCs, lower $\bar{n}$ values, and greater axial ratios than the corresponding micelles of pure G_{m1} gangliosides. These results are analogous to other studies on soluble amphiphile mixtures [5,255].

(5) Bile salt–swelling amphiphile–insoluble amphiphile micelles

The classic biological example of these systems is bile salt (BS)–lecithin (L)–cholesterol (Ch) micelles which have been studied in detail by QLS [239]. In TC–L–Ch systems, particle size and polydispersity were studied as functions of Ch mole fraction ($X_{Ch} = 0$–15%), L/TC molar ratio (0–1.6), temperature (5–85°C), and total lipid concentration (3 and 10 g/dl) in 0.15 M NaCl. For X_{Ch} values below the established solubilization limits (X_{Ch}^{max}), added Ch has little influence on the size of simple TC micelles, on the coexistence of simple and mixed TC–L micelles, or on the growth of "mixed disk" TC–L micelles. For supersaturated systems ($X_{Ch}/X_{Ch}^{max} > 1$), 10 g/dl simple micellar systems (L/TC = 0) exist as metastable micellar solutions even at $X_{Ch}/X_{Ch}^{max} = 5.3$. Metastability is decreased in coexisting systems ($0 < L/TC < 0.6$), and "labile" microprecipitation occurs when X_{Ch}/X_{Ch}^{max} exceeds ~ 1.6. In 10 g/dl mixtures, the microprecipitates initially range in size from 500 to 20000 Å and later coalesce to form a buoyant macroscopic precipitate phase. In 3 g/dl mixtures, the microprecipitates are smaller (200–400 Å) and remain as a stable, non-coalesced microdispersion. Transmission electron microscopy of the microprecipitates formed at both concentrations indicates a globular non-crystalline structure, and lipid analysis reveals the presence of Ch and L in a molar ratio of approximately 2/1, suggesting that the microprecipitates represent a metastable Ch-supersaturated liquid-crystalline phase. In supersaturated mixed micellar systems ($0.6 < L/TC < 2.0$), the precipitate phase is an L-rich liquid-crystalline structure which likewise coalesces in a 10 g/dl system but forms stable vesicle structures (600–800 Å radius) in 3 g/dl systems. Homogeneous nucleation theory was satisfactorily employed to analyze the origin of the metastable/labile limit in supersaturated systems and to deduce the interfacial tension between microprecipitates and solution [239]. On the basis of these experimental data and theoretical analyses, it was suggested that the "stable" microprecipitates observed in 3 g/dl coexistence systems may provide a secondary vehicle (in addition to micelles) for cholesterol transport in supersaturated hepatic bile [239].

With regard to the microenvironment of such mixed systems, a study with the use of fluorescent probes [238] demonstrated that the effect of Ch was to greatly decrease L fluidity, suggesting that the added Ch was indeed incorporated within the micelle and interacted with L in a manner similar to its influence in lamellar liquid-crystalline bilayers of L [209]. Thus, as discussed earlier, the incorporation of BS to form "mixed disk" micelles fluidizes the phospholipid matrix irrespective of whether the phospholipid is saturated or unsaturated. In contrast, solubilization of Ch into these mixed micelles leads to a reduction in fluidity. Ch also leads to a reduction in the number of bound cationic and anionic fluorophors in such systems [238], suggesting that the binding of these molecules, and perhaps others of biological interest, is extremely sensitive to changes in lipid packing induced by the addition of Ch, and apparently not to any electrostatic effects.

(6) Mixed micelle–unilamellar vesicle transition

The binary phase diagram shown in Fig. 19 displays coexistence and micellar phase boundaries as functions of TC and L concentrations. The diagram defines the areas where simple plus mixed micelles, mixed micelles alone, and liposomes are formed [102]. By diluting a mixture within the first micellar region, each of these phase boundaries is crossed, with eventual divergence in micellar growth at the phase limit and upon further dilution the system is transformed into unilamellar vesicles [102,251]. The size of the vesicles decreases monotonically with increasing dilution and approaches a minimum radius of ~ 120 Å in the GC–L system [251]. However, sizes can vary from ~ 120 to 500 Å depending upon total lipid concentration, L to BS ratio and temperature. Formation of the vesicles and their size are determined by the partitioning of BS molecules between the surrounding aqueous media and the particles. This is preceded by micellar growth which occurs from alteration of L/BS ratio in the "mixed disk" micelles secondary to the flow of BS monomers into the aqueous environment [102,251]. The formation of vesicles may be

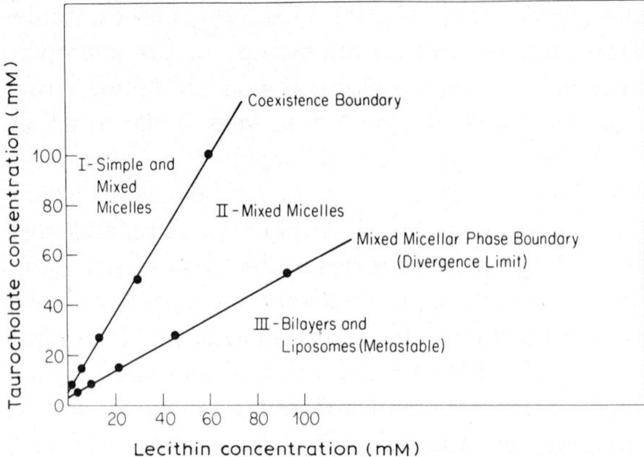

Fig. 19. Rectangular phase diagram of TC–L systems in 0.15 M NaCl at 20°C. Region I corresponds to concentrations where simple and mixed micelles coexist. In region II only mixed micelles are present, and in region III metastable vesicles and liposomes are found. (From ref. 102 with permission.)

either from the folding of micelles or from ab initio growth of vesicles since at the phase limit the monomeric aqueous L solubility is exceeded and now dominates the chemical activity of the system. By QLS these vesicles form a nearly monodisperse population [102,251] in contrast to large micelles [102]. Further, while mixed micelles are in thermodynamic equilibria, dilution vesicles are metastable, exhibiting a marked path dependence [251]. Upon changing temperature, which alters micellar phase limits, the micelle-to-vesicle transition is fast but the reverse is either very slow or does not occur [251]. Whereas the final unilamellar vesicles may be made to grow with experimental manipulations, they cannot be made to shrink [251].

(7) Native bile and intestinal content

Recent physical–chemical observations on native mammalian systems reveal that the proposed mixed micellar mechanism of lipid solubilization and transport in both bile and in upper small intestinal contents is incomplete [1,260–263]. Bile is predominantly a mixed micellar solution but, particularly when supersaturated with Ch, also contains small liquid-crystalline vesicles which, as suggested from model systems [239], are another vehicle for Ch and L transport. In dog bile which is markedly unsaturated with Ch [258], these vesicles exist in dilute concentrations and may be markers of the detergent properties of BS on the cells lining the biliary tree and/or related to the mode of bile formation at the level of the canaliculus. In human hepatic bile, which is generally dilute and markedly supersaturated with Ch, these vesicles may be the predominant form of Ch and L "solubilization" and transport [261]. If hepatic bile is extremely dilute, it is theoretically possible that no BS–L–Ch micelles may be present [268]; all of the lipid content may be aggregated in the form of liquid-crystalline vesicles, a paradigm which may be of particular relevance to the mechanism of secretion of bile lipids into the canalicular lumen.

Both micelles and unilamellar liquid-crystalline vesicles coexist during human fat digestion in the aqueous portions of upper intestinal content [262,263, Chapter 14]. In terms of composition and size, the micelles are not like biliary micelles, as has been traditionally believed, but are considerably larger ($\bar{R}_h \sim 100$ Å) with relative lipid compositions which fall on the limits of the mixed lipids/Ch–BS phase boundary. The liquid-crystalline vesicle (or liposomal) phase of upper small intestinal contents is less well defined physico-chemically [262,263]; its crucial importance in fat digestion and absorption is obvious in view of the fact that fat absorption proceeds efficiently in the total absence of BS micelles [262].

Acknowledgments

Supported in part by NIADDK (NIH) research grants AM 18559 and AM 34854.

The author is greatly indebted to Dr. S. Barnes (Birmingham, AL), Professor E. Giglio (Rome, Italy), Dr. E.N. Maslen (Nedlands, W. Australia), Dr. S.K. Arora (Austin, TX), Professor E.W.B. Einstein (Burnaby, Canada), Dr. V.M. Coiro (Rome, Italy), and Dr. John P. Schaefer (Tucson, AZ) for supplying crystallographic illustrations, and to Ms. Rebecca Ankener for editorial and bibliographic assistance.

References

1 Carey, M.C. (1982) in: The Liver: Biology and Pathobiology (Arias, I.M., Popper, H., Schacter, D. and Shafritz, D., Eds.) pp. 429–465, Raven Press, New York.
2 Hofmann, A.F. and Small, D.M. (1967) Annu. Rev. Med. 18, 333–376.
3 Carey, M.C. and Small, D.M. (1970) Am. J. Med. 49, 590–608.
4 Carey, M.C. and Small, D.M. (1972) Arch. Intern. Med. 130, 506–527.
5 Small, D.M. (1971) in: The Bile Acids (Nair, P.P. and Kritchevsky, D., Eds.) pp. 249–356, Plenum Press, New York.
6 Carey, M.C. (1983) in: Bile Acids in Gastroenterology (Barbara, L., Dowling, R.H., Hofmann, A.F. and Roda, E., Eds.) pp. 19–56, MTP Press, Boston, MA.
7 Cobbledick, R.E. and Einstein, F.W.B. (1980) Acta Cryst. B36, 287–292.
8 Haslewood, G.A.D. (1967)Bile Salts, pp. 1–116, Methuen, London.
9 Barnes, S. and Geckle, J.M. (1982) J. Lipid Res. 23, 161–170.
10 Small, D.M., Penkett, S.A. and Chapman, D. (1969) Biochim. Biophys. Acta 176,178–189.
11 Martis, L., Hall, N.A. and Thakkar, A.L. (1972) J. Pharm. Sci. 61, 1757–1761.
12 Carey, M.C., Montet, J.-C., Phillips, M.C., Armstrong, M.J. and Mazer, N.A. (1981) Biochemistry 20, 3637–3648.
13 Joos, P. and Ruyssen, R. (1969) Chem. Phys. Lipids 3, 83–90.
14 Barnes, S. (1984) Hepatology 4, 98S–102S.
15 Pauling, L. (1964) College Chemistry, 3rd Edn., pp. 1–832, Freeman, San Francisco, CA.
16 Ryu, K., Lowery, J.M., Evans, D.F. and Cussler, E.L. (1983) J. Phys. Chem. 87, 5015–5019.
17 Norman, A. (1960) Acta Chem. Scand. 14, 1300–1309.
18 Evans, D.F., DePalma, R., Nadas, J. and Thomas, J. (1972) J. Soln. Chem. 1, 377–386.

19 Moore, E.W., Celic, L. and Ostrow, J.D. (1982) Gastroenterology 83, 1079–1089.
20 Lindman, B., Kamenka, N., Fabre, H., Ulmius, J. and Wieloch, T. (1980) J. Colloid Interface Sci. 73, 556–565.
21 Lindman, B., Puyal, M.-C., Kamenka, N., Brun, B. and Gunnarsson, G. (1982) J. Phys. Chem. 86, 1702–1711.
22 Smith, W.B. and Barnard, G.D. (1981) Can. J. Chem. 59, 1602–1606.
23 Haslewood, G.A.D. (1978) The Biological Importance of Bile Salts, pp. 1–206, North-Holland, Amsterdam.
24 Heaton, K.W. (1972) Bile Salts in Health and Disease, pp. 1–252, Churchill-Livingstone, London.
25 Donovan, J.M., Yousef, I.M. and Carey, M.C. (1984) Gastroenterology (Abstr.) 86, 1064.
26 Armstrong, M.J. and Carey, M.C. (1982) J. Lipid Res. 23, 70–80.
27 Igimi, H. and Carey, M.C. (1981) J. Lipid Res. 22, 254–270.
28 Salvioli, G., Igimi, H. and Carey, M.C. (1983) J. Lipid Res. 24, 701–720.
29 Rajagopalan, N. and Lindenbaum, S. (1984) J. Lipid Res. 25, 135–147.
30 Elliott, W.H. and Shaw, R. (1981) in: Steroid Analysis by HPLC (Kautsky, M.P., Ed.) pp. 1–40, Marcel Dekker, New York.
31 Schubert, R., Jaroni, H., Schoelmerich, J. and Schmidt, K.H. (1983) Digestion 28, 181–190.
32 Gordon, G.S., Moses, A.C., Silver, R.D., Flier, J.S. and Carey, M.C. (1985) Proc. Natl. Acad. Sci. (U.S.A.) in press.
33 Roda, A., Hofmann, A.F. and Mysels, K.J. (1983) J. Biol. Chem. 258, 6362–6370.
34 Windholz, M. (Ed.) (1983) The Merck Index, 10th Edn., pp. 4–1463, Merck, Rahway, NJ.
35 Igimi, H. and Carey, M.C. (1980) J. Lipid Res. 21, 72–90.
36 Hofmann, A.F. (1963) Acta Chem. Scand. 171, 173–186.
37 Iida, T. and Chang, F.C. (1981) J. Org. Chem. 13, 2786–2788.
38 Van Berge-Henegouwen, G.P., Hofmann, A.F. and Gaginella, T.S. (1977) Gastroenterology 73, 291–299.
39 Iida, T. and Chang, F.C. (1982) J. Org. Chem. 47, 2966–2972.
40 Chang, F.C., Wood, N.F. and Holton, W.G. (1965) J. Org. Chem. 30, 1718–1723.
41 Iida, T., Taneja, H.R. and Chang, F.C. (1981) Lipids 16, 863–865.
42 Sobotka, H. (1938) The Chemistry of the Steroids, pp. 109–125, Williams and Wilkins, Baltimore, MD.
43 Lindley, P.F., Mahmoud, M.M., Watson, F.E. and Jones, W.A. (1980) Acta Cryst. B36, 1893–1897.
44 Arora, S.K., Germain, G. and Declercq, J.P. (1976) Acta Cryst. B32, 415–419.
45 Johnson, P. and Schaefer, J.P. (1972) Acta Cryst. B28, 3083–3088.
46 Tang, C.P., Popovitz-Biro, R., Lahav, M. and Leiserowitz, L. (1979) Israel J. Chem. 18, 385–389.
47 Candeloro de Sanctis, S., Coiro, V.M., Giglio, E., Pagliuca, S., Pavel, N.V. and Quagliata, C. (1978) Acta Cryst. B34, 1928–1933.
48 Batta, A.K., Salen, G., Blount, J.F. and Shefer, S. (1979) J. Lipid Res. 20, 935–940.
49 Hall, S.R., Maslen, E.N. and Cooper, A. (1974) Acta Cryst. B30, 1441–1447.
50 Vadnere, M., Natarajan, R. and Lindenbaum, S. (1980) J. Phys. Chem. 84, 1900–1903.
51 Coiro, V.M., Giglio, E., Morosetti, S. and Palleschi, A. (1980) Acta Cryst. B36, 1478–1480.
52 Djavanbakht, A., Kale, K.M. and Zana, R. (1977) J. Colloid Interface Sci. 59, 139–148.
53 Hogan, A., Ealick, S.E., Bugg, C.E. and Barnes, S. (1984) J. Lipid Res. 25, 791–798.
54 Schaefer, J.P. and Reed, L.L. (1972) Acta Cryst. B28, 1743–1748.
55 Sobotka, H. (1934) Chem. Rev. 15, 311–375.
56 Fieser, L.F. and Fieser, M. (1959) Steroids, pp. 115–118, Reinhold, New York.
57 Herndon, W.C. (1967) J. Chem. Educ. 44, 724–728.
58 Jones, J.G., Schwerzbaum, S., Lessinger, L. and Low, B.W. (1982) Acta Cryst. B38, 1207–1215.
59 D'Andrea, A., Fedeli, W., Giglio, E., Mazza, F. and Pavel, N.V. (1981) Acta Cryst. B37, 368–372.
60 Friedman, N., Lahav, M., Leiserowitz, L., Popovitz-Biro, R., Tang, C.-P. and Zaretzkii, Z. (1975) J. Chem. Soc. Chem. Commun., 864–865.
61 Candeloro de Sanctis, S., Giglio, E., Pavel, V. and Quagliata, C. (1972) Acta Cryst. B28, 3656–3661.
62 Craven, B.M. and DeTitta, G.T. (1972) J. Chem. Soc. Chem. Commun., 530–531.

63 Wieland, H. and Sorge, H. (1916) Z. Physiol. Chem. 97, 1–27.
64 Fowweather, F.S. (1949) Biochem. J. 44, 607–610.
65 Sobotka, H. (1937) Physiological Chemistry of the Bile, pp. 1–202, Williams and Wilkins, Baltimore, MD.
66 Ekwall, P. and Ekholm, R. (1957) in: Proc. Int. Congr. Surface Activity, Vol. I (Schulman, J.H., Ed.) pp. 23–30, Butterworths, London.
67 Crisp, D.J. (1949) in: Surface Chemistry, pp. 17–22, Butterworths, London.
68 Crisp, D.J. (1949) in: Surface Chemistry, pp. 23–35, Butterworths, London.
69 Cadenhead, D.A. and Phillips, M.C. (1967) J. Colloid Interface Sci. 24, 491–499.
70 Kratohvil, J.P. and DelliColli, H.T. (1968) Can. J. Biochem. 46, 945–952.
71 Furusawa, T. (1962) Fukuoka Acta Med. 53, 124–165.
72 Yoshimuta, S. (1960) Fukuoka Acta Med. 51, 510–528.
73 Hisadome, T., Nakama, T., Itoh, H. and Furasawa, T. (1980) Gastroenterol. Jpn. 15, 257–263.
74 Thomas, D.C. and Christian, S.D. (1980) J. Colloid Interface Sci. 78, 466–478.
75 Dasher, G.F. (1952) Science 116, 660–663.
76 Baret, J.F., Bois, A.G. and Benzonana, G. (1972) Kolloid Z.v.Z. Polymere 250, 352–355.
77 Gupta, P.M., Bahadur, P. and Singh, S.P. (1979) Indian J. Biochem. Biophys. 16, 336–337.
78 Haller, W. (1981) Ber. Bunsengas Phys. Chem. 85, 846–851.
79 Joos, P., Rosseneu-Motreff, M.Y. and Ruyssen, R. (1968) J. Chim. Phys. (Paris) 65, 951–958.
80 Joos, P., Ruyssen, R., Miñones Trillo, J., Garcia-Fernandez, S. and Sans Pedrero, P. (1969) J. Chim. Phys. (Paris) 66, 1665–1669.
81 Vochten, R. and Joos, P. (1970) J. Chim. Phys. (Paris) 67, 1360–1371.
82 Miñones Trillo, J., Garcia-Fernandez, S. and Sanz Pedrero, P. (1968) J. Colloid Interface Sci. 26, 518–531.
83 Llopis, J., Albert, A., Saiz, J.L. and Alonso, D. (1973) in: Chemistry, Physical Chemistry and Applications of Surface Active Substances, Vol. 2, pp. 339–350, Carl Hanser, Munich.
84 Miñones Trillo, J., Garcia Fernandez, S. and Sanz Pedrero, P. (1968) in: Chemistry, Physics and Practical Applications of Surface Active Substances, Vol. 2, Part 1 (P. Desnuelle, Ed.), pp. 405–411, Unidas, Barcelona.
85 Small, D.M. (1968) J. Am. Oil Chem. Soc. 45, 108–119.
86 Carey, M.C., Wu, S.-F. and Watkins, J.B. (1979) Biochim. Biophys. Acta 575, 16–26.
87 Small, D.M. and Admirand, W.H. (1969) Nature (London) 221, 265–267.
88 Fini, A., Roda, A. and DeMaria, P. (1982) Eur. J. Med. Chem. 17, 467–470.
89 Irving, C.S., Hammer, B.E., Danyluk, S.S. and Klein, P.D. (1982) in: Taurine in Nutrition and Neurology (Huxtable, R.J. and Pasantes-Morales, H., Eds.) pp. 5–17, Plenum Press, New York.
90 Roda, A., Fini, A., Fugazza, R. and Grigolo, B. (1985) J. Soln. Chem., 14, 595–604.
91 Dervichian, D.G. (1964) in: Progress in Biophysics and Molecular Biology (Butler, J.A.V. and Huxley, H.E., Eds.) Vol. 14, pp. 265–342, Pergamon, New York.
92 Hjelmeland, L.M., Nebert, D.W. and Osborne, J.C. (1983) Anal. Biochem. 130, 72–82.
93 Murray, R.C. and Hartley, G.S. (1935) Trans. Faraday Soc. 31, 183–189.
94 Mazer, N.A., Benedek, G.B. and Carey, M.C. (1976) J. Phys. Chem. 80, 1075–1085.
95 Krafft, F. and Wiglow, H. (1895) Ber. Dtsch. Chem. Ges. 28, 2566–2573.
96 Krafft, F. and Wiglow, H. (1895) Ber. Dtsch. Chem. Ges. 28, 2573–2582.
97 Hartley, G.S. (1936) Aqueous Solution of Paraffin-Chain Salts, pp. 4–69, Hermann, Paris.
98 Mukerjee, P. and Cardinal, J.R. (1976) J. Pharm. Sci. 65, 882–886.
99 Duane, W.C. (1977) Biochem. Biophys. Res. Commun. 74, 223–229.
100 Borgström, B. (1978) Lipids 13, 187–189.
101 Ammon, H.V. and Walter, L.G. (1982) Anal. Chem. 54, 2079–2082.
102 Mazer, N.A., Benedek, G.B. and Carey, M.C. (1980) Biochemistry 19, 601–615.
103 Ekwall, P., Fontell, K. and Sten, A. (1957) in: Proc. Second Int. Congr. Surface Activity (Schulman, J.H., Ed.), Vol. 1, pp. 357–373, Butterworths, London.
104 Norman, A. (1960) Acta Chem. Scand. 14, 1295–1299.
105 DeMoerloose, P. and Ruyssen, R. (1959) J. Pharm. Belg. 14, 95–105.

106 Miyake, H., Murakoshi, T. and Hisatsuga, T. (1962) Fukuoka Acta Med. 53, 695–702.
107 Carey, M.C., Montet, J.-C. and Small, D.M. (1975) Biochemistry 14, 4896–4905.
108 Fisher, L. and Oakenfull, D. (1979) Aust. J. Chem. 32, 31–39.
109 Paul, R., Mathew, M.K., Narayanan, R. and Balaram, P. (1979) Chem. Phys. Lipids 25, 345–356.
110 DeVendittis, E., Palumbo, G., Parlato, G. and Bocchini, V. (1981) Anal. Biochem. 115, 278–286.
111 Borgström, B. and Erlanson, C. (1973) Eur. J. Biochem. 37, 60–68.
112 Roe, J.M. and Barry, B.W. (1985) J. Colloid Interface Sci., 107, 398–404.
113 Roe, J.M. and Barry, B.W. (1983) J. Colloid Interface Sci. 94, 580–583.
114 Helenius, A., McCaslin, D.R., Fries, E. and Tanford, C. (1979) Methods in Enzymology Vol. LVI, pp. 734–749, Academic Press, New York.
115 Carpenter, P. and Lindenbaum, S. (1979) J. Soln. Chem. 8, 347–357.
116 Rajogopalan, N., Vadnere, M. and Lindenbaum, S. (1981) J. Soln. Chem. 10, 785–801.
117 O'Connor, C.J., Ch'ng, B.T. and Wallace, R.G. (1983) J. Colloid Interface Sci. 95, 410–419.
118 Pal, S., Das, A.R. and Moulik, S.P. (1982) Indian J. Biochem. Biophys. 19, 295–300.
119 Vadnere, M. and Lindenbaum, S. (1982) J. Pharm. Sci. 71, 875–881.
120 Roepke, R.R. and Mason, H.L. (1940) J. Biol. Chem. 133, 103–108.
121 Kretschmer, K., Koelsch, R., Bernhardt, M. and Berdichevsky, V.R. (1982) Studia Biophys. 91, 103–106.
122 Campanella, L., Sorrentino, L. and Tomassetti, M. (1983) Analyst 108, 1490–1494.
123 Ekwall, P., Rosendahl, T. and Löfman, N. (1957) Acta Chem. Scand. 11, 590–598.
124 Ekwall, P. (1953) in: Proc. First Int. Conf. on Biochem. Problems of Lipids (Ruyssen, R., Ed.), pp. 103–119, Kon. Vlaam. Acad. Wetensch., Brussels.
125 Ekwall, P. (1954) J. Colloid Sci. Suppl. 1, 66–80.
126 Vochten, R. and Joos, P. (1970) J. Chim. Phys. (Paris) 67, 1372–1379.
127 Shankland, W. (1970) Chem. Phys. Lipids 4, 109–130.
128 Juna, K. and Sugano, T. (1969) Nippon Kagaku Zasshi 90, 463–466.
129 Markina, Z.N., Tsirkurina, N.N., Bovkun, O.P., Kopeina, A.D. and Rebinder, P.A. (1967) Doklady Akad. Nauk. S.S.S.R. 173, 1132–1135.
130 Markina, Z.N., Tsikurina, N.N. and Rebinder, P.A. (1966) Doklady Akad. Nauk. S.S.S.R. 172, 1376–1379.
131 Tsikurina, N.N., Markina, Z.N., Chirova, G.A. and Rebinder, P.A. (1968) Kolloignyi Zh. 30, 292–298.
132 Rains, A.J.H. and Crawford, M. (1953) Nature (London) 171, 829–831.
133 Fontell, K. (1971) Kolloid Z. v. Z. Polymere 244, 246–252.
134 Fontell, K. (1971) Kolloid Z. v. Z. Polymere 244, 253–257.
135 Fontell, K. (1972) Kolloid Z. v. Z. Polymere 250, 333–343.
136 Bates, T.R., Gibaldi, M. and Kanig, M.L. (1966) J. Pharm. Sci. 55, 191–199.
137 Menger, F.M. and McCreery, M.J. (1974) J. Am. Chem. Soc. 96, 121–126.
138 Chang, Y. and Cardinal, J.R. (1978) J. Pharm. Sci. 67, 174–181.
139 Hofmann, A.F. (1963) Biochem. J. 89, 57–68.
140 Kratohvil, J.P., Hsu, W.P., Jacobs, M.A., Aminabhavi, T.M. and Mukunoki, Y. (1983) Colloid Polymer Sci. 261, 781–785.
141 DelliColli, H.T. (1970) Ph.D. Thesis, pp. 1–205, Clarkson College, Potsdam, New York.
142 Carey, M.C. and Small, D.M. (1969) J. Colloid Interface Sci. 31, 383–396.
143 Gatt, S., Gazit, B. and Barenholz, Y. (1981) Biochem. J. 193, 267–273.
144 Gilligan III, T.J., Cussler, E.L. and Evans, D.F. (1977) Biochim. Biophys. Acta 497, 627–630.
145 Chang, Y. and Cardinal, J.R. (1978) J. Pharm. Sci. 67, 994–999.
146 Mazer, N.A., Carey, M.C., Kwasnick, R.F. and Benedek, G.B. (1979) Biochemistry 18, 3064–3075.
147 Small, D.M. (1968) Adv. Chem. Ser. 84, 31–52.
148 Smith, E.L. and Pickels, E.G. (1940) Proc. Natl. Acad. Sci. (U.S.A.) 26, 272–277.
149 Olsen, J.A. and Herron, J.S. (1964) Sixth Int. Congr. Biochem. (Abstr.) No. VIII-112, 588.
150 Oeswein, J.Q., Hall, R.J., Kim, J.H., Cantarini, W.F. and Chun, P.W. (1983) J. Biol. Chem. 258, 3645–3654.

151 Rich, A. and Blow, D.M. (1958) Nature (London) 182, 423–426.
152 Sobotka, H. and Czeczowieczka, N. (1958) J. Colloid Sci. 13, 188–191.
153 Sugihara, G., Tanaka, M. and Matuura, R. (1977) Bull. Chem. Soc. Jpn. 50, 2542–2547.
154 D'Arrigo, G., Sesta, B. and LaMesa, C. (1980) J. Chem. Phys. 73, 4562–4568.
155 Sugihara, G. and Tanaka, M. (1976) Bull. Chem. Soc. Jpn. 49, 3457–3460.
156 Murata, Y., Akisada, H., Yoshida, M., Sugihara, G. and Tanaka, M. (1979) Fukuoka Daigaku Kenkyujo 9, 41–45.
157 Murata, Y., Sugihara, G., Nishikido, N. and Tanaka, M. (1982) in: Solution Behavior of Surfactants (Mittal, K.L. and Fendler, E.J., Eds.) Vol. 1, pp. 611–627, Plenum Press, New York.
158 Murata, Y., Sugihara, G., Fukushima, K., Tanaka, M. and Matsushita, K. (1982) J. Phys. Chem. 86, 4690–4694.
159 Sesta, B., LaMesa, C., Bonincontro, A., Cimetti, C. and DiBiasio, A. (1981) Ber. Bunsengas Phys. Chem. 85, 798–803.
160 Laurent, T.C. and Persson, H. (1965) Biochim. Biphys. Acta 106, 616–624.
161 Schurtenberger, P., Mazer, N. and Känzig, W. (1983) J. Phys. Chem. 87, 308–315.
162 Vitello, L.B. (1973) Ph.D. Dissertation, pp. 1–128, Clarkson College, New York.
163 Lindheimer, M., Montet, J-C., Molenat, J., Bontemps, R. and Brun, B. (1981) J. Chim. Phys. (Paris) 78, 447–455.
164 Woodford, F.P. (1969) J. Lipid Res. 10, 539–545.
165 Sehlin, R.C., Cussler, E.L. and Evans, D.F. (1975) Biochim. Biophys. Acta 388, 385–396.
166 Borgström, B. (1965) Biochim. Biophys. Acta 106, 171–183.
167 Phillies, G.D.J. (1981) J. Phys. Chem. 85, 3540–3541.
168 Phillies, G.D.J. (1982) J. Colloid Interface Sci. 86, 226–233.
169 Weinheimer, R.M., Evans, D.F. and Cussler, E.L. (1981) J. Colloid Interface Sci. 80, 357–368.
170 Fontell, K. (1971) Kolloid Z. v. Z. Polymere 246, 614–625.
171 Cussler, E.L. and Duncan, G.L. (1972) J. Soln. Chem. 1, 269–277.
172 Jacobs, M.A. (1976) M.S. Dissertation, pp. 1–48, Clarkson College, New York.
173 Lindman, B., Kamenka, N. and Brun, B. (1976) J. Colloid Interface Sci. 56, 328–336.
174 Zana, R. and Cuveli, D. (1985) J. Phys. Chem., 89, 1687–1690.
175 Smith, C.M., Williams, G.C., Krivit, W., White, J.G. and Hanson, R.F. (1979) J. Lab. Clin. Med. 94, 624–632.
176 Shinoda, K., Nakagawa, T., Tamamushi, B.-T. and Isemura, T. (1963) Colloidal Surfactants, pp. 1–310, Academic Press, New York.
177 Robb, I.D. and Smith, R. (1974) J. Chem. Soc. Faraday I 70, 287–292.
178 Beunsen, J.A. and Ruckenstein, E. (1983) J. Colloid Interface Sci. 96, 469–487.
179 Lindman, B. and Brun, B. (1973) J. Colloid Interface Sci. 42, 388–399.
180 Kamenka, N., Lindman, B., Fontell, K., Chorro, M. and Brun, B. (1977) C.R. Acad. Sci. Paris 284, 403–406.
181 Kale, K.M. and Zana, R. (1977) J. Colloid Interface Sci. 61, 312–322.
182 Démarq, M. and Dervichian, D.G. (1945) Bull. Soc. Chim. France 12, 939–945.
183 Koshinuma, M. (1981) Bull. Chem. Soc. Jpn. 54, 3128–3132.
184 Miyamoto, S. (1960) Bull. Chem. Soc. Jpn. 33, 371–375.
185 Miyamoto, S. (1960) Bull. Chem. Soc. Jpn. 33, 375–379.
186 Satake, I., Iwamatsu, I., Hosokawa, S. and Matuura, R. (1963) Bull. Chem. Soc. Jpn. 36, 204–209.
187 Mellander, O. and Stenhagen, E. (1942) Acta Physiol. Scand. 4, 349–361.
188 Moore, E.W. and Dietschy, J.M. (1964) Am. J. Physiol. 206, 1111–1117.
189 Rajogopalan, N. and Lindenbaum, S. (1982) Biochim. Biophys. Acta 711, 66–74.
190 Gustavsson, H. and Lindman, B. (1975) J. Am. Chem. Soc. 94, 3923–3930.
191 Hewish, N.A., Neilson, G.W. and Enderby, J.E. (1982) Nature (London) 297, 138–139.
192 Moore, E.W. (1984) Hepatology 4, 228S–243S.
193 Lang, J., Tondre, C., Zana, R., Bauer, R., Hoffmann, H. and Ulbricht, W. (1975) J. Phys. Chem. 79, 276–283.

194 Zana, R. (1975) in: Chemical and Biological Application of Relaxation Spectroscopy (Wyn-Jones, E., Ed.), pp. 133–138, Dordrecht, Amsterdam.
195 Mukerjee, P. (1974) J. Pharm. Sci. 63, 972–981.
196 Bennet, W.S., Eglinton, G. and Kovac, S. (1967) Nature (London) 214, 776–780.
197 Kovac, S. and Eglinton, G. (1969) Tetrahedron 25, 3609–3616.
198 Smith, W.B. (1978) J. Phys. Chem. 82, 234–238.
199 Fendler, E.J. and Rosenthal, S.N. (1979) in: Solution Chemistry of Surfactants (Mittal, K.L., Ed), Vol. 1, pp. 455–472, Plenum Press, New York.
200 Robeson, J., Foster, B.W., Rosenthal, S.W., Adams Jr., E.T. and Fendler, E.J. (1981) J. Phys. Chem. 85, 1254–1261.
201 Mittal, K.L. and Fendler, E.J. (Eds.) (1982) Solution Behavior of Surfactants, Vol. 2, pp. 743–884, Plenum Press, New York.
202 Foster, B.W., Huggins, R.L., Robeson, J. and Adams Jr., E.T. (1982) Biophys. Chem. 16, 317–328.
203 Foster, B.W., Robeson, J., Tagata, N., Beckerdite, J.M., Huggins, R.L. and Adams Jr., E.T. (1981) J. Phys. Chem. 85, 3715–3720.
204 Vadnere, M. and Lindenbaum, S. (1982) J. Pharm. Sci. 71, 881–883.
205 Fontell, K. (1972) Kolloid Z. v. Z. Polymere 250, 825–835.
206 Fabre, H., Kamenka, N. and Lindman, B. (1981) J. Phys. Chem. 85, 3493–3501.
207 Small, D.M. and Bourgès, M. (1966) Mol. Cryst. 1, 541–561.
208 Small, D.M., Bourgès, M.C. and Dervichian, D.G. (1966) Biochim. Biophys. Acta 125, 563–580.
209 Shipley, G.G. (1973) in: Biological Membranes (Chapman, D. and Wallach, D.F.H., Eds.), Vol. 2, pp. 1–89, Academic Press, New York.
210 Bourgès, M., Small, D.M. and Dervichian, D.G. (1967) Biochim. Biophys. Acta 144, 189–201.
211 Ulmius, J., Lindblom, G., Wennerstrom, H., Johansson, L.B.-Å., Fontell, K., Söderman, O. and Arvidson, G. (1982) Biochemistry 21, 1553–1560.
212 Pink, D.A., Georgallas, A. and Chapman, D. (1981) Biochemistry 20, 7152–7157.
213 Lindblom, G., Johansson, L.B.-Å. and Arvidson, G. (1981) Biochemistry 20, 2204–2207.
214 Saitô, H., Sugimoto, Y., Tabeta, R., Suzuki, S., Izumi, G., Kodama, M., Toyoshima, S. and Nagata, C. (1983) J. Biochem. (Tokyo) 94, 1877–1887.
215 Madden, T.D. and Cullis, P.R. (1982) Biochim. Biophys. Acta 684, 149–153.
216 Persson, M.-O., Lindblom, G. and Lindman, B. (1974) Chem. Phys. Lipids 12, 261–270.
217 Lindblom, G., Wennerström, H., Arvidson, G. and Lindman, B. (1976) Biophys. J. 16, 1287–1295.
218 Stark, R.E. and Roberts, M.F. (1984) Biochim. Biophys. Acta 770, 115–121.
219 Bangham, J.A. and Lea, E.J.A. (1978) Biochim. Biophys. Acta 511, 388–396.
220 Abramson, J.J. and Shamoo, A.E. (1979) J. Membrane Biol. 50, 241–255.
221 Hunt, G.R.A. and Jawaharlal, K. (1980) Biochim. Biophys. Acta 601, 678–684.
222 Hunt, G.R.A. (1980) FEBS Lett. 119, 132–136.
223 Castellino, F.J. and Violand, B.N. (1979) Arch. Biochem. Biophys. 193, 543–550.
224 Helenius, A. and Simons, K. (1975) Biochim. Biophys. Acta 415, 29–79.
225 Brunner, J., Skrabal, P. and Hauser, H. (1976) Biochim. Biophys. Acta 455, 322–331.
226 Billington, D. and Coleman, R. (1978) Biochim. Biophys. Acta 509, 33–47.
227 Gaginella, T.S., Lewis, J.C. and Phillips, S.F. (1977) Am. J. Dig. Dis. 22, 781–790.
228 Schoenfield, L.J. and Lachin, J.M., the Steering Committee and the National Cooperative Gallstone Study Group (1981) Ann. Intern. Med. 95, 257–282.
229 Mikkelson, R.B. (1976) in: Biological Membranes (Chapman, D. and Wallach, D.F.H., Eds.) pp. 153–190, Academic Press, New York.
230 Kramer, R.M., Hasselbach, H.J. and Semenza, G. (1981) Biochim. Biophys. Acta 643, 233–242.
231 Zimmerer Jr., R.O. and Lindenbaum, S. (1979) J. Pharm. Sci. 68, 581–585.
232 Gähwiller, Ch., von Planta, C., Schmidt, D. and Steffen, H. (1977) Z. Naturforsch. 32c, 748–755.
233 Müller, K. (1981) Biochemistry 20, 404–414.
234 Banerjee, S. and Chatterjee, S.N. (1983) Z. Naturforsch. 38c, 302–306.
235 Eriksson, P.-O., Arvidson, G. and Lindblom, G. (1983) Israel J. Chem. 23, 353–355.
236 Spink, C.H., Müller, K. and Sturtevant, J.M. (1982) Biochemistry 24, 6598–6605.

237 Stark, R.E., Manstein, J.L., Curatolo, W. and Sears, B. (1983) Biochemistry 22, 2486–2490.
238 Narayanan, R., Paul, R. and Balaram, P. (1980) Biochim. Biophys. Acta 597, 70–82.
239 Mazer, N.A. and Carey, M.C. (1983) Biochemistry 22, 426–442.
240 Montet, J.-C., Merienne, C. and Bram, C. (1982) Tetrahedron 38, 1159–1162.
241 Leibfritz, D. and Roberts, J.D. (1973) J. Am. Chem. Soc. 95, 4996–5003.
242 Fung, B.M. and Thomas Jr., L. (1979) Chem. Phys. Lipids 25, 141–148.
243 Mukerjee, P. (1978) Ber. Bunsengas Phys. Chem. 82, 931–937.
244 Mukerjee, P. (1980) Pure Applied Chem. 52, 1317–1321.
245 Fung, B.M. and Peden, M.C. (1976) Biochim. Biophys. Acta 437, 273–279.
246 Christian, S.D., Smith, L.S., Bushong, D.S. and Tucker, E.E. (1982) J. Colloid Interface Sci. 89, 514–522.
247 Thomas, D.C. and Christian, S.D. (1981) J. Colloid Interface Sci. 82, 430–438.
248 Spink, C.H. and Colgan, S. (1984) J. Colloid Interface Sci. 97, 41–47.
249 Yedgar, S. and Gatt, S. (1980) Biochem. J. 185, 749–754.
250 Montet, J.-C., Lindheimer, M., Reynier, M.-O., Crotte, C., Bontemps, R. and Gerolami, A. (1982) Biochimie (Paris) 64, 255–261.
251 Schurtenberger, P., Mazer, N.A., Känig, W. and Preisig, R. (1984) in: Proc. Int. Symp. on Surfactants in Solution (Mittal, K.L. and Lindman, B., Eds.) Vol. 2, pp. 841–855, Plenum Press, New York.
252 Claffey, W.J. and Holzbach, R.T. (1981) Biochemistry 20, 415–418.
253 Higuchi, W.I., Su, C.C., Park, J.Y., Alkan, M.H. and Gulari, E. (1981) J. Phys. Chem. 85, 127–129.
254 Higuchi, W.I. (1985) Hepatology 4, 161S–165S.
255 Lake, M. and Organisciak, D.T. (1984) Lipids 19, 553–557.
256 Barry, B.W. and Gray, G.M.T. (1975) J. Colloid Interface Sci. 52, 314–326.
257 Barry, B.W. and Gray, G.M.T. (1975) J. Colloid Interface Sci. 52, 327–339.
258 Kellaway, I.W. and Marriott, C. (1977) Can. J. Pharm. Sci. 12, 70–73.
259 Kellaway, I.W. and Marriott, C. (1977) Can. J. Pharm. Sci. 12, 74–76.
260 Mazer, N.A., Schurtenberger, P., Carey, M.C., Preisig, R., Weigand, K. and Känzig, W. (1984) Biochemistry 23, 1994–2005.
261 Sömjen, G.J. and Gilat, T. (1983) FEBS Lett. 156, 265–268.
262 Carey, M.C., Small, D.M. and Bliss, C.M. (1983) Annu. Rev. Physiol. 45, 651–677.
263 Carey, M.C. (1984) in: Liver and Lipid Metabolism (Calandra, S., Carulli, N. and Salvioli, G., Eds.) pp. 145–161, Elsevier, Amsterdam.

H. Danielsson and J. Sjövall (Eds.), *Sterols and Bile Acids*

CHAPTER 14

Roles of bile acids in intestinal lipid digestion and absorption

B. BORGSTRÖM, J.A. BARROWMAN and M. LINDSTRÖM

Department of Physiological Chemistry, University of Lund, Lund (Sweden)

(I) Introduction

(1) Historical remarks

Bile has long been attributed an important role in medicine [1]. The effect of an impaired bile flow to the intestine has been known to result in steatorrhea — fat malabsorption — and defective absorption of fat-soluble vitamins, notably vitamin K [2]. Thus, it is obvious that bile is important for fat assimilation from the intestine. However, it is equally apparent that when fat absorption after bile obstruction or diversion could be studied by quantitative methods, the malabsorption was found to be only partial [3]. In fact, it has seemed surprising that some 60–70% of a normal fat load is absorbed in man and the experimental animal in the absence of bile in the intestine. The absorption of nonpolar lipids, however, is much less efficient, and cholesterol absorption has been reported to have an absolute requirement for the presence of bile salts [4]. Of the bile components important for fat absorption bile salts have been ascribed the main role although experimental results are accumulating regarding the role of bile phospholipids in the specific uptake of sterols by the intestine [5].

(2) Brief outline of intestinal lipid digestion and absorption

The bulk of dietary fat consists of long-chain triglycerides with minor amounts of other lipids of varying polarity from the more polar phospholipids and sterols to highly nonpolar compounds. This latter group includes biologically important compounds such as the fat-soluble vitamins, sterol esters, biota of various sources and industrial pollutants including toxic, procarcinogenic and carcinogenic compounds. From a physical point of view dietary fat is an emulsion of oil in water, stabilized with phospholipids and other amphiphilic compounds such as protein at the aqueous/lipid interface. The nonpolar lipids stay in the interior of the fat droplets mainly made up of triglyceride fat. In a phospholipid-stabilized fat emulsion only some 3% of the interfacial molecules are made up by triglycerides [6].

The relative content of the dietary fat components varies with different sources but generally the physico-chemical properties are rather similar. For absorption to take place the physico-chemical properties of the fat have to be changed. This takes place as a consequence of the lipolytic activity in the intestinal tract and the addition of bile to chyme. Through lipolytic enzymes the dietary lipids are converted to more polar products. Bile contributes bile salt–phospholipid–cholesterol aggregates to the intestinal content (cf. Chapter 13). The concerted action of these agents is the formation of lipid products in a physical state which allows them to be transported into the enterocyte membrane and onwards for further metabolism in the cell. Bile salts are involved in the proper function of some of these enzymatic reactions and in the formation of product phases on which a normal uptake process is based. Little is known at present of the importance of bile salts for the intracellular reactions following uptake of fat into the enterocyte. Different aspects of intestinal lipid absorption have been reviewed in recent years by Patton [7], Thomson and Dietschy [8], Carey [9], Carey et al. [10], Wells and Direnzo [11], and Grundy [12]. The role of bile acids in fat absorption has been discussed by Holt [13].

(II) Roles of bile salts in the intestinal lumen

Most higher animals have a gallbladder in which the bile secreted from the liver is stored when the gastrointestinal tract is at rest, i.e. in between meals. Among laboratory species, only the rat lacks a gallbladder. The bile is concentrated in the gallbladder some 10 times and at rest the gallbladder contains the major part of the bile salt pool. When food is ingested the gallbladder starts to empty as a consequence of hormonal [14] and nervous mechanisms [15]. The gallbladder bile comes into circulation and undergoes enterohepatic circulation [9] as long as digestion continues. Due to these effects, intestinal bile salt concentration usually shows a peak value during the first 0.5 h after intake of a meal followed by a rather steady concentration at a lower level indicating secretion into the intestine of the more dilute liver bile. The postprandial bile salt concentration in man is in the order of 5–15 mM [16]. Similar figures have also been measured in the rat [17].

(1) What is the physical state of the lipids in the intestinal contents?

Bile is a mixed micellar solution of bile salt–lecithin–cholesterol which on dilution forms aggregates of much larger size than micelles indicating the formation at the phase limits of liposome-like bodies [9]. In intestinal content during lipid digestion in man, saturated mixed micelles and vesicles or liposomes containing the same product lipids coexist [18]. The concentration of monomeric bile salts in intestinal content is probably low and no simple bile salt micelles may exist [19]. These factors and the fact that bile salts are actively absorbed distally provide for the maintenance of a rather constant bile salt concentration in the upper small intestine during digestion with a concentration of monomeric bile salt below that of the critical micellar concentration in a pure bile salt solution.

(2) Bile salts are bad emulsifiers!

Emulsification is generally thought to be important for lipolysis since it increases the surface area to volume ratio and thus increases the rate of lipolysis catalyzed by pancreatic lipase [20]. Emulsification is achieved by mechanical energy in the form of shearing forces breaking up the oil phase into droplets. Amphiphiles decrease the surface tension and thereby decrease the energy needed for emulsification and also stabilize the emulsion formed by preventing coalescence. Dietary fat is triglyceride oil stabilized by phospholipids, proteins and added surfactants with a varying degree of emulsification depending on source and handling before intake. The shear forces occurring in the gastrointestinal tract by churning in the stomach and small intestine are considered to be low [21].

Bile salts have been shown to be bad emulsifiers at any concentration and the resulting emulsions are quite unstable [22]. They are less efficient than phospholipids and sodium oleate and this is probably related to the unique planar structure of the bile salt molecule. Bile salts induce an equilibrium surface pressure in monolayer that is 26 dynes/cm. This is low compared to most aliphatic detergents. For sodium dodecyl sulfate it is 40 dynes/cm and for phosphatidylcholine 45 dynes/cm (B. Borgström, unpublished). Bile salts above the critical micellar concentration reduce the surfactant properties of other amphiphiles by displacing them from the interface forming mixed micelles. Bile salts also compete favorably with other detergents for the interface by forming mixed detergent micelles [23] decreasing the monomer concentration of the detergent (cf. Chapter 13). The importance thereof may be to make the substrate interface available for the lipase–colipase system in the intestinal contents [24]. The price to be paid for this destabilization, a reduced interfacial area, is normally well compensated for by a high enzyme concentration. Bile salts thus have very special detergent properties of importance for their function in the intestinal lumen.

(3) What is the importance of bile salts for the function of the lipolytic enzymes?

Four different lipolytic enzymes and one coenzyme have been recognized that are secreted into the gastrointestinal lumen during digestion. The lingual lipase, also named pharyngeal lipase, is secreted from glands at the base of the tongue and catalyzes preferentially the conversion of triglyceride to diglyceride. It seems to function mainly in the stomach content. Its activity is not stimulated by bile salts in vitro, an inhibition being seen in the concentration range 2.5–7.5 mM with less inhibition as the bile salt concentration increases. The enzyme is probably important for a limited lipolysis prior to subsequent pancreatic lipolysis. Its relative importance may increase in pancreatic lipase deficiency. It is not known if it is active in the intestinal lumen [25].

The classical pancreatic lipase has been called the bile-salt-independent lipase indicating that it does not need bile salt for its function in contrast to the bile-salt-dependent lipase of pancreatic juice (carboxyl ester lipase, see below). In fact, pancreatic lipase is fully catalytically active in the absence of bile salts, though product formation is affected by the presence of bile salts. Furthermore, pancreatic lipase is completely inhibited by bile salts above their critical micellar concentration. The physiological substrate for lipase, a triglyceride emulsion covered at the oil/aqueous interface by amphiphilic proteins and lipids, is not available to lipase. An important function for bile salts is to clear the interface of the lipid droplets of these substances. This can be regarded as a competition for the interface [24]. The surface layer of bile salts has a surface pressure in the range of 26 dynes/cm which is higher than that of most proteins including lipase. A coenzyme for lipase, colipase, which is also secreted in the pancreatic juice, enables lipase to reach its substrate interface in the presence of bile salt. The mechanism of function of colipase in this process is not fully clarified. One hypothesis is that lipase and colipase form a complex in which the conformation of lipase has been changed so as to allow the penetration to the substrate interface in the presence of bile salts [26]. Bile salts have been shown to bind to colipase in a cooperative manner at the critical micellar concentration. Whether this binding is important for colipase function is not known; results indicate that the simultaneous presence of amphiphiles such as phospholipids prevents such binding [19].

The bile-salt-dependent lipase of pancreatic juice has many names such as cholesterol esterase, nonspecific lipase, the most rational being carboxyl ester lipase [27]. In the case of water-insoluble substrates this enzyme has an absolute requirement for bile salts specifically having hydroxyl groups in the 3α and 7α positions [28,29]. The best documented role for this enzyme is to allow the absorption of dietary cholesterol, through hydrolysis of cholesterol esters in the lumen. The enzyme also catalyzes the esterification of cholesterol and a role for it has been proposed in cholesterol absorption [30]. In addition, a wide range of primary and secondary fatty acyl esters including glycerides, vitamin A and E esters are hydrolyzed by this enzyme.

The enzyme aggregates in the presence of physiological concentrations of bile salt; in the presence of α-trihydroxy bile salts the rat enzyme forms hexamers [31,32] and with dihydroxy bile salts more complex aggregates are formed [32]. Cholate induces dimerization of the porcine [33] and human enzyme [29].

It has been suggested that carboxyl ester lipase has two different bile-salt-binding sites [34–36], one nonspecific for the bile salt structure and one specific for primary bile salts causing the di(poly)merization. An interesting question is whether the bile salts regulate substrate specificity not only by bile salt–enzyme interactions but also by forming the appropriate substrate surface structure [27].

The physiological substrate for carboxyl ester lipase thus may be a wide variety of esters occurring in the diet and it has been suggested that lipolysis is a 2-stage process. In the first stage, the classical lipase generates a product phase that, in the presence of bile salts, forms a substrate for carboxyl ester lipase [27]. Human milk, like that of some other primates has been shown to contain an enzyme functionally and immunologically indistinguishable from pancreatic carboxyl ester lipase [37]. This milk enzyme, which is dependent on bile salts, has been ascribed an important function in intestinal lipolysis in the newborn [38,39].

Phospholipase A_2 is another enzyme of pancreatic juice that has no absolute requirement for bile salt. It is catalytically active against short-chain phospholipids in the absence of bile salt but with long-chain phospholipids bile salts are necessary. It seems that as for carboxyl ester lipase, bile salts are necessary for the proper configuration of the substrate and that in the case of pancreatic phospholipase A_2, mixed bile salt (BS)/phospholipid micelles are the proper substrate [40]. No hydrolysis of phosphatidylcholine (PC) is seen at a BS/PC ratio lower than 1 : 1 and higher than 5 : 1 [41]. If PC-stabilized triglyceride emulsions are mixed with a bile salt micellar solution the PC is desorbed to mixed micelles which are the substrate for the enzyme. Phospholipase A_2 has also been shown to partition to the micellar phase in such complex systems [42]. Although most probably both biliary and dietary phospholipids are hydrolyzed in intestinal contents to lysophospholipid it is not clear how this rate is regulated by the BS/PC ratio. At the BS/PC ratio occurring in bile, PC is a bad substrate for phospholipase A_2 Dilution of bile in intestinal content and addition of dietary PC would be expected to lower the ratio and consequently change the availability of the substrate for phospholipase A_2. The formation of product, i.e. lysophospholipids, may affect the organization of the structure of the phospholipid aggregates and make them available for the enzyme [43]. As a whole, the hydrolysis of phospholipids of either biliary or dietary origin in the intestinal tract is not well documented.

(4) What is the composition of the luminal contents after a fat meal?

Stomach content has been known for a long time to contain appreciable quantities of free fatty acid now known to be the result of the activity of lingual lipase [25]. Due to the acid pH these acids are present mostly in the oil phase of the dietary fat as non-ionized fatty acids [44]. The dietary fat, partly hydrolyzed, reaches the duodenal content where it is mixed with bile and pancreatic juice. Analysis of duodenal contents has shown the presence of varying quantities of fat split products with a rather high content of free fatty acid [45]. With the high levels of lipolytic enzymes and the time factor necessary to collect contents it is difficult to say how representative the samples are for the actual composition. Of more interest are the physical forms of the lipids present. Hofmann and Borgström [45] centrifuged human intestinal contents and isolated an oil phase and a micellar phase, the latter representing lipolytic products of triglycerides, mainly monoglyceride and fatty acid in mixed bile salt micellar solution. Further work has shown the presence of other lipid phases [46]. The elegant work of Patton and Carey [47] has defined two more product phases during lipolysis in vitro, a crystalline phase containing calcium and ionized fatty acid and a "viscous isotropic phase" composed predominantly of monoglycerides and fatty acids. Monoglycerides and fatty acids in combination with bile salts and/or triglycerides can, depending on the relative proportions, also form reverse hexagonal, lamellar as well as L_2-phases (an inverse micellar phase); all of which can be expected to obtain in intestinal contents in addition to the oil and micellar phases. Intestinal lipolysis is a dynamic process, the concentration and composition of its products depending on several factors such as rate of formation, rate of uptake by the enterocyte, and the total concentration of fat and of bile salts. With the relatively low bile salt concentration ($\simeq$ 5–10 mM) of intestinal content, formation of liquid crystalline and/or inverse phases can temporarily be expected in addition to the mixed micellar and oil phases. The occurrence and importance of such phases for fat uptake are not well documented. They may represent a transition from one phase to the other without importance per se for the uptake.

In the lumen of the small intestine, dietary fat does not only meet bile salt but the much more complex bile in which bile salts are about half saturated with lecithin in a mixed micellar system of bile salt–lecithin–cholesterol. On dilution in the intestinal content, the micelles grow in size as the phase limit is approached and large disk-like micelles form which fold into vesicles [49]. These changes are due to the phase transition that occurs when the bile salt concentration is decreased and the solubility limit for lecithin in the mixed micelles is exceeded. The information is mostly derived from in vitro studies with model systems but most probably is applicable to the in vivo situation. What in fact takes place when the bile-derived lamellar bile salt–lecithin–cholesterol system meets the partly digested dietary fat can only be pictured. Most probably it involves an exchange of surface components, a continuous lipolysis at the interphase by pancreatic enzymes and the formation of amphiphilic products which go into different lamellar systems for further uptake by the enterocyte. Due to the relatively low bile salt concentration and the potentially high concentration of product phases in intestinal content early in fat digestion, the micellar and monomeric concentration of bile salt can be expected to be low but to increase towards the end of absorption.

The importance of bile salts therefore may not so much be to solubilize the lipolytic products into micelles as to break them up in lamellar systems which can interact with the aqueous phase.

(III) Roles of bile salts in transport of lipolytic products from lumen to cytosol through mucosal diffusion barriers and plasma membrane

(1) Methods employed in the study of lipid absorption

To study intestinal absorption of lipids, several different experimental models have been used. They include systems of varying degree of complexity ranging from brush border vesicles to human beings fed a test meal. The process of transport of lipids from the luminal contents to the mesenteric lymph includes several independent steps, and the established experimental models are designed to study one or several of these steps.

The isolated brush border vesicles from the plasma membrane of the microvilli is the simplest in vitro system used so far. The interaction of lipid with rabbit intestinal brush border vesicles has been investigated by Proulx et al. [50] who found that PC, phosphatidylethanolamine, cholesterol, diglyceride as well as fatty acids were taken up by vesicles. Barsukov et al. [51] have shown that transfer of PC from PC vesicles to isolated brush border vesicles can occur in the presence of PC-exchange protein. The use of brush border vesicles is an interesting new approach that permits detailed studies of rate of transfer of specific lipids into the plasma membrane of the enterocyte. The model is seriously limited by the fact that incubation with solutions containing bile salts at a concentration above the critical micellar concentration will result in partial or total solubilization of the membrane vesicles.

The enterocytes of the small intestine can be isolated and used for study of intracellular aspects of intestinal lipid transport like triglyceride synthesis [52]. The disappearance of the mucus barrier during isolation of the epithelial cells results in plasma membrane disintegration and loss of cellular integrity when the cells are exposed to bile salts. As is the case for brush border vesicles, the system of isolated cells does not allow study of interaction between enterocytes and lipids dispersed in a form that resembles physiological conditions, i.e. solubilized in mixed bile salt micelles.

The most commonly employed in vitro technique for study of lipid uptake into the cell is the use of segments of small intestine in the form of biopsies, disks, slices or everted sacs. Thomson and O'Brien [53] found that although the rate of lipid uptake was not the same for different types of in vitro preparations, they all gave similar results as far as the qualitative role of bile salts for lipid uptake was concerned.

The lack of blood supply restricts the use of in vitro preparations to short-time incubation studies only. Long-time experiments which allow determination of lipid absorption under steady-state conditions can be performed by perfusion of an intestinal segment in situ or by infusion of lipids into the duodenum of a rat with a lymph fistula. A comparison of in vitro and in vivo techniques has been made by Clark [54].

Collection of duodenal contents through a duodenal tube after feeding a test meal containing a non-absorbable marker is a commonly used technique for studies of lipid digestion and absorption in man [55]. Using a multilumen tube, Simmonds et al. [56] were able to study in detail in man the absorption kinetics of cholesterol from a micellar solution.

(2) Which are the barriers for lipid transport from lumen to cytosol?

The lipid solutes in the bulk phase of the intestinal contents are considered to form a relatively homogeneous dispersion of lipids in the aqueous phase. However, the concentration of a solute in the bulk phase does not necessarily have to be the same as in the aqueous environment adjacent to the plasma membrane of the enterocytes. This concentration gradient is a result of the unstirred water layer which is a diffusion barrier between the luminal contents and the brush border membrane. The unstirred water layer consists of an infinite number of water lamellae arranged in parallel with the enterocyte membrane. The closer the water lamellae are situated to the enterocyte membrane, the lower the relative rate of stirring will be. Since the relative rate of stirring of the lamellae increases in direction towards the lumen, it is impossible to define an exact limit of the unstirred water layer. The functional thickness of the unstirred water layer can be measured [57] and can be used as a relative indicator of the depth of the luminal phase through which molecules and aggregates can travel by passive diffusion only [58,59].

The thickness of the unstirred water layer of rabbit intestine in vitro has been found to vary between 115 and 334 μm depending on the rate of stirring of the bulk phase [58]. The thickness of the unstirred water layer of the rat small intestine in vivo has been reported to be even greater [60]. If the effective thickness of the unstirred water layer can reach values of around 500 μm, then it is evident that it is a far from negligible compartment of the total luminal volume at least in the case of the rat.

It has recently been discussed [61–63] whether the diffusional barrier at the intestinal surface can be accounted for solely by an unstirred water layer. It has been proposed that the mucus layer overlying the enterocytes should be regarded as an important diffusion barrier for uptake of lipid solutes from the luminal contents. The mucus adherent to the rat duodenal wall has been found to be approximately 80 μm thick in the fasted state [64]. The intestinal mucus coat is formed by proteoglycans produced by goblet cells, but so far very little is known about the molecular structure of the mucus layer [65]. The possible interaction between mucus constituents and luminal lipid solutes needs to be investigated in detail, since it might reveal key factors which constitute the diffusional barrier of the small intestine.

One should also consider the glycocalyx, a carbohydrate-containing polymer network between the microvilli and the mucus gel coat. It probably consists mainly of oligosaccharide chains that are covalently linked to the lipids and proteins of the brush border membrane. The definite structure of the glycocalyx is not yet available, and nothing can be said about its possible importance as an absorption barrier.

The plasma membrane of the brush border microvilli is characterized by certain distinctive structural features, which may be related to the specialized functional properties that distinguish it from plasma membranes of other cells. The width of the microvillus membrane (measured by electron microscopy) is 10–11 nm, whereas the average eukaryotic plasma membrane is only 7–9 nm. This is probably due to the biochemical composition of the membrane, which is characterized by a high protein to lipid ratio (1.7 : 1) and a unique lipid composition. The cholesterol–phospholipid ratio and the molar ratio of glycolipid to phospholipid are both about 1 : 1, which is consistent with the low values for membrane fluidity determined in microvillus membranes. This should be compared with the corresponding ratios found in the plasma membrane of other cells including the basolateral portion of the enterocyte membrane which are less than 0.5 : 1 [66]. The permeability characteristics of the microvillus membrane have been studied by determination of the change in the permeability coefficient when a specific substituent group is added to the lipid probe molecule. The general conclusion was that the plasma membrane of the brush border microvilli is a structure of relatively high polarity [58].

The concept of an unstirred water layer is relevant to the process of intracellular lipid solute transport as well. The cytosol adjacent to the inside of the brush border plasma membrane comprises an unstirred water layer extending into the intracellular compartment. The dimensions are not known but this diffusional barrier has also to be accounted for when considering the rate-limiting step for transport of lipids. However, lipid transfer through the aqueous phase might be affected by a factor that is present in the cytosol but not on the luminal side of the microvillus membrane. Ockner and Manning [67] have isolated and characterized a water-soluble protein in the cytosol of small intestinal mucosa, which binds long-chain fatty acids. It has been proposed that this fatty-acid-binding protein participates in transport of fatty acids from plasma membrane to endoplasmic reticulum during fat absorption.

In summary, a lipid molecule on its route from the luminal bulk phase into the intracellular compartment of an enterocyte has to overcome two unstirred water layers and one plasma membrane of lipid bilayer structure. The unstirred water layer on the luminal side partly coincides with the mucus gel and the glycocalyx; relatively little is known of the importance of these diffusional barriers.

(3) What factors determine the rate of transport across the intestinal diffusion barriers?

The uptake of lipids across the brush border plasma membrane into the enterocyte is considered to be a transport process that requires no energy [8]. The route of transfer of lipids thus has to take place via a process of passive diffusion. A theoretical model for passive lipid solute transfer that takes into account the different factors that affect the rate of transport has been worked out by Dietschy and collaborators [8,68] (cf. Chapter 5).

Passive transport can take place only in the direction of an existing concentration gradient. This is the case for lipolytic products which form a gradient across the brush border membrane with a high concentration in the luminal contents during the digestion of a fat-containing meal and a relatively low concentration in the cytosol of the enterocytes.

The factors that are mainly responsible for the relative rate of uptake of a particular lipid are the resistance of the luminal unstirred water layer and the permeability of the plasma membrane of the enterocyte. Depending on the properties of a specific lipid, the relative importance of these two factors can be predicted. If a lipid is rapidly transported across the luminal unstirred water layer, i.e. it has a relatively high aqueous diffusion constant, then the permeability of the membrane will be the key factor determining the rate of transport into the cytosol. The concentration gradient will be high across the lipid membrane, whereas the con-

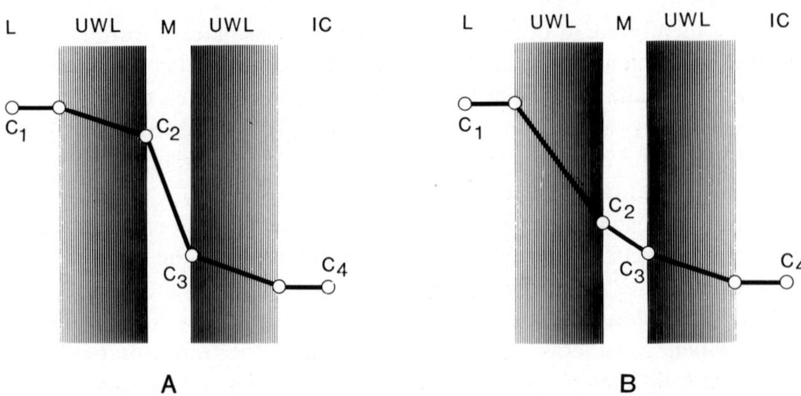

Fig. 1. Profile of the concentration gradient (C_1–C_4) from the luminal bulk phase (L) across the brush border plasma membrane (M) to the intracellular compartment (IC) of the enterocyte. Adjacent to the membrane, on both the luminal and the intracellular side there is an unstirred water layer (UWL). It should be noted that this diagram does not attempt to present the relative dimensions of the two unstirred water layers and the plasma membrane. The concentration gradient will have a different appearance in the case of a lipid towards which the membrane permeability is low (panel A) compared to the case where the resistance of the unstirred water layer against diffusion of the lipid is high while the lipid readily transverses the plasma membrane (panel B). After Thomson and Dietschy [8].

centration of the lipid solute adjacent to the membrane will approach the luminal bulk concentration as is shown in Fig. 1A.

On the other hand, if diffusion from luminal bulk phase to the surface of the membrane is slow and the membrane permeability towards the lipid solute is relatively high, then the resistance of the unstirred water layer will represent the factor that is rate limiting for uptake into the cytosol. As a consequence the concentration gradient will be large across the luminal unstirred water layer while the gradient across the membrane will be shallow as depicted in Fig. 1B.

The relative importance of the diffusion barriers for different lipids has been studied by Westergaard and Dietschy [58] by comparing the uptake of fatty acids of different chain lengths. They found that passage through the unstirred water layer was the rate-limiting step for long-chain fatty acids. Uptake of short-chain and medium-chain fatty acids with relatively high diffusion coefficients compared to those of long-chain species was restricted by transport across the plasma membrane, since permeability of the membrane towards these fatty acids is relatively lower.

(4) What is the role of micellar solubilization for intestinal lipid absorption?

The work of Hofmann and Borgström [45] showed that lipids in luminal contents during digestion of a fatty meal could be separated into an oil phase and an aqueous micellar phase. It became evident that micellar solubilization of lipolytic products is a significant process, and its possible effect on transport of lipids across the brush border membrane has been an area of intense research since.

TABLE 1

The efficiency of lipid transport of micellar compared to monomer solutions [69]

	Concentration (C) (mM)	Diffusion coefficient (D) (cm^2/sec)	$C \times D$ (μmoles/cm/sec)
Fatty acid in monomer solution	$1 \cdot 10^{-5}$	$8 \cdot 10^{-6}$	$8 \cdot 10^{-11}$
Fatty acid in micellar solution	$1 \cdot 10^{-2}$	$1.2 \cdot 10^{-6}$	$1200 \cdot 10^{-11}$

The diffusion constant for a fatty acid monomer in aqueous solution is much greater than the corresponding value for a mixed bile salt micelle containing fatty acids. The monomer concentration of a fatty acid is on the other hand so low that the large capacity of a mixed micelle for fatty acid solubilization compensates for the smaller diffusion coefficient and makes the micellar aggregate an important vehicle for diffusion of fatty acids through the unstirred water layer. A quantitative estimate of the effect of micellar solubilization on transport of long-chain fatty acids has been made by Hofmann [69] who calculated that the product of concentration gradient and aqueous diffusion coefficient was approximately 150 times higher for micellar aggregates compared to a monomer solution (Table 1).

A detailed investigation of the effect of micellar solubilization on the transport of lipids has been made by Westergaard and Dietschy [59]. They studied in vitro uptake of lipids into rabbit intestinal disks by varying the proportions of lipid and bile salts in mixed micelles in 3 different ways. Either lipid concentration was increased with bile salts kept at a constant level, lipid concentration was unchanged while bile salt concentration was varied, or both lipid and bile salt concentration was increased with the molar ratio kept constant. Theoretical calculations of how the mass of the lipid probe was distributed between the aqueous and the micellar compartment showed that there was a good correlation between calculated aqueous monomer concentration and experimentally obtained values for lipid uptake. The rate of uptake is thus proportional to the aqueous monomer concentration of a particular lipid. The conclusion drawn was that diffusion of the lipid molecules in monomeric form through the aqueous phase is an obligatory step before uptake into the plasma membrane, and that the role of bile salt is therefore to overcome the resistance of the unstirred water layer by micellar solubilization.

By comparing the relative rate of uptake of two different lipid probe molecules, another piece of evidence for a monomeric mechanism in lipid uptake by membranes has been found. Hoffman [70] and Hoffman and Yeoh [71] have determined the relationship between micellar concentration and uptake by rat small intestine in vitro for oleic acid and a monoglyceride analog, a 1-monoether. They found that the rate of uptake for both of the two micellar solutes was linearly dependent on the micellar concentration, but that the ratio of rate of uptake was different from the molar ratio of the two lipids in the micellar phase. Oleic acid was absorbed more rapidly than the monoether, probably due to a higher monomer concentration in the aqueous phase. This suggests that single molecules rather than intact micelles are taken up by the membrane. However, experiments by Hoffman et al. [72] performed in vivo with lymph fistula rats showed no difference in absorption of oleic acid and monoether from a micellar solution infused intraduodenally. Only when they were given as an emulsion in the absence of a micellar phase were the rates of uptake of the two lipids different. Thus, it is important to bear in mind that rate-controlling factors in uptake may be different in vivo and in vitro.

Different small intestinal sites of absorption for different micellar constituents have also been an argument for uptake of monomers instead of micelles. Whereas the major part of the lipolytic products are absorbed in the proximal part of jejunum, the site of bile salt uptake has been said to be the distal ileum. Recent investigations of the quantitative role of different parts of the small intestine for bile salt absorption suggest that the role of the distal ileum has been overestimated. Sklan et al. [73] found that about 50% of bile salts of endogenous origin were absorbed in the proximal half of the rat small intestine in vivo. A similar investigation was performed by McClintock and Shiau [74], who injected a bolus dose of bile salts into the jejunum of rats with a bile fistula. They found that 60% of taurocholate was absorbed before the bolus reached distal ileum.

A direct effect of luminal lipids on the absorption of bile salts has been found by Sklan and Budowski [75]. Taurocholate uptake was determined in situ in segments of rat small intestine, and jejunal absorption increased when taurocholate was injected together with oleic acid, monoolein, PC or lyso-PC. For each lipid a certain molar ratio of lipid to bile salt was found that resulted in an optimal uptake of taurocholate. In contrast, the active uptake of bile salts by isolated intestinal villi preparations of hamster distal ileum has been found to be inhibited by dietary lipids [76].

These data were interpreted as indicating (a) that in the rat the proximal small intestine has a dominating role in the quantitative uptake of bile salts, and (b) that the lipid constituents of the mixed bile salt micelles affect the rate of uptake of bile salts. The possibility of lipid uptake through direct contact between micellar aggregates and the plasma membrane coexisting with monomeric uptake thus cannot be completely ruled out. Despite the data regarding bile salt absorption referred to above, the bulk of experimental evidence suggests that in most species including man [77] the major absorptive site of bile salts is in the distal ileum. The relative contribution of each part of the small intestine in bile salt absorption is dependent on several factors, such as prevailing intraluminal pH, dissociation constants of the various bile salts — conjugated and unconjugated — concentration of lipids, transit time, etc. [9].

(5) Absorption of lipids from non-micellar phases

Up till now intestinal lipid absorption from mixed micellar solutions has been studied in detail. The existence of non-micellar dispersions of lipolytic products in intestinal contents during fat digestion has recently been proposed [18,47], but so far only little information regarding the importance of these phases for the lipid absorption process is available. Other than in monomolecular or micellar form, lipids can exist either in an emulsified oil phase, or in a thermodynamically stable dispersion of non-micellar lipid aggregates. The aggregates are likely to be formed in the presence of bile salts when the amount of lipids is too large to allow complete micellar solubilization.

It is well established that uptake of oleic acid from an emulsion is significantly reduced compared to uptake from a micellar solution. This has been shown in vitro with everted sacs of rat jejunum [78] as well as in vivo with lymph fistula rats [72].

Data on absorption of non-micellar lipids in the presence of bile salts is available from the study by Knoebel [79]. The lymphatic transport of absorbed oleic acid and site of uptake from the intestinal lumen was measured in bile fistula rats. It was found that the concentration of bile salts in a continuous intraduodenal infusion did not affect the steady-state level of lipid appearing in the lymph until the bile salt concentration was as low as 1 mM, which represented a molar ratio of 20 : 1 of lipid to bile salt. In the case of infusates with relatively low concentrations of bile salts it was found that a larger part of the available surface area of the small intestine was utilized. The main conclusion is that lipids are equally well absorbed in vivo from non-micellar dispersions of lipids and bile salts as from solutions where the lipids are completely solubilized by bile salt mixed micelles. However, a detailed analysis of kinetics of uptake from non-micellar phases in vitro with isolated intestinal segments has not yet been done.

(IV) Roles of bile salts in intracellular events in lipid absorption

Passive absorption of bile salts in the upper small intestine, a component of their enterohepatic circulation, results in a flux of bile salt through the enterocyte, particularly during digestion and absorption. Do these bile salts have an influence on metabolic activity in the cell with respect to absorbed lipids? It was first proposed by Dawson and Isselbacher in 1960 [80] that bile salts stimulate the re-esterification of fatty acids in the intestinal mucosa. This is a subject of some controversy still.

There is no doubt that in the absence of luminal bile salts there is diminished transport of long-chain fatty acids in intestinal lymph and there is evidence that a greater proportion of absorbed long-chain fatty acid is transported in portal venous blood [81,82]. Such observations have been interpreted to show diminished fatty acid esterification by the enterocyte. A similar re-routing of absorbed vitamin A in the bile-diverted animal from the lymphatic to the portal venous route has also been ascribed to defective esterification [83].

Many studies report decreased mucosal levels of di- and triglycerides with increased concentrations of unesterified fatty acids in bile salt deficiency [8]. One possible explanation for this could be diminished monoglyceride solubilization and absorption and a consequent reduction in available monoglyceride for esterification. However, a reduced esterifying capacity is also possible. This could be the result of lack of activation of pre-existing enzymes in the mucosa by bile salts or a lack of stimulation of synthesis of these enzymes by bile salts. There is some evidence for the latter. In rats, bile diversion produces a significant reduction in lipid re-esterifying capacity (acyl-CoA synthetase, acyl-CoA: monoglyceride acyl transferase and diglyceride: acyl transferase) in the jejunal mucosa [84,85]. The concentrations of re-esterifying enzymes in the mucosa of bile-diverted rats can be restored by duodenal infusion of physiological concentrations of sodium taurocholate, suggesting a role for intracellular bile salts in maintaining normal levels of lipid re-esterifying enzymes [84]. On the other hand, enterocytes from rats after 1 day's biliary diversion show diminished synthesis of phosphatidylcholine and protein, attributed to a lack of choline normally derived from biliary phospholipid, but no change in the capacity to synthesize triglycerides [86].

Enzymic processes in the enterocyte which handle a number of lipid species other than triglycerides are also known to be influenced by bile salts. For example, it has been postulated that pancreatic cholesterol esterase is absorbed by the mucosal cells and catalyzes the esterification of cholesterol in the cell [87]. This postulate has been challenged by Watt and Simmonds [88] although Bhat and Brockman [30] recently produced evidence for the importance of pancreatic cholesterol esterase for transport across the enterocyte membrane. Another enzyme, acyl-CoA : cholesterol acyltransferase (ACAT) of microsomal origin, has been ascribed a major role in mucosal esterification of cholesterol [89]. Unlike pancreatic cholesterol esterase, this enzyme is inhibited by taurocholate in vitro.

The provitamin A, β-carotene, is cleaved in the enterocyte by a soluble oxygenase which requires bile salts for its activity [90]. The product, retinal, is reduced by another soluble enzyme to retinol which is esterified chiefly with palmitic acid by a microsomal enzyme, acyl-CoA: retinol acyltransferase which is inhibited by taurocholate in vitro; this enzyme is very similar to ACAT [91]. Since β-carotene is taken up by the intestine and rather efficiently converted to retinyl esters which appear in lymph, it must be inferred that the cytosolic oxygenase is exposed to sufficiently high concentrations of bile salts for the cleavage to occur.

Tocopheryl acetate is hydrolyzed in the mucosa by an esterase associated with the endoplasmic reticulum [92]. This enzymic activity is enhanced by taurocholate; the concentrations required for this effect, however, are similar to or greater than those in the intestinal lumen and would not be encountered in the enterocyte.

These examples illustrate interactions of bile salts with cellular lipid-metabolizing enzymes which have been demonstrated in vitro. However, without information regarding the concentrations of bile salts in the cellular compartments where the reactions are occurring, the physiological role of intracellular bile salts in the handling of these various lipids cannot be determined. It is likely that bile salts exist largely within the cell in protein-bound form or associated with membranes. In these situations, local concentrations might be achieved sufficient to affect enzymic activities. At present, the role of bile salts in lipid metabolism in the enterocyte is far from clear.

(V) Roles of bile salts in the absorption of specific lipid classes

(1) Triglycerides

As already discussed, long-chain triglyceride fat is absorbed to some 60–70% in the absence of bile in the intestine. The role of bile salts in long-chain absorption of triglycerides is to provide for the formation of a mixed micellar phase that effectively allows for the transport of the lipolytic products over the unstirred water layer. In the absence of bile salts the transport has to be achieved by a less efficient lamellar monoglyceride: fatty acid soap system. Medium-chain triglycerides are absorbed efficiently in the absence of bile due to the higher monomeric solubility of their lipolytic products, the medium-chain fatty acids and monoglycerides.

(2) Phospholipids

In 1955 Blomstrand [93] fed phospholipids labeled with [^{14}C]palmitic acid to rats with both the bile and thoracic duct cannulated. The results indicated that in this situation 68% of the fatty acids were absorbed and that bile was not obligatory for absorption of phospholipid fatty acid. The distribution of the labeled fatty acid in the thoracic duct lipids showed the same pattern as after feeding the free fatty acid, indicating that the phospholipids had been hydrolyzed before absorption. The mechanism responsible for the hydrolysis of phospholipid in bile fistula rats is not obvious. A novel enzyme with phospholipase A_1 activity has been demonstrated in the rat intestine [94]. This enzyme has its highest specificity for phosphatidyl glycerol and its role for the hydrolysis of dietary PC is unclear.

(3) Cholesterol

It is established from the early isotope era that bile is necessary for sterol absorption in the rat [4] and bile salts, specifically cholic acid, were later shown to be the essential constituent of bile in mediating absorption of cholesterol [95]. The mechanism by which bile salts assist cholesterol absorption has been investigated in some detail. Watt and Simmonds [96] compared the uptake of cholesterol in vivo from a micellar bile salt solution and from a solution in the non-ionic detergent Pluronic F68. No mucosal uptake of cholesterol occurred in the absence of bile salts. A measurable uptake could be seen, however, from the non-ionic mixed micelles in vitro. Their conclusion was that micellar solubilization in a detergent solution is necessary for uptake into the cell in vitro but that there is a specific requirement for bile salt for absorption (lumen to lymph). These authors found no difference in the initial uptake from trihydroxy bile salt mixed micelles compared with dihydroxy; taurocholate, however, promoted a significantly greater output of absorbed cholesterol into the lymph draining the intestine. Possibly, the diverse effects of specific bile salts on cholesterol absorption in the intact rat [97] can be explained through the specificity of cholesterol esterase (see also ref. 8 and Chapter 5).

The only detergent so far shown to replace bile salts in cholesterol absorption is the closely structurally related taurofusidate, a steroid antibiotic [96]. The mechanism of the absolute requirement of bile salts for sterol absorption is presently not understood.

(4) Fat-soluble vitamins

Like cholesterol, fat-soluble vitamins are strongly dependent on the presence of bile salts in the intestinal lumen for their absorption. Using thoracic duct lymph samples to estimate their absorption, Forsgren [98] showed marked depression of absorption of radiolabeled vitamins A, D, E and K in patients with total biliary obstruction. Intraluminal bile salt deficiency probably also contributes to impaired vitamin D absorption in primary biliary cirrhosis [99]. When exocrine pancreatic insufficiency is also present, absorption of vitamin K is even more markedly impaired [98]. More polar subspecies of the fat-soluble vitamins such as vitamin K_3 [100] and 25-hydroxyvitamin D_3 [101] depend much less on bile salts for their absorption.

In animal studies, absorption of vitamin D [102] and E [103] has been shown to depend on the presence of bile salts in the intestine. In rats, a polar lipid, oleic acid, is absorbed almost as well from an emulsion as from a micellar solution while α-tocopherol uptake from an emulsion was much less than from a micellar solution [104].

How bile salts promote fat-soluble absorption of vitamins is not fully understood. It is likely that several mechanisms are involved. For example, there is evidence that handling of certain of the fat-soluble vitamins in the enterocyte is influenced by bile salts. In the intestinal lumen, it is likely that a suitable solubilizing phase, liposomal or micellar, involving bile salts, monoglycerides and fatty acids creates a sufficiently high concentration of such lipids of low polarity close to the brush border membrane of the enterocyte.

Fat-soluble vitamins such as retinol and β-carotene are readily dissolved in mixed lipid–bile salt micelles in vitro. Retinol is approximately 10 times more readily dissolved in such micelles than β-carotene [105]. It is likely that these two substances occupy different regions of the micelle. The difference in solubility, therefore, may reflect the limited capacity of the nonpolar core of the micelle for the relatively bulky β-carotene molecule. Retinol, on the other hand, may occupy a more hydrophilic region of the micelle. In a mixed oil/micellar system, α-tocopherol distributes between the two phases, its concentration in the micellar phase being enhanced by expansion of the micelles with monoglycerides and lecithin of long-chain fatty acids. However, lipids containing medium-chain fatty acids do not expand the micelles as effectively as their long-chain counterparts such that there is less solubilization of α-tocopherol in the micellar phase [106].

Studies in vivo have also demonstrated that fat-soluble vitamins are solutes in bile salt micelles. For example, David and Ganguly [107] showed that when rats are fed retinyl acetate in ground nut oil, the vitamin distributes between the oil and micellar phases of the intestinal content with the retinyl ester predominantly in the oil phase and free retinol favoring the micellar phase. In man, vitamin D_3 fed in a test meal is subsequently found in mixed lipid–bile salt micelles in intestinal content [108].

In a number of in vivo studies by Hollander and co-workers the concurrent feeding of polyunsaturated fatty acids has been shown to depress absorption of all species of fat-soluble vitamin [109]. How this comes about is not clear; it does not depend on displacement of the vitamins from bile salt micelles but presumably involves an interaction at the cell membrane or at some later step in absorption such as the binding to intracellular transport proteins.

In clinical terms, intraluminal bile salt deficiency such as occurs in various forms of cholestasis, can clearly lead to impaired assimilation of fat-soluble vitamins. When the bile-salt-binding resin cholestyramine is given on a long-term basis in the treatment of hypercholesterolemia there is some risk of malabsorption of fat-soluble vitamins though in clinical practice this is not common.

(5) Other nonpolar compounds

A heterogeneous group of lipids of low polarity is found in the diet. Some of these, e.g. squalene, enter normal biochemical processes in the body. Others are of no nutritional advantage and may in some cases be toxic. Hexadecane [110], octadecane [111], polynuclear aromatic hydrocarbons such as 3-methylcholanthrene and 7,12-dimethylbenzanthracene, and polychlorinated biphenyls [112] have all been shown in vitro to dissolve in mixed bile salt micelles. 7,12-Dimethylbenzanthracene in solution in long-chain or medium-chain triglyceride oils is absorbed to a small extent in the absence of bile. When dissolved in long-chain triglyceride, this absorption is markedly enhanced when bile is present. On the other hand, bile has no effect on the absorption of the compound from a medium-chain triglyceride solution [113]. This may reflect the fact that in contrast to long-chain triglyceride lipolytic products, medium-chain monoglycerides and fatty acids form inadequate mixed micelles. Some of the nonpolar lipids may be partly metabolized in the enterocyte to more polar compounds which are transported to the liver in the portal vein. In contrast cholesterol and retinol are largely esterified to more nonpolar compounds which are obliged to travel exclusively as chylomicron solutes in lymph.

Lastly, mention should be made of a recent study of the possible co-carcinogenic effects of bile salts in which enhanced uptake by the colon of 7,12-dimethylbenzanthracene was demonstrated in the presence of deoxycholic acid [114]. It is very likely that this reflects an increase in mucosal permeability caused by this secondary bile acid.

(VI) Are bile salts necessary for lipid absorption?

The answer to this question has already been given above. Bile salts are not necessary for absorption of triglycerides but may be necessary for absorption of other lipids such as cholesterol and some nonpolar lipids. Bile salts can, however, be said to be necessary for a normal absorption, meaning that fat absorption in the absence of bile salt is different mechanistically from that in the presence of bile salts. Fat absorption is impaired at suboptimal bile salt concentration [115,116] possibly due to a reduced micellar phase in intestinal content. In bile fistula man, lipolysis is unimpaired but the concentration of fatty acids in the "aqueous phase" is reduced 100-fold [117].

It thus is generally accepted that "micellar dispersion" rather than lipolysis is the rate-limiting step in bile deficiency that results in partial malabsorption.

Bile salts have some special properties as detergents depending on the rigid and planar geometry of the steroid structure with the polar groups on one side. This leads among other things to a more complex pattern of self-association with an extended concentration range of aggregation rather than a sharp critical micellar concentration. Infusion experiments indicate that oleic acid can be taken up from the intestine of the rat and esterified when dispersed in synthetic non-ionic detergents [118]. However, as previously discussed, bile salts seem to be specific for the uptake of cholesterol [96]. In animal experiments Pluronic F68 but not Tween was found to improve malabsorption of fat caused by dietary cholestyramine [119]. In other experiments, the feeding of Pluronic L-81 was shown to cause malabsorption in animals with normal bile flow [120,121]. Such malabsorption, however, was found to be due to defective discharge of resynthesized triglyceride from the enterocyte rather than to impaired digestion and absorption [122]. In vitro experiments indicate that most detergents inhibit pancreatic lipolysis and that this inhibition is reversed to some extent by bile salt in the presence of colipase [123].

References

1 Heaton, K.W. (1972) Bile Salts in Health and Disease, Churchill Livingstone, Edinburgh.
2 Dam, H. (1943) Lancet 63, 353.
3 Shapiro, A., Koster, H., Rittenberg, D. and Schoenheimer, R. (1936) Am. J. Physiol. 117, 525–528.
4 Siperstein, M.B., Chaikoff, I.L. and Reinhardt, W.O. (1952) J. Biol. Chem. 198, 111–114.
5 Child, P. and Kuksis, A. (1981) in: 72nd Annual Meeting of American Oil Chemists' Society, New Orleans, p. 26.
6 Hamilton, J.A. and Small, D.M. (1981) Proc. Natl. Acad. Sci. (U.S.A.) 78, 6878–6882.
7 Patton, J. (1981) in: Physiology of the Gastrointestinal Tract (Johnson, L.R., Ed.) pp. 1123–1146, Raven Press, New York.
8 Thomson, A.B.R. and Dietschy, J.M. (1981) in: Physiology of the Gastrointestinal Tract (Johnson, L.R., Ed.) pp. 1147–1220, Raven Press, New York.
9 Carey, M.C. (1982) in: The Liver: Biology and Pathobiology (Arias, I., Popper, H., Schachter, D. and Shafritz, D.A., Eds.) pp. 429–465, Raven Press, New York.
10 Carey, M.C., Small, D.M. and Bliss, C.M. (1983) Annu. Rev. Physiol. 45, 651–677.
11 Wells, M.A. and Direnzo, N.A. (1983) The Enzymes, Vol. XVI, pp. 113–139, Academic Press, New York.
12 Grundy, S.M. (1983) Annu. Rev. Nutr. 3, 71–96.
13 Holt, P.R. (1972) Arch. Intern. Med. 130, 574–583.
14 Spellman, S.J., Shaffer, E.A. and Rosenthal, L. (1979) Gastroenterology 77, 115–120.
15 Roch, E., Malmud, L. and Fisher, R.S. (1981) Gastroenterology 80, 1263.

16 Regan, P.T., Malagelada, J.-R., Di Magno, E.P. and Go, V.L.W. (1979) Gastroenterology 77, 285–289.

17 Dietschy, J.M. (1968) J. Lipid Res. 9, 297–309.

18 Stafford, R.J., Donovan, J.M., Benedek, G.B. and Carey, M.C. (1981) Gastroenterology 80, 1291.

19 Borgström, B. (1978) Lipids 13, 187–189.

20 Benzonana, G. and Desnuelle, P. (1965) Biochim. Biophys. Acta 105, 121–136.

21 Linthorst, J., Tepper, M. and Holt, P.R. (1974) Fed. Proc. 33, 259.

22 Linthorst, J.M., Bennett Clark, S. and Holt, P.R. (1977) J. Colloid Interface Sci. 60, 1–10.

23 Borgström, B. and Donnér, J. (1976) J. Lipid Res. 17, 491–497.

24 Borgström, B. and Erlanson, C. (1978) Gastroenterology 75, 382–386.

25 Hamosh, M. (1984) in: Lipases (Borgström, B. and Brockman, H.C., Eds.) pp. 50–77, Elsevier, Amsterdam.

26 Erlanson-Albertsson, C. and Åkerlund, H.E. (1982) FEBS Lett. 144, 38–42.

27 Rudd, E.A. and Brockman, H.L. (1984) in: Lipases (Borgström, B. and Brockman, H.L., Eds.) pp. 185–204, Elsevier, Amsterdam.

28 Hyun, J., Kothari, H., Herm, E., Mortenson, J., Treadwell, C.R. and Vahouny, G. (1969) J. Biol. Chem. 244, 1937–1945.

29 Lombardo, D. and Guy, O. (1980) Biochim. Biophys. Acta 611, 147–155.

30 Bhat, S.G. and Brockman, H.L. (1982) Biochem. Biophys. Res. Commun. 109, 486–492.

31 Calame, K.B., Gallo, L., Cheriathundam, E., Vahouny, G.V. and Treadwell, C.R. (1975) Arch. Biochem. Biophys. 168, 57–65.

32 Hyun, J., Treadwell, C.R. and Vahouny, G.V. (1972) Arch. Biochem. Biophys. 152, 233–242.

33 Momsen, W.E. and Brockman, H.L. (1977) Biochim. Biophys. Acta 486, 103–113.

34 Lombardo, D., Campese, D., Multigner, L., Lafont, H. and de Caro, A. (1983) Eur. J. Biochem. 133, 327–333.

35 Campese, D., Lombardo, D., Multigner, L., Lafont, H. and de Caro, A. (1984) Biochim. Biophys. Acta 784, 147–157.

36 Erlanson-Albertsson, C. (1986) in: Molecular and Cellular Basis of Digestion (Desnuelle, P., Sjöström, H. and Norén, C., Eds.) Elsevier, Amsterdam, pp. 297–307.

37 Bläckberg, L., Lombardo, D., Hernell, O., Guy, O. and Olivecrona, T. (1981) FEBS Lett. 136, 284–288.

38 Hernell, O. (1975) Eur. J. Clin. Invest. 5, 267–272.

39 Fredrikzon, B., Hernell, O., Bläckberg, L. and Olivecrona, T. (1978) Pediat. Res. 12, 1048–1052.

40 Hoffman, W.J., Vahey, M. and Hagder, J. (1983) Arch. Biochem. Biophys. 221, 361–370.

41 Nalbone, G.D., Lairon, M., Charbonnier-Augeire, M., Vigne, J.L., Leonardi, J., Chabert, C., Hauton, J.C. and Verger, R. (1980) Biochim. Biophys. Acta 620, 612–625.

42 Nalbone, G., Charbonnier-Augeire, M., Lafont, H., Grataroli, R., Vigne, J.L., Lairon, D., Chabert, C., Leonardi, J., Hauton, J.C. and Verger, R. (1983) J. Lipid Res. 24, 1441–1450.

43 Jain, M.K. and De Haas, G.H. (1983) Biochim. Biophys. Acta 736, 157–162.

44 Patton, J.S., Rigler, M.W., Liao, T.H., Hamosh, P. and Hamosh, M. (1982) Biochim. Biophys. Acta 712, 400–407.

45 Hofmann, A.F. and Borgström, B. (1964) J. Clin. Invest. 43, 247–257.

46 Mansbach, C.M., Cohen, R.S. and Leff, P.B. (1975) J. Clin. Invest. 56, 781–791.

47 Patton, J.S. and Carey, M.C. (1979) Science 204, 145–148.

48 Lindström, M., Ljusberg-Wahren, H., Larsson, K. and Borgström, B. (1981) Lipids 16, 749–754.

49 Mazer, N., Schurtenberger, P., Kanzig, W., Carey, M. and Preisig, R. (1981) Gastroenterology 80, 1341.

50 Proulx, P., McNeil, J., Brglez, I. and Williamson, D.G. (1982) Can. J. Biochem. 60, 904–909.

51 Barsukov, L.I., Hauser, H., Hasselbach, H.-J. and Semenza, G. (1980) FEBS Lett. 115, 189–192.

52 Yousef, I.M. and Kuksis, A. (1972) Lipids 7, 380–386.

53 Thomson, A.B.R. and O'Brien, B.D. (1981) Am. J. Physiol. 241, G270–G274.

54 Clark, S.B. (1971) J. Lipid Res. 12, 43–55.

55 Borgström, B., Dahlqvist, A., Lundh, G. and Sjövall, J. (1957) J. Clin. Invest. 36, 1521–1536.

56 Simmonds, W.J., Hofmann, A.F. and Theodor, E. (1967) J. Clin. Invest. 46, 874–890.
57 Diamond, J.M. (1966) J. Physiol. 183, 83–100.
58 Westergaard, H. and Dietschy, J.M. (1974) J. Clin. Invest. 54, 718–732.
59 Westergaard, H. and Dietschy, J.M. (1976) J. Clin Invest. 58, 97–108.
60 Winne, D. (1976) Experientia 32, 1278–1279.
61 Smithson, K.W., Millar, D.B., Jacobs, L.R. and Gray, G.M. (1981) Science 214, 1241–1244.
62 DeSimone, J.A. (1983) Science 220, 221–222.
63 Smithson, K.W. (1983) Science 220, 222.
64 Allen, A., Garner, A., Hutton, D. and McQueen, S. (1983) Proc. Physiol. Soc. 341, 66P–67P.
65 Allen, A. (1981) in: Physiology of the Gastrointestinal Tract (Johnson, L.R., Ed.) pp. 617–639, Raven Press, New York.
66 Trier, S.J. and Madara, J.L. (1981) in: Physiology of the Gastrointestinal Tract (Johnson, L.R., Ed.) pp. 925–961, Raven Press, New York.
67 Ockner, R.K. and Manning, J.A. (1974) J. Clin. Invest. 54, 326–338.
68 Dietschy, J.M. (1978) in: Disturbances in Lipid and Lipoprotein Metabolism (Dietschy, J.M., Gotto, A.M. and Ontko, J.A., Eds.) pp. 1–28, Amer. Physiol. Soc., Bethesda, MD.
69 Hofmann, A.F. (1976) in: Lipid Absorption: Biochemical and Clinical Aspects (Rommel, K., Goebell, H. and Böhmer, R., Eds.) pp. 3–21, MTP Press, Lancaster.
70 Hoffman, N.E. (1970) Biochim. Biophys. Acta 196, 193–203.
71 Hoffman, N.E. and Yeoh, V.J. (1971) Biochim. Biophys. Acta 233, 49–52.
72 Hoffman, N.E., Simmonds, W.J. and Morgan, R.G.H. (1971) Biochim. Biophys. Acta 231, 487–495.
73 Sklan, D., Budowski, P. and Hurwitz, S. (1976) Lipids 11, 467–471.
74 McClintock, C. and Shiau, Y.-F. (1983) Am. J. Physiol. 244, G507–G514.
75 Sklan, D. and Budowski, P. (1977) Lipids 12, 193–197.
76 Fondacaro, J.D. (1983) Proc. Soc. Exp. Biol. Med. 173, 118–124.
77 Borgström, B., Lundh, G. and Hofmann, A.F. (1963) Gastroenterology 45, 229–238.
78 Lee, K.Y., Hoffman, N.E. and Simmonds, W.J. (1971) Biochim. Biophys. Acta 249, 548–555.
79 Knoebel, L.K. (1972) Am. J. Physiol. 223, 255–261.
80 Dawson, A.M. and Isselbacher, K.J. (1960) J. Clin. Invest. 39, 730–740.
81 Borgström, B. (1953) Acta Physiol. Scand. 28, 279–286.
82 Blomstrand, R., Carlberger, G. and Forsgren, L. (1969) Acta Chir. Scand. 135, 329–339.
83 Gagnon, M. and Dawson, A.M. (1968) Proc. Soc. Exp. Biol. Med. 127, 99–102.
84 Rodgers, J.B., Tandon, R. and O'Brien, R.J. (1973) Biochim. Biophys. Acta 326, 345–354.
85 O'Doherty, P.J.A. Yousef, I.M. and Kuksis, A. (1974) Can. J. Biochem. 52, 726–733.
86 O'Doherty, P.J.A., Yousef, I.M., Kakis, G. and Kuksis, A. (1975) Arch. Biochem. Biophys. 169, 252–261.
87 Treadwell, C.R. and Vahouny, G.V. (1968) in: Handbook of Physiology, Alimentary Canal (Code, C.F., Ed.) Vol. 3, pp. 1407–1438, American Physiological Society, Washington, DC.
88 Watt, S.M. and Simmonds, W.J. (1981) J. Lipid Res. 22, 157–165.
89 Norum, K.R., Helgerud, P. and Lilljeqvist, A.-C. (1981) Scand. J. Gastroenterol. 16, 401–410.
90 Goodman, D.S. and Huang, H.S. (1965) Science 149, 879–880.
91 Helgerud, P., Petersen, L.B. and Norum, K.R. (1982) J. Lipid Res. 23, 609–618.
92 Mathias, P.M., Harries, J.T., Peters, T.J. and Muller, D.P.R. (1981) J. Lipid Res. 22, 829–837.
93 Blomstrand, R. (1955) Acta Physiol. Scand. 34, 158–161.
94 Mansbach, C., Pieroni, G. and Verger, R. (1982) J. Clin. Invest. 69, 368–376.
95 Swell, L., Trout, E.C., Hopper, J.R., Field Jr., H. and Treadwell, C.R. (1958) J. Biol. Chem. 232, 1–8.
96 Watt, S.M. and Simmonds, W.J. (1976) Clin. Exp. Pharmacol. Physiol. 3, 305–322.
97 Gallo-Torris, H.E., Miller, D.W. and Hamilton, J.G. (1971) Arch. Biochem. Biophys. 143, 22–36.
98 Forsgren, L. (1969) Acta Chir. Scand. Suppl. 399.
99 Danielsson, A., Lorentzon, R. and Larsson, S.E. (1982) Scand. J. Gastroenterol. 17, 349–355.
100 Jaques, L.B., Millar, G.J. and Spinks, J.W.T. (1954) Schweiz. Med. Wochenschr. 84, 792–796.
101 Bengoa, J.M., Sitrin, M.D. and Rosenberg, I.H. (1983) Gastroenterology 84, 1102.
102 Schachter, D., Finkelstein, J.D. and Kowarski, S. (1964) J. Clin. Invest. 43, 787–796.

103 Gallo-Torres, H. (1970) Lipids 5, 379–384.
104 MacMahon, M.T. and Thompson, G.R. (1970) Eur. J. Clin. Invest. 1, 288–294.
105 El-Gorab, M. and Underwood, B.A. (1973) Biochim. Biophys. Acta 306, 58–66.
106 Takahashi, Y.I. and Underwood, B.A. (1974) Lipids 9, 855–859.
107 David, J.S.K. and Ganguly, J. (1967) Indian J. Biochem. Biophys. 4, 14–17.
108 Rautureau, M. and Rambaud, J.C. (1981) Gut 22, 393–397.
109 Hollander, D. (1981) J. Lab. Clin. Med. 97, 449–462.
110 Savary, P. and Constantin, M.J. (1967) Biochim. Biophys. Acta 137, 264–276.
111 Borgström, B. (1967) J. Lipid Res. 8, 598–608.
112 Laher, J.M. and Barrowman, J.A. (1983) Lipids 18, 216–222.
113 Laher, J.M., Chernenko, G.A. and Barrowman, J.A. (1983) Can. J. Physiol. Pharmacol. 61, 1368–1373.
114 Rose, R.C. and Nahrwold, D.L. (1982) J. Natl. Cancer Inst. 68, 619–622.
115 Badley, B.W.D., Murphy, G.M., Bouchier, H.D. and Sherlock, S. (1970) Gastroenterology 58, 781–789.
116 Hofmann, A.F. (1972) Arch. Intern. Med. 13, 597–605.
117 Porter, H.P., Saunders, D.R., Tytgat, G., Brunser, O. and Rubin, C.E. (1971) Gastroenterology 60, 1008–1019.
118 Simmonds, W.J., Redgrave, T.G. and Willix, R.C. (1968) J. Clin. Invest. 47, 1015–1025.
119 Sheltaway, M.J. and Losowsky, M.S. (1975) Nutr. Metabol. 18, 265–271.
120 Bochenek, W.J. and Rodgers, J.B. (1977) Biochim. Biophys. Acta 489, 503–506.
121 Brunelle, C.W., Bochenek, W.J., Abraham, R., Kim, D.N. and Rodgers, J.B. (1979) Dig. Dis. Sci. 24, 718–726.
122 Tso, P., Balint, J.A. and Rodgers, J.B. (1980) Am. J. Physiol. 239, G348–353.
123 Borgström, B. (1977) Biochim. Biophys. Acta 488, 381–391.

H. Danielsson and J. Sjövall (Eds.), *Sterols and Bile Acids*

Subject Index

For practical reasons, sterols and bile acids are normally listed under their trivial names. In most instances, a page is referred to where the structure of the compound is described.